BEST PRACTICES FOR
Occupational Therapy in Early Childhood

Gloria Frolek Clark, PhD, OTR/L, BCP, FAOTA, and Stephanie Parks, PhD, OT/L

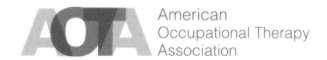

American
Occupational Therapy
Association

AOTA Vision 2025
Occupational therapy maximizes health, well-being, and quality of life for all people, populations, and communities through effective solutions that facilitate participation in everyday living.

Mission Statement
The American Occupational Therapy Association advances occupational therapy practice, education, and research through standard-setting and advocacy on behalf of its members, the profession, and the public.

AOTA Staff
Sherry Keramidas, *Executive Director*
Matthew Clark, *Chief Officer, Innovation & Engagement*

Elizabeth Dooley, *Vice President, Strategic Marketing & Communications*
Laura Collins, *Director of Communications and Publications*
Caroline Polk, *Digital Manager and* AJOT *Managing Editor*
Ashley Hofmann, *Acquisitions & Development Manager, AOTA Press*
Barbara Dickson, *Production & Business Manager, AOTA Press*

Rebecca Rutberg, *Director, Marketing*
Amanda Goldman, *Marketing Manager*
Jennifer Folden, *Brand Designer*

American Occupational Therapy Association, Inc.
6116 Executive Boulevard, Suite 200
North Bethesda, MD 20852-4929
Phone: 301-652-AOTA (2682)
Fax: 301-652-7711
www.aota.org
To order: 1-877-404-AOTA or store.aota.org

Disclaimers
This publication is designed to provide accurate and authoritative information in regard to the subject matter covered. It is sold or distributed with the understanding that the publisher is not engaged in rendering legal, accounting, or other professional service. If legal advice or other expert assistance is required, the services of a competent professional person should be sought.
—*From the Declaration of Principles jointly adopted by the American Bar Association and a Committee of Publishers and Associations*

It is the objective of the American Occupational Therapy Association to be a forum for free expression and interchange of ideas. The opinions expressed by the contributors to this work are their own and not necessarily those of the American Occupational Therapy Association.

ISBN: 978-1-56900-498-2
Ebook ISBN: 978-1-56900610-8
Library of Congress Control Number: 2020946680

Cover design by Debra Naylor, Naylor Design, Inc., Washington, DC
Composition by Manila Typesetting Company, Manila, Philippines
Printed by Versa Press, Inc., East Peoria, IL

Suggested Citation
Frolek Clark, G., & Parks, S. (Eds.). *Best practices for occupational therapy in early childhood*. AOTA Press.

Contents

List of Figures, Tables, Exhibits, and Case Examples vii

About the Editors xi

Contributors xiii

Foreword..xvii
    Barbara E. Chandler, PhD, FAOTA

Introduction xix
    Gloria Frolek Clark, PhD, OTR/L, BCP, FAOTA, and Stephanie Parks, PhD, OT/L

Section I. Foundation: Understanding Early Childhood and the Role of Occupational Therapy   1

Chapter 1. History of Occupational Therapy Services in Early Childhood.................................3
Joyce Rioux, EdD, OTR/L, SCSS, FAOTA, and Gloria Frolek Clark, PhD, OTR/L, BCP, FAOTA, with contributions from Barbara Hanft, MA, OTR/L

Chapter 2. Influences From Early Childhood Professional Organizations and Technical Assistance Centers.....13
Susan P. Maude, PhD, and Stephanie Parks, PhD, OT/L

Chapter 3. Best Practices in Personnel Preparation for Occupational Therapists and Occupational Therapy Assistants...23
Sarah Fabrizi, PhD, OTR/L, and Kris Pizur-Barnekow, PhD, OTR/L, IMH–E®

Chapter 4. Best Practices for Occupational Therapy Assistants in Early Childhood..........................31
Sarah Heldmann, BS, COTA/L

Chapter 5. Best Practices for Occupational Therapy Practitioners in Leadership Roles 39
Lesly Wilson James, PhD, MPA, OTR/L, FAOTA, and Sandra Schefkind, OTD, OTR/L, FAOTA

Chapter 6. Best Practices in Data-Based Decision Making...47
Gloria Frolek Clark, PhD, OTR/L, BCP, FAOTA

Chapter 7. Best Practices in the Use of Assistive Technology to Enhance Participation...................55
Judith Schoonover, MEd, OTR/L, ATP, FAOTA

Chapter 8. Best Practices in Supporting Family Partnerships...63
Anna Wallisch, PhD, OTR/L, and Lauren M. Little, PhD, OTR/L

Chapter 9. Best Practices in Collaborating With Community, School, and Health Care Partners 71
Lea Ann Lowery, OTD, OTR/L

Chapter 10. Best Practices in Early Childhood Transitions...79
Joanne Jackson Foss, PhD, OTR, FAOTA, and Christine T. Myers, PhD, OTR/L

Section II. Knowledge Essential to Early Development   87

Chapter 11. Brain Development in the Early Years..89
Stefanie C. Bodison, OTD, OTR/L

Chapter 12. Early Childhood Mental Health...99
Kris Pizur-Barnekow, PhD, OTR/L, IMH–E®, and Stephan Viehweg, LCSW, ACSW, IMH–E®, CYC–P

Chapter 13. Understanding Early Literacy Development 109
Stephanie Parks, PhD, OT/L, and Gloria Frolek Clark, PhD, OTR/L, BCP, FAOTA

Section III. Considerations for Early Intervention: IDEA Part C   **117**

Chapter 14. Understanding Part C: Early Intervention Law and the Individualized Family Service Plan (IFSP) Process 119
Anne Lucas, MS, OTR/L

Chapter 15. Best Practices in Early Intervention Screening and Evaluation..................129
Beth Elenko, PhD, OTR/L, BCP, CLA

Chapter 16. Best Practices in Intervention Under Part C 137
Pam Stephenson, OTD, OTR/L

Chapter 17. Best Practices in Documenting Early Intervention Services and Outcomes..................145
Ashley Stoffel, OTD, OTR/L, FAOTA, and Lesly Wilson James, PhD, MPA, OTR/L, FAOTA

Section IV. Considerations for Preschool: IDEA Part B   **155**

Chapter 18. Understanding Preschool Laws and the Individualized Education Program Process..................157
Rebecca E. Argabrite Grove, MS, OTR/L, FAOTA

Chapter 19. Best Practices in Preschool Screening and Evaluation..................165
Debi Hinerfeld, PhD, OTR/L, FAOTA

Chapter 20. Best Practices in Intervention in Preschool..................173
Terry Giese, MBA, OT/L, FAOTA

Chapter 21. Best Practices in Documentation of Preschool Services and Outcomes..................181
Francine Seruya, PhD, OTR/L, FAOTA

Section V. Considerations for Medical and Health Care   **191**

Chapter 22. Understanding Health Care Requirements, Process, and Billing..................193
Janice Flegle, MA, OTR/L, BCP, and Sara O'Rourke, MOT, OTR/L, BCP

Chapter 23. Best Practices in Evaluation in Health Care Settings 199
Kaitlin Hagen, MOT, OTR/L; Alaena McCool, MS, OTR/L, CPAM; and Rebecca Martin, OTR/L, OTD

Chapter 24. Best Practices in Health Care Interventions for Developmental Conditions..................207
Bonnie Riley, OTD, OTR/L, and Molly Connor-Hall, MS, OTR/L

Chapter 25. Best Practices in Health Care Intervention for Acquired Conditions..................215
Kaitlin Hagen, MOT, OTR/L; Rebecca Martin, OTR/L, OTD; and Alaena McCool, MS, OTR/L, CPAM

Chapter 26. Best Practices in Documentation of Health Care Services and Outcomes..................225
Stephanie L. de Sam Lazaro, OTD, OTR/L

Section VI. Evidence-Guided Practice: Addressing Evaluation and Intervention   **233**

Chapter 27. Best Practices in Supporting Activities of Daily Living and Sleep (Adaptive Skills) 235
Meredith Gronski, OTD, OTR/L, CLA

Chapter 28. Best Practices in Supporting Mealtimes and Nutritional Needs (Adaptive Skills) 243
Winifred Schultz-Krohn, PhD, OTR/L, BCP, SWC, FAOTA, and Ashwini Wagle, EdD, MS, RD

Chapter 29. Best Practices in Supporting Learning and Early Literacy Skills (Cognitive Skills)..................257
Gloria Frolek Clark, PhD, OTR/L, BCP; Jayna Niblock, PhD, OTD, OTR/L, BCP; and Taylor Crane Vos, OTD, OTR/L

Chapter 30. Best Practices in Supporting Development of Fine and Visual–Motor Coordination (Physical Skills) 265
Elizabeth Koss Schmidt, MOT, OTR/L; Kristen Martin, MOT, OTR/L; Margaret Bassi, OTD, OTR/L; and Kelly Tanner, PhD, OTR/L, BCP

Chapter 31. Best Practices in Supporting Large Motor Coordination (Physical Skills) 273
Elizabeth Koss Schmidt, MOT, OTR/L; Kristen Martin, MOT, OTR/L; Margaret Bassi, OTD, OTR/L; and Kelly Tanner, PhD, OTR/L, BCP

Chapter 32. Best Practices in Supporting Social Participation (Communication)..................281
Kris Pedersen, SLPD, CCC-SLP, and Stephanie Parks, PhD, OT/L

Chapter 33. Best Practices in Supporting Social, Emotional, and Self-Regulation Skills (Social–Emotional Skills)...291
Karrie Kingsley, OTD, OTR/L

Chapter 34. Best Practices in Supporting Play and Leisure Activities..301
Bonnie Riley, OTD, OTR/L

Chapter 35. Best Practices in Supporting Children Who Are Deaf and Hard of Hearing...................309
Meredith Gronski, OTD, OTR/L, CLA

Chapter 36. Best Practices in Supporting Children With Visual Impairments 319
Tammy Bruegger, OTD, MSE, OTR/L, ATP

Chapter 37. Best Practices in Supporting Children With Health Needs 329
Julie Jones, OTD, OTR/L, BCP

Chapter 38. Best Practices in Supporting Children With Autism Spectrum Disorder and Attention Deficit Hyperactivity Disorder..337
Lesly Wilson James, PhD, MPA, OTR/L, FAOTA; Ashley Stoffel, OTD, OTR/L, FAOTA; and Kris Pizur-Barnekow, PhD, OTR/L, IMH–E®

Chapter 39. Best Practices Supporting Families of Children With Prenatal Substance Exposure and Postnatal Trauma 347
Yvonne Swinth, PhD, OTR/L, FAOTA, and Jennifer S. Pitonyak, PhD, OTR/L, SCFES

Appendixes   **359**

Appendix A. Guidelines for Occupational Therapy Services in Early Intervention and Schools..............361

Appendix B. Evidence-Based Practice and Occupational Therapy..371
Elizabeth G. Hunter, PhD, OTR/L, and Deborah Lieberman, MHSA, OTR/L, FAOTA

Appendix C. AOTA Occupational Profile Template 377

Appendix D. Occupational Therapy Intervention Plan 381

Appendix E. AOTA Resources for Practitioners and Families..383

Appendix F. Examples of Assessments for Early Childhood (Birth–5 Years) 385

Appendix G. Sample Early Intervention Team Report 391

Appendix H. Sample Initial Preschool Team Evaluation Report...393

Appendix I. Sample Occupational Therapy Evaluation in Health Care 397
Stephanie L. de Sam Lazaro, OTD, OTR/L

Appendix J. Occupational Therapy Telehealth Practices in Early Childhood...................................399
Stephanie Parks, PhD, OT/L, and Gloria Frolek Clark, PhD, OTR/L, BCP, FAOTA

Index 403

List of Figures, Tables, Exhibits, and Case Examples

Figures

Figure 6.1. Graph template for monitoring Sofia's progress with baseline and goal 48

Figure 6.2. Mastery monitoring template 49

Figure 10.1. Early childhood transition timeline for SPP/APR indicators C-8A, 8B, 8C, B-11, and B-12 for Part C children determined to be eligible at least 90 days prior to their third birthday.. 80

Figure 14.1. The early intervention and individualized family service plan process 122

Figure 35.1. Familiar sounds audiogram........................... 311

Figure 35.2. Ear with a cochlear implant........................... 312

Figure 39.1. ACE pyramid........................... 349

Figure B.1. *Evidence-based practice* is the use of the best available research evidence combined with the practitioner's expertise and the client's needs and preferences 372

Tables

Table I.1. Overview of Contents xx

Table 1.1. AOTA Resources for Early Childhood Practitioners 8

Table 2.1. Selected EC, EI, and ECSE Organizations........ 15

Table 2.2. Primary National Technical Assistance Centers 16

Table 2.3. Comparison of Selected EC Education and ECSE Approaches 19

Table 3.1. Examples of Learning Activities for Occupational Therapy Early Childhood Curriculum 25

Table 3.2. Examples of Interprofessional Practice in Education—Evidence Briefs 26

Table 3.3. Core Competency Crosswalk From Professional Early Childhood Organizations 27

Table 3.4. Interprofessional Concept With Course Objectives... 28

Table 4.1. Examples of the AOTA *Code of Ethics* for OTAs Working in Early Childhood............................. 33

Table 5.1. AOTA Early Childhood Resources 44

Table 6.1. Evaluation: Qualitative vs. Quantitative Data Gathered During Interview 53

Table 8.1. Ecology of Human Performance Interventions and Examples.. 65

Table 8.2. Make the Switch to Strengths-Based Language 67

Table 9.1. Conceptual Framework for Collaboration and Examples of Collaborative Practice................... 72

Table 9.2. Similarities and Differences Between Work Settings Influence Collaboration 73

Table 10.1. Family-Centered Approaches and Examples.. 82

Table 12.1. Factors Influencing Relationships 101

Table 13.1. Skills That Predict Literacy Achievement..... 111

Table 15.1. Examples of Assessment Tools Used in Early Intervention.. 134

Table 16.1. Summary of Best Practices in the Natural Environment.. 139

Table 17.1. Tips for Participating in the Child Outcomes Summary Process.. 148

Table 17.2. Reflective Questions for Writing an IFSP Outcome.. 150

Table 17.3. Examples of IFSP Outcomes 151

Table 18.1. Office of Special Education Programs Annual Preschool Performance Indicators 158

Table 19.1. Common Assessment Tools 169

Table 22.1. Contact Information for Major Health Care Provider Networks.. 194

Table 22.2. *CPT* Evaluation Codes and Descriptors 195

Table 22.3. Common *CPT* Codes for Occupational Therapy Treatment.. 196

Table 23.1. Commonly Used Assessments in Pediatric Health Care Practice.. 203

Table 24.1. Contributions of Interprofessional Team Members in Health Care................................ 208

Table 24.2. Key Concepts in Delivering Health Care Services.. 208

Table 24.3. Occupations to Consider During Program Planning With Families 210

Table 24.4. Theories for Addressing Performance Skills.. 211

Table 26.1. Common *CPT* Codes Used in Early Childhood Health Care Settings.. 227

Table 26.2. Documentation Descriptions and Practice Settings.. 228

Table 26.3. Long- and Short-Term Goal Examples by Setting.. 230

Table 27.1. Amount of Sleep Needed by Child's Age 237

Table 27.2. Assessment Tools for ADLs 237

Table 28.1. Food Groups 244

Table 28.2. Religion-Based Dietary Practices and Restrictions 248

Table 29.1. Examples of Assessment Tools to Identify Cognitive Skills in Early Childhood 259

Table 30.1. Phases of Fine and Visual–Motor Development 266

Table 30.2. Grasp Pattern Development 266

Table 30.3. Examples of Assessment Tools Used for Occupational Performance and Fine and Visual–Motor Skills 267

Table 30.4. Fine Motor and Visual–Motor Activities 269

Table 31.1. Movement and Large Motor Development Milestones 274

Table 31.2. Examples of Assessment Tools Used for Large Motor Skills 276

Table 31.3. Motor Learning Principles 277

Table 31.4. Motor Components 278

Table 32.1. Social Communication Development Milestones 282

Table 32.2. Strategies to Promote Social Participation and Examples 284

Table 33.1. Commonly Used Assessments for Social–Emotional Skills in Early Childhood 294

Table 34.1. Social Behaviors of Play and Strategies to Promote Social Interaction 303

Table 34.2. Play Assessments Commonly Used by Occupational Therapists 304

Table 34.3. Play Outcomes in Early Childhood Settings 304

Table 35.1. Definitions of Hearing Loss 310

Table 35.2. Communication Approaches 313

Table 36.1. Visual Conditions and Interventions (General, Medical, and Occupational Therapy) 322

Table 36.2. Assessment Tools Designed or Adapted for Children With Visual Impairments 323

Table 36.3. Comparing Strategies for Ocular Visual Impairment and Cortical Visual Impairment 324

Table 37.1. Resources for Families 330

Table 37.2. Diagnoses and Health Care Considerations and Impact on Participation 331

Table 37.3. Types of Feeding Tubes 332

Table 38.1. Therapeutic Process for Children With ASD and ADHD 340

Table A.1. Legislative Influences on Occupational Therapy Practice in EI and Schools 362

Table A.2. Examples of Occupational Therapy Practitioner Roles Under ESSA (General Education) 366

Table A.3. Examples of Occupational Therapy Practitioner Roles in Part C and Part B of IDEA 336

Table B.1. Strength of Evidence (Level of Certainty) 373

Table B.2. U.S. Department of Education (2016) Criteria Recommended in ESSA for the Identification of Evidence 374

Exhibits

Exhibit 1.1. A Sibling's Perspective: Joyce Rioux 5

Exhibit 2.1. Examples of Guidelines Based on DAP Principles 17

Exhibit 2.2. Multicultural Principles for Head Start Programs Serving Children Ages Birth–5 Years 18

Exhibit 3.1. Examples of ACOTE® Requirements for Entry-Level Occupational Therapy Practitioners 25

Exhibit 3.2. Action Examples for Early Childhood 29

Exhibit 4.1. Clearly Communicating the Occupational Therapy Practitioner's Role 36

Exhibit 6.1. Mastery Monitoring Subskills and Criteria ... 49

Exhibit 6.2. Goal Attainment Scaling Template Sample ... 50

Exhibit 6.3. Toileting Checklist 51

Exhibit 6.4. Frequency Chart 51

Exhibit 6.5. Duration Chart 52

Exhibit 6.6. Rubric Template Example 52

Exhibit 6.7. Fidelity of Implementation Sample 54

Exhibit 7.1. Myths Regarding Assistive Technology and Young Children 56

Exhibit 9.1. Situation–Background–Assessment–Recommendation Manualized Communication Strategy 74

Exhibit 9.2. Benefits of Community Partnerships 74

Exhibit 9.3. Tips for Supporting Communication in Collaborative Practice 76

Exhibit 15.1. Salient Features of Family-Centered Practice 131

Exhibit 17.1. Common Types of Professional Documentation in Early Intervention 146

Exhibit 17.2. Tips for Documentation 146

Exhibit 17.3. Strategies to Improve the Family's Use of IFSP Outcome Pages 147

Exhibit 17.4. Collecting Data on Child IFSP Outcomes 152

Exhibit 20.1. Guiding Principles of Universal Design for Learning 174

Exhibit 20.2. Examples of Occupational Therapy Intervention Approaches 175

Exhibit 20.3. Exhibit of an Embedded Learning Opportunity Activity Matrix 177

Exhibit 20.4. Comparing Coaching and Consulting Models 178

Exhibit 21.1. Fundamentals of Documentation 182

Exhibit 21.2. Individualized Education Program Goal Samples 185

Exhibit 21.3. Sample Occupational Therapy Contact Report 186

Exhibit 21.4. Sample Quarterly Individualized Education Program Progress Report 187

Exhibit 23.1. Sample Questions for Gathering the Occupational Profile 202

Exhibit 26.1. Sample Daily Note Grid 231

Exhibit 26.2. Progress Report Template Example 231

Exhibit 31.1. Influence of Underlying Factors on Children's Occupations 278

Exhibit 33.1. Example Language for Addressing Social–Emotional Development and Self-Regulation 296

Exhibit 34.1. Key Features and Qualitative Aspects of Play to Note During Authentic Observations of Play 303

Exhibit 35.1. Examples of Intervention and Supports for Children Who Are Deaf or Hard of Hearing 314

Exhibit 36.1. Early Signs of a Visual Impairment 322

Exhibit 36.2. Strategies for Working With Children With Deaf-Blindness 325

Exhibit 37.1. Evaluation Considerations 333

Exhibit 38.1. Types of ADHD Based on Symptoms 338

Case Examples

Case Example 3.1. Alex: Interprofessional Teamwork in an Autism Diagnostic Clinic 28

Case Example 8.1. Alex: Early Intervention (Home) 68

Case Example 8.2. Emily: Preschool 68

Case Example 8.3. Maria: Outpatient Clinic 68

Case Example 8.4. Daniel: Early Intervention Telehealth 69

Case Example 12.1. Joshua: Using the PAUSE Method ... 102

Case Example 35.1. Nicholas: A Collaborative Approach to Intervention in an Early Childhood School for the Deaf 316

About the Editors

Gloria Frolek Clark, PhD, OTR/L, BCP, FAOTA, received a bachelor's degree in occupational therapy from the University of North Dakota and a doctorate in human development and family studies (early childhood special education) from Iowa State University (ISU). She was part of ISU's early childhood special education leadership grant program, funded through the U.S. Office of Special Education Programs. Dr. Frolek Clark has worked more than 40 years in early intervention and school practice, including 15 years as a state consultant at the Iowa Department of Education. She was cofounder and first chairperson of the American Occupational Therapy Association's (AOTA) Early Intervention and School Special Interest Section, member of the Commission on Practice, member of the Pediatric Specialty Board, liaison to the School System Specialty Certification Panel, and past AOTA Board Director.

Dr. Frolek Clark has coauthored multiple book chapters, AOTA official documents, and systematic reviews. She is coeditor of *Best Practices for Occupational Therapy Services in Schools* (2013, 2019), *Occupational Therapy Practice Guidelines for Early Childhood: Birth to 5* (2013, 2020), and *Best Practices for Documenting Occupational Therapy Services in Schools* (2017).

Currently, Dr. Frolek Clark works with children and families through her private practice, teaches classes at Drake University in Des Moines, presents nationally on a variety of topics, and consults with education agencies to enhance effectiveness of services. She is a proud mother of three children and a grandmother of seven.

Stephanie Parks, PhD, OT/L, is an assistant professor of practice in the Department of Special Education at the University of Kansas. She teaches coursework in early childhood and early childhood special education undergraduate and graduate unified licensure programs, and she supervises students in the field. Dr. Parks and colleagues are currently developing an Early Intervention Interdisciplinary Certificate program focusing on interdisciplinary intervention in natural and inclusive settings for the graduate level.

Dr. Parks received her bachelor's degree in early childhood education from Graceland University in Lamoni, Iowa; advanced degrees in early childhood special education at the University of Missouri, Columbia; and occupational therapy degree at the University of Kansas Medical Center. Dr. Parks earned her doctoral degree in special education with an emphasis in early childhood/early childhood special education from the University of Kansas, Lawrence.

Since receiving her doctorate, she worked for a national professional development center, Early Childhood Personnel Center, to provide technical assistance to states in developing their interdisciplinary early childhood personnel development systems. Dr. Parks has also worked in school districts as a consultant and professional development specialist. As a practitioner, she has served young children and families in Part C and 619 programs as an occupational therapist and early childhood special educator for more than 20 years in the Kansas City metropolitan area.

Contributors

REBECCA E. ARGABRITE GROVE, MS, OTR/L, FAOTA
Practice Associate & Manager: Governance, Ethics &
   International
American Occupational Therapy Association
North Bethesda, MD

MARGARET BASSI, OTD, OTR/L
Occupational Therapist
Nationwide Children's Hospital
Columbus, OH

STEFANIE C. BODISON, OTD, OTR/L
Assistant Professor
University of Southern California
Los Angeles

TAMMY BRUEGGER, OTD, MSE, OTR/L, ATP
Assistant Professor of Occupational Therapy
Rockhurst University
Kansas City, MO

Assistive Technology Practitioner
The Children's Center for the Visually Impaired
Kansas City, MO

MOLLY CONNOR-HALL, MS, OTR/L
Occupational Therapist
Valley Health
Winchester, VA

STEPHANIE L. DE SAM LAZARO, OTD, OTR/L
Associate Professor and Director
Graduate Programs in Occupational Therapy
St. Catherine University
Saint Paul, MN

BETH ELENKO, PHD, OTR/L, BCP, CLA
Associate Professor
New York Institute of Technology
Old Westbury

SARAH FABRIZI, PHD, OTR/L
Assistant Professor
Florida Gulf Coast University
Ft. Myers

JANICE FLEGLE, MA, OTR/L, BCP
Retired Director Occupational Therapy; Emeritus Faculty
Munroe-Meyer Institute, University of Nebraska Medical
   Center
Omaha

GLORIA FROLEK CLARK, PHD, OTR/L, BCP, FAOTA
Owner
Gloria Frolek Clark, LLC
Adel, IA

Adjunct Professor of Occupational Therapy
Drake University
Des Moines, IA

TERRY GIESE, MBA, OT/L, FAOTA
Chair Emeritus
Naperville Mayor's Advisory Commission on Disabilities
Naperville, IL

MEREDITH GRONSKI, OTD, OTR/L, CLA
Assistant Professor and Chair
Doctor of Occupational Therapy Program
Methodist University
Fayetteville, NC

KAITLIN HAGEN, MOT, OTR/L
Manager, Therapy Services
International Center for Spinal Cord Injury, Kennedy
   Krieger Institute
Baltimore

BARBARA HANFT, MA, OTR, FAOTA
Developmental Consultant
Kill Devil Hills, NC

SARAH HELDMANN, BS, COTA/L
Adjunct Faculty & Occupational Therapy Assistant
Owens Community College
Toledo, OH

DEBI HINERFELD, PHD, OTR/L, FAOTA
Occupational Therapy Practitioner
Private Practice Owner
Adjunct Professor of Occupational Therapy
Roswell, GA

JOANNE JACKSON FOSS, PHD, OTR, FAOTA
Professor Emerita
University of Florida
Gainesville

LESLY WILSON JAMES, PHD, MPA, OTR/L, FAOTA
Assistant Professor
Lenoir-Rhyne University
Columbia, SC

JULIE JONES, OTD, OTR/L, BCP
Assistant Professor
St. Ambrose University
Davenport, IA

KARRIE KINGSLEY, OTD, OTR/L
Associate Professor of Clinical Occupational Therapy
University of Southern California
Los Angeles

LAUREN M. LITTLE, PHD, OTR/L
Associate Professor
Rush University
Chicago

LEA ANN LOWERY, OTD, OTR/L
Clinical Professor
University of Missouri
Columbia

ANNE LUCAS, MS, OTR/L
Technical Assistance Specialist
Early Childhood Technical Assistance Center
University of North Carolina at Chapel Hill
Center for IDEA Early Childhood Data Systems, SRI
    International
Chapel Hill

KRISTEN MARTIN, MOT, OTR/L
Occupational Therapy Clinical Leader
Nationwide Children's Hospital
Columbus, OH

REBECCA MARTIN, OTR/L, OTD
Manager of Clinical Education and Training & Assistant
    Professor
International Center for Spinal Cord Injury, Kennedy
    Krieger Institute
Baltimore, Maryland

SUSAN P. MAUDE, PHD
Credential Specialist
Georgia Department of Early Care and Learning
Atlanta, GA

ALAENA MCCOOL, MS, OTR/L, CPAM
Occupational Therapist II
International Center for Spinal Cord Injury, Kennedy
    Krieger Institute
Baltimore

CHRISTINE T. MYERS, PHD, OTR/L
Clinical Associate Professor & Program Director
Department of occupational Therapy
University of Florida
Gainesville

JAYNA NIBLOCK, PHD, OTD, OTR/L, BCP
Pediatric Occupational Therapist
Blank Children's Hospital
Des Moines, IA

SARA O'ROURKE, MOT, OTR/L, BCP
Program Manager
Nationwide Children's Hospital
Columbus, OH

STEPHANIE PARKS, PHD, OT/L
Assistant Professor of Practice
Department of Special Education
University of Kansas
Lawrence

KRISTIN PEDERSEN, SLPD, CCC–SLP
Clinical Associate Professor
Department of Speech-Language-Hearing
University of Kansas
Lawrence

JENNIFER S. PITONYAK, PHD, OTR/L, SCFES
Associate Professor & Associate Director
School of Occupational Therapy
University of Puget Sound
Tacoma, WA

KRIS PIZUR-BARNEKOW, PHD, OTR/L, IMH–E®
Associate Professor
University of Wisconsin–Milwaukee
Milwaukee

BONNIE RILEY, OTD, OTR/L
Assistant Professor
St. Catherine University
St. Paul, MN

JOYCE RIOUX, EDD, OTR/L, SCSS, FAOTA
Assistant Director of Therapies
Capitol Region Education Council
Windsor, CT

SANDRA SCHEFKIND, OTD, OTR/L, FAOTA
Consultant
Early Childhood Personnel Center
Farmington, CT

ELIZABETH KOSS SCHMIDT, PHD, OTR/L
Postdoctoral Fellow
Boston University Department of Occupational Therapy
Boston

JUDITH SCHOONOVER, MED, OTR/L, ATP, FAOTA
Occupational Therapist & Assistive Technology Professional
Independent Consultant
Holland, MI

WINIFRED SCHULTZ-KROHN, PHD, OTR/L, BCP, SWC, FAOTA
Professor & Chair of Occupational Therapy
San Jose State University
San Jose, CA

FRANCINE SERUYA, PHD, OTR/L, FAOTA
Professor & Program Director
Occupational Therapy Program
Mercy College
Dobbs Ferry, NY

PAM STEPHENSON, OTD, OTR/L
Assistant Professor
Occupational Therapy Program
Mary Baldwin University
Fishersville, VA

ASHLEY STOFFEL, OTD, OTR/L, FAOTA
Clinical Associate Professor
University of Illinois at Chicago
Chicago

YVONNE SWINTH, PHD, OTR/L, FAOTA
Professor
School of Occupational Therapy
University of Puget Sound
Tacoma, WA

KELLY TANNER, PHD, OTR/L, BCP
Director of Occupational Therapy Research
Nationwide Children's Hospital
Columbus, OH

STEPHAN VIEHWEG, I.CSW, ACSW, IMH-E(R), CYC-P
Assistant Scientist & Scholar
Department of Pediatrics
Indiana University School of Medicine
Indianapolis

TAYLOR CRANE VOS, OTD, OTR/L
Occupational Therapist
Outpatient Pediatrics: Metro West Learning Center, LLC
Clive, IA

ASHWINI WAGLE, EDD, MS, RD
Department Chair
Department of Nutrition, Food Science, and Packaging
San Jose State University
San Jose, CA

ANNA WALLISCH, PHD, OTR/L
Postdoctoral Researcher
Juniper Gardens Children's Project
University of Kansas
Kansas City

Foreword

Best Practices for Occupational Therapy in Early Childhood provides important information and assistance to occupational therapy practitioners as well as parents, educators, child care providers, and other professionals. It expands and deepens the information from an earlier book, *Early Childhood: Occupational Therapy Services for Children Birth to Five* (Chandler, 2010). This new content articulates occupational therapy's evidence-based practices in working with young children and their families.

The occupational therapy perspective is to help others "achieve health, well-being, and participation in life" (AOTA, 2020, p. 73). Using a family-centered approach, occupational therapy practitioners partner with families to enhance the child's early development, health, and family resources. With other professionals, occupational therapy practitioners identify and develop programs to produce positive outcomes for children and their families.

Occupational therapy practitioners must understand the federal and state legislation that has been enacted to address the needs of young children and their families, education laws, and public health laws relating to children and families. Legislation is subject to political perspectives which may change. Joining your state occupational therapy association and lobbying your state representatives is essential as an advocate for children and families.

Challenges continue. Services readily found in one part of the country may be more difficult to access in areas. The early detection, treatment, intervention, and ongoing monitoring of outcomes is extremely important in a young child's development. Our roles as occupational therapy professionals continue to grow, including our responsibility to advocate for effective and evidence-based interventions.

We have all come a long way—but there is more to go.

—Barbara E. Chandler, PhD, FAOTA
Retired to her home in the mountains of Virginia

REFERENCES

American Occupational Therapy Association. (2020). Occupational therapy practice framework: Domain and process (4th ed.). *American Journal of Occupational Therapy, 74,* 7412410010. https://doi.org/10.5014/ajot.2020.74S2001

Chandler, B. E. (Ed.). *Early childhood: Occupational therapy services for children birth to five.* AOTA Press.

Introduction

Gloria Frolek Clark, PhD, OTR/L, BCP, FAOTA, and Stephanie Parks, PhD, OT/L

> *"A person's a person, no matter how small."*
> —Dr. Seuss (1954)

Staying current on new evidence and practice across the field of early childhood can be challenging and time consuming—especially for occupational therapy practitioners with high workloads working across multiple settings. (*Note.* The term *occupational therapy practitioner* is used to refer to both occupational therapists and occupational therapy assistants). The purpose of *Best Practices for Occupational Therapy in Early Childhood* is to weave the influences (e.g., legislative, professional, contextual) and roles of occupational therapy practitioners into one source to present the most effective evidence-guided practices for practitioners, researchers, educators, and colleagues working with young children in early intervention, preschools, and health care. We chose to include all aspects of early childhood (e.g., early intervention, preschools, health care) to increase knowledge about each setting and coordinate occupational therapy services across these settings.

Throughout this text, we follow American Occupational Therapy Association's (AOTA) official documents, including the supervision guidelines (2020a), which state "the occupational therapist is responsible for all aspects of occupational therapy service delivery and is accountable for the safety and effectiveness of the occupational therapy service delivery process" (p. 1) and "must be directly involved in the delivery of services during the initial evaluation and regularly throughout the course of intervention" (p. 3). In addition, "the occupational therapy assistant delivers safe and effective occupational therapy services under the supervision of and in partnership with the occupational therapist" (p. 3). Information from the newly revised *Occupational Therapy Practice Framework, 4th Edition* (AOTA, 2020b) is infused throughout the book to guide occupational therapy practices. The *Guidelines for Occupational Therapy Services in Early Intervention and Schools* (AOTA, 2017) also provides guidance regarding the role of occupational therapy in these settings (see Appendix A, "Guidelines for Occupational Therapy Services in Early Intervention and Schools").

Occupational therapy practitioners working in early childhood must implement current evidence-based practices to guide decisions about services. AOTA synthesizes the strength of evidence on the basis of the guidelines of the U.S. Preventive Services Task Force (2016). However, the U.S. Department of Education (2016) uses a different set of guidelines for synthesizing evidence for school settings under the Every Student Succeeds Act (2015).

The similarities and differences can be found in Appendix B, "Evidence-Based Practice and Occupational Therapy."

Best Practices for Occupational Therapy in Early Childhood focuses on occupation, development, participation, principles of family-centered practice, client-centered practices, and community partnerships across various settings. Chapters break topics into short, stand-alone resources with essential information and best practices in evaluation and intervention. Many chapters include resources that guide readers to additional information or materials. The chapters are organized by sections (see Table I.1) and present information in various "chunks," such as occupational therapy's role, settings, developmental information, and evidence-guided practices, to enable readers to access information easily. Table I.1 also includes information on this text's ten appendixes.

Authenticity of information is provided by evidence-based research as well as each authors' knowledge, skills, and experience on the various topics in early childhood. Both editors have strong knowledge and experience in early childhood. Dr. Parks began her career as an early childhood special education preschool teacher, became an occupational therapist, worked in early intervention and early childhood special education for more than 20 years, and now serves as practice faculty in the early childhood and early childhood special education undergraduate and graduate programs at the University of Kansas. Dr. Frolek Clark is an occupational therapist who has worked in early intervention, preschool, and school settings for more than 40 years while working as a consultant at the Iowa Department of Education Bureaus of Special Education and Early Childhood for 15 years. She received her doctoral degree from the Iowa State University in human development and family studies with emphasis on early childhood special education. Currently, she has a private practice and teaches a class at Drake University.

In addition to working in early childhood, many of the authors are occupational therapy practitioners with degrees in other disciplines and additional certifications such as assistive technology professional, specialty and board certifications, or endorsement in infant mental health. We sought multidisciplinary authors for several chapters to provide a broad perspective on topics. The voices of early childhood special educators, social workers, dietitians, speech-language pathologists, and practitioners who are also parents of children with special needs can be "heard" throughout this book. Together with the chapter authors from across the United States, we hope this book will promote enhanced outcomes for young children and their families across all settings.

Table I.1. Overview of Contents

SECTION	SUMMARY OF CONTENT
Section I. Understanding Early Childhood and Occupational Therapy's Role	History of occupational therapy services in early childhood; influences form other professional organizations; personnel preparation; role of OTAs; leadership roles; data collection; assistive technology; supporting family, community, school, and health care partnerships; and transitions.
Section II. Early Development	Brain development, mental health, development of early and emergent literacy.
Section III. Considerations for Early Intervention: IDEA Part C	Law and IFSP process; screening and evaluation, intervention in natural environment; and documentation.
Section IV. Considerations for Preschool: IDEA Part B	Law and IEP process; screening and evaluation, intervention in preschools; and documentation.
Section V. Considerations for Medical and Health Care Settings	Requirements, process, and billing; screening and evaluation, intervention for developmental and acquired conditions; and documentation.
Section VI. Evidence-Guided Practice: Addressing Evaluation and Intervention	Address evaluation and intervention related to adaptive (ADLs, mealtimes) and cognitive skills (learning and literacy); physical skills (fine and visual–motor coordination, large motor); social and communication skills; social–emotional skills; and play and leisure. Also includes specific topics on children with hearing and visual impairments, health needs, ASD and ADHD, and prenatal substance exposure and postnatal trauma.
Appendices A–J	Includes AOTA official documents; the AOTA Occupational Profile Template; an intervention plan template; AOTA resources in early childhood; a list of assessment tools commonly used in EC; examples of EI, PS, and health care evaluation reports; and information about using telehealth in EC settings.

Note. ADHD = attention deficit hyperactivity disorder; ADLs = activities of daily living; AOTA = American Occupational Therapy Association; ASD = autism spectrum disorder; EC = early childhood; EI = early intervention; IDEA = Individuals with Disabilities Education Improvement Act; IEP = individualized education program; IFSP = individualized family service plan; OTAs = occupational therapy assistants; PS = preschool.

REFERENCES

American Occupational Therapy Association. (2017). Guidelines for occupational therapy services in early intervention and schools. *American Journal of Occupational Therapy, 71*(Suppl. 2), 7112410010. https://doi.org/10.5014/ajot.2017.716S01

American Occupational Therapy Association. (2020a). Guidelines for supervision, roles, and responsibilities during the delivery of occupational therapy services. *American Journal of Occupational Therapy, 74,* 7413410020. https://doi.org/10.5014/ajot.2020.74S3004

American Occupational Therapy Association. (2020b). Occupational therapy practice framework: Domain and process (4th ed.). *American Journal of Occupational Therapy, 74,* 7412410010. https://doi.org/10.5014/ajot.2020.74S2001

Every Student Succeeds Act of 2015, Pub. L. No. 114-95 § 114 Stat. 1177.

Seuss, Dr. (1954). *Horton hears a who.* Random House.

U.S. Department of Education. (2016). *Non-regulatory guidance: Using evidence to strengthen education investments.* https://ed.gov/policy/elsec/leg/essa/guidanceuseseinvestment.pdf

U.S. Preventive Services Task Force. (2016). *Grade definitions.* https://www.uspreventiveservicestaskforce.org/Page/Name/grade-definitions

Section I.

Foundation: Understanding Early Childhood and the Role of Occupational Therapy

History of Occupational Therapy Services in Early Childhood

1

Joyce Rioux, EdD, OTR/L, SCSS, FAOTA, and Gloria Frolek Clark, PhD, OTR/L, BCP, FAOTA
With contributions from Barbara Hanft, MA, OTR, FAOTA

KEY TERMS AND CONCEPTS

- The Arc
- Child saving movement
- Community Mental Health Act of 1963
- Easterseals
- Education of the Handicapped Act of 1970
- Elementary and Secondary Education Act of 1965

- *Guidelines for Occupational Therapy Services in School Systems*
- Individuals with Disabilities Education Act of 1997
- *Occupational Therapy Practice Framework: Domain and Process*
- Promoting Partners: Leadership Training for Therapists in Education and Early Intervention

- Section 504 of the Rehabilitation Act
- Social Security Act of 1935
- Training Occupational Therapists in Educational Management Systems

OVERVIEW

The history of early childhood education is about people— ordinary people and powerful people—living in ordinary and extraordinary times. It is a history of adults working with and for children from the dawn of the United States of America to the modern era, even in the most challenging of circumstances. (Hinitz, 2013, p. 1)

The early childhood programs and services of today evolved from their historical predecessors (Hinitz, 2013). With each passing decade, notable political, social, and economic underpinnings have influenced changes in the approach, availability, and focus on young children, including young children with disabilities. Bettye Caldwell, an educator and steadfast supporter of early enrichment for children, described the "1950s as . . . *forget and hide,* . . . [the] 1960s as a time to *screen and segregate,* and the 1970s as a time to *identify and help*" (Lascarides & Hinitz, 2000, p. 442). Continuing with this theme, the authors of this chapter would label the 1980s as *train and deliver;* the 1990s as *collaboration and accountability;* the 2000s as *family centered, child focused, and collaborative partnerships;* and the 2010s as *participation, parent coaching,* and *interprofessional collaboration.*

This chapter explores the history of programs and services for young children and families across the decades and the interconnections with occupational therapy in shaping the field. The chapter will conclude with a summary of considerations for occupational therapy practitioners' future role in early childhood practice. (*Note.* Occupational *therapy practitioner* refers to both occupational therapists and occupational therapy assistants.)

HISTORY OF EARLY CHILDHOOD PROGRAMS AND SERVICES

Early Perspectives on Children With Disabilities

In the 1920s, a variety of residential schools and institutions in the United States—public and private—existed to address the needs of different categories of disabling conditions (e.g., deafness, blindness, mental retardation, epilepsy; Lascarides & Hinitz, 2000). Psychologist Alfred Binet in France was working to develop a measure to differentiate between students who would be successful in public school and those who would not. The impetus of this work defines the mindset of the times: that children with limitations were destined to fail and would require special attention outside the mainstream. Many schools started separate classes for people with single disabilities versus those with multiple disabilities. People with multiple disabilities and severe cognitive limitations were often removed from society and sent to institutions at the recommendation of their physicians. In addition, several states had laws that allowed them to assume temporary custody of children with disabilities from poor families who could not afford to pay for schooling or services and committed them to institutions. Therefore, the state became responsible for the child's placement and services without input from a parent. The Children's Bureau (now known as the Maternal and Child Health Bureau) worked with states in the early 1940s to abolish these commitment laws.

Early Social Resources and Programs

In the late 19th and early 20th centuries, the **child saving movement**, a movement credited to a group of upper middle class women concerned with children, increased public awareness about childhood problems (e.g., infant mortality, child labor; Hitchcock, 2009). In 1912, the U.S. government established the Children's Bureau to examine health and well-being concerns for all children (Hanft, 1988). During this time, children were recruited for manual labor, infant mortality was high, most family incomes were low, and living conditions were often unsanitary. The bureau's investigation resulted in the Public Protection of Maternity and Infancy Plan being presented to Congress in 1917. A primary emphasis of this plan centered on early intervention services inclusive of centers for well-baby care, distribution of educational materials, and nursing visits aimed at infant and maternal health.

Federal support and funding (i.e., state grants for health services) for these programs were gained in 1921 with the passage of the Sheppard–Towner Maternity and Infancy Protection Act (P. L. 67-97). The passage of this act occurred as a result of the Children's Bureau research, advocacy parties lobbying for support, and women being armed with the right to vote, which worried many politicians in how a "nay" vote would affect their career (Rodems et al., 2011).

Although the Sheppard–Towner Maternity and Infancy Protection Act was repealed 5 years later, the services afforded for infant and maternal health were influential in later legislation, including the **Social Security Act of 1935** (P. L. 74-271; Rodems et al., 2011). Title V of the Social Security Act introduced special grants to states to fund the Maternal and Child Health Services and Services for Crippled Children programs, which were aimed at improving services for dependent children and mothers and children with physical disabilities (e.g., orthopedic problems, rheumatic heart disease, congenital heart disease; Hanft, 1988; Madgett, 2017). The term *crippled children* (now referred to as children and youth with special health care needs; Genetic Alliance & Family Voices, 2013) was used to describe those with physical handicaps because professionals and reformers believed that these children could be cured with proper medical treatment and education, unlike children who were blind, deaf, or intellectually disabled (Hitchcock, 2009).

The enactment of the Social Security Act of 1935 was the first time that the federal government extended support for children with disabilities (Hitchcock, 2009). Mandates required that children receive aftercare services (e.g., nursing, occupational therapy, social services, physical therapy) following a medical procedure. Aftercare services could occur in homes, schools, or other facilities and required interdisciplinary cooperation among education, health, and welfare services. At this time, occupational therapists worked in 13 pediatric hospitals across the nation, providing services to children with cerebral palsy, orthopedically handicapping conditions, and infantile paralysis (i.e., poliomyelitis; Anderson & Reed, 2017).

By 1941, some consistency among state services and services for children with disabilities was present through children's hospitals, outpatient services, and residential homes (Hitchcock, 2009). However, during World War II, a decline in the level of services for children occurred when many medical professionals were deployed. Over the next several decades, medical services for children slowly increased as more states developed programs for children with cerebral palsy, epilepsy, and congenital heart disease.

Family Support, Advocacy, and Philanthropy

Parents of children with disabilities and members of fraternal organizations initiated many early programs and services centered on children's health care and educational needs. One such example occurred in 1907, when Ohio businessman Edgar Allen could not find adequate medical services to save his son after a streetcar accident. In turn, he sold his business and built a hospital (Easterseals, 2019). During this process, he discovered that children with disabilities were often hidden from the public. To remedy this, he collaborated with members of the Ohio Rotary Club and began the National Society for Crippled Children (now known as **Easterseals**).

The Cuyahoga County Council for the Retarded Child in Ohio was established by a group of mothers in 1933 in an effort to advocate for their children's inclusion in public schools (The Arc, 2019). This small grassroots effort grew as they banded together with similar groups across the nation and eventually became **The Arc.** Other organizations were formed through philanthropic work, including the United Cerebral Palsy Association, founded in 1949 (Jansheski, 2019); the National Society for Autistic Children (now called Autism Society of America), developed in 1965 (Autism Society, 2011); and the Association for Children with Learning Disabilities (now called the Learning Disabilities Association of America [LDAA]), started in 1964 (LDAA, n.d.). Each of these organizations, along with other private and nonprofit organizations, provided families with a voice to drive change and advocate for children with special needs at local, state, and federal levels.

The Kennedy family, including Eunice Kennedy Shriver, was politically influential in changing the conversation on and calling attention to the needs of children with disabilities (John F. Kennedy Presidential Library and Museum, n.d.). A direct outcome of Shriver's influence included the formation of the President's Panel on Mental Retardation to investigate and propose solutions to address the needs of people with cognitive limitations (Harris, 2006). The panel proposed 95 recommendations, which were mostly incorporated into future legislation and included further research, civil rights advocacy, institution downsizing, an increase in community services, and a focus on normalization principles (e.g., normal routines; opportunities; standards; respect for choices, wishes, and desires).

Early Childhood Education

Bridging into the 20th century, two tracks of early childhood programs existed for any child, irrelevant of diagnostic concerns (Cahan, 1989). One track focused on basic custodial care for children from low socioeconomic families, such as single mothers working to support their families. The programs were often deplorable, with one adult to 30 or more children in a room, poor nutritional options, and limited resources. The second track afforded preparatory education for children from middle and high socioeconomic families. These programs even offered additional resources for parent education and social exchanges.

As time evolved, some programs accessed charity workers to expand their program and attempted to address children's educational, developmental, social, and health care needs. The 1920s were marked with the formation of kindergarten and primary grade lab schools—that is, early childhood programs—formed on college campuses or training schools (Lascarides & Hinitz, 2000). The intent was to provide an environment in which teachers could acquire training and study children's development.

1950s: Forget and Hide

The 1950s saw a growing dissonance between parents of children with disabilities and negative societal views of people with disabilities (Lascarides & Hinitz, 2000; Minnesota Governor's Council on Developmental Disabilities, n.d.). Parent groups were frustrated with the poor living conditions and lack of community supports for their children. Society, in general, accepted an out-of-sight, out-of-mind attitude and rationalized the placement of children with disabilities in institutions (Lascarides & Hinitz, 2000). Occupational therapists were often hired by institutions or through community agencies such as Easterseals and crippled children's centers to provide services to children with physical disabilities.

With the 1954 landmark Brown v. Board of Education of Topeka ruling that children cannot be segregated based solely on their race, the doors opened for parents of children with disabilities to advocate for their civil rights (Lascarides & Hinitz, 2000). Grants to higher education institutions were enacted in the late 1950s to promote training for teachers and professionals in educating children with cognitive disabilities (labeled as *mental retardation* during this time period). Unfortunately, little focus was given to preschool and early childhood programs, let alone a focus on young children with disabilities. In addition, women with children younger than 6 years old were expected to stay home and out of the workforce unless financially burdened.

1960s: Screen and Segregate

In 1963, the *Community Mental Health Act* (P. L. 88-164) outlined project grants for construction of University Affiliated Facilities for the Mentally Retarded (UAF; now known as University Centers for Excellence in Developmental Disabilities [UCEDDs]). These centers came at a time when parents usually either placed their children with disabilities in institutions based on a physician's recommendation or opted to keep such children at home, where resources and supports outside of the family were very limited. Leadership Education in Neurodevelopmental and Related Disabilities (LEND) programs funded through the Maternal and Child Health Bureau were rolled out to operate within the UAF. LEND programs were developed to train health professionals (e.g., occupational therapists) in becoming leaders to improve the health of infants, children, and youth with disabilities (or suspected of having a disability) through interdisciplinary practice. Today, the Association

of University Centers on Disabilities (AUCD, 2011) represents 67 UCEDDs, LEND programs, and Intellectual and Developmental Disabilities Research Centers. The primary focus of AUCD is to advance policy and practice for people with disabilities.

In 1965, the *Elementary and Secondary Education Act* (ESEA; P. L. 89-10) offered subsidies for direct public education services for select populations of children with disabilities ages 3–21 years (Lascarides & Hinitz, 2000; Exhibit 1.1). That same year, the Office of Economic Opportunity started an 8-week pilot summer program called Head Start designed for preschool children from families of low socioeconomic status (Early Childhood Learning and Knowledge Center, 2018). This comprehensive program did not target children with diagnosed disabilities; instead, it was launched as a stopgap measure in the war on poverty and aimed to meet the social, emotional, physical, general health, and nutritional needs of young children. Based on the program's success, funding was provided and the first school year program was begun in the fall of that same year.

With the passing of the ESEA, the Bureau of Education for the Handicapped (now known as the Office of Special Education Programs) was created to allocate incentive funding for research and projects aimed to improve special education, set up regional resource centers, and provide assistance to state and local educational agencies to support activities on behalf of children with disabilities. In 1968, the Handicapped Children's Early Education Assistance Act (P. L. 90-538) was the first federal legislation that acknowledged the importance of early education. Public and private agencies or organizations could pursue grants to establish experimental preschool programs (First Chance projects) to uncover positive procedures and methods for use with this population (Hanft, 1988; LaVor & Krivit, 1969).

1970s: Identify and Help

The *Education of the Handicapped Act of 1970* (P. L. 91-230) established a national advisory committee and provided assistance to interested state educational agencies

---

EXHIBIT 1.1. A Sibling's Perspective: Joyce Rioux

In 1965, my parents sent my 6-year-old brother off to school, only to have him returned with the message that the school could not educate him. Public preschool and kindergarten programs, let alone special education, did not exist in our tiny town. My brother was born with a heart defect and identified with mental retardation. Sending him to school at age 6 years allowed him a gap year to catch up developmentally with typically developing students—an observed belief at that time.

When he was turned away from this public school educational opportunity, my parents advocated for his inclusion, armed with the knowledge that they gained during his many doctor and medical visits to Boston Children's Hospital and from the work done through the Kennedy Administration. Within a short time, the school district set up a class consisting of my brother, children in wheelchairs, and children with behavior difficulties, all led by a teacher with no special education training or experience. Initially, the program was very custodial in nature—it did not take on an educational direction until a teacher trained in special education was hired.

to design and implement special education and related services for children with disabilities between the ages of 3 years and 21 years. Although related services were not defined, in 1971, 20% of occupational therapists and 6% of occupational therapy assistants polled by the American Occupational Therapy Association (AOTA) identified pediatrics as their practice setting (Anderson & Reed, 2017). Common pediatric settings at that time were hospitals or maternal child health and crippled children's service clinics. In 1972, Congress set a mandate in which 10% of the Head Start enrollment by fiscal year 1976 would include children with disabilities (Cohen et al., 1979; Lacarides & Hinitz, 2000).

The year 1973 was pivotal for the approval of *Section 504 of the Rehabilitation Act* (P. L. 93-112). This civil rights law outlined that any program—including preschool programs—receiving federal financial assistance that is offered to people without disabilities must also be offered to people with disabilities. The language of a free appropriate public education was introduced with this legislation. *Appropriate* meant that people with disabilities would be provided a comparable education similar to those without disabilities and be provided special education, related aids, and related services to access that education. Failure to provide these services would jeopardize federal funding. In 1974, Education Amendments (P. L. 93-380) were made to the ESEA that outlined support for state and local educational agencies to develop and implement public preschool education for children with disabilities at their discretion.

Before 1975, Iowa, Maryland, Michigan, Minnesota, and Nebraska were providing a free appropriate public education to all children younger than age 21 years and became known as birth mandate states. In 1975, the Education for All Handicapped Children Act (P. L. 94-142) established that all states must provide a free appropriate public education (FAPE) to children from ages 5 to 18 years by 1980 (U.S. Department of Education, 2010). This meant that more than 1 million children with disabilities who were previously excluded now had a legal right to FAPE. At that time, 13 states provided a preschool education for children ages 3–5 years and began to include children with disabilities (although not all disabilities). With the implementation of the Education for All Handicapped Children Act, occupational therapy was recognized as a related service. Therefore, occupational therapy practitioners needed to establish their role and educate others as they moved from a health care focus to educational settings (Anderson & Reed, 2017).

1980s: Train and Deliver

In 1980, AOTA provided a national training on school practice, *Training Occupational Therapists in Educational Management Systems* (TOTEMS; Gilfoyle & Hays, 1980). Although the training did not contain specific information about early childhood, therapists were beginning to understand educational versus medical services. After federal amendments to the Education for All Handicapped Children Act, the *Guidelines for Occupational Therapy Services in School Systems* (AOTA, 1987), written specifically

to assist occupational therapy practitioners in schools, were quickly revised 2 years later (AOTA, 1989).

In the early 1980s, Barbara Hanft, an occupational therapist, transitioned from managing an early childhood center and was hired by AOTA in the Government and Legal Affairs Division. In her new role, she actively lobbied Congress on behalf of 65 national organizations regarding the benefits of providing family-centered, interdisciplinary, and interagency services for families with infants and toddlers with disabilities. She also advocated for occupational therapy, physical therapy, and speech–language pathology to be primary services from birth to age 3 years versus a related service as defined under the *Individuals with Disabilities Education Act* (IDEA, 1986 [99-457], Part B).

In 1985, 8 states extended special education and related services to children from birth to age 3 years; 31 states plus the District of Columbia provided services for children ages 3–5 years (Hanft, 1988). In the majority of states, there was little overlap between health (under the Department of Health and Human Services) and education (under the Department of Education) programs. This division affected the expectations and understanding of families and legislators regarding the services being offered and the distinction between medical and educational services.

When the Education for All Handicapped Children Act was amended in 1986 (P. L. 99-457), 17% of AOTA members surveyed worked in schools (Anderson & Reed, 2017). Under IDEA (1990), Part B, Section 619, states and local educational agencies were required to have available special education and related services for preschool children with disabilities. Amendments also required states to establish an interagency coordinating council of early intervention (i.e., including education, social services, and health services) to enhance the development of infants and toddlers with disabilities or at risk for delay. The primary intent of Part H was to minimize the cost of future education and probability of institutionalization (Part H was later named Part C in *IDEA, 1997*). To prepare for this mandate, states had the autonomy to develop a timetable for providing early intervention services by 1991 that outlined how they would meet the specific requirements.

In 1987, AOTA was one of the first organizations to be awarded a family-centered grant called the Family-Centered Care Project to support in-service training. Hanft, in collaboration with Jane Acquaviva, AOTA's director for the Division of Education, drafted a 3-day training that required a team of 12 occupational therapists and 6 parents to train in 40 states. The inclusion of parents as trainers was innovative and brought positive attention on a national level. In partnership with other state agencies, state occupational therapy associations hosted the trainings, which covered understanding natural environments, how to work with families, and how to reflectively listen.

Because of confusion between educational versus medical service delivery, some insurance companies were refusing health care services to young children because they assumed that services in schools would cover all areas. Many states developed brochures to educate parents and providers on the emphasis of these two settings. Local education agencies were beginning to bill Medicaid for IDEA services, as legislated by the Medicare Catastrophic Coverage Act of 1988 (P. L. 100-360). Occupational therapy services provided at schools were eligible for reimbursement, causing further confusion as well as reimbursement denials for health care agencies if occupational therapy services occurred in these agencies and in schools on the same day.

1990s: Collaboration and Accountability

AOTA received national attention for its wealth of published guideline documents covering pediatrics, training programs to prepare entry-level occupational therapists, and planned professional development programs focused on early intervention (Hinojosa et al., 1994; Humphry & Link, 1990). Early intervention was being acknowledged as a specialty area, and AOTA responded to the call to support practitioners in best practice.

In 1990, the Education for All Handicapped Children Act Amendments (P. L. 101-476) set forth priorities for preparing personnel. Barbara Chandler, AOTA's pediatric manager, saw an opportunity to encourage a group of practitioners in early intervention and schools to form a special interest section (SIS). In 1994, after securing the needed signatures, the School System SIS was created to address the needs of occupational therapy practitioners working with children from birth to graduation. The name was later changed in 2008 to the Early Intervention & School SIS, and in 2018, to the Children and Youth SIS to encompass all pediatric settings.

In 1994, Leslie Jackson, a pediatric occupational therapist who worked at AOTA, coordinated with Hanft on an AOTA grant-funded program, *Promoting Partners: Leadership Training for Therapists in Education and Early Intervention,* which brought together occupational therapy providers, state educational agencies (e.g., Departments of Education), and occupational therapy preparatory programs to address shared practice concerns.

In 1997, the Education for All Handicapped Children Act was reauthorized as the IDEA (P. L. 101-476), with a stronger emphasis on the importance of early intervention services occurring in natural environments. Part B established preschool educational services for children ages 3–5 years with disabilities. With this legislation, developmental delay was added as a disability category. By the 1998–1999 school year, 574,000 preschool children with disabilities (4.8% of the population; U.S. Department of Education, 2000), and 187,000 infants and toddlers (1.6% of the population; Early Childhood Technical Assistance Center, 2019) received special education and early intervention services in preschool classrooms, family child care centers, private homes, nursery schools, and residential facilities.

To implement IDEA 1997 reforms, AOTA became a primary partner of the Associations of Service Providers Implementing IDEA Reforms in Education (ASPIIRE; Jackson, 2001). ASPIIRE was one of four IDEA Partnership projects focused on bringing people together to raise issues; share concerns; and work together to develop materials, resources, and trainings. With Jackson as AOTA's ASPIIRE liaison, an occupational therapy workgroup was formed to focus on children's social–emotional needs in educational programs and an ASPIIRE cadre was established to represent special education and early childhood professionals. Thirty-four occupational therapists served on the cadre to represent and address the needs of school and early intervention practitioners, researchers, program administrators, and educators.

2000–2010: Family-Centered, Child-Focused, Collaborative Partnerships

At the beginning of the millennium, early intervention services emphasized being family centered and child focused, building collaborative partnerships, and using best practices.

With the first publication of AOTA's *Occupational Therapy Practice Framework: Domain and Process* (OTPF; AOTA, 2002), occupational therapy practitioners could more clearly articulate their contribution to persons, groups, and populations to promote health and participation through engagement in occupations. In 2002–2003, the possibility of an early intervention specialty certification was studied; however, certification for this area was not chosen at that time. Board certification in pediatrics was popular with occupational therapists in pediatrics and a specialty certification for occupational therapy practitioners in schools was recommended and established in 2014.

2010–Present: Participation, Parent Coaching, Interprofessional Collaboration

From 2017 to 2018, under IDEA of 2004 (P. L. 108-446), more than 388,000 infants and toddlers (3.26% of the population; Early Childhood Technical Assistance Center, 2019) received early intervention (Part C) and 774,000 preschoolers (6.44% of the population; U.S. Department of Education, 2018) received special education (Part B).

Using the *OTPF* (AOTA, 2014, 2020) and emphasizing natural environments and least restrictive programming, occupational therapy practitioners have focused more on occupations within the natural routines of children and families. Coaching and strategies for involving families during early intervention have emerged as important methods for supporting family engagement and targeting positive outcomes for children.

Providing opportunities for professional development, AOTA has hosted several specialty conferences through the years. AOTA has also joined other professional organizations and education associations to produce interprofessional standards (Early Childhood Personnel Center, 2017). Members of AOTA can access online recent evidence-based practice resources (e.g., social–emotional, motor, self-care, and cognitive development to support early childhood programs and services). AOTA has also published practice guidelines and systematic reviews in the *American Journal of Occupational Therapy* on early childhood topics (see Frolek Clark & Kingsley, 2020). Table 1.1 outlines these AOTA resources for early childhood occupational therapy practitioners that have been published since 2010.

TABLE 1.1.   AOTA Resources for Early Childhood Practitioners

YEAR	AUTHOR OR EDITOR	TITLE
2010	Chandler	*Occupational Therapy in Early Childhood*
2011	AOTA	*Occupational Therapy Services in Early Intervention and School-Based Settings*
2011	Watling et al.	*Occupational Therapy Practice Guidelines for Children and Adolescents With Challenges in Sensory Processing and Sensory Integration*
2013	Gutman	*American Journal of Occupational Therapy, 67*(4). Special issue on occupational therapy and early intervention/early childhood
2013	Bazyk & Arbesman	*Occupational Therapy Practice Guidelines for Mental Health Promotion, Prevention, and Intervention for Children and Youth*
2013	Frolek Clark & Kingsley	*Occupational Therapy Practice Guidelines for Early Childhood: Birth Through 5 Years*
2015	Orentlicher et al.	*Transitions Across the Lifespan*
2016	Hanft & Shepherd	*Collaborating for Student Success* (2nd ed.)
2016	Tomchek & Koenig	*Occupational Therapy Practice Guidelines for Children and Adolescents With Autism*
2017	AOTA	*Guidelines for Occupational Therapy Services in Early Intervention and Schools*
2017	Frolek Clark & Handley-More	*Best Practices for Documenting Occupational Therapy Services in Schools*
2018	Watling et al.	*Occupational Therapy Practice Guidelines for Children and Adolescents With Challenges in Sensory Integration and Sensory Processing*
2019	Frolek Clark et al.	*Best Practices for Occupational Therapy in Schools* (2nd ed.)
2020	Frolek Clark & Kingsley	*Occupational Therapy Practice Guidelines for Early Childhood: Birth Through 5 Years* (2nd ed.)
2020	Frolek Clark & Parks	*Best Practices for Occupational Therapy in Early Childhood*
2020	Richards	*American Journal of Occupational Therapy, 74*(2). Special issue on occupational therapy interventions for children and youth

Note. AOTA = American Occupational Therapy Association.

PREPARING FOR THE FUTURE

What do occupational therapy practitioners in early childhood practice need to consider for the future? Based on the profession's history and looking forward, we offer the following list of the 10 most important actions:

1. *Appreciate our history.* From 1917 to today, occupational therapy has undergone a dramatic transformation while maintaining the core values and beliefs surrounding the power of engaging in occupation. Today, practitioners collaborate with families, analyze the activity and environment to promote occupational engagement and performance, effectively problem solve to enhance participation, collect data to monitor progress, coserve with team members, and contemplate future actions in the ever evolving system of early childhood.

2. *Embrace being a health care professional.* Occupational therapy practitioners are distinctly positioned to bring a health care lens to early childhood discussions. In accordance with the Centers for Disease Control and Prevention's (CDC; 2016) *Health in All Policies,* we can promote health equity (i.e., physical, mental, and social well-being) in policies and programs. We can also remind others that education and health correspond closely and influence each other in both directions.

When children are healthy, they are more available to engage, learn, and develop.

3. *Have an operational definition of* occupational therapy *in early childhood.* Early intervention services and preschool activities require slightly different definitions. As occupational therapy practitioners in early childhood, we create and facilitate opportunities for preschoolers to engage in occupations—those meaningful and important preschool activities that put them on a path to success, to learn, to grow, and to develop into contributing members of society. In early intervention, our focus is on the child participating in family occupations and routines.

4. *Work to your full scope of practice.* AOTA's *Vision 2025* (AOTA, 2017b) sets forth that occupational therapy will be known for promoting mental health, being inclusive, using evidence-based practices, and more. Occupational therapy practitioners in early childhood need to be cautious that their practice does not become narrowed but rather broadened to always consider the child through a holistic occupation-based perspective. Directly and immediately linking preparatory interventions to occupations allows us to better use our full scope of practice.

5. *Know laws, regulations, and operational systems.* Our roles and foci change under different laws and systems.

We can be early interventionists, service coordinators, related service providers, health care providers, specialized instruction support personnel, and so much more. Understanding the parameters that we operate under, and being able to articulate that to others, is critical. Advocating for inclusive practices is also critical.

6. *Apply multitiered systems of support (MTSS) starting at the population level.* In schools, occupational therapy practitioners are familiar with educational MTSS models under the Every Student Succeeds Act (P. L. 114-95; 2015): response to intervention and positive behavioral interventions and supports. By adding the multitiered public health model (CDC, 2018) and the *OTPF-4* definition of *client* (i.e., person, group, population; AOTA, 2020) to the MTSS mix, occupational therapy practitioners will become well positioned to address and target early childhood needs at the population level before problems surface.

7. *Develop an occupational profile with the population in mind.* Uncover the strengths and barriers of the population you serve. Current data from the CDC and the National Survey of Children's Health report the following challenges that young children are facing:
   - About 1 in 6 children ages 3–17 years have one or more developmental disabilities (CDC, 2019).
   - One in 10 children from birth to age 17 years experienced three or more adverse childhood experiences (Child Trends, 2018).
   - One in 59 children at age 8 years had a diagnosis of autism (CDC, 2014).
   - Every day, 250 preschoolers are suspended or expelled from preschool (Center for American Progress, 2017).

8. *Monitor intervention to support outcomes.* States report annual data to the federal government on their compliance with IDEA (2004) Part B and Part C indicators. Part B, Indicator 6 requires reporting preschool children's time spent in the general education setting (i.e., least restrictive environment). Part B, Indicator 7 requires reporting preschool children's improved outcomes in the areas of social–emotional skills, early literacy, and appropriate behaviors to meet their needs. Part C has similar monitoring priorities and indicators associated with services provided in natural environments and positive social–emotional skills, acquisition and use of knowledge skills, and use of appropriate behaviors to meet their needs. Clearly, these are all areas that occupational therapy practitioners can support.

9. *Know your why.* This phrase means that you understand and can explain to others your rationale for providing services in a particular way. When you know your why, you can drive change. You can help others understand the pivotal role of occupational therapy in school and curriculum teams, promote family–school–community partnerships, and make a difference for all children.

10. *Make better associations.* As practitioners, we have greater impact in association than in isolation. Joining professional associations at the local, state, and national level makes us stronger together. For more information about professional associations, see Chapter 2,

"Influences From Early Childhood Professional Organizations and Technical Assistance Centers."

SUMMARY

Peeling back the layers of history and identifying key parties and figures who stood against injustices and drove change in early childhood services and programs provides the foundation of current approaches. Today, these services and programs are making a difference in preparing children for engaging in primary occupations—play, movement, feeding, social participation, and more. Looking ahead, occupational therapy practitioners are well positioned to continue the charge and positively impact services and programs in early childhood.

REFERENCES

American Occupational Therapy Association. (1987). *Guidelines for occupational therapy services in school systems.* Rockville, MD: Author.

American Occupational Therapy Association. (1989). *Guidelines for occupational therapy services in school systems* (2nd ed.). Rockville, MD: Author.

American Occupational Therapy Association. (2002). Occupational therapy practice framework: Domain and process. *American Journal of Occupational Therapy, 56,* 609–639. https://doi.org/10.5014/ajot.56.6.609

American Occupational Therapy Association. (2011). Occupational therapy services in early intervention and school-based settings. *American Journal of Occupational Therapy, 65,* S46–S54. https://doi.org/10.5014/ajot.2011.65S46

American Occupational Therapy Association. (2014). Occupational therapy practice framework: Domain and process (3rd ed.). *American Journal of Occupational Therapy, 68*(Suppl. 1), S1–S48. https://doi.org/10.5014/ajot.2014.682006

American Occupational Therapy Association. (2017a). Guidelines for occupational therapy services in early intervention and schools. *American Journal of Occupational Therapy, 71*(Suppl. 2), 7112410010. https://doi.org/10.5014/ajot.2017.716S01

American Occupational Therapy Association. (2017b). Vision 2025. *American Journal of Occupational Therapy, 71,* 7103420010. https://doi.org/10.5014/ajot.2017.713002

American Occupational Therapy Association. (2020). Occupational therapy practice framework: Domain and process (4th ed.). *American Journal of Occupational Therapy, 74*(Suppl. 2), 7412410010. https://doi.org/10.5014/ajot.2020.74S2001

Anderson, L. T., & Reed, K. L. (2017). *The history of occupational therapy: The first century.* Slack.

Association of University Centers on Disabilities. (2011). *History.* https://www.aucd.org/template/page.cfm?id=156

Autism Society. (2011). Where we've been and where we're going: The Autism Society's proud history. *Autism Advocate, 61*(3), 7–11. https://www.autism-society.org/wp-content/uploads/2014/04/autism-society-history.pdf

Bazyk, S., & Arbesman, M. (2013). *Occupational therapy practice guidelines for mental health promotion, prevention, and intervention for children and youth.* AOTA Press.

Brown v. Board of Education of Topeka, 347 U.S. 483 (1954).

Cahan, E. D. (1989). *Past caring: A history of U.S. preschool care and education for the poor, 1820–1965.* https://www.research-connections.org/childcare/resources/2088/pdf

Center for American Progress. (2017). *New data reveal 250 preschoolers are suspended or expelled every day.* https://www.americanprogress.org/issues/early-childhood/news/2017/11/06/442280/new-data-reveal-250-preschoolers-suspended-expelled-every-day/

Centers for Disease Control and Prevention. (2014). *Autism spectrum disorder.* https://www.cdc.gov/ncbddd/autism/addm.html

Centers for Disease Control and Prevention. (2016). *Health in all policies.* https://www.cdc.gov/policy/hiap/index.html

Centers for Disease Control and Prevention. (2018). *Health impact in 5 years.* https://www.cdc.gov/policy/hst/hi5/index.html

Centers for Disease Control and Prevention. (2019). *CDC's work on developmental disabilities.* https://www.cdc.gov/ncbddd/developmentaldisabilities/about.html

Chandler, B. (2010). *Occupational therapy in early childhood.* AOTA Press.

Child Trends. (2018). *The prevalence of adverse childhood experiences, nationally, by state, and by race or ethnicity.* https://www.childtrends.org/publications/prevalence-adverse-childhood-experiences-nationally-state-race-ethnicity

Cohen, S., Semmes, M., & Guralnick, M. J. (1979). Pub. L. 94-142 and the education of preschool handicapped children. *Exceptional Children, 45,* 279–285. https://doi.org/10.1177/001440297904500406

Community Mental Health Act of 1963, Pub. L. 88-164.

Early Childhood Learning and Knowledge Center. (2018). *Head Start history.* https://eclkc.ohs.acf.hhs.gov/about-us/article/head-start-history

Early Childhood Personnel Center. (2017). *Cross-disciplinary personnel competencies.* https://ecpcta.org/cross-disciplinary-competencies/

Early Childhood Technical Assistance Center. (2019). *Part C national program data.* https://ectacenter.org/partc/partcdata.asp

Easterseals. (2019). *The story of Easterseals.* https://www.easterseals.com/who-we-are/history/

Education of the Handicapped Act of 1970, Pub. L. 91-230.

Education for All Handicapped Children Act of 1975, Pub. L. 94-142, reauthorized as the Individuals With Disabilities Education Improvement Act, codified at 20 U.S.C. §§ 1400–1482.

Education for All Handicapped Children Act Amendments of 1986, Pub. L. 99-457.

Education for All Handicapped Children Act Amendments of 1990, Pub. L. 101-476.

Elementary and Secondary Education Act of 1965, Pub. L. 89-10.

Elementary and Secondary Education Act Amendments of 1974, Pub. L. 93-380.

Every Student Succeeds Act, Pub. L. 114-95, 129 Stat. 1802 (2015).

Frolek Clark, G., & Handley-More, D. (2017). *Best practices for documenting occupational therapy services in schools.* AOTA Press.

Frolek Clark, G., & Kingsley, K. (Eds.). (2013). *Occupational therapy practice guidelines for early childhood: Birth through 5 years.* AOTA Press.

Frolek Clark, G., & Kingsley, K. (2020). Occupational therapy practice guidelines for early childhood: Birth through 5 years. *American Journal of Occupational Therapy, 74,* 7403397010. https://doi.org/10.5014/ajot.2020.743001

Frolek Clark, G., & Parks, S. (Eds.). (2020). *Best practices for occupational therapy in early childhood.* AOTA Press.

Frolek Clark, G., Rioux, J., & Chandler, B. E. (Eds.). (2019). *Best practices for occupational therapy in schools* (2nd ed.) AOTA Press.

Genetic Alliance & Family Voices. (2013). *Children and youth with special healthcare needs in Healthy People 2020: A consumer perspective.* https://www.ncbi.nlm.nih.gov/books/NBK132165/pdf/Bookshelf_NBK132165.pdf

Gilfoyle, E., & Hays, C. (1980). *Training occupational therapists in educational management systems (TOTEMS).* American Occupational Therapy Association.

Gutman, S. A. (Ed.). (2013). Occupational therapy and early intervention/early childhood [Special Issue]. *American Journal of Occupational Therapy, 67,* 379–489.

Handicapped Children's Early Education Assistance Act, Pub. L. 90-538 (1968).

Hanft, B. (1988). The changing environment of early intervention services: Implications for practice. *American Journal of Occupational Therapy, 42,* 724–731. https://doi.org/10.5014/ajot.42.11.724

Hanft, B., & Shepherd, J. (Eds.). (2016). *Collaborating for student success* (2nd ed.). AOTA Press.

Harris, J. C. (2006). *Intellectual disability: Understanding its development, causes, classification, evaluation, and treatment.* Oxford University Press.

Hinitz, B. F. (Ed.). (2013). *The hidden history of early childhood education.* Routledge.

Hinojosa, J., Moore, D. S., Sabari, J. S., & Doctor, R. G. (1994). A competency-based training program in early intervention. *American Journal of Occupational Therapy, 48,* 361. https://doi.org/10.5014/ajot.48.4.361

Hitchcock, L. (2009). *The creation of federal services for crippled children, 1890–1941* (Doctoral dissertation, The University of Alabama). https://ir.ua.edu/handle/123456789/675

Humphry, R., & Link, S. (1990). Preparation of occupational therapists to work in early intervention programs. *American Journal of Occupational Therapy, 44,* 828. https://doi.org/10.5014/ajot.44.9.828

Individuals With Disabilities Education Act of 1990, Pub. L. 101-476, renamed the Individuals With Disabilities Education Improvement Act, codified at 20 U.S.C. §§ 1400–1482.

Individuals With Disabilities Education Act Amendments of 1997, Pub. L. 105-117, 20 U.S.C. § 1400 *et seq.*

Individuals With Disabilities Education Improvement Act of 2004, Pub. L. 108-446, 20 U.S.C. §§ 1400–1482.

Jackson, L. (2001). The ASPIIRE project. *OT Practice, 6*(11), 10.

Jansheski, G. (2019). *United Cerebral Palsy Association.* https://www.cerebralpalsyguidance.com/cerebral-palsy/united-cerebral-palsy-association/

John F. Kennedy Presidential Library and Museum. (n.d.). *John F. Kennedy and people with intellectual disabilities.* https://www.jfklibrary.org/learn/about-jfk/jfk-in-history/john-f-kennedy-and-people-with-intellectual-disabilities

Lascarides, V. C., & Hinitz, B. F. (2000). *History of early childhood education.* Falmer Press.

LaVor, M., & Krivit, D. (1969). The Handicapped Children's Early Education Assistance Act Public Law 90-538. *Exceptional Children, 35,* 379–383. https://doi.org/10.1177/001440296903500506

Learning Disabilities Association of America. (n.d.). *History.* https://ldaamerica.org/about-us/history/

Madgett, K. (2017). *Sheppard–Towner Maternity and Infancy Protection Act (1921).* https://embryo.asu.edu/pages/sheppard-towner-maternity-and-infancy-protection-act-1921

Medicare Catastrophic Coverage Act of 1988, Pub. L. 100-360, 102 Stat. 683.

Minnesota Governor's Council on Developmental Disabilities. (n.d.). *Parallels in time: A history of developmental disabilities.* https://mn.gov/mnddc/parallels/five/5a/1.html

Orentlicher, M., Schefkind, S., & Gibson, R. (Eds.). (2015). *Transitions across the lifespan.* AOTA Press.

Rehabilitation Act of 1973, Pub. L. 93-112, 29 U.S.C. §701 *et seq.*

Richards, L. G. (Ed.). (2020). Occupational therapy interventions for children and youth [Special Issue]. *American Journal of Occupational Therapy, 74*(2).

Rodems, E. S., Shaefer, H. L., & Ybarra, M. (2011). The Children's Bureau and passage of the Sheppard–Towner Act of 1921: Early social work macro practice in action. *Families in Society: The Journal of Contemporary Social Services, 92,* 358–363. https://doi.org/10.1606/1044-3894.4146

Sheppard–Towner Maternity and Infancy Protection Act, Pub. L. 67-97 (1921). https://embryo.asu.edu/pages/sheppard-towner-maternity-and-infancy-protection-act-1921

Social Security Act of 1935, Pub. L. 74-271, 42 U.S.C. §§ 301–1397mm.

The Arc. (2019). *About us: Our history.* https://thearc.org/about-us/history/

Tomchek, S., & Koenig, K. (2016). *Occupational therapy practice guidelines for children and adolescents with autism.* AOTA Press.

U.S. Department of Education. (2000). *To assure the free appropriate public education of all children with disabilities: Individuals With Disabilities Education Act, Section 618.* Editorial Publications Center.

U.S. Department of Education. (2010). *Thirty-five years of progress in educating children with disabilities through IDEA.* https://www2.ed.gov/about/offices/list/osers/idea35/history/index.html

U.S. Department of Education. (2018). *IDEA Section 618 data products: Static tables.* https://www2.ed.gov/programs/osepidea/618-data/static-tables/index.html

Watling, R., Koenig, K., Davies, P., & Schaaf, R. (2011). *Occupational therapy practice guidelines for children and adolescents with challenges in sensory processing and sensory integration.* AOTA Press.

Watling, R., Miller Kuhaneck, H., Parham, D., & Schaaf, R. (2018). *Occupational therapy practice guidelines for children and adolescents with challenges in sensory integration and sensory processing.* AOTA Press.

Influences From Early Childhood Professional Organizations and Technical Assistance Centers

2

Susan P. Maude, PhD, and Stephanie Parks, PhD, OT/L

KEY TERMS AND CONCEPTS

- Behavior approach
- Compensatory education
- Comprehensive commercially available curricula
- Cross-disciplinary competencies
- Developmentally appropriate practice
- Early childhood education
- Early childhood inclusion
- Early childhood special education
- Early Head Start
- Early intervention
- Early learning and development standards
- Embedded learning opportunities
- Head Start
- HighScope approach
- Montessori approach
- National technical assistance centers
- Reggio Emilia approach

OVERVIEW

Professional organizations provide practitioners with several benefits, including legislation, research, networking, employment, and ongoing professional development. Although occupational therapy practitioners have a "professional home" within the American Occupational Therapy Association (AOTA), key early childhood (EC) professional organizations provide age-specific (birth to age 5 or 8 years) resources. (*Note. Occupational therapy practitioner* refers to both occupational therapists and occupational therapy assistants.) While exploring professional organizations in EC, one needs to understand that three unique and separate fields have influenced and still influence the birth to age 5 population. These three key fields include early childhood education (ECE), special education (SPED), and compensatory education.

Early Childhood Education

ECE for young children under school age has its roots originally in practices in Europe and include nursery, preschool, child, or family care settings. Although the original kindergarten programs started with education theorist Friedrich Froebel's work in Germany (Bruce, 2015), such programs are also underpinned by the work of other European theorists and philosophers such as Maria Montessori and, more recently, Loris Malaguzzi from Reggio Emilia, Italy (Cagliari et al., 2016; Lillard, 2016). In any infant, toddler, or preschool program in the United States, practices observed can range from play based and child driven to more academic and teacher directed. Occupational therapy practitioners working in ECE settings will want to better understand where on the continuum each family, center, or classroom lies because of the contextual features, specific materials, and unique practices and routines associated with each approach.

Although diverse in practice, the field of ECE typically follows the philosophy of *developmentally appropriate practice* (DAP), which is defined and described in the National Association for the Education of Young Children's (NAEYC, 2019a) *Developmentally Appropriate Practice Position Statement* (Bredekamp, 1987; Copple & Bredekamp, 2009), as requiring that curricula, the environment, and interventions match the child's development. Using DAP, practitioners or child caregivers nurture a child's social–emotional, physical, and cognitive development by basing all practices and decisions on

- Theories of child development;
- Individually identified strengths and needs of each child uncovered through authentic assessment; and
- The child's cultural background as defined by his or her community and family structure.

Special Education

Federal laws support special education for children. Services for infants and toddlers, ages birth–3 years, and their families are called *early intervention* (EI) and are driven by Part C of the Individuals with Disabilities Education Improvement Act of 2004 (IDEA; P. L. 108-446). Services for preschoolers, ages 3–5 years, are called *early childhood special education* (ECSE) and are driven by Part B, Section 619, of IDEA. EI provides services and supports to eligible infants and toddlers as well as their family members, and then ECSE shifts to services and supports directly to eligible preschoolers with less direct parent involvement than under Part C.

Each state has defined eligibility requirements for children with developmental delays or disabilities or

---

who may be at risk. Chapter 14, "Understanding Part C: Early Intervention Law and the Individualized Family Service Plan (IFSP) Process," and Chapter 18, "Understanding Preschool Laws and the Individualized Education Program Process," of this book further identify the services and supports for EI- and ECSE-eligible children and their families. Historically, EI and ECSE were "downward" extensions of SPED (for ages 5–21 years) and focused solely on atypical development. In the past 2 decades, EI and ECSE have recognized the importance of typical child development as a foundational principle while building strategies and supports for individual growth and development.

Similar to EC education, there is a continuum of philosophy and approaches within and across EI and ECSE programs. Philosophies range from behavioral (e.g., applied behavior analysis) to play based, and approaches range from one-on-one or self-contained settings to support of full inclusion and services provided within natural environments. Although the fields of EI and ECSE are diverse in practice, the underpinnings of both involve individual supports and strategies built around typical and atypical development.

Compensatory Education (Programs for Children at Risk)

Federal programs targeted to support children and families who are 100% at or below the federal poverty level include *compensatory education* programs such as *Head Start,* established in 1965, for children ages 3–5 years, and *Early Head Start,* established in 1995, for children ages birth–5 years. These programs were created to serve children who were considered at risk for academic success yet were not eligible for SPED. Both programs provide a multicomponent and multidisciplinary intervention that includes medical–dental, nutrition, social services, psychological, and educational programs as well as strong parent involvement in interventions and policy (Epstein & Barnett, 2012).

In 1962, David Weikart, a U.S. school psychologist in Michigan, in collaboration with a local educational committee, designed a key compensatory study, the Perry Preschool Project, for Black children who were considered disadvantaged (Schweinhart et al., 2005). Much of the EC curriculum used was based on the work of Jean Piaget, a Swiss psychologist who focused on cognitive development, and Lev Vygotsky, a Russian psychologist who coined the term *zone of proximal development* and emphasized the importance of adults in scaffolding a child's development (Vygotsky, 1978). The HighScope Educational Research Foundation was founded in 1970 upon the results from the Perry Preschool Project, and its curriculum is still practiced nationally using the Plan–Do–Review format (Epstein, 2007). The goal of compensatory education programs is to give children who may be at risk for academic success a head start that they would not typically have.

In the past 2 decades, there has been considerable discussion about and development toward ECE opportunities for all 3- and 4-year-olds, often referred to as *universal prekindergarten* (or *universal preschool*). These public-funded ECE programs across the United States may be located within public schools or community-based settings that have been expanded for this purpose.

ESSENTIAL CONSIDERATIONS

To provide best practice for children and their families who participate in ECE, SPED, and compensatory education programs, occupational therapy practitioners need to have a working understanding of the foundations of these programs, the contextual landscape of program systems and the communities served, and the diversity of the children and families. Professional organizations can offer key resources and support background knowledge. A variety of EC professional organizations and technical assistance centers offer key resources and background knowledge for occupational therapy practitioners working in EC.

Professional Organizations

Professional organizations provide leadership that assists in aligning and unifying efforts for policy, accreditation and licensing, advocacy, and practice. These organizations guide the profession by disseminating information on current evidence-based practices led by research, establishing regulations and program standards that are often used by state departments and agencies, instituting personnel standards that drive higher education or in-service efforts, producing white papers and other similar resources, and offering ongoing professional development for licensing.

Table 2.1 provides information about selected EC, EI, and ECSE professional organizations and federal programs that can assist practitioners when serving and supporting young children with diverse abilities and their families. Note that this list is not exhaustive. In addition, not all information that occupational therapy practitioners need can be provided through a national professional organization.

Technical Assistance Centers

Funded by the U.S. Department of Education's Office of Special Education Programs, *national technical assistance centers* help support state agencies that provide EI and ECSE services. Although occupational therapy practitioners would not contact these centers directly, center websites provide information that is applicable to practice. Table 2.2 provides information about the primary centers.

BEST PRACTICES

Two major EC professional organizations have published extensively on the professional standards, position statements, and recommended practices that guide the practices of practitioners across disciplines who work in EI and ECSE: NAEYC and the Division for Early Childhood (DEC) of the Council for Exceptional Children (CEC). Significant contributions to best practices from these and other professional organizations of EC, EI, and ECSE are discussed here. These best practices include

- Follow DAP
- Implement DEC-recommended practices

TABLE 2.1.   Selected EC, EI, and ECSE Organizations

PROFESSIONAL ORGANIZATION/WEBSITE	DESCRIPTION
American Montessori International (AMI) and American Montessori Society (AMS) https://montessori-ami.org/ and https://amshq.org/	AMI and AMS are dedicated to the work of Maria Montessori. The ***Montessori approach*** is based on self-directed activity and hands-on sensory-based learning. In Montessori classrooms, children make choices of materials in their learning while the classroom and the highly trained guide (teacher) offer age-appropriate activities to support learning.
American Occupational Therapy Association (AOTA) https://www.aota.org/	AOTA is the national professional association that represents the interests and concerns of occupational therapy practitioners and students and advances occupational therapy practice, education, and research.
American Physical Therapy Association (APTA) https://www.apta.org/	APTA is the national association for physical therapists, physical therapist assistants, and students.
American Speech-Language-Hearing Association (ASHA) https://www.asha.org/	ASHA is the national professional, scientific, and credentialing association for audiologists; speech–language pathologists; speech, language, and hearing scientists; audiology and speech–language pathology support personnel; and students.
Association for Childhood Education International (ACEI), now CEI or CE International https://acei.org/	CE International's stakeholders and partners are schools, nonprofit organizations, international nongovernmental organizations, universities, foundations, governments, and other groups that value education.
Association of State and Tribal Home Visiting Initiatives (ASTHVI) http://asthvi.org/	ASTHVI supports effective implementation and improvement of home visiting programs at the state, territory, and tribal levels through the use of evidence-based approaches focused on pregnant women and families with children ages birth–5 years.
Child Care Aware® of America https://usa.childcareaware.org/	Child Care Aware of America works to advance affordability, accessibility, development, and learning of children in child care, with more than 400 state and local child care resource and referral agencies nationwide.
Child Care Services Association (CCSA) https://www.childcareservices.org/	CCSA works to ensure affordable, accessible, high-quality child care for all families through research, services, and advocacy.
Council for Exceptional Children (CEC) https://www.cec.sped.org/	CEC is the leading voice for special and gifted education (ages birth through adult). The CEC is recognized as the source for special education professional standards, ethics and practices, and guidelines to ensure that individuals with exceptionalities have well-prepared, career-oriented special educators.
Division for Early Childhood (DEC) https://www.dec-sped.org/	DEC, a subdivision of CEC, is an international membership organization for those who work with or on behalf of children (ages birth–8 years) who have or are at risk for developmental delays and disabilities to enhance their optimal development. It promotes policies and advances evidence-based practices that support these children and their families.
HighScope Educational Research Foundation https://highscope.org/	The ***HighScope approach*** is a research-supported curriculum based on the belief that children construct their own knowledge of the world with the support of intentional teachers who shape and encourage their individual learning experiences. Children make their own discoveries and build their own initiatives by creating plans, following through on their intentions, and reflecting on their learning. This Plan–Do–Review process is a trademark of the HighScope approach.
Maternal, Infant, and Early Childhood Home Visiting (MIECHV) https://mchb.hrsa.gov/maternal-child-health-initiatives/home-visiting-overview	MIECHV gives pregnant women and families, particularly those considered at risk, necessary resources and skills to raise children who are physically, socially, and emotionally healthy and ready to learn.
Military Child Education Coalition (MCEC) https://www.militarychild.org/	MCEC consists of public school districts, private schools, colleges and universities, small businesses and corporations, organizations, military commands and installations, military families, and individuals from local communities.
National Association for Bilingual Education (NABE) http://www.nabe.org/	NABE advocates for educational equity and academic excellence for bilingual and multilingual students in a global society. Priorities include improving instructional programs and practices for linguistically and culturally diverse children; providing bilingual and dual-language educators with high-quality professional development opportunities; securing adequate funding for quality dual-language programs serving English learners (ELs); and keeping the rights of ELs clearly in focus as states and communities move forward with sustainable educational reforms.

(Continued)

TABLE 2.1.   Selected EC, EI, and ECSE Organizations *(Cont.)*

PROFESSIONAL ORGANIZATION/WEBSITE	DESCRIPTION
National Association for the Education of Young Children (NAEYC) https://www.naeyc.org/	NAEYC is a professional membership organization with nearly 60,000 individual members and more than 50 affiliates of the early childhood community who work to promote high-quality early learning for all young children, ages birth–8 years, by connecting early childhood practice, policy, and research.
National Association for Family Child Care (NAFCC) https://www.nafcc.org/	NAFCC is dedicated to promoting high-quality early childhood experiences on behalf of the 1 million family child care providers operating nationwide.
National Association for Family, School, and Community Engagement (NAFSCE) https://nafsce.org/	NAFSCE is focused on advancing family, school, and community engagement. Its mission is to advance high-impact policies and practices for family, school, and community engagement to promote child development and improve student achievement.
National Association on Mental Illness (NAMI) https://www.nami.org/	NAMI is the nation's largest grassroots mental health organization dedicated to building better lives for the millions of Americans affected by mental illness.
National Black Child Development Institute (NBCDI) https://www.nbcdi.org/	NBCDI engages leaders, policymakers, professionals, and parents around critical and timely issues that directly affect Black children and their families, including early childhood education, health, child welfare, literacy, and family engagement.
National Head Start Association (NHSA) https://www.nhsa.org/	NHSA is a program of the U.S. Department of Health and Human Services that provides comprehensive early childhood education, health, nutrition, and parent involvement services to low-income children and their families. The Knowledge Center helps curate, communicate, and connect knowledge about Head Start to the world. These resources are used by families, communities, programs, researchers, and policymakers to support the future of our nation's most at-risk children.
World Organization for Early Childhood Education (Organisation Mondiale Pour L'Education Préscolaire [OMEP]) United States National Committee (OMEP-USNC) http://worldomep.org/	OMEP is a worldwide nongovernmental organization that focuses on the education and welfare of young children, ages birth–8 years. The USNC works to educate its members and the public about issues regarding young children throughout the world.
Reggio Emilia Approach https://www.reggiochildren.it/ North American Reggio Emilia Alliance (NAREA) https://www.reggioalliance.org/narea/	The Reggio Emilia approach is a pedagogy first developed in the municipality of Reggio Emilia, Italy, at the end of World War II. This approach, now seen worldwide, is described as student centered and constructivist using self-directed, experiential learning in relationship-driven environments. NAREA exists to connect together early childhood educators and advocates in discovering, interpreting, and promoting Reggio Emilia–inspired education across North America.
United Nations Children's Fund (UNICEF) https://www.unicef.org/	Formerly known as United Nations International Children's Emergency Fund, UNICEF works in more than 190 countries and territories to save children's lives, defend their rights, and help them fulfill their potential, from early childhood through adolescence.
World Health Organization (WHO) https://www.who.int/	WHO works worldwide to promote health, keep the world safe, and serve the vulnerable. The goal of WHO is to ensure that a billion more people have universal health coverage, protect a billion more people from health emergencies, and provide a further billion people with better health and well-being.
Zero to Three (ZTT) https://www.zerotothree.org/	ZTT Policy Center is a nonpartisan, research-based resource for federal and state policymakers and advocates on the unique developmental needs of infants and toddlers.

TABLE 2.2.   Primary National Technical Assistance Centers

CENTER	DESCRIPTION
Center for IDEA Early Childhood Data Systems https://dasycenter.org	Assists state agencies with early childhood data systems
Early Childhood Personnel Center https://ecpcta.org	Assists states to develop and implement comprehensive personnel development and training systems
Early Childhood Technical Assistance Center https://ectacenter.org	Supports state early intervention and preschool programs to develop high-quality programs and enhance outcomes for children with disabilities and their families
National Center for Pyramid Model Innovations https://challengingbehavior.cbcs.usf.edu/	Assists states and programs to implement the Pyramid Model for Supporting Social Emotional Competence in Infants and Young Children to support social, emotional, and behavioral outcomes

- Follow your state's early learning standards and guidelines
- Demonstrate cross-disciplinary competencies
- Advocate for inclusion and natural environments
- Embrace equity, inclusion, and diversity.

Follow Developmentally Appropriate Practice

Based on research about development, learning, effective practices, and teaching intentionally, the NAEYC (2019a) position statement on DAP articulates 12 principles that should guide EC practitioners. DAP was first introduced in the United States in the late 1980s through Bredekamp's (1987) seminal work, *Developmentally Appropriate Practice in Early Childhood Programs Serving Children from Birth Through Age 8.* After several revisions to date, DAP continues to be regarded as the salient foundation upon which most Western-based EC approaches are built.

The core of DAP lies in understanding children's learning and development as well as intentional decision making. As practitioners make decisions, they should consider three areas of knowledge: knowing about child development and learning, knowing what is individually appropriate, and knowing what is culturally important. Exhibit 2.1 provides examples of guidelines based on some of the 12 DAP principles.

Implement Division for Early Childhood–Recommended Practices

DEC acknowledges that DAP should be the foundation of quality EC programs for all children and families; however, young children who have or are at risk for developmental delays or disabilities need more specialized practices to promote participation and provide meaningful opportunities for engagement (i.e., occupational performance). Therefore, DEC (2014) developed recommended practices to provide guidance to educators, related service personnel, and families about the most effective ways to improve the learning outcomes and promote the development of these young children, ages birth–5 years. These practices are organized into eight topics: leadership, assessment, environment, family, instruction, interaction, teaming and collaboration, and transition. More information can be found at https://www.dec-sped.org/dec-recommended-practices/.

Follow Your State's Early Learning Standards and Guidelines

In the past decade, many states have focused on promoting high-quality *early learning and development standards,* also referred to as *early learning guidelines* (ELG). Currently, all U.S. states and territories have developed and implemented ELGs for preschool-age children, and nearly all have ELGs for infants and toddlers. ELGs are intended to cover a range of domains across physical, cognitive, and social–emotional development and are aligned with standards for other systems, including Head Start. For more information and links to state-specific ELGs, see https://bit.ly/2O0gZBM (National Center on Early Childhood Quality Assurance, 2016).

Demonstrate Cross-Disciplinary Competencies

A work group from the Early Childhood Personnel Center (ECPC) studied discipline-specific personnel standards and competency areas from the national professional organizations, along with each state's EC, EI, and ECSE personnel standards, and developed a crosswalk of EC literature from the various professional associations. *Cross-disciplinary competencies* refer to the skills, abilities, and traits agreed upon as needed for all personnel disciplines working in EC, EI, and ECSE. Along with national association personnel and leaders from EC therapy and education disciplines, the group used these data to identify four core cross-disciplinary EC competency areas shared by all practitioners working with very young children, their families, and caregivers:

- Coordination and collaboration
- Family-centered practice
- Evidence-based intervention
- Professionalism.

In 2017, AOTA, the American Physical Therapy Association, and the American Speech-Language-Hearing Association, along with four national EC, ECSE, and SPED associations (CEC, DEC, NAEYC, and Zero to Three) formally endorsed these four areas (ECPC, 2017). ECPC and this cross-disciplinary team further analyzed the data and have identified 38 indicators across the four competency areas as follows: coordination and collaboration (9 indicators), family-centered practice (11 indicators), evidence-based intervention (8 indicators), and professionalism (10 indicators; Bruder et al., 2019).

EXHIBIT 2.1.   Examples of Guidelines Based on DAP Principles

- Children must be met where they are, which means that practitioners must get to know them well, and must be provided with opportunities to reach goals that are both challenging and achievable.
- All practices should be appropriate to children's age and developmental status, attuned to them as unique individuals, and responsive to the social and cultural contexts in which they live.
- Children's goals and experiences should not be made too easy. Practitioners should ensure that goals and experiences are suited to their learning and development and are challenging enough to promote their progress and interest.
- Practitioners must base best practice on knowledge—not on assumptions—of how children learn and develop. The research base yields major principles in human development and learning.

Advocate for Inclusion and Natural Environments

In April 2009, DEC and NAEYC released a joint position statement on EC inclusion, providing this definition of EC inclusion:

> *Early childhood inclusion* embodies the values, policies, and practices that support the right of every infant and young child and his or her family, regardless of ability, to participate in a broad range of activities and contexts as full members of families, communities, and society. The desired results of inclusive experiences for children with and without disabilities and their families include a sense of belonging and membership, positive social relationships and friendships, and development and learning to reach their full potential. The defining features of inclusion that can be used to identify high quality early childhood programs and services are access, participation, and supports. (p. 2)

Recommendations from the joint position statement include
- Creating high expectations for every child to reach their full potential,
- Developing a program philosophy on inclusion,
- Establishing a system of services and support,
- Revising program and professional standards,
- Achieving an integrated professional development system, and
- Revising federal and state accountability systems.

Embrace Equity, Inclusion, and Diversity

AOTA's (2017) *Vision 2025* states: "As an inclusive profession, occupational therapy maximizes health, well-being, and quality of life for all people, populations, and communities through effective solutions that facilitate participation in everyday living" (p. 1). One of the pillars of this vision—Equity, Inclusion, and Diversity—states, "We are intentionally inclusive and equitable and embrace diversity in all its forms" (AOTA, 2018, p. 1). During service delivery, occupational therapy practitioners should adhere to these values.

NAEYC (2019b) recently released a position statement, *Advancing Equity in Early Childhood Education,* and incorporated it as one of its foundational documents. Recommendations and evidence are available for practitioners, administrators, and professional development providers at the in-service and preservice levels and for policymakers.

This position statement further expands NAEYC's practices for embracing diversity and full inclusion:

> All children have the right to equitable learning opportunities that help them achieve their full potential as engaged learners and valued members of society. Thus, all early childhood educators have a professional obligation to advance equity. They can do this best when they are effectively supported by the early learning settings in which they work and when they and their wider communities embrace diversity and full inclusion as strengths, uphold fundamental principles of fairness and justice, and work to eliminate structural inequities that limit equitable learning opportunities. (p. 2)

In 2009, the Office of Head Start (2009) published an updated and revised *Multicultural Principles for Head Start Programs,* initially published 18 years earlier. This updated version provided a selective review of research conducted since the first publication and is centered around 10 principles (Exhibit 2.2). For more research-based information, practices, tools, resources, and strategies to ensure optimal services for linguistically and culturally diverse children and their families, see the Head Start National Center on Cultural and Linguistic Responsiveness (https://eclkc.ohs .acf.hhs.gov/culture-language).

EXHIBIT 2.2.   Multicultural Principles for Head Start Programs Serving Children Ages Birth–5 Years

Principle 1. Every individual is rooted in culture.

Principle 2. The cultural groups represented in the communities and families of each Head Start program are the primary sources for culturally relevant programming.

Principle 3. Culturally relevant and diverse programming requires learning accurate information about the cultures of different groups and discarding stereotypes.

Principle 4. Addressing cultural relevance in making curriculum choices and adaptation is a necessary, developmentally appropriate practice.

Principle 5. Every individual has the right to maintain his or her own identity while acquiring the skills required to function in our diverse society.

Principle 6. Effective programs for children who speak languages other than English require continued development of the first language while the acquisition of English is facilitated.

Principle 7. Culturally relevant programming requires staff who both reflect and are responsive to the community and families served.

Principle 8. Multicultural programming for children enables children to develop an awareness of, respect for, and appreciation of individual cultural differences.

Principle 9. Culturally relevant and diverse programming examines and challenges institutional and personal biases.

Principle 10. Culturally relevant and diverse programming and practices are incorporated in all systems and services and are beneficial to all adults and children.

Source. Reprinted from *Multicultural Principles for Head Start Programs Serving Children Ages Birth to Five: Addressing Culture and Home Language in Head Start Program Systems & Services,* by Early Head Start National Resource Center @ ZERO TO THREE, 2009, pp. 1–2. https://eclkc.ohs.acf.hhs.gov/sites/default/files/pdf/ principles-01-10-revisiting-multicultural-principles-hs-english_0.pdf

TABLE 2.3. Comparison of Selected EC Education and ECSE Approaches

APPROACH	KEY COMPONENTS	ROLE OF ADULTS/TEACHERS	ENVIRONMENT/CONTEXT
Behavior approach	▪ Is often used when providing special instruction for children with delays/disabilities (e.g., autism spectrum disorder) ▪ Is based on behaviorism ▪ Includes brief periods of one-on-one instruction	▪ Cue a behavior, prompt the appropriate response, and provide reinforcement ▪ Address isolated skills with frequent and detailed progress monitoring	▪ Initially, "learning to learn" behaviors addressed at small tables/cubbies to reduce distractions ▪ Skills generalized to facilitate peer play, and inclusive early childhood education settings supported
Comprehensive commercially available curricula	▪ Includes theme/project-based investigations ▪ Addresses the following areas of development: social–emotional, physical, cognition, and language ▪ Includes scope and sequence, daily activity guides, and ongoing assessments	▪ Lead small and large group activities centered around interest areas	▪ 10+ classroom interest areas, often referred to as "centers" (e.g., blocks, dramatic play, toys and games, art, library, discovery, music and movement, sand and water, cooking, computers, outdoors)
Embedded learning opportunities (naturalistic instruction)	▪ Provides specialized instruction during everyday learning opportunities ▪ Uses typically occurring activities and authentic materials across any curricular approach ▪ Uses an activity matrix to plan what, when, and how to teach a specific learning objective throughout naturally occurring daily routines	▪ Plan for and implement individualized instructional sequences within routines ▪ Teach through short interactions embedded within routine activities instead of pulling a child out or aside to address skills ▪ Use own priorities to drive goals and activities (i.e., family or caregiver role in early intervention)	▪ Natural environments, including homes, preschools, and child care contexts
HighScope curriculum	▪ Involves children learning by interacting with people, materials, and the environment ▪ Focuses on executive function via "plan-do-review" methods ▪ Uses consistent routines	▪ Facilitate "key experiences" with time for active exploration and learning ▪ Document learning through child observation records	▪ Well-defined areas, and easily accessible materials labeled at child's level ▪ Purposefully set up classroom areas to explore and build social relationships
Montessori approach	▪ Is based on children learning best by doing, through their senses ▪ Groups together children of multiple ages ▪ Offers long periods of individual work time (often 2–3 hours at a time) ▪ Focuses on independence, autonomy, and choice	▪ Systematically demonstrate use of learning materials (i.e., task) ▪ Instruct didactically ▪ Ensure that setting is prepared and aesthetically pleasing	▪ Specifically designed, often "errorless" learning materials ▪ Mats or rugs to designate space for children to work
Reggio Emilia Approach	▪ Focuses on social learning, collaboration, community, and democracy ▪ Considers children with disabilities to have "special rights"	▪ Serve as "guides" ▪ Emphasize documentation through portfolio data collection ▪ Use long-term meaningful projects to teach across domains as opposed to using short weekly themes	▪ Aesthetically pleasing with a focus on open-ended child art and easily accessible materials ▪ Environment considered the "third teacher" in the classroom ▪ Use of "provocations" (experiences set up to encourage a child's interests or ideas such as photo, picture, book) and "loose parts" (natural and manufactured materials that can be used in a variety of ways including moved, combined, and taken apart) to facilitate open-ended play

Note. EC = early childhood; ECSE = early childhood special education.

Understand Approaches Commonly Used in Early Intervention and Early Childhood Programs

Although many EI and EC learning approaches have fundamental commonalities, some have distinct features and reflect the developmental theorists and educational philosophies or tenets they are based on. Therefore, occupational therapy practitioners working with young children and their families need to understand the salient components, roles of adults, and contextual features of various approaches prevalent in EI, child care, preschool, or home-based programs. Table 2.3 provides an overview of selected ECE and ECSE approaches, including key components, the role of adults or teachers, and the role of the environment or context in those approaches.

SUMMARY

Professional organizations for EC, EI, and ECSE guide practitioners in these settings. Occupational therapy practitioners should be aware of and implement the guidance from these organizations, as well as from AOTA, to ensure that their interactions, recommendations, and interventions are responsive to the philosophical values and beliefs that undergird the settings and are reflective of current evidence-based practices. Occupational therapy practitioners must consider the primary funding source responsible (e.g., federal, state, local) to understand the philosophical and contextual foundations of the EC program.

Occupational therapy practitioners need to consider the diversity of the population they serve, which may include children and families who are culturally and linguistically diverse (Kidd et al., 2008), immigrants or refugees, or communities with dual-language learners. In addition, new approaches and practices, such as trauma-informed care, are emerging from neuroscience. Practitioners must be aware of the impact of state early learning standards for guiding individual development, state mandates, and regional initiatives on services and supports. Moreover, information accessed through professional organizations at the national and state levels can facilitate practitioners to be "cultural mediators" among diverse populations and practices.

REFERENCES

American Occupational Therapy Association. (2017). Vision 2025. *American Journal of Occupational Therapy, 71*, 7103420010. https://doi.org/10.5014/ajot.2017.713002

Bredekamp, S. (1987). *NAEYC position statement on developmentally appropriate practice in programs for 4- and 5-year-olds*. National Association for the Education of Young Children.

Bruce, T. (2015). Friedrich Froebel. In *The Routledge International Handbook of Philosophies and Theories of Early Childhood Education and Care* (pp. 43–49). Routledge.

Bruder, M. B., Catalino, T., Chiarello, L. A., Cox Mitchell, M., Deppe, J., Gundler, . . . Ziegler, D. (2019). Finding a common lens: Competencies across professional disciplines providing early intervention. *Infants and Young Children, 32*, 280–293. https://doi.org/10.1097/IYC.0000000000000153

Cagliari, P., Castagnetti, M., Giudici, C., Rinaldi, C., Vecchi, V., & Moss, P. (Eds.). (2016). *Loris Malaguzzi and the schools of Reggio Emilia: A selection of his writings and speeches, 1945–1993*. Routledge.

Copple, C., & Bredekamp, S. (2009). *Developmentally appropriate practice in early childhood programs serving children from birth through age 8*. National Association for the Education of Young Children.

Division for Early Childhood. (2014). *DEC recommended practices in early intervention/early childhood special education 2014*. http://www.dec-sped.org/recommendedpractices

Division for Early Childhood & National Association for the Education of Young Children. (2009). *Early childhood inclusion: A joint position statement of the Division for Early Childhood (DEC) and the National Association for the Education of Young Children (NAEYC)*. The University of North Carolina, FPG Child Development Institute.

Early Childhood Personnel Center. (2017). *Cross-disciplinary personnel competencies*. https://ecpcta.org/cross-disciplinary-competencies/

Early Head Start National Resource Center. (2009). *Revisiting and updating the multicultural principles for Head Start programs serving children ages birth to five: Addressing culture and home language in Head Start program systems & services*. https://eclkc.ohs.acf.hhs.gov/sites/default/files/pdf/principles-01-10-revisiting-multicultural-principles-hs-english_0.pdf

Epstein, A. S. (2007). *Essentials of active learning in preschool: Getting to know the High/Scope curriculum*. High/Scope Educational Research Foundation.

Epstein, D. J., & Barnett, W. S. (2012). Early education in the United States: Programs and access. In R. C. Pianta (Ed.), *Handbook of early childhood teacher education* (pp. 3–21). Guilford Press.

Individuals With Disabilities Education Improvement Act of 2004, Pub. L. 108-446, 20 U.S.C. §§ 1400–1482.

Kidd, J. K., Sánchez, S. Y., & Thorp, E. K. (2008). Defining moments: Developing culturally responsive dispositions and teaching practices in early childhood preservice teachers. *Teaching and Teacher Education, 24*, 316–329. https://doi.org/10.1016/j.tate.2007.06.003

Lillard, A. S. (2016). *Montessori: The science behind the genius*. Oxford University Press.

National Association for the Education of Young Children. (2019a). *NAEYC position statement on developmentally appropriate practice: 2019*. https://www.naeyc.org/sites/default/files/globally-shared/downloads/PDFs/get-involved/leadership/initial_public_draft_dap_2019.pdf

National Association for the Education of Young Children. (2019b). *Advancing equity in early childhood education: A position statement of the National Association for the Education of Young Children*. https://www.naeyc.org/sites/default/files/globally-shared/downloads/PDFs/resources/position-statements/naeycadvancingequitypositionstatement.pdf

National Center on Early Childhood Quality Assurance. (2016). *Early learning standards and guidelines*. https://childcareta.acf.hhs.gov/sites/default/files/public/state_elgs_web_final_2.pdf

Office of Head Start. (2009). *Revisiting and updating the multicultural principles for Head Start programs serving children ages birth to five*. https://eclkc.ohs.acf.hhs.gov/sites/default/

files/pdf/principles-01-10-revisiting-multicultural-princi-ples-hs-english_0.pdf

Schweinhart, L. J., Montie, J., Zongping, X., Barnett, W. S., Bel-field, C. R., & Nores, M. (2005). *The High/Scope Preschool Project through age 40: Summary, conclusions, and frequently* *asked questions*. High/Scope Educational Research Foundation. http://nieer.org/wp-content/uploads/2014/09/specialsum-mary_rev2011_02_2.pdf

Vygotsky, L. S. (1978). *Mind in society: The development of higher psychological processes*. Harvard University Press.

Best Practices in Personnel Preparation for Occupational Therapists and Occupational Therapy Assistants

3

Sarah Fabrizi, PhD, OTR/L, and Kris Pizur-Barnekow, PhD, OTR/L, IMH–E

KEY TERMS AND CONCEPTS

- Accreditation Council for Occupational Therapy Education®
- Family-centered practice
- Fieldwork educators
- Interprofessional communication
- Interprofessional education
- Interprofessional practice
- LEND
- Mentors
- Preservice fieldwork
- Roles and responsibilities
- Teams and teamwork
- Values and ethics

OVERVIEW

Occupational therapy practitioners use specific knowledge and skills to promote the participation and engagement of families and their young children in everyday occupations (American Occupational Therapy Association [AOTA], 2020b). (*Note. Occupational therapy practitioner* refers to both occupational therapists and occupational therapy assistants.) Practitioners engage family members and their children through the promotion of participation in the ordinary routines of everyday life (Muhlenhaupt et al., 2015) and have the knowledge, training, and expertise to enhance developmental skills and parent–child relationships that promote optimal development. Through activity analysis and grading of activities, occupational therapy practitioners identify opportunities that build family capacity, improve outcomes, and enhance school readiness.

The preparation of occupational therapy practitioners to provide services to families and young children influences both the quality of the services and the family and child outcomes. One major contributor to the provision of these services is a well-prepared workforce that includes an interprofessional team of early childhood providers (Stayton, 2015). AOTA recognizes that interprofessional education and collaborative practice are key to building family capacity, improving outcomes, and enhancing school readiness, because they develop the skills needed for early intervention and early childhood service delivery. *Interprofessional education* (IPE) occurs when two or more professions are given the opportunity to learn together (World Health Organization [WHO], 2010). Multiple resources about interprofessional practice may be found at the AOTA website (www.aota.org). As an advocate for occupational therapy practitioners, AOTA continually represents the membership on a national stage, and this work is supported through AOTA membership.

The Division for Early Childhood (DEC), a subsection of the Council for Exceptional Children for those who work with young children with disabilities and their families, recommended practices identify eight domains for professionals who serve families and young children ages birth–5 years (DEC, 2014): assessment, environment, family, instruction, interactions, leadership, teaming, and transition. In addition, scholars in the field of early childhood have elaborated on family-centered practices, documentation, natural environments, and inclusion (Bruder & Dunst, 2015). *Family-centered practice* follows the belief that a child's needs are best met through their family, and services are provided to strengthen and support the family unit. Although these recommended practices are relatively well known, Bruder and Dunst (2015) suggested that professional competence and confidence in providing services that incorporate these practices are not straightforward and that family engagement is key to providing effective service delivery.

In the literature, information regarding the educational preparation of professionals for early childhood practice is mixed. Although some sources describe curriculum content as lacking, others note course work and fieldwork as adequate. AOTA states that entry-level qualifications provide occupational therapy practitioners with preparation for early intervention practice through course work, fieldwork experiences, passing national board certification, and state licensure (AOTA, 2019). Around 4.6% of occupational therapists and 2.8% of occupational therapy assistants in the workforce practice in early intervention, and 5.2% of new graduates work in early intervention as the setting of their choice (AOTA, 2015a). However, these figures do not include the practitioners who work with children and families in hospital-based settings or early childhood programs in schools.

This chapter describes the need to place continued emphasis on high-quality preparation in education, fieldwork experiences, interprofessional collaboration in education and practice, and leadership and advocacy in early childhood to provide best practice and outcomes for young children and their families.

Copyright © 2021 by the American Occupational Therapy Association. For permission to reuse, contact www.copyright.com.
https://doi.org/10.7139/2021.978-1-56900-610-8.003

ESSENTIAL CONSIDERATIONS

Occupational therapy educational institutions should consider the unique settings in early childhood and embed learning opportunities throughout the curriculum that include accreditation requirements. They should also include activities that incorporate both the distinct role of the occupational therapy practitioner and how to integrate that knowledge as a member of the interprofessional early childhood team.

Educational Preparation for Early Childhood Practice

The academic preparation needed for occupational therapy practitioners to work with families and children with special needs has been an important topic of discussion in the profession for decades. In 1990, an expert panel of occupational therapists made curricular recommendations, including

- An increase in knowledge and skills to work within the family system,
- Theories and models of development of infants and families,
- The role of occupational therapy in working with families,
- Opportunities to practice skills for consultation and indirect services,
- An appreciation of culture and its effect on the service provision process, and
- An understanding of the theory of play and incorporating family play (Humphry & Link, 1990).

A decade later, a national survey was conducted to identify occupational therapists' current values and attitudes in working with parents of preschool children with developmental disabilities. Results indicated that efforts to support family-centered intervention in occupational therapy education programs did increase therapists' confidence. At the time of the survey, almost three-quarters of the respondents (72.5%) reported that their basic professional education adequately prepared them to work with parents (Hinojosa et al., 2002).

This study was a replication of an earlier survey (Hinojosa et al., 1988) in which 85% of occupational therapist respondents reported that they did not believe that their basic professional education had prepared them to work with families. In the 12 years between the surveys, the study suggested, occupational therapists recognized the importance of working with parents and felt more confident about the skill preparation they received in education.

A potential area for increased focus in occupational therapy educational preparation for early childhood practice remains play and the role of play in occupational therapy intervention. In the results from two survey studies, one in 1998 (Couch et al., 1998) and a replication in 2013 (Kuhaneck et al., 2013), the majority of occupational therapy practitioners reported that they most often used play as a means in intervention and that entry-level occupational therapy course work had not prepared them to use play assessments. A study examining entry-level occupational therapy programs' emphasis on play in their curricula, as reported by faculty, described that only about one-third

of reporting faculty provided students practice with play assessments (Mitchell et al., 2018).

Education programs did, in fact, report teaching a variety of approaches to the use of play in intervention, including practicing play, addressing play skills, and promoting playfulness. Suggestions for educational programs include practice and feedback in writing play goals, documenting outcomes of play interventions, and advocating for the role of occupational therapy in play and reimbursement related to play.

Entry-level requirements

The **Accreditation Council for Occupational Therapy Education®** (ACOTE®; 2018) develops entry-level standards for occupational therapy practitioners. A selection of the standards pertaining to practice in early childhood are listed in Exhibit 3.1.

Learning activities

In addition to the minimum standards developed by ACOTE, preparation for early childhood practice must include scaffolded opportunities throughout the occupational therapy and occupational therapy assistant program curricula. Students benefit from a variety of embedded learning activities with a specific focus on early childhood practice; see Table 3.1 for examples of possible learning activities.

Fieldwork

Fieldwork represents an important piece of occupational therapy practitioner education where classroom learning is applied. In both the occupational therapy and the occupational therapy assistant curricula, the Level I and Level II fieldwork experience introduces students to early childhood settings and provides them with an opportunity to apply classroom learning to working with early childhood teams, including young children and their families. Although there is no specific information about fieldwork placement in early childhood settings, collaboration and coordination between the educational institution and early childhood settings, along with the early childhood professionals working in those settings, are essential.

Experienced occupational therapy practitioners in early childhood settings can engage in this learning process as fieldwork educators and mentors to support both students' and early-career occupational therapy practitioners' ability to apply academic knowledge as well as identify resources valuable to early childhood practice. **Fieldwork educators** collaborate with academic institutions by providing a structured evaluation of student performance in a practice setting. Fieldwork educators provide students with knowledge of their specific practice setting, model clinical reasoning and professional judgment, collaborate both with the student and the interprofessional team, and demonstrate their unique role. **Mentors** are more experienced practitioners who guide new or less experienced practitioners. Mentors are dedicated to promoting and enhancing the profession and often have strong leadership and advocacy or advanced practice skills.

EXHIBIT 3.1. Examples of ACOTE® Requirements for Entry-Level Occupational Therapy Practitioners

An occupational therapy practitioner must, per the Preamble,
- "Be educated as a generalist with a broad exposure to the delivery models and systems used in settings where occupational therapy is currently practiced and where it is emerging as a service" (p. 2).
- "Be prepared to be a lifelong learner to keep current with evidence-based professional practice" (p. 3).
- "Be prepared to effectively communicate and work interprofessionally with all who provide services and programs for persons, groups, and populations" (p. 4).
- "Demonstrate active involvement in professional development, leadership, and advocacy" (p. 4).

Requirements are included in Section B: Content Requirements—in particular, Section B.1.0: Foundational Content Requirements and Section B.4.0: Referral, Screening, Evaluation, and Intervention Plan. Occupational therapy practitioners must demonstrate knowledge in
- "Human development throughout the lifespan (infants, children, adolescents, adults, and older adults). Course content must include, but is not limited to, developmental psychology" (Section B.1.1; p. 38).
- "The role of sociocultural, socioeconomic, and diversity factors, as well as lifestyle choices in contemporary society to meet the needs of persons, groups, and populations (e.g., principles of psychology, sociology, and abnormal psychology)" (Section B.1.2; p. 39).
- "The therapeutic use of self, including one's personality, insights, perceptions, and judgments, as part of the therapeutic process in both individual and group interaction" (Section B.4.1; p. 43).
- "The ability to identify occupational needs through effective communication with patients, families, communities, and members of the interprofessional team in a responsive and responsible manner that supports a team approach to the promotion of health and wellness" (Section B.4.23; p. 51).

Source. Reprinted from "2018 Accreditation Council for Occupational Therapy Education (ACOTE®) Standards and Interpretive Guide," by the Accreditation Council for Occupational Therapy Education, 2018, *American Journal of Occupational Therapy, 72*(Suppl. 2), 7212410005. Copyright © 2018 by the American Occupational Therapy Association. Reprinted with permission.

TABLE 3.1. Examples of Learning Activities for Occupational Therapy Early Childhood Curriculum

CURRICULUM CONTENT	LEARNING ACTIVITIES
Working with the family system	- Invite a family to share their story, in person or by video. - Provide suggestions of developmentally appropriate activities that fit in a family's routine. - Practice gathering an occupational profile with a family with children of various ages and needs. - Reflect on an existing individualized family service plan (IFSP) or individualized education program (IEP).
Working on the early childhood team	- Schedule guest lectures from other disciplines that work with occupational therapy practitioners in early childhood settings. - Implement a role-play of an IFSP or IEP meeting. - Cocreate a group intervention with a student from another discipline on the early childhood team. - Share ideas and activity suggestions with the family, child, and interprofessional team.
Play as a unique contribution of early childhood occupational therapy practitioners	- Conduct an assessment of play with a child. - Implement a case-based intervention plan with play goals. - Document a play-based session with specific outcomes related to play. - Discuss how to advocate for the inclusion of play opportunities embedded in the child's or family's routine.
Research and fieldwork	- Schedule guest lectures from occupational therapy practitioners who work in early childhood settings (e.g., hospital, early intervention, outpatient, schools). - Shadow practitioners in a variety of services and programs for young children and their families. - Discuss program options and set specific skill training. - Review early childhood program collaboration, development, and outcome measurement.

Additionally, occupational therapy programs must include key content and skills relevant to the early intervention and early childhood population. Knowledge of the role of occupational therapy practitioners in early childhood is important, but knowledge of shared and overlapping roles can support respect, coordination of services, and collaboration between professionals. One important consideration is the inclusion of opportunities for students from different disciplines to interact and learn together.

Interprofessional Practice

Interprofessional education (IPE) provides an opportunity for students from different disciplines to interact and learn together. The definition of *IPE* is enhancement of students' ability to learn from, with, and about disciplines that are different from their own (Interprofessional Education Collaborative [IPEC], 2016). The goal of IPE is to enhance *interprofessional practice* (IPP), in which groups of individuals work collaboratively to achieve the best outcomes for the people they serve.

IPP is recognized as best practice in health care settings (WHO, 2010) and has more recently been called *interprofessional collaborative practice* (IPCP) by IPEC (2016). WHO and IPEC promote the importance of IPCP in health care, and AOTA advocates for the inclusion of interprofessional practices and competencies in early childhood settings (Muhlenhaupt et al., 2015), because these competencies recognize the distinct value of all professions in enhancing child outcomes.

The following four core competencies of IPCP are adapted here to be relevant for early childhood practice:
1. *Values and ethics:* Work with individuals of other professions to maintain a climate of mutual respect and shared values.
2. *Roles and responsibilities:* "Use the knowledge of one's own role and those of other professions to appropriately assess and address the needs of" children and families (IPEC, 2016, p. 10).
3. *Interprofessional communication:* "Communicate with . . . children, families, communities, and professionals" in a responsive and responsible manner that supports a team approach to the promotion of developmental outcomes (IPEC, 2016, p. 10).
4. *Teams and teamwork:* Apply relationship-building values and the principles of team dynamics to perform effectively in different team roles to plan, deliver, and evaluate family-centered programs that are safe, timely, efficient, effective, and equitable. (IPEC, 2016)

The services that occupational therapy practitioners provide are changing as new models (e.g., transdisciplinary, primary service provider, coaching) are implemented. To demonstrate competence and feel confident in their role, students in occupational therapy and occupational therapy assistant programs must have access to families of young children. It is important to include opportunities to hear firsthand the family perspectives, begin to use the therapeutic use of self to establish relationships with families, and work alongside families as a member of the team.

Preservice fieldwork, course-related experiences in community-based settings, is an important consideration because students are strongly influenced by what they observe and what they are required to do in specific settings. See Table 3.2 for examples of interprofessional practice in education.

BEST PRACTICES

To prepare students to use evidence-based practice in early childhood settings, educational preparation needs to include
- Up-to-date information on federal and state laws affecting early childhood,
- National and state collaborations that support interprofessional skills,
- Active learning that incorporates the distinct role of occupational therapy in early childhood, and
- Support for building advocacy and leadership in early childhood settings.

Regardless of service delivery setting, occupational therapy practitioners are well prepared to deliver services that follow recommended practices in early childhood (AOTA, 2019).

Understand Influence of Federal and State Laws

Occupational therapy practitioners provide effective services when they understand the critical influence of federal policies on pediatric practice (AOTA, 2017). These include education, public health, and human service laws. For more information, refer to Chapter 14, "Understanding Part C: Early Intervention Law and the Individualized Family Service Plan (IFSP) Process"; Chapter 18, "Understanding Preschool Laws and the Individualized Education Program Process"; and Chapter 22, "Understanding Health Care Requirements, Process, and Billing."

Apply Knowledge From National Collaborations in Early Childhood

Knowledge from national professional organizations and associations informs occupational therapy practice. Table 3.3

TABLE 3.2.   Examples of Interprofessional Practice in Education—Evidence Briefs

EDUCATIONAL ACTIVITY	DESCRIPTION OF ACTIVITY	OUTCOMES
Partnering with a medical facility's children's medical services (CMS) clinic serving children with disabilities (Shaffer, 2018).	Students attended a child's annual checkup (6–7 hours) held every other Friday. The interprofessional team at the CMS clinic included a nurse practitioner, dietitian, orthotist, psychologist, social worker, speech–language pathologist, occupational therapist, and physical therapist, as well as 68 early childhood teachers and students.	Significant findings from students (preservice early childhood educators) included ▪ A broader understanding of partnering with families and professionals across disciplines and ▪ A deeper understanding of disability from a family's perspective.
Stay 'n' Play Parents Interacting With Infants (PIWI): Relationship-based, inclusive parent–child playgroup practicum (McCollum et al., 2018).	Families attend a weekly playgroup with their young child. Students from three different educational programs (early childhood special education, speech and hearing science, and human development and family studies) work as a team with a consistent group of families over an 8-week period with training and consistent supervision.	Students who participated reported increased knowledge of strategies for collaborating with families in ways that support and enhance their competence and confidence in interacting with their children. Students also became aware of their primary role of supporting parent–child interactions and relationships.

TABLE 3.3.   Core Competency Crosswalk From Professional Early Childhood Organizations

DESCRIPTION OF COMPETENCY	CORE COMPETENCIES IDENTIFIED BY ORGANIZATIONS		
	INTERPROFESSIONAL COLLABORATIVE PRACTICE	EARLY CHILDHOOD PERSONNEL CENTER	DIVISION OF EARLY CHILDHOOD
Team communication and collaboration	Interprofessional communication	Collaboration and coordination	Teaming and collaboration
Addressing the child and family's needs through family-centered or client-centered teamwork	Roles and responsibilities	Family-centered practices	Family-centered practices, family capacity-building practices, family and professional collaboration
Effective teamwork and interventions to improve outcomes	Teams and teamwork	Interventions as informed by evidence	Assessment, environment, instructional practices, interaction, transition
Values and ethics	Values and respect for ethical practice	Professionalism and ethics	Leadership

illustrates the crosswalk comparing core competencies that are identified by three primary national groups: Interprofessional Collaborative Practice, the Early Childhood Personnel Center (ECPC), and DEC.

Over the past several years, ECPC has been working with national organizations to build alignment of their personnel standards:

- AOTA
- American Physical Therapy Association
- American Speech-Language-Hearing Association
- DEC
- National Association for the Education of Young Children
- ZERO TO THREE.

The organizations agreed on four common core areas of competence:

1. Coordination and collaboration,
2. Family-centered practice,
3. Instruction and interventions as informed by evidence, and
4. Professionalism and ethics.

These course objectives can guide preparation for practice in early childhood, and practitioners new to early childhood practice can use them to determine areas appropriate for mentorship and professional development (see Table 3.4).

Address the Distinct Value and Role of Occupational Therapy Practitioners in Early Childhood Practice

The social construction and identity of occupational therapy as a profession are grounded in history and context (Clouston & Whitcombe, 2008). This is also true in certain practice areas, such as early childhood. When practicing in early childhood, occupational therapy practitioners are guided by the *Occupational Therapy Practice Framework* (4th ed.; AOTA, 2020b) and the *Guidelines for Occupational Therapy in Early Intervention and Schools* (AOTA, 2017). These documents guide professional reasoning while

describing practitioner roles in various settings (e.g., home, school, community, and health care).

In addition, occupational therapy practitioners are guided by theoretical models and practice frameworks that demonstrate occupational therapy's distinct value when serving children and families. Occupation-based models, including Kielhofner's Model of Human Occupation (Taylor, 2017), the Person–Environment–Occupation–Participation Model (Christiansen et al., 2005), the Cognitive Orientation to daily Occupational Performance Model (Polatajko et al., 2001), and the Model of Co-Occupation (Pizur-Barnekow & Jacques, 2019), are just a few examples of models that highlight occupational and social participation and demonstrate occupational therapy's distinct value when serving children and families.

Advocacy in occupational therapy practice is grounded in theory and includes initiatives taken by occupational therapy practitioners "to pursue a change in the environment that will ultimately enhance occupation" (McColl, 2003, p. 5). Occupational therapy practitioners should advocate for health promotion initiatives, policy changes, and evidence-supported research and programs that will improve the health and well-being of young children and their families. Advocacy can also include representation of oneself or the profession, such as the case of an early childhood team or involvement with a national organization.

Explore Additional Opportunities for Learning in Early Childhood

Although occupational therapy practitioners are well prepared to engage in interprofessional collaborative practice, carry out DEC-recommended practices, and demonstrate the core competencies as outlined by ECPC, there are additional learning opportunities for preservice and professional preparation that can enhance and enrich the background of occupational therapy students and professionals. One example of an opportunity that promotes leadership development for those who serve children with

TABLE 3.4.   Interprofessional Concept With Course Objectives

INTERPROFESSIONAL CONCEPT	COURSE OBJECTIVES
Coordination and collaboration	Occupational therapy practitioners ▪ Can collaborate and coordinate services with family and service providers across disciplines and agencies throughout the occupational therapy process. ▪ Will demonstrate a range of effective communication skills and use methods preferred by families if indicated. ▪ Will select and share resources with the early childhood team. ▪ Can facilitate and support the team approach to early childhood service provision.
Family-centered practice	Occupational therapy practitioners ▪ Can establish a therapeutic relationship with the family and child to support engagement. ▪ Will support the development of family competence and confidence in the caregiving role. ▪ Will use an individualized and effective approach across all cultural, linguistic, and socioeconomic backgrounds. ▪ Will explain child development to families in a way that promotes participation and engagement in everyday activities.
Evidence-based practice	Occupational therapy practitioners ▪ Will select and use valid and reliable assessments to determine eligibility for services, child and family strengths, and outcomes of intervention. ▪ Will apply evidence-based interventions with proven efficacy and effectiveness throughout the occupational therapy process. ▪ Will summarize data collected to help families make informed decisions and document the progress of the child. ▪ Will use environmental adaptations and modifications to maximize inclusion and participation.
Professionalism	Occupational therapy practitioners ▪ Will follow all *Standards of Practice for Occupational Therapy* (AOTA, 2015b), the *2020 Occupational Therapy Code of Ethics* (AOTA, 2020a) and federal guidelines outlined in the Individuals with Disabilities Education Act of 1990 (P. L. 101-476) for practice in early childhood. ▪ Will be knowledgeable in and use evidence-based disciplinary and interdisciplinary practice. ▪ Can collaborate, consult, and reflect with families and other service providers in early childhood. ▪ Will advocate at the local, state, and national levels for effective and high-quality services to achieve best outcomes for children and families.

Source: Adapted from Bruder et al. (2019).

CASE EXAMPLE 3.1. ALEX: INTERPROFESSIONAL TEAMWORK IN AN AUTISM DIAGNOSTIC CLINIC

To develop his leadership skills in occupational therapy, **Alex** applied to be a LEND fellow. In the LEND program, he participates in an autism diagnostic clinic that specializes in an IPP approach to evaluation of children at risk for autism. Nicholai, a boy age 3 years, was referred for evaluation because of his parents' concerns about his play skills.

The clinical psychologist administers the Autism Diagnostic Observation Schedule—2 (ADOS–2; Lord et al., 2012) and completes a comprehensive developmental history and testing for adaptive and cognitive functioning. As the occupational therapist, Alex administers assessments evaluating Nicholai's occupational performance, including ADLs, play, rest and sleep, and performance skills (e.g., sensory, motor, adaptive, psychosocial) and offers his observations while observing administration of the ADOS–2. Because of the parents' concerns about play, Alex uses Kielhofner's Model of Human Occupation (MOHO; Taylor, 2017) to describe volitional aspects during play. The speech–language pathology trainee administers assessments evaluating speech and language expression and comprehension.

The interprofessional team meets with the family to discuss observations and test results. Nicholai meets the criteria for autism on the basis of the evaluation results. He covers his ears frequently during the evaluation, and Alex explains to the parents how performance capacities (e.g., auditory hypersensitivity) may affect play. Alex utilizes MOHO to describe the challenges their son had transitioning from one activity to the next. Alex suggests that routines may be comforting to Nicolai and preparing him for transitions through verbal cues or pictures may help Nicolai transition from one activity to the next more readily.

Then Alex introduces Lia, an occupational therapy assistant, to the parents as Lia will be working in collaboration with Nicolai's parents.

After describing the role of occupational therapy, Lia shares resources for playgroups in the area that are inclusive and support children with autism. She explains that play is a strong treatment modality and that she will be incorporating sensorimotor activities along with strategies to help Nicholai transition from one activity to another. A visual schedule will be created for Nicholai to assist with transitions (e.g., which activities he will be doing next).

disabilities and their families is the Leadership Education in Neurodevelopmental and Related Disabilities (LEND) training program.

LEND, funded through the Autism Collaboration, Accountability, Research, Education and Support (CARES) Act of 2019 (P. L. 116-60), is a specialized training program that is interprofessional in nature. Occupational therapy graduate students or fellows learn with, about, and from trainees from other disciplines, including (but not limited to) physical therapy, speech–language pathology, clinical psychology, and special education students and self-advocates. LEND programs are designed to promote leadership skills and clinical expertise for professionals who will be or who are serving children with neurodevelopmental disabilities. They provide trainees with additional preparation in family-centered care, cultural humility, leadership, and advocacy through didactics and clinical practicum experiences (Human Resources and Services Administration, 2018).

Professional preparation and training programs like LEND are recognized by AOTA as specialized opportunities that enhance occupational therapy's visibility on interprofessional teams (Loukas et al., 2019). Case Example 3.1 illustrates how LEND addresses core competencies of family-centered care, teamwork, and advocacy and presents collaborative efforts between a LEND fellow and Lia, an occupational therapy assistant, as they plan intervention for a child.

SUMMARY

Occupational therapy education programs have the opportunity to prepare students for practice in early childhood settings. Occupational therapy students and new practitioners can explore additional opportunities to build competence in working with young children and their families by becoming familiar with early childhood professional organizations and recent publications. As service providers in early childhood, practitioners must understand the importance of family-centered care, inclusive practices, and interprofessional teamwork. In addition, a well-prepared workforce is familiar with federal and state laws that guide service delivery and professional resources that enhance knowledge about occupational therapy's distinct value in early childhood practice settings. Exhibit 3.2 provides some "next step" suggestions for action planning.

REFERENCES

Accreditation Council for Occupational Therapy Education. (2018). 2018 Accreditation Council for Occupational Therapy Education (ACOTE®) standards and interpretive guide. *American Journal of Occupational Therapy, 72*(Suppl. 2), 7212410005. https://doi.org/10.5014/ajot.2018.72S217

American Occupational Therapy Association. (2015a). *2015 salary and workforce survey: Executive summary.* Author.

American Occupational Therapy Association. (2015b). Standards of practice for occupational therapy. *American Journal of Occupational Therapy, 69,* 6913410057. https://doi.org/10.5014/ajot.2015.696S06

American Occupational Therapy Association. (2017). Guidelines for occupational therapy services in early intervention and schools. *American Journal of Occupational Therapy, 71,* 7112410010. https://doi.org/10.5014/ajot.2017.716S01

American Occupational Therapy Association. (2019). *AOTA practice advisory: Occupational therapy practitioners in early intervention.* https://www.aota.org/~/media/Corporate/Files/Practice/Children/Practice-Advisory-Early-Intervention.pdf

American Occupational Therapy Association. (2020a). 2020 occupational therapy code of ethics. *American Journal of Occupational Therapy, 74*(Suppl. 3), 7413410005. https://doi.org/10.5014/ajot.2020.74S3006

American Occupational Therapy Association. (2020b). Occupational therapy practice framework: Domain and process (4th ed.). *American Journal of Occupational Therapy, 74*(Suppl. 2), 7412410010. https://doi.org/10.5014/ajot.2020.74S2001

Autism Collaboration, Accountability, Research, Education and Support (CARES) Act of 2019, Pub. L. 116-60, 42 U.S.C. §§ 201.

Bruder, M. B., Catalino, T., Chiarello, L. A., Mitchell, M. C., Deppe, J., Gundler, D., . . . Ziegler, D. (2019). Finding a common lens: Competencies across professional disciplines providing early childhood intervention. *Infants & Young Children, 32,* 280–293. https://doi.org/10.1097/IYC.0000000000000153

Bruder, M. B., & Dunst, C. J. (2015). Parental judgments of early childhood intervention personnel practices: Applying a consumer science perspective. *Topics in Early Childhood Special Education, 34,* 200–210. https://doi.org/10.1177/0271121414522527

Christiansen, C. H., Baum, C. M., & Haugen, J. B. (2005). *Occupational therapy: Performance, participation, and well-being.* Slack.

Clouston, T. J., & Whitcombe, S. W. (2008). The professionalisation of occupational therapy: A continuing challenge. *British Journal of Occupational Therapy, 71,* 314–320. https://doi.org/10.1177/030802260807100802

Couch, K., Dietz, J., & Kanny, E. (1998). The role of play in pediatric occupational therapy. *American Journal of Occupational Therapy, 52,* 111–117. https://doi.org/10.5014/ajot.52.2.111

EXHIBIT 3.2.   Action Examples for Early Childhood

Be a member!
- Join your state occupational therapy association and AOTA.
- Join state and national early childhood organizations.
- Follow and advocate for early childhood policy and programs of interest to you.
- Collaborate with early childhood services and programs in your area.

Stay connected with the occupational therapy education programs around you.
- Be a fieldwork educator—take Fieldwork I and II students.
- Collaborate in student fieldwork and research projects.

Communicate with families and children that you are already working with.
- Cocreate programs.
- Find out what the families need are and share them.
- Provide evidence-based interventions.

Know competencies.
- Explore each set of competencies by other professional early childhood associations (e.g., IPEC, ECPC, DEC) and relate to a situation you have encountered in practice.

Division for Early Childhood. (2014). *DEC recommended practices in early intervention/early childhood special education 2014.* http://www.dec-sped.org/recommendedpractices

Hinojosa, J., Anderson, J., & Ranum, G. W. (1988). Relationships between therapists and parents of preschool children with cerebral palsy: A survey. *OTJR: Occupation, Participation and Health, 8,* 285–297. https://doi.org/10.1177/153944928800800504

Hinojosa, J., Sproat, C. T., Mankhetwit, S., & Anderson, J. (2002). Shifts in parent–therapist partnerships: Twelve years of change. *American Journal of Occupational Therapy, 56,* 556–563. https://doi.org/10.5014/ajot.56.5.556

Human Resources and Services Administration. (2018). *Leadership Education in Neurodevelopmental and Related Disabilities (LEND)* [Fact Sheet]. https://mchb.hrsa.gov/training/documents/fs/factsheet-LEND.pdf

Humphry, R., & Link, S. (1990). Preparation of occupational therapists to work in early intervention programs. *American Journal of Occupational Therapy, 44,* 828–833. https://doi.org/10.5014/ajot.44.9.828

Individuals with Disabilities Education Act of 1990, Pub. L. 101-476, renamed the Individuals with Disabilities Education Improvement Act, codified at 20 U.S.C. §§ 1400–1482.

Interprofessional Education Collaborative. (2016). *Core competencies for interprofessional collaborative practice: 2016 update.* Author.

Kuhaneck, H. M., Tanta, K. J., Coombs A. K., & Pannone, H. (2013). A survey of pediatric occupational therapists' use of play. *Journal of Occupational Therapy, Schools, & Early Intervention, 6,* 213–227. https://doi.org/10.1080/19411243.2013.850940

Lord, C., Rutter, M., DiLavore, P. C., Risi, S., Gotham, K., & Bishop, S. (2012). *Autism Diagnostic Observation Schedule* (2nd ed.). Western Psychological Services.

Loukas, K., Cahill, T., & Spencer, L. (2019). Occupational therapy and Leadership Education in Neurodevelopmental and Related Disabilities: Developing leaders and enhancing participation. *OT Practice, 24*(4), 20–23.

McColl, M. A. (2003). Introduction: A basis for theory of occupational therapy. In M. A. McColl, M. Law, D. Stewart, L. Doubt, N. Pollock, & T. Krupa (Eds.), *Theoretical basis of occupational therapy* (2nd ed., pp. 1–6). Slack.

McCollum, J. A., Santos, R. M., & Weglarz-Ward, J. M. (Eds.). (2018). *Interaction: Enhancing children's access to responsive interactions* (DEC Recommended Practices Monograph Series No. 5). Division for Early Childhood of the Council for Exceptional Children.

Mitchell, A. W., Hale, J., Lawrence, M., Murillo, E., Newman, K., & Smith, H. (2018). Entry-level occupational therapy programs' emphasis on play: A survey. *Journal of Occupational Therapy Education, 2*(1). https://doi.org/10.26681/jote.2018.020105

Muhlenhaupt, M., Pizur-Barnekow, K., Schefkind, S., Chandler, B., & Harvison, N. (2015). Occupational therapy contributions in early intervention: Implications for personnel preparation and interprofessional practice. *Infants and Young Children, 28,* 123–132. https://doi.org/10.1097/IYC.0000000000000031

Pizur-Barnekow, K., & Jacques, N. (2019). Introduction to occupation and co-occupation. In V. C Stoffel & C. Brown (Eds.), *Mental health in occupational therapy: A vision for the future* (2nd ed.). F.A. Davis.

Polatajko, H. J., Mandich, A. D., Miller, L. T., & Macnab, J. (2001). Cognitive Orientation to Daily Occupational Performance (CO-OP)—Part II: The evidence. *Physical and Occupational Therapy in Pediatrics, 20*(2–3), 83–106. https://doi.org/10.1080/J006v20n02_06

Shaffer, L. (2018). Training early childhood professionals using an interprofessional practice field experience. *Journal of Interprofessional Education & Practice, 10,* 47–50. https://doi.org/10.1016/j.xjep.2017.12.002

Stayton, V. D. (2015). Preparation of early childhood special educators for inclusive and interdisciplinary settings. *Infants & Young Children, 28,* 113–122. https://doi.org/10.1097/IYC.0000000000000030

Taylor, R. (2017). *Kielhofner's Model of Human Occupation: Theory and application* (5th ed.) Wolters Kluwer Health.

World Health Organization. (2010). *Framework for action on interprofessional education & collaborative practice.* Author.

Best Practices for Occupational Therapy Assistants in Early Childhood

4

Sarah Heldmann, BS, COTA/L

KEY TERMS AND CONCEPTS

- Close supervision
- Developmentally appropriate
- General supervision
- Interprofessional collaboration
- Minimum supervision
- Occupational therapy assistants
- Routine supervision
- Service competency
- Supervision
- Supervision log

OVERVIEW

Occupational therapy assistants (OTAs), who work with and are supervised by occupational therapists, have been an important part of the occupational therapy profession for more than 60 years. There is an upward trend of OTAs working in early intervention. In 2014, 2.8% of OTAs reported working in early intervention, as compared with 1.8% in 2010 (American Occupational Therapy Association [AOTA], 2015b). In the early intervention setting, occupational therapy practitioners reported that they spend 66.5% of their time on direct client intervention, 22.6% on indirect or administrative tasks, 5.9% on consultation, 1.5% on research, and 3.5% on other functions (AOTA, 2015b). (*Note. Occupational therapy practitioner* refers to both occupational therapists and occupational therapy assistants.) As the demand for occupational therapy practitioners in early childhood settings increases, additional OTAs will be essential.

Education Requirements

To become an entry-level occupational therapy assistant, an individual must undergo a rigorous process, including
- Graduate from an OTA program accredited by the Accreditation Counsel for Occupational Therapy Education (ACOTE®),
- Complete supervised fieldwork required by the educational institution where the student met academic requirements,
- Pass a national examination conducted by the National Board for Certification in Occupational Therapy (NBCOT®), and
- Complete state requirements for licensure, certification, or registration (AOTA, 2020b).

After completing this process, the OTA is able to work in any setting, including early childhood, under the supervision of an occupational therapist (OT). State licensure boards, with one exception, do not require OTAs to be certified to practice, making certification from NBCOT optional after the student passes the national examination.

The course work included in the current ACOTE standards to prepare the OTAs for early childhood settings includes typical and atypical child development, assessment, evidence-based interventions, and working with families and other team members. As of 2020, there are currently more than 220 accredited OTA programs in the United States, with more than a dozen new programs beginning the accreditation process (AOTA, n.d.). For additional information on personnel preparation for OTAs, see Chapter 3, "Best Practices in Personnel Preparation for Occupational Therapists and Occupational Therapy Assistants."

Benefits of an Occupational Therapy Assistant on the Team

OTAs bring unique skills sets and experiences to the occupational therapy process, helping create a more diverse team of practitioners. Younesi (2019) summarized the value of OTAs:

> OTAs exemplify that they are an integral part of the team by performing treatment in a fast-paced environment, displaying vast knowledge about the occupational therapy process and intervention, and demonstrating the ability to collaborate with multiple practitioners, all while facilitating a positive therapeutic relationship with the client. OTAs increase their knowledge by juggling various caseloads of clients, working with multiple OTs, and at times helping clinicians who are entering the field. (para. 5)

Additionally, OTAs are a cost-effective solution to therapy staffing, allowing for focus on direct client service. Although OTAs can contribute to each part of the occupational therapy process, their primary role is to provide direct

---

treatment interventions, which, in most settings, are billable and contribute to the profitability of the therapy team.

ESSENTIAL CONSIDERATIONS

In all states, OTAs are required to work under the supervision of an OT (Thomas, 2019). Understanding this dynamic collaborative partnership is essential. The following section addresses supervision, code of ethics, regulations, and the role of occupational therapy assistants.

Supervision

Supervision is an interactive and dynamic process intended to provide safe and effective occupational therapy services for clients and promote professional development and competency for practitioners (AOTA, 2020b). The process should be cooperative and collaborative, with the intention of professional growth and an understanding of the competence, experience, and education of the other. The dynamic relationship between OT and OTA requires mutual responsibility, respect, and open communication. Communication must be timely, open, honest, and appreciative of the other practitioner.

Both practitioners must understand their role as defined by AOTA official documents (AOTA, 2015a, 2020b). State practice laws should be reviewed and understood, because they determine the legal aspect of the relationship between occupational therapy practitioners. If necessary, clarification should be sought through AOTA and state occupational therapy associations or members of licensure boards.

Although the OT is responsible for all aspects of occupational therapy service delivery, both practitioners are responsible for the supervision process. Both should keep a record of supervision, including date, form of contact, time, and topics discussed. Both practitioners should be open to learning from each other, embracing their own individual strengths and weaknesses, and making efforts to grow professionally.

Methods of supervision

Supervision can be completed through a variety of means, including face-to-face meetings, video, electronic communication, written documentation, and phone conversations. OTAs may require varying levels of supervision, including close, routine, general, or minimum (Solomon & O'Brien, 2016). *Close supervision* refers to on-site, direct, and daily contact between the OTA and OT. *Routine supervision* consists of on-site, regularly scheduled contact between the practitioners. *General supervision* between an OTA and OT occurs as needed, with direct contact monthly or as mandated by state regulations. *Minimum supervision* is direct or indirect supervision as needed or as mandated by the state regulations. The level of supervision required between an OTA and OT varies on the basis of a number of factors, including

- Level of expertise of both practitioners,
- Type of practice setting,
- Complexity of client needs, and
- Requirements of practice setting and regulating bodies (AOTA, 2014a).

Establish service competence

The level of expertise is not solely based on number of years of experience but also considers skills, knowledge, and proficiency. OTAs should establish *service competency,* determining that two individuals can perform the same task and achieve the same result, to assure their supervising OT that they can complete delegated assessments or interventions in the same manner as the OT. Service competency can be established through the use of videotaping, cotreatment, and direct observation.

Documentation of supervision

The supervisory process between OTA and OT must be supported by documentation, regardless of the frequency of supervision. Both practitioners are responsible for maintaining records of the supervisory process as outlined in state practice acts. The OT simply cosigning treatment notes is not evidence of supervision. Practitioners should consider documenting the date, time, and type of supervision (e.g., in person, electronic, phone) on a *supervision log.* The log should also briefly describe what was discussed and be signed by both practitioners.

Topics for consideration may include the child's evaluation or reevaluation, plan of care, treatment interventions, data collection and progress, and client discharge from services. Additionally, practitioners may discuss and document service competency and review evidence-based practice and setting policies and procedures. Documentation that provides proof of the supervisory process should be stored in a safe location that is accessible to both practitioners.

Building strong OT–OTA relationships across early childhood settings

The supervisory process should be one of mutual respect between practitioners. Like any dynamic relationship in life, the supervisory relationship between OT and OTA can be challenging. Both practitioners can take steps to eliminate challenges and build strong partnerships. Rowe (2019) identified 10 strategies for building strong relationships between OTs and OTAs:

1. *Use AOTA official documents.* These resources can help clarify roles and facilitate appropriate relationship dynamics. Reviewing the difference between the roles of the two practitioners and discussing the supervisory process can lead to mutual respect and understanding.

2. *Understand state laws relevant to the location of your practice.* In addition to guidelines set forth by AOTA, it is important to understand the laws and regulations regarding occupational therapy in your state. State associations and licensure boards provide state-specific education and are a source for information when questions arise.

3. *Understand that the relationship is collaborative.* Both the OT and OTA are responsible for contributing to the supervisory relationship.

4. *Exercise humility.* Both the OT and OTA bring unique skill sets to the relationship and should be open to learning from the other.

5. *Embrace one another's strengths and weaknesses.* Each practitioner should be self-aware of their strengths and weaknesses and make efforts to improve weak areas. In addition to acknowledging their own strengths and weaknesses, they must consider how these interact with the strengths and weaknesses of other occupational therapy practitioners.
6. *Build trust.* Practitioners must be open and honest with one another to build trusting relationships that lead to the best occupational therapy services. For example, if the OTA does not understand a concept or goal, they must ask for clarification from the OT. In return, the OT must provide clarification.
7. *Appreciate one another.* Show recognition to other practitioners for their efforts and the skills they bring to the intraprofessional relationship.
8. *Develop strong communication.* Make efforts to understand how the other practitioner communicates best (written, in person, auditory, etc.), and adjust your communication style to match.
9. *Do not infer dominance or possession.* Although the OT and OTA work closely together, they are partners and should not refer to each other as "my occupational therapist" and vice versa.
10. *Celebrate your mutual love for occupation therapy and early childhood.* When challenges arise and other strategies are not working, it is important to reflect on your mutual love of occupational therapy and early childhood.

Practice Guided by AOTA's *2020 Occupational Therapy Code of Ethics*

AOTA's *2020 Occupational Therapy Code of Ethics* (2020a) guides members toward ethical actions in professional roles, provides a guide for enforceable conduct, and protects consumers receiving occupational therapy services. The *Code of Ethics* is based on six principles:

1. Beneficence
2. Nonmaleficence
3. Autonomy
4. Justice
5. Veracity
6. Fidelity.

Table 4.1 provides examples of how OTAs can use each of these principles in early childhood practice.

Knowledge of Federal, State, and Local Laws and Policies in Early Childhood

It is important for OTAs to understand federal, state, and local laws and policies regarding early childhood. These laws and policies may affect level of supervision, type and frequency of documentation, and the location and nature of services provided. In the medical setting, medical insurance will likely be the payer and influence policies and procedures. Collaboration with a case manager or social worker can help determine requirements for various medical insurances and their impact on occupational therapy treatment.

In a preschool, occupational therapy practitioners work under the Individuals with Disabilities Education Improvement Act of 2004 (IDEA) Part B (P. L. 108-446). IDEA Part C (early intervention) addresses services to children ages birth–3 years. Children who are eligible for IDEA services have an individualized family service plan (IFSP) or individualized education program (IEP) developed by a team, including the parent or guardian of the child. These legal plans document and summarize the child's levels of development and performance; evaluation results; family

TABLE 4.1.   Examples of the AOTA *Code of Ethics* for OTAs Working in Early Childhood

PRINCIPLE	DEFINITION	EARLY CHILDHOOD EXAMPLE
Beneficence	"Occupational therapy personnel shall demonstrate a concern for the well-being and safety of persons" (p. 3).	An OTA completes a review of evidence-based practice for a diagnosis they are unfamiliar with to best serve her client.
Nonmaleficence	"Occupational therapy personnel shall refrain from actions that cause harm" (p. 3).	An OTA informs the boss that they cannot treat a new client because they are neighbors.
Autonomy	"Occupational therapy personnel shall respect the right of the person to self-determination, privacy, confidentiality, and consent" (p. 3).	An OTA allows the child to choose from among a variety of occupation-based interventions to be used in treatment.
Justice	"Occupational therapy personnel shall promote equity, inclusion, and objectivity in the provision of occupational therapy services" (p. 4).	An OTA advocates to implement an adapted-toy lending service for families who are unable to afford toys for their children.
Veracity	"Occupational therapy personnel shall provide comprehensive, accurate, and objective information when representing the profession" (p. 4).	An OTA is introduced at a meeting as being an OT and politely corrects the individual making the introductions.
Fidelity	"Occupational therapy personnel shall treat clients (persons, groups, or populations), colleagues, and other professionals with respect, fairness, discretion, and integrity" (p. 4).	An OTA disagrees with the goals written by a supervising OT and takes action to discuss them with the OT in a professional manner.

Note. Principle definitions from AOTA (2020a). OT = occupational therapist; OTA = occupational therapy assistant.

concerns; the child's strengths and needs; IFSP outcomes or IEP goals; and services needed, including the frequency, payment arrangements (if any), and transition plans.

Children may also receive occupational therapy services in health care and community systems. In these systems, factors such as site policies, grant funding, and donations may influence the service and delivery of occupational services. For more information regarding laws and policies, see Chapter 14, "Understanding Part C: Early Intervention Law and the Individualized Family Service Plan (IFSP) Process"; Chapter 18, "Understanding Preschool Laws and the Individualized Education Program Process"; and Chapter 22, "Understanding Health Care Requirements, Process, and Billing."

Role of Occupational Therapy Assistants in Early Childhood

OTAs work in a variety of early childhood settings, including home, community, educational, preschool, and health care settings. OTAs must consider the effects each of these settings has on the delivery of occupational therapy, including the primary occupations of early childhood.

Home settings

OTAs working in a home setting must consider the needs of both the child and the family. Solomon and O'Brien (2016) outlined essential skills for successful intervention with families.

- *Solution-focused curiosity and interest.* Practitioners who are nonjudgmental and focus on strengths of the family and realistic solutions generally have better receptiveness with families. For example, practitioners should ask families questions that focus on what is going well rather than what is wrong, and ask families for input on implementing adaptations, equipment, or interventions that will have to be carried over by the family.
- *Collaborative goal setting.* Occupational therapy practitioners must consider input from the family when establishing a plan of care and also at each therapy session. For example, during the home visit, practitioners should ask the family whether there are any specific concerns, what has gone well since the last visit, and whether any clarification of the home program activities is needed.
- *Acknowlegment.* Occupational therapy practitioners must communicate effectively with families and provide acknowledgment of their input. They can do this by verbally repeating what families have said, rephrasing, asking for clarification, or using nonverbal communication (e.g., nodding).
- *Continuity.* Occupational therapy practitioners must build a positive rapport with families. The beginning and end of a therapy session are essential times to build this rapport. OTAs who are solution oriented and future focused will develop a positive rapport with families.

Community settings

In the community, OTAs may work in a variety of settings, including afterschool programs, child care, faith-based programs, recreational centers, community health clinics, homeless shelters, and so forth. The community service delivery models "may include approaches such as individual therapy, group therapy, skill-building, coaching, mentoring, family education and training, teacher or caretaker education and training, and program consultation" (Solomon & O'Brien, 2016, p. 61). Therapy practitioners should be mindful of opportunities to develop community-based programming to meet the needs of consumers by enhancing occupational performance.

Education settings

Under IDEA, occupational therapy practitioners support engagement and participation in daily living activities (AOTA, 2017a). In the preschool setting, OTAs work with children and other educational staff to meet educational and IEP goals. The focus of interventions is on functional skills and adaptations to increase participation in the occupation of education. For example, a child struggling with cutting skills may work to increase hand strength for scissor use (functional skill) or be provided with looped, spring-loaded scissors as an alternative (adaptation). OTAs working in preschools should gain knowledge of laws, regulations, and policies surrounded this setting.

Additionally, OTAs must work to achieve effective relationships with classroom teachers and paraeducators. Much like the relationship between OT and OTA, the partnership with classroom staff is collaborative and should be based on mutual respect. The tips for effective OT/OTA relationships described previously can be applied to this relationship as well.

Health care settings

OTAs working in the health care setting (e.g., hospitals, outpatient clinics) must understand the roles of interdisciplinary team members involved in the care of the young child, medical equipment, levels of care in the medical system, and the impact on occupation that involvement in the medical system may have on the child. ***Interprofessional collaboration,*** collaboration between professionals of different disciplines, is essential in the medical system because of significant health concerns (e.g., contraindications to therapeutic interventions, vital signs, medical equipment monitoring). The OTA may need to communicate with other health care team members before each treatment session to ensure the child is cleared for therapeutic intervention.

An OTA in health care settings may encounter children who use medical equipment (e.g., ventilation, oxygen tubing, supplemental nutrition tubing). OTAs should gain a basic understanding of how such equipment works through on-the-job training and collaboration with other health care professionals. They must understand the body systems to observe the changing medical needs of the child before, during, and after occupational therapy intervention. OTAs can use their skill set of activity analysis and creativity to help children engage in primary occupations (e.g., play participation) while they are in the medical system.

BEST PRACTICES

The OT is responsible for all aspects of the occupational therapy process and supervises the OTA. The OTA can, however, complete aspects of each part of the occupational therapy process, as delegated and as permitted by state licensure (e.g., regulatory act).

Assist With Screening and Evaluations

AOTA (2015a, 2020b) states that the OT must be directly involved in and initiate the screening and evaluation process. The OTA may assist in screening, evaluation, and reevaluation by conducting a file review, collecting work samples, and administering delegated assessments. The OTA reports observations to the OT as allowed by federal and state regulations.

Although the OTA can contribute, they may not work independently; the OT must analyze and synthesize the information to determine the need for services. The OTA may contribute to the intervention plan. When delegated, the OTA may share with the appropriate individuals the results of an evaluation and the OT's recommendations regarding potential services or referrals. An OTA may share information at meetings but may not make alterations to the recommendations without approval from the supervising OT.

Provide Evidence-Based Interventions

In collaboration with the OT, the OTA can use professional reasoning, knowledge of evidence-based practice, and therapeutic use of self to determine the best types of interventions to implement the intervention plan and address the goals and outcomes in the IFSP or IEP, or the therapy goals set out by the supervising OT in a health care treatment plan. An OTA can grade and adapt therapeutic interventions to fit the needs of children and families, report to the OT the need to modify the intervention plan, and effectively document occupational therapy services delivered.

OTAs may also contribute to the transition, discharge, and outcome assessment process. The child's needs, goals, performance, and any additional resources needed should be communicated to the OT. Additionally, the OTA communicates available resources to children and their families as well as collaborates with other professionals (e.g., social worker, special education teacher, nurse) when appropriate.

Use developmentally appropriate, occupation-based interventions

OTAs may spend a significant amount of their time engaged in direct intervention with children, their families, or educational staff. Developmentally appropriate practices and occupation-based interventions are the core of occupational therapy in early childhood. First, OTAs must understand what is ***developmentally appropriate***: occupations that align with the child's chronological age as well as their sequential and predictable cognitive and physical development. Although occupational therapy practitioners learn this skill set in school, development charts are also readily available as a quick reference guide.

It may also be beneficial to share these resources with families and caregivers to foster their understanding of developmental milestones. OTAs should use their knowledge of developmental milestones as well as task and environmental analysis to help determine performance skills to be addressed in interventions. OTAs must also understand the developmental progression of occupations relevant to early childhood: ADLs, IADLs, sleep, play, leisure, social participation, and education.

After determining what is developmentally appropriate and which skill sets to address, the OTA must creatively use occupations in providing intervention. Depending on the practice setting, the OTA may address some or all of these areas of occupation. For example, in a home-based setting, the focus may be more on ADLs (e.g., brushing teeth) and play (e.g., standing while pulling a toy or stacking blocks), whereas in a school setting the focus may be on social participation (e.g., taking turns with a peer) and education (e.g., using classroom materials appropriately).

Effectively Document Services

It is essential to provide accurate, skilled documentation. Additionally, reviewing the *Occupational Therapy Practice Framework* (AOTA, 2020c) for performance skills and proper language to use can increase the effectiveness of documentation in articulating the distinct value of occupational therapy. Documentation varies depending on the setting and payer source; nevertheless, all documentation must justify the need for skilled occupational therapy services.

Most often, an OTA will write a contact note for services with the child. The contact note typically follows the "subjective, objective, assessment, and plan" (SOAP) format regarding the contact provided. Contact with the child for direct therapy sessions, phone calls, and meetings should all be recorded. In other situations, occupational therapy practitioners may keep only an attendance sheet, informal log, or observations that will later contribute to a progress report (Morreale & Borcherding, 2017). Payer sources, facility procedures, laws, and state practice acts influence the type and frequency of documentation. Regardless of the type, documentation completed by an OTA must also be co-signed by an OT.

Promote Leadership in Early Childhood

Leadership is important for the profession. OTAs should be encouraged to demonstrate leadership skills. They can do this by serving as fieldwork educators, presenting at staff meetings, writing articles highlighting occupational therapy for a staff newsletter, presenting at state or national conferences, serving on an occupational therapy board, conducting research, mentoring new graduates, and so forth.

Advocacy is also a leadership action. Advocacy is important both for the clients and for ongoing services from occupational therapy practitioners. Practitioners should be able to easily describe and define occupational therapy by providing a quick but concise definition that is specific to their credentials, practice setting, and client needs. Practitioners should consider the developmental level of the child they are working with when providing a definition and focus on the needs of the child when giving a definition to caregivers (see Exhibit 4.1).

Clearly Communicating the Occupational Therapy Practitioner's Role

Clear descriptions of occupational therapy should be based on the audience.

To a 3-year-old: "My name is Sarah; I heard you love trains, and I am here to help you play with them."

To a child's parent: "My name is Sarah, and I am an occupational therapy assistant. As you know, Ty has difficulty reaching for objects, like the trains he loves to play with. He has a goal to improve his hand skills. We will do this through the use of play—for example, having him reach for his trains. When you think of occupations, think of anything that takes up your time during the day. For you or me, it might be work, driving, or making dinner, but for your son one of his primary occupations is play. There are some strategies to increase his arm use while playing, if you are interested. This will make it motivating and fun for both of you."

Occupational therapy practitioners must advocate for the children and families they serve to overcome barriers for participation in meaningful occupations. Creating resource guides, securing necessary equipment, starting a lending service of switch-adapted toys, and stocking brochures and handouts for children and their families are all examples of ways OTAs can advocate (Moreno & Pelham-Foster, 2017). OTAs can participate on local, states, and federal levels to improve accessibility of public spaces, including playgrounds, airports, and schools, to help children participate in meaningful occupations. For example, the Wood County Board of Developmental Disabilities in Ohio developed a multi-agency team (including occupational therapy practitioners) to fund, design, and build an inclusive playground to meet the needs of their clients (https://www.wcplays.org).

OTAs often have success stories to share about the children and families they serve. Sharing these (while maintaining confidentiality) can be a powerful tool when lobbying for occupational therapy with local, state, and federal government officials. These advocacy efforts often require one willing individual to start the project and inspire others to join.

It is important for occupational therapy practitioners to advocate for their role. There are many ways to do this. First, use inclusive language, such as "occupational therapy practitioners." Use the *Standard of Practice for Occupational Therapy* (AOTA, 2015a) and *Guidelines for Supervision, Roles, and Responsibilities During the Delivery of Occupational Therapy Services* (2020b) to ensure OTAs are included when appropriate.

Pursue Lifelong Learning

Occupational therapy practitioners must commit to being lifelong learners. OTAs must stay up to date on advancements and new evidence-based interventions to ensure effectiveness of practice. AOTA offers board certification and specialty certification areas for continuing education, and specialty certification areas are available for OTAs. Many areas are relevant to early childhood occupational therapy, including environmental modification; feeding, eating, and swallowing; low vision; and school systems.

These specialty certifications require extensive course work in the subject area and are moving from a portfolio to an exam-based certification in 2020.

OTAs may also choose to advance their career by obtaining a certificate in infant massage or another appropriate modality, taking courses in early childhood development, or collaborating with other researchers and participating in research studies. OTAs should encourage the use of evidence-based practice at their work setting by starting a journal club or reviewing an evidence-based case study with coworkers (Davis, 2014).

SUMMARY

In partnership with occupational therapists, occupational therapy assistants advance practice in early childhood settings. They are trained in early childhood development, task and environmental analysis, and using creativity to meet the diverse needs of children and their families. They provide effective occupational therapy services in early childhood. Advocating for children and families and for the profession of occupational therapy, OTAs demonstrate leadership and initiative. OTAs will continue to be essential members of the early childhood team as the occupational therapy profession works toward AOTA's *Vision 2025:* "As an inclusive profession, occupational therapy maximizes health, well-being, and quality of life for all people, populations, and communities through effective solutions that facilitate participation in everyday living" (AOTA, 2017b, p. 1).

REFERENCES

American Occupational Therapy Association. (n.d.). *ACOTE accreditation.* https://www.aota.org/Education-Careers/Accreditation.aspx

American Occupational Therapy Association. (2015a). Standards of practice for occupational therapy. *American Journal of Occupational Therapy, 69,* 6913410057. https://doi.org/10.5014/ajot.2015.696S06

American Occupational Therapy Association. (2015b). *Work setting trends for occupational therapy: How to choose a setting.* https://www.aota.org/Education-Careers/Advance-Career/Salary-Workforce-Survey/work-setting-trends-how-to-pick-choose.aspx

American Occupational Therapy Association. (2017a). Guidelines for occupational therapy services in early intervention and schools. *American Journal of Occupational Therapy, 71*(Suppl. 2), 7112410010. https://doi.org/10.5014/ajot.2017.716S01

American Occupational Therapy Association. (2017b). Vision 2025. *American Journal of Occupational Therapy, 71,* 7103420010. https://doi.org/10.5014/ajot.2017.713002

American Occupational Therapy Association. (2020a). 2020 occupational therapy code of ethics. *American Journal of Occupational Therapy, 74*(Suppl. 3), 7413410005. https://doi.org/10.5014/ajot.2020.74S3006

American Occupational Therapy Association. (2020b). Guidelines for supervision, roles, and responsibilities during the delivery of occupational therapy services. *American Journal of Occupational Therapy, 74,* 7413410020. https://doi.org/10.5014/ajot.2020.74S3004

American Occupational Therapy Association. (2020c). Occupational therapy practice framework: Domain and process (4th ed.). *American Journal of Occupational Therapy, 74*(Suppl. 2), 7412410010. https://doi.org/10.5014/ajot.2020.74S2001

Davis, S. (2014). Evidence based practice and the new practitioner. *OT Practice, 19*(22), 17–18.

Individuals With Disabilities Education Improvement Act of 2004, Pub. L. 108-446, 20 U.S.C. §§ 1400–1482.

Moreno, S. A., & Pelham-Foster, S. (2017). Online resource guides: Facilitating return to play and leisure activities. *OT Practice, 22*(18), 14–17.

Morreale, M., & Borcherding, S. (2017). *The OTA's guide to documentation: Writing SOAP notes* (4th ed.). Slack.

Rowe, N. (2019). *10 tips to build a strong OT/OTA relationship.* https://www.aota.org/Education-Careers/Students/Pulse/Archive/career-advice/OT-OTA-Relationship.aspx

Solomon, J. W., & O'Brien. J. C. (2016). *Pediatric skills for occupational therapy assistants* (4th ed.). Elsevier.

Thomas, H. (2019). Working with occupational therapy assistants. In K. Jacobs & G. L. McCormack (Eds.), *The occupational therapy manager* (pp. 385–391). AOTA Press.

Younesi, S. (2019). *Perks of OTA leadership.* https://www.aota.org/Education-Careers/Students/Pulse/Archive/student-leadership-advocacy/Perks-of-OTA-Leadership.aspx

Best Practices for Occupational Therapy Practitioners in Leadership Roles

Lesly Wilson James, PhD, MPA, OTR/L, FAOTA, and Sandra Schefkind, OTD, OTR/L, FAOTA

KEY TERMS AND CONCEPTS

- Adverse childhood experiences
- Communities of practice
- Culturally competent practice
- Education
- Family engagement
- Interprofessional collaborative practice
- Leadership
- Occupational deprivation
- Physical health
- Socialization

OVERVIEW

Although there is no one agreed-on definition of **leadership,** it is widely accepted that it includes a process of influencing others to work together toward a common goal. Leadership can be viewed "as a process of motivating people to work together collaboratively to accomplish great things" (Vroom & Jago, 2007, p. 18). Leadership is one of the five pillars of the American Occupational Therapy Association's (AOTA) *Vision 2025,* which states, "As an inclusive profession, occupational therapy maximizes health, well-being, and quality of life for all people, populations, and communities through effective solutions that facilitate participation in everyday living" (AOTA, 2017c, p. 1). The other four pillars are effective; collaborative; accessible; and equity, inclusion, and diversity.

Leadership typically develops through a complex internal process and may occur outside of formal leadership roles in an organization. Garbarini and Winston (2015) wrote that "anyone who has a vision, engenders trust, and is respected can create change through leadership" (p. 62). Leaders in formal positions of authority often create policy, but, of equal importance, occupational therapy practitioners in informal leadership roles offer mentorship and acceptance. They can become key problem solvers and innovators (Heard, 2018). (*Note. Occupational therapy practitioner* refers to both occupational therapists and occupational therapy assistants.)

Leaders are willing to take risks to build leadership for themselves and others. Kouzes and Posner (2013) noted, "Great leaders are great learners. They stay open to new information and to the ideas of others, and aren't afraid to experiment and make mistakes" (p. 8). Leaders must be willing to demonstrate five exemplary practices:
1. Model a way toward collective leadership
2. Inspire a shared vision
3. Challenge the process
4. Enable others to act
5. Encourage the heart (Kouzes & Posner, 2017).

In so doing, they reveal their personal leadership skills and, in turn, build leadership in others. These exemplary practices are discussed throughout this chapter.

Effective teaming is a key leadership skill in occupational therapy early childhood practice. *Interprofessional collaborative practice* is defined as "when multiple health workers from different professional backgrounds work together with patients, families, carers, and communities to deliver the highest quality of care" (World Health Organization, 2010, p. 7). Occupational therapy practitioners must continuously apply leadership theories to their interprofessional practices (Karmali, 2018) and be able to articulate the distinct value of their service within the team.

Some research suggests that an occupational therapy practitioner's personal leadership identity develops over time and requires either internal or external recognition of leadership ability or outcome (Truskowski, 2018). However, there are barriers in formal training and credentialing for practitioners to assume special education formal leadership roles. Greater advocacy, policy changes, and additional preparatory course work are needed to address these barriers (Sauvigne-Kirsch, 2017).

Demographics and Workforce

Although occupational therapy is identified in the Individuals with Disabilities Education Improvement Act of 2004 (IDEA; P. L. 108-446), there are limited data focused on identifying and building this workforce. Limited data exist specific to personnel shortages in occupational therapy in early childhood, and few studies have been conducted regarding leadership positions. The *2015 AOTA Salary & Workforce Survey* (2015c) revealed that 4.6% of occupational therapists and 2.8% of occupational therapy assistants work in an early intervention (EI) setting. Additionally, the survey revealed that 19.9% of occupational therapists and 15% of occupational therapy assistants work in a school-based setting (the study did not specifically identify practitioners in preschools or other pediatric settings).

In areas of personnel shortages, benefits and incentives, such as loan forgiveness programs and free continuing education opportunities, should be offered. Limited employment changes may suggest that occupational therapy practitioners are generally satisfied or may indicate that there are a lack of alternative positions for job change or advancement. Practitioners working in early childhood settings should advocate for opportunities for professional and personal growth. This is a leadership action to support and promote occupational therapy early childhood service.

Relevant Background

If there is agreement that "the early childhood workforce constitutes a group of professionals who are widely diverse with respect to their roles . . . qualifications, education, and experience; and racial, ethnic, socio-economic, cultural, and linguistic characteristics" (National Professional Development Center on Inclusion, 2008, p. 1), then occupational therapy practitioners should be viewed as an added value to any leadership team. However, historically, only a limited number of occupational therapy practitioners have served in these formal state leadership roles (Case-Smith, 2013). Coordinated state efforts are needed to build a pipeline for occupational therapy's leadership role and visibility in and through the EI and childhood sector. Some strategies include increasing occupational therapy participation in interdisciplinary learning opportunities, lobbying, testifying at hearings, presenting at early childhood conferences, and networking.

ESSENTIAL CONSIDERATIONS

To assume a leadership role, occupational therapy practitioners must be responsive to key trends in population health. Using a public health approach, practitioners can engage in prevention, promotion, and interventions to address mental and physical health. Below are several areas for consideration within population health where occupational therapy practitioners can apply their advocacy, planning, and service.

Mental Health

Adverse childhood experiences (ACEs) is the term used "to describe all types of abuse, neglect, and other potentially traumatic experiences that occur to people under the age of 18" (Centers for Disease Control and Prevention [CDC], 2019, p. 1). Occupational therapy practitioners must be aware of the significance of the findings of the CDC–Kaiser Permanente ACE Study (Felitti et al., 1998), which suggests that higher exposure to early adversity experiences, such as trauma and neglect, has been correlated with negative health and well-being outcomes. Early adversity leads to disease, risky behaviors, early morbidity, injury, depression, and the development of chronic conditions (CDC, 2019).

Occupational therapy practitioners can lead by preventing violence through the therapeutic use of occupation and by supporting healthy and safe family routines. They must

offer trauma-informed strategies across settings (Fette et al., 2019) and address mental health conditions (e.g., depression, anxiety) and compounding influences (e.g., foster care) that affect children and families. One leadership action is reading and distributing materials found in the *School Mental Health Toolkit* (AOTA, 2019). Screening children for signs of autism is another example of a leadership action that results in early referral and treatment and has been associated with more positive outcomes (James et al., 2014). These actions exhibit practitioners' ability to "inspire a shared vision" (Kouzes & Posner, 2017) by being "an effective leader who gathers information central to promoting positive forces and movement toward possibilities" (Garbarini & Winston, 2015, p. 65).

Physical Health

Early childhood leadership capitalizes on applying a holistic, occupational lens to service. ***Physical health*** connects to an optimal level of activity and correlates to mental health (U.S. Department of Health & Human Services [DHHS], 2018). Signs of physical health can be monitored at the population level, such as number of preschoolers who meet the criteria for childhood obesity. Occupational therapy practitioners can identify patterns of inactivity and suggest customized routines to promote health and well-being through the primary occupation of play (Persch & Reifenberg, 2018). Examples include promoting and customizing recess as an important healthy routine for all preschoolers and encouraging community outings, such as walks and park visits, for the family's growth and development.

Occupational therapy practitioner leaders can also quantify authentic participation outcomes (e.g., frequency of peer interactions, level of attendance) and benefit to both physical and mental health (e.g., feelings of belonging, level of pain) as well as early childhood indicators (e.g., early literacy, transition, socioemotional outcomes). These actions also exhibit practitioners' leadership ability to "challenge the process" (Kouzes & Posner, 2017) by promoting an environment that welcomes taking risks, seizing opportunities, and confronting challenges (Garbarini & Winston, 2015).

Poverty

Nineteen percent of children (14.1 million) in the United States live in families with incomes below the poverty line (Annie E. Casey Foundation, 2018). Families who live in concentrated high-poverty neighborhoods—where poverty rates for the total population are 30% or more—face more health challenges, higher crime rates, subpar schools, and limited access to support networks and jobs (Annie E. Casey Foundation, 2018). Poverty may be associated with ***occupational deprivation,*** where illness or disability inhibits engagement in meaningful occupations (Fabrizi & Ponsolle-Mays, 2018).

Promoting safe and healthy early childhood occupations in our communities, such as access to neighborhood playgrounds, proper car seat installation, and healthy mealtime and sleep routines, is an example of leadership. Any occupational therapy practitioner can demonstrate leadership by exploring ways to work together with community partners, such as librarians, city planners, and paramedics, to enhance the community, such as conducting developmental screenings during community health fairs. These actions, including acknowledgment of cultural considerations, exhibit practitioners' ability to "enable others to act" (Kouzes & Posner, 2017) by promoting collaborative efforts and instilling confidence and trust in others, which fosters their capabilities (Garbarini & Winston, 2015).

Education

In the field of early childhood, *education* is a broad term used to describe any type of program that facilitates learning for young children, including preschool. There is a long history of evidence showing that high-quality preschool programs promote readiness and are correlated to later school literacy and academic success, especially for children at risk (Center on the Developing Child, 2007). More than half of all children ages 3–4 years—4.3 million total—were not in preschool between 2014 and 2016. Students who reach fourth grade without being able to read proficiently are more likely to struggle academically and eventually drop out of school (Hernandez, 2011). In 2017, 65% of fourth graders in public schools nationwide were reading below proficiency (Annie E. Casey Foundation, 2018).

To provide best practice for children and their families who participate in early childhood education, special education, and education programs for children at risk, occupational therapy practitioners need to have a working understanding of the foundations of these programs, the contextual landscape of program systems and the communities served, and the diversity of the children and families. Practitioners must understand the features of a program's curriculum and approach used for the child's learning (i.e., philosphical foundation, routines, materials, playful experiences) to promote access and participation while addressing the child's needs. For example, in a Montessori-based approach, a calm yet focused environment is fostered with a 2- to 3-hour block of individualized "work time" incorporated into the daily schedule, during which children learn concepts through specially designed "errorless" learning materials. In contrast, in programs that use a HighScope curriculum, an emphasis is placed on on the Plan–Do–Review format to promote self-initiated play and task completion.

It is essential to promote achievement toward academics and early literacy through activity and environmental analysis and modifications in homes, child care, and preschools and through adoption of literacy-rich play opportunities. Occupational therapy practitioners should demonstrate leadership to improve educational participation, accommodate diverse learners, and prepare staff and families to receive children transitioning to school. Practitioners can demonstrate leadership by applying universal design for learning principles and by improving participation of children and families in community settings, such as schools, preschools, libraries, and museums (AOTA, 2015a).

Promoting social and occupational justice during conversations with a preschool director highlights the role of occupational therapy in creating more inclusive activities and environments. Sharing materials such as AOTA's (2017a) early childhood inclusion brochure can promote the role of occupational therapy practitioners. These actions exhibit the practitioner's ability to "model the way" (Kouzes & Posner, 2017), which involves leaders illuminating and discussing perceived values and beliefs and gathering momentum by promoting agreement and consensus that represents members of the organization (Garbarini & Winston, 2015).

Family Engagement and Cultural Competency

Family engagement is the "systematic inclusion of families in activities and programs that promote children's development, learning, and wellness, including in the planning, development, and evaluation of such activities, programs, and systems" (DHHS & U.S. Department of Education, 2016, p. 1). *Culturally competent practice* uses the experiences and perspectives of children and families as a tool to support them more effectively. It might involve an occupational therapy practitioner, for example, informing a family that, as a service provider, they may be unaware of but are willing to learn about the family's values and beliefs. Information about a family's culture is essential when practitioners develop a service plan generated by and with family (Augustyn & Wallisch, 2017). Grounded in evidence, building family and caregiver capacity through coaching is an essential leadership skill for practitioners (Little et al., 2018). Only with cultural humility can practitioners customize a service plan that builds capacity of the family to care for the unique needs of their child.

The occupational profile provides an essential opportunity to engage with families as they articulate their needs and wants (AOTA, 2020). Posing guiding questions about a family's EI experiences may reveal ways to improve service delivery, which is a leadership action for occupational therapy practitioners to implement (Stoffel et al., 2017). These actions also exhibit practitioners' ability to "encourage the heart" (Kouzes & Posner, 2017) and facilitate a cohesive team by welcoming challenges, acknowledging accomplishments, and celebrating the successes of both an individual and the team (Garbarini & Winston, 2015).

BEST PRACTICES

There are two main leadership areas—technical and adaptive (Heifetz & Laurie, 2001)—that can be applied to occupational therapy early childhood services. Each area is defined and detailed in the following sections.

Assume Technical Leadership

Occupational therapy practitioners must assume a leadership role in the technical aspects of their practices across various settings. This includes collecting data, measuring effectiveness, applying research to practice, citing literature, and monitoring trends. This promotes occupational therapy leadership and active participation in the individualized family service plan or individualized education program team process. Practitioners report on effective interventions to match family priorities and state improvement plans and priorities for early literacy, social–emotional skills, and early childhood transitions.

Occupational therapists can participate in local and state-level data teams to "analyze, explore, and interpret data to support program improvement" (DaSy, 2017). They can participate by "investigating critical questions," "engaging families [and] other stakeholders," "monitoring trends," and "celebrating successes" on local and state levels (DaSy, 2017). Such participation can assist practitioners to be better advocates for the collection, analysis, and dissemination of high-quality data that capture the impact of occupational therapy services in early childhood systems.

Supervision is often conducted by staff members who are unfamiliar with occupational therapy practices, so practitioners must share their professional standards for practice (AOTA, 2015b) and evidence-based research with the early childhood leadership and key stakeholders. Sharing information about the young child and their family's everyday routines, culture, areas of interest, and prioritized family-centered outcomes demonstrates leadership and promotes others to advocate their value. Occupational therapy practitioners should strive to enhance current research efforts in early childhood by assuming leadership roles in scholarship through conducting research related to family-centered, routine-based interventions that focus on the child's participation in their natural environments.

Occupational therapy practitioners build knowledge and skills through continuous learning, a form of technical leadership. They can achieve this by accessing technical assistance and training opportunities offered through their state's Part C Comprehensive Systems of Professional Development and through AOTA's and their state occupational therapy association's continuing education opportunities.

Use Adaptive (Social) Leadership

Occupational therapy practitioners must assume a leadership role by harnessing their social (adaptive) prowess. *Socialization* is "the process by which individuals acquire and internalize the values, norms, roles, and skills that enable them to function as members of their cultural group" (Sabari, 1985, p. 96). Social power involves recognizing one's contributions and potential impact within a larger context. Practitioners must continuously inform and engage as a demonstration of social leadership. Social actions include conducting in-services, hosting brown bags, networking at professional meetings, creating tools to share stories, and launching journal clubs. Lamb (2017) noted that "the opportunities to act are all around us, often hidden in the routine of our daily work" (p. 4).

Social leaders use an ecological approach to conceptualize and deliver service. Occupational therapy practitioners consider their service within a dynamic system of shifting organizational, environmental, and activity demands (Bronfenbrenner & Morris, 2006). Cramm et al. (2013) asserted that "systems-level approaches are required if occupational therapy is to shift from the periphery and adequately position itself as a key player in knowledge translation" (p. 122). Practitioners advocate for their distinct value within the team and articulate their contributions toward achieving family, district, and state outcomes (AOTA, 2017b).

Apply social power across systems

Lamb (2017) wrote that as occupational therapy practitioners, "we have embraced our use of power, and we are no longer uncomfortable with it. Instead, it has proved pivotal in building occupational therapy's capacity as a profession" (p. 2). Social power can be harnessed across systems at the individual, group, or population level. When practitioners consider the sociocultural needs of a family during mealtime routines and adjust services accordingly, they meet social demands at the client level.

Social power can be applied at the group level, as well. When occupational therapy practitioners adjust their schedule to attend team meetings face to face whenever possible, they have more opportunities to connect formally and informally with key partners. Greater frequency of social interactions may lead to new programming opportunities, so the face-to-face time is a strategic social investment. In each example provided, practitioners demonstrate social leadership when considering relationships, contexts, and situations when planning or delivering early childhood occupational therapy services.

Build relationships in context

Hinojosa (2012) wrote that occupational therapy practitioners "need to focus on the totality of our practice—meaning that we need to examine not only what we do with clients, but also how we interact with professionals as part of our interventions" (p. e35). There is strategic value in building strong relationships with clients, administrators, and teams. Because early childhood services are based on team decision making, practitioners must be aware of Tuckman's five stages model of team development to inform expectations of the teaming process (MindTools, 2018; Smith, 2005).

The initial stage of team development is *forming*, which involves the team coming together. *Storming* is next and includes team conflict, confusion of roles or responsibilities, and the organization of the team. *Norming* follows and is when the team begins to develop a better understanding of roles and responsibilities. *Performing* occurs next and is when the team members begin to function well together and work toward their goal. The final stage is *adjourning*, when the team ends or the goals have been met (James & Walter, 2015).

Best practices in early childhood address common themes of family-centered and routine-based approaches, service setting, and the inclusion of parent participation and training (Kingsley & Mailloux, 2013). Occupational therapy services should be provided in the context of the naturally occurring routines of the child's day, which enables the practitioner to answer questions and offer solutions to everyday participation challenges, highlighting occupational therapy's value for problem solving and critical thinking. It creates more visibility and understanding of our professional domain and practice. For example, as a practitioner designs ways to make a preschool more inclusive for all students, they demonstrate value but also increase the likelihood that occupational therapy service is included in future programming. The team better understands the breadth and scope of occupational therapy service and its value for reaching family or state early childhood outcomes.

Initiate responsiveness

When using the occupational profile, occupational therapists can be predictive and responsive to family needs within a broader context. Whitney (2019) noted that "having the parents describe their experience of raising a child with developmental delay, and understanding their perception of how intervention would promote adaptation to their family routines, help(s) inform the quality of care within the larger, multidisciplinary team" (p. 6). Occupational therapy practitioners demonstrate social leadership in early childhood practice by contextualizing service within a larger system of care and considering the family's current and future needs.

At a systems level, occupational therapy practitioners can take the initiative to participate in the state's EI system public hearings and open comment opportunities. They can review and comment on the state's annual EI performance plan and any policy or procedure updates that affect occupational therapy. This is another example of social leadership.

Build networks

One of four unified early childhood personnel competencies is coordination and collaboration (Early Childhood Personnel Center [ECPC], 2019; Muhlenhaupt et al., 2019). Collaborations can be improved when discipline-specific and interprofessional networks are built. Network building can harness occupational therapy's power and strengthen its position; it is a strong form of social leadership.

Occupational therapy practitioners can join rotary clubs or local chapters of disability groups and become active in state occupational therapy associations as well as AOTA. Participating in one of AOTA's *communities of practice* (CoPs), defined as "groups of people who share a concern, a set of problems, or a passion about a topic, and who deepen their knowledge and expertise in this area by interacting on an ongoing basis" (Wenger et al., 2002, p. 4), provides an effective model for knowledge translation (Cramm et al., 2013). AOTA CoP members have become social learning leaders by conducting shared work and by becoming champions for the profession and for the clients they serve.

Demonstrate Everyday Leadership

Practitioners can take a number of everyday occupational therapy leadership actions:
- Know where you are headed by creating your own mission statement.
- Be a good communicator and active listener.
- Invest in the future by mentoring others.
- Support evidence-based practice.
- Promote our profession through professional membership activities.
- Offer servant leadership by helping others.
- Promote a diverse workforce by volunteering at health fairs (Zachry & Flick, 2015).

Some specific early childhood leadership actions include sharing a resource with a parent, introducing oneself to preschool office staff, meeting with an administrator to discuss launching a pilot program, copresenting with a colleague at a conference, and applying to become an Act Early ambassador (CDC, 2019) or a Leadership Education in Neurodevelopmental and Related Disabilities grantee (Association of University Centers on Disabilities, 2011).

One important leadership strategy is communicating and customizing key messages in a succinct and clear manner. AOTA offers numerous early childhood practice resources (see Table 5.1). AOTA also offers many volunteer leadership opportunities, including CoPs, institutes, and a Volunteer Leadership Development Committee. In addition to this book, AOTA has published a practice guideline to summarize recent systematic reviews in early childhood (Frolek Clark & Kingsley, 2020).

Understand Interprofessional Early Childhood Practices

Several national early childhood associations provide knowledge and guidance for practitioners. The Division of Early Childhood has worked collaboratively with the Early Childhood Technical Assistance Center to identify three early childhood leadership components, along with companion checklists for self-reflection and analysis:
1. Collaboration
2. Motivation and guidance
3. Vision and direction.

The ECPC, established by the U.S. Office of Special Education Programs in 2013, provides knowledge generation, technical assistance, and dissemination that addresses challenges faced in the early childhood workforce. An interprofessional ECPC work group composed of project staff, national association personnel, and leaders from early childhood therapy and education disciplines identified four unified personnel competencies shared by all providers during interprofessional early childhood practices:
1. Coordination and collaboration
2. Family-centered practice
3. Instruction and intervention, as informed by evidence
4. Professionalism and ethics (ECPC, 2019).

AOTA has formally endorsed these four competency areas (ECPC, 2019). See Chapter 2, "Influences From Early Childhood Professional Organizations and Technical Assistance Centers," for more information.

SUMMARY

Early childhood services are ever changing while children and families face new challenges. Occupational therapy practitioners must continuously adapt and assume new leadership roles as leadership advocates for our profession and our role as key providers in this area. We must share our evidence and effectiveness, build relationships, and grasp new opportunities offered through seed grants and other local ventures. To champion the role of occupational therapy and support families and children to improve their performance and overall quality of life, occupational therapy practitioners need to share information about our

TABLE 5.1.   AOTA Early Childhood Resources

AOTA RESOURCE	AOTA WEBSITE LINK	PURPOSE AND TARGET AUDIENCE
Frequently asked questions on role of occupational therapy in early intervention	https://bit.ly/2W6fuGw	Internal audience (for occupational therapy practitioners) to reflect on our practices
PowerPoint presentation on role of occupational therapy in early intervention*	https://bit.ly/2AM3RgF	Provides a packaged in-service to external audiences (for other providers, administrators) to understand our role
Fact sheet on role of occupational therapy with children and youth	https://bit.ly/2O92StU	External audience (for other providers, policymakers, and administrators) to understand our role
Special Interest Section Q&A on early intervention*	https://bit.ly/3eiooqS	Internal audience (for occupational therapy practitioners) to reflect on our practices
Trifold on inclusion and early intervention	https://bit.ly/3gM43Md	External audience (for other providers, administrators) to understand our role in promoting inclusion
Official document: Guidelines on role of occupational therapy in early intervention and schools*	https://bit.ly/2BYAqbB	Internal audience (for occupational therapy practitioners) to reflect on our practices
Early intervention evidence-based practice reviews and research	https://bit.ly/2W5D1Hz	Provides a systematic review of the evidence and practice guidelines for internal audience (occupational therapy practitioners)
Occupational Therapy Practice Guidelines for Early Childhood: Birth Through 5 *	https://bit.ly/3eevVGX	Based on a systematic review of literature; lists interventions for cognitive–literacy, mental health, motor, and self-care development
Childhood occupations toolkit	https://bit.ly/2BYAMir	Provides tips for families on everyday routines and illustrates our role to our partners (target is external audience)
School mental health toolkit	https://bit.ly/3iOMugm	Reviews issues such as depression, foster care, trauma, and recess time
Occupational therapy's distinct value for children and youth*	https://bit.ly/325cM7W	Synthesizes advocacy, practice, and evidence into a usable form for discussions with external audiences
Practice advisory on early intervention	https://bit.ly/2ZiOLJ4	For external audiences and for self-reflection
AOTA volunteer leadership opportunities*	https://bit.ly/2Du0Z9c	Members can apply to join councils, committees, and commissions

Resource is only available to AOTA members.

profession as providing effective solutions to the essential daily occupations of our family experiences while collecting data through ongoing needs assessments and surveillance.

RESOURCES

- **Collaboration in Leadership Checklist:** https://bit.ly/32223eE
  Self-evaluation (team or individual) tool to determine whether collaboration is being incorporated at all levels
- **Motivation and Guidance in Leadership Checklist:** https://bit.ly/2W7yrsp
  Self-evaluation (team or individual) to determine whether occupational therapy practitioners are practicing and promoting values and beliefs on a daily basis
- **Vision and Direction in Leadership Checklist:** https://bit.ly/3034QBQ
  Self-evaluation (team or individual) to ensure that state and local levels are articulating and using the vision and mission of the organization
- **Child Outcomes Summary (COS) Process:** https://bit.ly/38R4DFO

Key information about the COS process and meaningful COS decision making

- **COS form and 7-point rating scale:** https://bit.ly/2W6SqYb
  For providers to summarize information collected from multiple sources to provide a 7-point rating for the three child outcomes
- **COS process decision tree:** https://bit.ly/2WmSgwf
  Series of questions about the extent to which a child exhibits age-appropriate skills and behaviors to guide a specific 7-point rating
- **Families Are Full Team Members Checklist:** https://bit.ly/3ffFuac
  Steps and actions teams can take to ensure that families are included as full team members
- **Communication for Teaming and Collaboration Checklist:** https://bit.ly/3iPxjn7
  Indicators that team members can use to assess whether quality communication is taking place during all formal and informal team interactions
- **Collaboration to Learn and Grow Checklist:** https://bit.ly/3263Yii

Steps and actions team members can take to share and gain expertise to provide effective interventions that meet the child's and family's needs
- **Seven Key Principles: Looks Like/Doesn't Look Like:** https://bit.ly/2ZVaPsd
Foundations necessary to support family-centered services

REFERENCES

American Occupational Therapy Association. (2015a). *Occupational therapy and universal design for learning.* https://www.aota.org/~/media/Corporate/Files/AboutOT/Professionals/WhatIsOT/CY/Fact-Sheets/UDL%20fact%20sheet.pdf

American Occupational Therapy Association. (2015b). Standards of practice for occupational therapy. *American Journal of Occupational Therapy, 69,* 6913410057. https://doi.org/10.5014/ajot.2015.696S06

American Occupational Therapy Association. (2015c). Surveying the profession: The 2015 AOTA salary & workforce survey. *OT Practice 20*(11), 7–11.

American Occupational Therapy Association. (2017a). *Early childhood inclusion and occupational therapy (OT): Maximizing participation for young children and their families.* Retrieved from https://www.aota.org/~/media/Corporate/Files/AboutOT/consumers/Youth/EC-Inclusion-and-OT-brochure-20171108.pdf

American Occupational Therapy Association. (2017b). Guidelines for occupational therapy services in early intervention and schools. *American Journal of Occupational Therapy, 71*(Suppl. 2), 7112410010. https://doi.org/10.5014/ajot.2017.716S01

American Occupational Therapy Association. (2017c). Vision 2025. *American Journal of Occupational Therapy, 71,* 7103420010. https://doi.org/10.5014/ajot.2017.713002

American Occupational Therapy Association. (2019). *School mental health toolkit.* http://www.aota.org/Practice/Children-Youth/Mental%20Health/School-Mental-Health.aspx

American Occupational Therapy Association. (2020). Occupational therapy practice framework: Domain and process (4th ed.). *American Journal of Occupational Therapy, 74*(Suppl. 2), 7412410010. https://doi.org/10.5014/ajot.2020.74S2001

Annie E. Casey Foundation. (2018). *2018 KIDS COUNT data book: 2018 state trends in child well-being.* https://www.aecf.org/resources/2018-kids-count-data-book/

Association of University Centers on Disabilities. (2011). *About LEND.* https://www.aucd.org/template/page.cfm?id=473

Augustyn, J., & Wallisch, A. (2017). Occupational therapy in early intervention: Supporting families and children through cultural competency and coaching. *OT Practice, 22*(6), 14–17.

Bronfenbrenner, U., & Morris, P. (2006). The bioecological model of human development. In W. Damon & R. M. Lerner (Eds.), *Handbook of child psychology: Vol. 1. Theoretical models of human development* (6th ed., pp. 793–828). Wiley.

Case-Smith, J. (2013). Systematic reviews of the effectiveness of interventions used in occupational therapy early childhood services. *American Journal of Occupational Therapy, 67,* 379–382. https://doi.org/10.5014/ajot.2013.007872

Centers for Disease Control and Prevention. (2019). *About adverse childhood experiences.* https://www.cdc.gov/violenceprevention/acestudy/

Center on the Developing Child. (2007). *Early childhood program effectiveness* (InBrief). https://developingchild.harvard.edu/resources/inbrief-early-childhood-program-effectiveness-video/

Cramm, H., White, C., & Krupa, T. (2013). From periphery to player: Strategically positioning occupational therapy within the knowledge translation landscape. *American Journal of Occupational Therapy, 67,* 119–125. https://doi.org/10.5014/ajot.2013.005678

DaSy. (2017). *What are data teams?* https://dasycenter.org/wp-content/uploads/2018/07/Data_Teams_infographic_.png

Early Childhood Personnel Center. (2019). *Cross-disciplinary personnel competencies alignment.* https://ecpcta.org/cross-disciplinary-competencies/

Fabrizi, S. E., & Ponsolle-Mays, M. (2018). Enriching kids' lives: Addressing the effects of poverty on the health and well-being of school-aged children and their families. *OT Practice, 23*(9), 8–12.

Felitti, V. J., Anda, R. F., Nordenberg, D., Williamson, D. F., Spitz, A. M., Edwards, V., . . . Marks, J. S. (1998). Relationship of childhood abuse and household dysfunction to many of the leading causes of death in adults: The Adverse Childhood Experiences (ACE) Study. *American Journal of Preventive Medicine, 14,* 245–258. https://doi.org/10.1016/j.amepre.2019.04.001

Fette, C., Lambdin-Pattavina, C., & Weaver, L. (2019). *Understanding and applying trauma-informed approaches across occupational therapy settings.* https://www.aota.org/~/media/Corporate/Files/Publications/CE-Articles/CE-Article-May-2019-Trauma.pdf

Frolek Clark, G., & Kingsley, K. (2020). Occupational therapy practice guidelines for early childhood: Birth–5 years. *American Journal of Occupational Therapy, 74,* 7403397010. https://doi.org/10.5014/ajot.2020.743001

Garbarini, J. G., & Winston, K. (2015). Exploring the leader in you. In S. B. Dunbar & K. Winston (Eds.), *An occupation perspective on leadership: Theoretical and practical dimensions* (2nd ed., pp. 61–74). Slack.

Heard, C. P. (2018). Informal leadership in the clinical setting: Occupational therapist perspectives. *American Journal of Occupational Therapy, 72*(Suppl. 1), 7211510179. https://doi.org/10.5014/ajot.2018.72S1-PO4018

Heifetz, R. A., & Laurie, D. L. (2001, December). The work of leadership. *Harvard Business Review.* https://hbr.org/2001/12/the-work-of-leadership

Hernandez, D. J. (2011). *Double jeopardy: How third grade reading skills and poverty influence high school graduation.* Annie E. Casey Foundation. https://files.eric.ed.gov/fulltext/ED518818.pdf

Hinojosa, J. (2012). Personal strategic plan development: Getting ready for changes in our professional and personal lives. *American Journal of Occupational Therapy, 66,* e34–e38. https://doi.org/10.5014/ajot.2012.002360

Individuals With Disabilities Education Improvement Act of 2004, Pub. L. 108-446, 20 U.S.C. §§ 1400–1482.

James, L. W., Pizur-Barnekow, K. A., & Schefkind, S. (2014). Online survey examining practitioners' perceived preparedness in the early identification of autism. *American Journal of Occupational Therapy, 68,* e13–e20. https://doi.org/10.5014/ajot.2014.009027

James, L. W., & Walter, J. R. (2015). Teams and occupational therapy practitioner leadership. In S. B. Dunbar & K. Winston (Eds.), *An occupational perspective on leadership: Theoretical and practical dimensions* (2nd ed., pp. 67–177). Slack.

Karmali, S. (2018). Using leadership theories to improve interprofessional communication and patient outcomes. *SIS Quarterly Practice Connections, 3*(1), 18–20.

Kingsley, K., & Mailloux, Z. (2013). Evidence for the effectiveness of different service delivery models in early intervention services. *American Journal of Occupational Therapy, 67*, 431–436. https://doi.org/10.5014/ajot.2013.006171

Kouzes, J. M., & Posner, B. Z. (2013). *Great leadership creates great workplaces*. Jossey-Bass.

Kouzes, J. M., & Posner, B. Z. (2017). *The leadership challenge: How to make extraordinary things happen in organizations* (6th ed.). Jossey-Bass.

Lamb, A. J. (2017). Unlocking the potential of everyday opportunities. *American Journal of Occupational Therapy, 71*, 7106140010. https://doi.org/10.5014/ajot.2017.716001

Little, L. M., Pope, E., Wallisch, A., & Dunn, W. (2018). Occupation-based coaching by means of telehealth for families of young children with autism spectrum disorder. *American Journal of Occupational Therapy, 72*, 7202205020. https://doi.org/10.5014/ajot.2018.024786

MindTools. (2018). *Forming, storming, norming and performing: Understanding the stages of team formation*. https://www.mindtools.com/pages/article/newLDR_86.htm

Muhlenhaupt, M., de Lazaro, S. L., Fabrizi, S., Schefkind, S., & Owens, A. (2019). Interprofessional core competencies to enhance occupational therapy services in early childhood settings. *OT Practice, 24*(3), 13–16.

National Professional Development Center on Inclusion. (2008). *What do we mean by professional development in the early childhood field?* https://npdci.fpg.unc.edu/resources/articles/NPDCI-ProfessionalDevelopment-03-04-08

Persch, A., & Reifenberg, G. (2018). Practical tools for addressing healthy habits in children. *OT Practice, 23*(1), 14–17.

Sabari, J. S. (1985). Professional socialization: Implications for occupational therapy education. *American Journal of Occupational Therapy, 39*, 96–102. https://doi.org/10.5014/ajot.39.2.96

Sauvigne-Kirsch, J. (2017). Examining occupational therapists as potential special education leaders. *American Journal of Occupational Therapy, 71*(Suppl. 1), 7111510185. https://doi.org/10.5014/ajot.2017.71S1-PO3128

Smith, M. K. (2005). *Bruce W. Tuckman—Forming, storming, norming and performing in groups*. https://infed.org/mobi/bruce-w-tuckman-forming-storming-norming-and-performing-in-groups/

Stoffel, A., Rhein, J., Khetani, M. A., Pizur-Barnekow, K., James, L. W., & Schefkind, S. (2017). Family centered: Occupational therapy's role in promoting meaningful family engagement in early intervention. *OT Practice, 22*(18), 8–13.

Truskowski, S. (2018). Use of a novel mixed methods approach to study leadership within occupational therapy. *American Journal of Occupational Therapy, 72*(Suppl. 1), 7211505139. https://doi.org/10.5014/ajot.2018.72S1-PO6044

U.S. Department of Health and Human Services. (2018). *Physical activity guidelines for Americans* (2nd ed.) Author.

U.S. Department of Health & Human Services & U.S. Department of Education. (2016). *Policy statement on family engagement from the early years to the early grades*. https://www2.ed.gov/about/inits/ed/earlylearning/files/policy-statement-on-family-engagement.pdf

Vroom, V. H., & Jago, A. G. (2007). The role of the situation in leadership. *American Psychologist, 62*, 17–24. https://doi.org/10.1037/0003-066X.62.1.17

Wenger, E., McDermott, R., & Snyder, W. M. (2002). *Cultivating communities of practice: A guide to managing knowledge*. Harvard Business School Press.

Whitney, R. (2019). *The occupational profile as a guide to clinical reasoning in early intervention: A detective's tale*. http://www.aota.org/~/media/Corporate/Files/Publications/CE-Articles/CE-article-April-2019-Occupational-Profile.pdf

World Health Organization. (2010). *Framework for action on interprofessional education and collaborative practice*. https://www.who.int/hrh/resources/framework_action/en/

Zachry, A., & Flick, J. (2015). Occupational therapy practitioners: Everyday leaders. *OT Practice, 20*(1), 19–20.

Best Practices in Data-Based Decision Making

6

Gloria Frolek Clark, PhD, OTR/L, BCP, FAOTA

KEY TERMS AND CONCEPTS

- Accountability
- Baseline data
- Checklists
- Data-based decision making
- Documentation
- Duration
- Frequency
- Goal
- Goal attainment scaling
- Goal line
- Mastery monitoring
- Performance-based measurement
- Rubrics
- Working hypothesis

OVERVIEW

"Occupational therapy practitioners must meet ever-increasing accountability demands in all service delivery environments" (Fawcett & Strickland, 1998, p. 737). (*Note. Occupational therapy practitioner* refers to both occupational therapists and occupational therapy assistants.) *Accountability* holds providers responsible for outcomes and continues to be critical no matter the practice setting. *Data-based decision making* in education refers to a process of ongoing data collection and analysis to improve student instruction or interventions. Decisions about eligibility, need for service, effectiveness of interventions, and ongoing service needs should be based on data collected through a rigorous process to ensure that data are reliable and valid.

Although both quantitative and qualitative data offer information about the child, quantitative data allow monitoring for effectiveness. Knowing the child is able to drink from a bottle is informative; however, quantitative data allow precise information (e.g., child increased fluid intake per feeding from 2–3 ounces to 6 ounces). There are challenges to collecting quantitative data when working with young children because most of these data must be collected through observation or permanent products (e.g., work or product samples, photos, video). Assessment tools designed to monitor progress may also be used. (*Note.* The American Occupational Therapy Association [AOTA; 2010] uses the term *evaluation* to describe the process, whereas *assessment* refers to specific tools or instruments.)

Data collection should be simple, and occupational therapy practitioners should enlist others in the process. Increased training is required to ensure reliable data if multiple people are collecting data (e.g., parents, child care providers, preschool teachers). These individuals know the child best and are typically the ones providing daily opportunities for the child to learn the skills or practice the performance in their natural environment.

ESSENTIAL CONSIDERATIONS

This section discusses the various expectations about accountability of professionals working in various settings and provides some methods for gathering data.

Expectations About Accountability

In addition to professional requirements, settings have various accountability requirements that must be followed. This section covers expectations from AOTA, education law, and health care settings.

AOTA accountability expectations

AOTA documents identify occupational therapy using terms such as *evidence based, client centered, cost-effective,* and *effectiveness of occupational therapy services* (AOTA, 2015, 2020). Professional documentation must communicate the child's needs and the reason for services, record their response to therapy intervention, identify progress on the child's outcomes, and provide justification for skilled occupational therapy service necessity and reimbursement (AOTA, 2018). *Documentation* (e.g., evaluation reports, contact reports, progress reports) should include data to link the child's evaluation results and intervention needs, identify the efficacy of intervention, and record the child's performance on measurable outcomes or goals.

Education law accountability expectations

The Every Student Succeeds Act of 2015 (ESSA; P. L. 114-95) holds schools accountable for student achievement. States are able to design their own accountability systems, must include a broad meaure of student performance, and can implement plans for low-performing schools (U.S. Department of Education, n.d.).

The Individuals With Disabilities Education Improvement Act of 2004 (IDEA; P. L. 108-446) requires accountability throughout the eligibility and progress reporting process, including evaluation, intervention, and outcomes and goals. Children eligible under Part C of IDEA (ages birth–3 years) or Part B of IDEA (ages 3–21 years) require an evaluation from professionals so these data can be used to determine eligibility and service needs. The individualized family service plan (IFSP) requires a statement of measurable family or child outcomes and the criteria, procedures, and timelines to determine progress, whereas the individualized education program (IEP) requires a statement of measurable goals for the child and a description of how progress is measured and reported to the family. Data may also be used to support or refute the need for Part B extended school year services.

Using measurable data in daily logs is necessary to identify the child's response to intervention and progress on their goals. A daily log entry might read, "During the toddler play group at the library, Sofia stayed in library for 6 minutes (last week she attempted to run outside after 3 minutes)," or, "During recess, Zane positively interacted with peers twice while on the monkey bars (yesterday he hit 3 peers)."

Health care accountability expectations

Accountability in health care billing is critical. Some payers request a copy of the occupational therapist's evaluation or contact records before issuing payment. Others require data be completed before authorizing service. Spontaneous requests about a child's progress may be made by payers, including private payers, such as the parents.

Using measurable data in daily logs shows medical necessity and ongoing changes to the child's performance. For example, the log might read, "Tabitha imitated a visual–motor design with 1 error, as compared to 4 errors during the previous session," or "Yesterday, Jacob needed maximum physical support to sit on the edge of the bed for 90 seconds; however, today he sat for 2 minutes with moderate physical assistance." For more information, see Chapter 22, "Understanding Health Care Requirements, Process, and Billing."

Data Collection Methods for Early Childhood

Occupational therapy practitioners can use many methods to gather data with early childhood clients to determine their progress on the outcome or goal and the effectiveness of services. This section highlights a few of them. Determining the level of support is important in all of these examples.

Progress monitoring: Performance-based measurement

Performance-based measurement is a systematic data collection method used to identify progress toward general outcomes and to determine the effectiveness of the intervention. The steps to this process are described below.

Step 1. Define the concern. The concern should be alterable, specific, observable, and measurable.

Step 2. Select the measurement strategy. The measurement strategy includes considerations such as the materials used, the setting where performance occurs, and the reliability and validity of data collected. If the concern is *frequency* (how often performance occurs), such as too often (decrease length of tantrums) or too little (difficulty using pincer grip to grasp items), then performance should be counted. If the concern is *duration* (length of time), such as whether performance takes too long (e.g., child requires 40 minutes to eat) or is too short (e.g., lack of attention), then performance should be timed.

Step 3. Determine current level of performance. The current level of performance is the **baseline data**, which are collected on the basis of the identified concern and measurement strategies. At least 3 stable data points are collected and summarized with the median score (some agencies require 4 data points). The baseline data are compared with appropriate standards and expectations, such as developmental standards, peer standards, family expectations, preschool requirements, or the occupational therapist's professional judgment.

Step 4. Set a goal. The **goal** may be on the occupational therapy medical treatment plan justifying services, the child's IFSP outcome, or the child's IEP goal. Generally, measurable goals are formatted as follows: conditions (location, time frame, assistance), child's name, performance desired, and criteria for mastery.

Step 5. Set up a chart. Visual graphs are critical to determine the child's rate of progress. A line connecting the child's baseline and ending (goal or outcome) point is known as the **goal line**. In Figure 6.1, the goal line connects

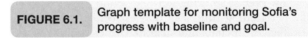

FIGURE 6.1. Graph template for monitoring Sofia's progress with baseline and goal.

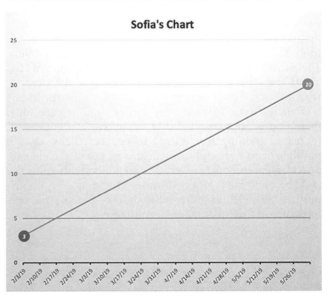

EXHIBIT 6.1.	Mastery Monitoring Subskills and Criteria

Definition of Child's Skill to Be Mastered: Self-feed using a spoon at least 5 times per meal

Subskill	Mastery Criterion
1. Pick up spoon	Within 6 seconds of adult verbal command
2. Scoop food on spoon	Independently with food on spoon
3. Bring spoon to mouth	Independently with minimal spillage
4. Use lips to clean spoon	Independently without using teeth
5. Lower spoon to plate	Independently
6. Repeat Steps 2–5	Independently, at least 4 times

Sofia's baseline (3) with her goal (20). This indicates the rate of progress she must make to meet this goal by the date set.

Step 6. Establish a decision-making plan. Determine the frequency of data collection during intervention and data review to determine effectiveness. The occupational therapist and team compare at least 3–4 consecutive data points (e.g., Sofia's performance) with the goal line to determine whether the intervention is effective. If all data points are below the line, the intervention is not working and should be changed; if data points are above and below the line, the intervention may be working; and if all data points are above the line, the child may meet their goal faster than expected (Frolek Clark & Handley-Moore, 2017).

Progress monitoring: Mastery monitoring

Mastery monitoring is a method of determining progress when skills are absent or not mastered. The steps are similar to performance-based measurement.

Step 1. Define the skill needed. Task analyze the skill and establish a sequence of subskills. Skills are listed in a hierarchy of subskills, with a mastery criterion listed for each subskill, on the basis of the individual child's needs and typical performance. The child must master all the subskills to meet the overall goal (see Exhibit 6.1).

Step 2. Select the measurement strategy. Establish a mastery criterion for each subskill. Define the procedure for collecting data (e.g., setting, routine, conditions, schedule for data collection).

Step 3. Determine current level of performance (i.e., baseline). The baseline is typically considered to be 0, because these subskills are not met. Begin intervention. After 3–5 sessions, determine whether the subskills are correct (e.g., are in the right order, need to be broken down). Draw a vertical review line on graph if changes are made.

Step 4. Set a goal. This may be a goal on the occupational therapy medical treatment plan justifying services, the child's IFSP outcome, or the child's IEP goal. Rather than, for example, a goal to complete all 6 of 6 subskills, the goal should reflect the functional performance expected (which is generally mastery of these subskills in order to achieve the goal).

Step 5. Set up a chart. Write subskills on the chart. The goal line is a flat line because all subskills must be met. (See the information below about quarter stars.)

Step 6. Establish a decision-making plan. Determine the frequency of data collection during intervention and data review to determine effectiveness.

Data are plotted on a graph with a plus sign if the child completed the subskill according to the mastery criterion. Rather than using a minus sign when a subskill was not

FIGURE 6.2.	Mastery monitoring template.

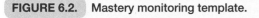

Subskills:	#																								
	10																								
	9																								
	8																								
	7						GOAL LINE																		★
Repeat steps 2-5	6																								
Lower spoon to plate	5	P	P	V	V	+	+											★							
Use lips to clean spoon	4	P	P	P	P	P	P																		
Bring spoon to mouth	3	P	V	V	+	+	+					★													
Scoop food on spoon	2	P	P	P	P	V	V ★																		
Pick up spoon	1	P	P	P	P	P	P																		
DATES (numbers used here for teaching purpose only-use actual dates)		1	2	3	4	5	6	7	8	9	10	11	12	13	14	15	16	17	18	19	20	21	22	23	24

Key: + completed; V-needed verbal cue; P-needed physical assistance; R-refused.

mastered, practitioners are encouraged to use informative codes, such as the following:

- PR: Parent reported child could complete this
- P: Child completed with physical assistance
- V: Child completed with a verbal cue.
- R: Child refused

If, after several days of requiring physical assistance to hold the spoon, the child can complete the task with verbal assistance, that is a positive change that can be easily seen with these informative codes. Figure 6.2 plots the child's 6 subskills. Goal lines are flat, because all of the subskills must be met first. The number of subskills achieved can be counted and used to determine whether progress is occurring.

Another method is to identify the number of weeks for the intervention (e.g., 24 weeks), determine the number of subskills (e.g., 8), and compute the halfway mark (e.g., in 12 weeks, approximately 4 subskills should be met). Stars called *quarter stars* can also be added to the chart to identify points across the chart. Do not connect the stars; they are markers in time, not a true slope. These are computed as follows:

- In 6 weeks, 2 subskills
- In 12 weeks, 4 subskills
- In 18 weeks, 6 subskills
- In 24 weeks, 8 subskills.

Sometimes the subskills do not divide easily into 4 and may result in "rough" numbers. For example, a total of 6 subskills in 24 weeks would be broken down as follows:

- In 6 weeks, 1.5 subskills
- In 12 weeks, 3 subskills
- In 18 weeks, 4.5 subskills
- In 24 weeks, 6 subskills.

Quarter stars indicate a stopping point to analyze the data to see if the child's rate of progress is increasing at a rate that they should have mastered this number of subskills. Using the data on the chart, the practitioner is able to target the subskills that are not mastered. While this is not exact, quarter stars provide the team with a way to more closely monitor the child's "rate of progress" toward meeting the goal. Young children's growth is not always linear but may occur in spurts and plateaus, so data should reflect professional judgment.

Goal attainment scaling

Goal attainment scaling (GAS) is a systematic method that can be used to describe the child's current and ongoing performance, identify outcomes and goals, and monitor performance. GAS scales vary in the number of score levels (typically 5 or 6) used, with 0 typically used to identify the expected level of outcome (see Exhibit 6.2). The sixth score is helpful because it denotes regression, which is common among children with medical conditions.

The 8 steps in the process, described by Ottenbacher and Cusick (1990), are

- *Step 1.* Identify the overall goals or outcomes.
- *Step 2.* Identify the problem areas.
- *Step 3.* Identify specific behaviors or events in problem areas that can be measured.
- *Step 4.* Determine how data will be collected.
- *Step 5.* Determine the expected level of performance.
- *Step 6.* Identify a continuum of outcomes (most to least favorable).
- *Step 7.* Review GAS to identify overlaps and gaps.
- *Step 8.* Determine when further evaluations will be conducted.

An advantage of GAS is that it can be used with young children who are learning a skill (e.g., skill emerging or not yet present). Because GAS is a criterion-referenced rather than a norm-referenced tool, it is responsive to minimal yet significant changes. The measurable goals should be individualized, realistic, and collaboratively established with others.

Checklists or rubrics with standards

Data collection in homes may be less formal than in preschool or health care settings; however, accountability remains essential. Checklists may be formal or informal lists of skills or tasks the child is expected to perform. Rubrics are tools that use gradations of criteria to assess performance.

Occupational therapists should identify a standard to use as a comparison. For example, the standard may be peer performance, the parent or preschool teacher's expectation, or the medical standard for nutrition. This avoids the trap of setting a goal of "scores 6/8 on a rubric" when

---

EXHIBIT 6.2.   Goal Attainment Scaling Template Sample

Goal: Child will play catch with classmates at recess for at least 5 minutes without dropping the ball. (Baseline: 1 minute)

Score	Description	Objective
+2	Much more than expected	Child plays catch with a classmate at recess for more than 10 minutes without dropping the ball.
+1	Somewhat more than expected	Child plays catch with a classmate at recess for more than 5 and less than 10 minutes without dropping the ball.
0	Expected level of outcome	Child plays catch with a classmate at recess for 5 minutes without dropping the ball.
−1	Progress	Child plays catch with a classmate at recess for more than 1 but less than 5 minutes without dropping the ball.
−2	Baseline (present level of performance)	Child plays catch with a classmate at recess for 1 minute without dropping the ball.
−3	Regression from baseline	Child plays catch with a classmate at recess for less than 1 minute without dropping the ball.

peers might actually score only 5/8 or 4/8 on the rubric if they were tested. Both offer easy documentation of children's performance.

Checklists. Checklists may be used to quickly document the child's performance during occupations such as eating, toileting, social participation, play, and work. In the home, parents may use scraps of paper to informally document their child's performance; the practitioner then collects the parents' results and graphs the data more formally (electronically or manually).

Exhibits 6.3 to 6.5 provide some examples of these checklists. Although Exhibit 6.3 is focused on toileting, the task could be changed to reflect eating or other activities. Exhibit 6.4 can be used to document the frequency (out of 10 trials or opportunities, 10 seconds, or 10 minutes) with which something occurs. This data collection checklist or sheet allows the practitioner to visually see progress by simply circling the frequency across data collection occurrences. Exhibit 6.5 can be used to document the duration (how long the performance lasted). Circling the data provides a graph that can offer a quick visual model of progress.

Rubrics. Rubrics can be used in multiple settings. **Rubrics** "specifically state the expectations for the task and are based on acceptable standards; however, occupational therapy practitioners should confirm the standard (expected performance)" with the parent, teacher, or others (Frolek Clark, 2019, p. 382). Exhibit 6.6 demonstrates a 4-point rubric scale. Using an even number tends to prevent people from favoring the midpoint score, such as the 3 in a 5-point scale.

EXHIBIT 6.4. Frequency Chart

Goal: During the first 10 spoonfuls of food at lunch, Stone will bring his spoon to his mouth 8 out of 10 times for 3 out of 5 consecutive days. (Note: Stone is alert at the beginning of the meal, so self-feeding is worked on then; he is fed for the remainder of the meal.)

Date 2/14 Time 11:32	Date 2/19 Time 11:35	Date 2/27 Time 11:35	Date 3/4 Time 11:40	Date Time	Date Time	Date Time	Date Time	Date Time	Date Time	Date Time	Date Time
10	10	10	10	10	10	10	10	10	10	10	10
9	9	9	9	9	9	9	9	9	9	9	9
8	8	8	8	8	8	8	8	8	8	8	8
7	7	7	7	7	7	7	7	7	7	7	7
6	6	6	6	6	6	6	6	6	6	6	6
5	5	5	5	5	5	5	5	5	5	5	5
4	4	4	④	4	4	4	4	4	4	4	4
3	③	3	3	3	3	3	3	3	3	3	3
2	2	②	2	2	2	2	2	2	2	2	2
①	1	1	1	1	1	1	1	1	1	1	1

Key:
◯ = number of bites without spilling

Canadian Occupational Performance Measure

The Canadian Occupational Performance Measure (COPM; Law et al., 2019) is designed to detect change by self-reporting. According to the authors, 5-year-olds who are self-assessing, self-aware, and self-understanding could use this tool. However, this tool may be used by parents and caregivers of young children to determine needs and

EXHIBIT 6.3. Toileting Checklist

Date each encounter and circle highest level achieved. See key below.

Task	Date Time	Date Time	Date Time	Date Time	Date Time	Date Time	Date Time	Date Time	Date Time
Goes to bathroom area	R, I, G, V P, FP	R, I, G, V P, FP	R, I, G, V P, FP	R, I, G, V P, FP	R, I, G, V P, FP	R, I, G, V P, FP	R, I, G, V P, FP	R, I, G, V P, FP	R, I, G, V P, FP
Pulls pants down	R, I, G, V P, FP	R, I, G, V P, FP	R, I, G, V P, FP	R, I, G, V P, FP	R, I, G, V P, FP	R, I, G, V P, FP	R, I, G, V P, FP	R, I, G, V P, FP	R, I, G, V P, FP
Uses toilet	R, BM, UR, PW, NS	R, BM, UR, PW,	R, BM, UR, PW,	R, BM, UR, PW,	R, BM, UR, PW,	R, BM, UR, PW,	R, BM, UR, PW,	R, BM, UR, PW,	R, BM, UR, PW,
Wipes	R, I, G, V P, FP	R, I, G, V P, FP	R, I, G, V P, FP	R, I, G, V P, FP	R, I, G, V P, FP	R, I, G, V P, FP	R, I, G, V P, FP	R, I, G, V P, FP	R, I, G, V P, FP
Flushes	R, I, G, V P, FP	R, I, G, V P, FP	R, I, G, V P, FP	R, I, G, V P, FP	R, I, G, V P, FP	R, I, G, V P, FP	R, I, G, V P, FP	R, I, G, V P, FP	R, I, G, V P, FP
Pulls pants up	R, I, G, V P, FP	R, I, G, V P, FP	R, I, G, V P, FP	R, I, G, V P, FP	R, I, G, V P, FP	R, I, G, V P, FP	R, I, G, V P, FP	R, I, G, V P, FP	R, I, G, V P, FP
Washes hands	R, I, G, V P, FP	R, I, G, V P, FP	R, I, G, V P, FP	R, I, G, V P, FP	R, I, G, V P, FP	R, I, G, V P, FP	R, I, G, V P, FP	R, I, G, V P, FP	R, I, G, V P, FP
Returns to classroom	R, I, G, V P, FP	R, I, G, V P, FP	R, I, G, V P, FP	R, I, G, V P, FP	R, I, G, V P, FP	R, I, G, V P, FP	R, I, G, V P, FP	R, I, G, V P, FP	R, I, G, V P, FP

Note. BM = bowel movement; FP = full physical; G = gestural; I = Independent; NS = not successful; P = physical; PW = pants wet; R = refusal; UR = urinated; V = verbal.

EXHIBIT 6.5. Duration Chart

Directions: Circle the number of minutes child maintains participation with familiar simple game.

Date 2/14/20	Date 2/19/20	Date 2/27/20	Date 3/4/20	Date	Date	Date	Date
15 min	15 min	15 min	15 min	15 min	15 min	15 min	15 min
14 min	14 min	14 min	14 min	14 min	14 min	14 min	14 min
13 min	13 min	13 min	13 min	13 min	13 min	13 min	13 min
12 min	12 min	12 min	12 min	12 min	12 min	12 min	12 min
11 min	11 min	11 min	11 min	11 min	11 min	11 min	11 min
10 min	10 min	10 min	10 min	10 min	10 min	10 min	10 min
9 min	9 min	9 min	9 min	9 min	9 min	9 min	9 min
8 min	8 min	8 min	8 min	8 min	8 min	8 min	8 min
7 min	7 min	7 min	7 min	7 min	7 min	7 min	7 min
6 min	6 min	6 min	6 min	6 min	6 min	6 min	6 min
5 min	5 min	5 min	(5) min	5 min	5 min	5 min	5 min
4 min	(4) min	4 min	4 min	4 min	4 min	4 min	4 min
3 min	3 min	(3) min	3 min	3 min	3 min	3 min	3 min
(2) min	2 min	2 min	2 min	2 min	2 min	2 min	2 min
1 min	1 min	1 min	1 min	1 min	1 min	1 min	1 min

EXHIBIT 6.6. Rubric Template Example

Description: Buzz is a child who hits and kicks peers. At the parents' request, the task is "plays with peers." Buzz's baseline is at 1 (has to be removed from play area); 3 is the expected outcome (10 minutes of positive interactions with an adult nearby).

Task component	1: Not acceptable	2: With assistance	3: Acceptable (expected)	4: Exceeds expectations
Plays with peers	Hits and kicks others; removed from play area	Positively interacts for 1–9 minutes with an adult nearby	Positively interacts for 10 minutes with an adult nearby	Positively interacts for 3–10 minutes without an adult nearby

goals. The COPM can be used across all developmental levels to measure progress in areas such as self-care, play, and socialization.

The 5 steps of the COPM include the following:

1. *Problem definition:* Occupations are self-identified through interviews (in the case of children, the parents identify the child's barriers with occupations).
2. *Rating importance:* In response to the question, "How important is it to you to be able to do this activity?" the parents rate each activity (on a 10-point scale) in terms of the importance for the family and child. Ten is the highest rating (*extremely important*).
3. *Scoring performance:* In response to the question, "How would you rate the way you do this activity now?" the parents rate each problem, using the 10-point scale.
4. *Scoring satisfaction:* In response to the question, "How satisfied are you with the way you do this activity now?" the parents rate each problem, using the 10-point scale.
5. *Reassessment:* After a previously determined timeframe, the parent are asked to evaluate each specific problem on the 10-point Performance and Satisfaction scales. The administrator calculates change in performance by subtracting Time 1 scores from Time 2 (reassessment) scores.

BEST PRACTICES

Occupational therapy practitioners should use data collected throughout service delivery (evaluation through discharge planning) to make decisions about the need and effectiveness of services and to evaluate the outcomes of their programs. Each of these is discussed in further detail in this section.

Gather Quantitative and Qualitative Data During the Evaluation

Across all settings, the occupational therapy evaluation consists of the occupational profile and the analysis of the results (AOTA, 2020). Data for the occupational profile provide an understanding of why the family is seeking an evaluation. Medical, health, developmental, and educational information; supports or barriers to occupational performance; and desired outcomes can be gathered through interviews with parents, teachers, caregivers, and appropriate others (AOTA, 2020). Record review and interview may be used to gather these data. During the interview, the client may provide qualitative information; however, the occupational therapist should try to quantify the data whenever possible to understand the significance of the performance. Table 6.1 provides examples of strategies for gathering measurable data.

While gathering data, the occupational therapist may begin developing a *working hypothesis,* or tentative reason for the identified concerns that is further explored as more data are gathered. If the interview focused on *occupations,* the therapist's hypothesis may reflect the occupations that should be addressed. For instance, if the child in Table 6.1 had a full night's sleep, maybe the tantrums would decrease. However, if the interview focuses on *performance skills,* the data collected influence the working hypothesis but may not reach the occupation level.

For example, if a child struggles with fine motor and visual–motor tasks, the occupational therapist may hypothesize that the child has a motor or sensory issue. However, guiding the interview to an occupation level (top down) may provide further information (e.g., this child has difficulty initiating and completing preschool work that involves coloring, cutting, and drawing). Discussion with the school nurse indicates that the child failed vision screening and has an eye examination scheduled for the following week. At that point, the therapist may hypothesize that vision could be an issue and will wait for results.

Observing the child in their natural environment is preferred because the occupational therapist can view the environmental and contextual influences (e.g., social interactions, space constraints). In the home setting, the therapist can observe the family interactions with the child and discuss areas where they may want more support or resources. In preschools or community child care programs, the therapist is able to observe the child's occupations, as well as motor, social, and sensory performance, while peers are nearby. Although health care settings do not offer the natural environment, the therapist is able to observe the child's responses and make modifications to challenge or support the child.

Depending on the setting, the occupational therapist may use data from assessment measures to identify the child's performance. When choosing a tool, therapists should identify what data they need. Occupation-based measures are preferred when possible, because they provide information about the child's occupational performance, but data from performance skill or environmental

measures may also be useful (e.g., visual–motor assessments, sensory environment).

Generally, young children do not sit for standardized measures, so alternative assessment methods are often used in early childhood. These may include

- The *embedded approach,* in which information is gathered while the child is in their environment or routine, such as an ecological-based assessment or play-based assessment;
- The *authentic approach,* in which children's abilities are documented in real-life contexts through videotapes, photos, work samples, and portfolios; and
- The *mediated approach,* in which guided teaching is used to assess children's responsivity to instruction, such as dynamic assessment (e.g., test–teach–retest model) and curriculum-based assessment, which links assessment to the curriculum and programming (Losardo & Notari-Syverson, 2011).

These methods produce data that can be used as baseline and ongoing data monitoring.

After all of the data are collected through record review, interview, observation, and assessments, the occupational therapist analyzes them to refine the hypothesis and create collaborative goals with the family and team. These data are used to determine eligibility (IDEA, 2004) and need for occupational therapy services. In all settings, the child's goals or outcomes should be directly linked to the evaluation findings and concerns expressed by the referring source (e.g., parent, school, physician).

Gather Data During Evidence-Based Interventions

Occupational therapy practitioners implement services documented on health care treatment plans, services documented on the IFSP and IEPs, or services reimbursed through other means. Gathering data to monitor the child's response to ongoing services is necessary to determine the effectiveness of therapy and make decisions about ongoing therapy needs.

Using the methods previously described, data should be collected on a systematic basis (e.g., same day and same time of day for comparison) and using a frequency based on the need. For example, safety and health situations (e.g., child who is aggressive toward self or others, infant who struggles sucking liquids from a bottle) should be monitored more frequently so that decisions can be made in a timely manner. In addition, reviewing the data on a consistent schedule is essential. In the case of health, decisions may be made sooner if the infant has minimal fluid intake. If data are gathered several times a day, decisions could be made within a few days (10 data points). If data are gathered weekly, decisions could be made in 4 weeks (4 consecutive data points).

Determine the Fidelity of the Implementation

When occupational therapy practitioners provide programs for others to implement, providing a quick checklist is critical to determining the fidelity of the implementation. For example, the family or child care staff is given a home

TABLE 6.1. Evaluation: Qualitative vs. Quantitative Data Gathered During Interview

AREA OF CONCERN	PARENT'S INITIAL STATEMENT (QUALITATIVE)	PARENT STATEMENT AFTER FOLLOW-UP QUESTIONS (QUANTITATIVE)
Self-care: Rest	"My son has a difficult time sleeping at night."	"He hasn't fallen asleep by himself before 11 p.m. since Sunday—8 days now!"
Self-care: Hygiene	"We have no specific bedtime routine, just whatever works."	"He screams for 10 minutes while I give him a bath and brush his teeth."
Self-regulation	"He has lots of tantrums and screams if he doesn't like something at school."	"Three tantrums occurred yesterday, and each lasted between 10 and 12 minutes."

EXHIBIT 6.7. Fidelity of Implementation Sample

Directions: Indicate (√) as you complete, and list approximate amount of time child was in each position

Task	Jan 20	Jan 21	Jan 22	Jan 23	Jan 24
Placed on stomach with entertaining object or person by face	√ 10 s	√ 15 s		√ 3 s	√ 4s
Placed in supported sitting with adult directly in front of child to stabilize as needed	√ 24 s	√ 24 s			√ 8 s

program that provides the child with additional work on tummy time and supported sitting. A week later, the child does not show any improvements. The occupational therapy practitioner now has two options.

The first option is to determine that the intervention was not effective and to change it. The second option is to review the implementation checklist (see Exhibit 6.7). The practitioner chooses this option and notices that the family implemented the home program with 60% to 80% frequency per task (4/5 days and 3/5 days), and the child's performance was improving during the beginning of the week (achieved 15 seconds and 24 seconds). Therefore, the intervention may be working, but something else occurred. Further discussion with the parent may indicate that the mother returned to work on January 22 and a new caregiver was implementing the program. The implementation checklist assists the parent and practitioner to identify the need for further training for the new caregiver.

There are many different methods that can be used to document data from evaluation and interventions. Practitioners should identify several that can be used easily in their setting.

SUMMARY

Regardless of the setting, occupational therapy practitioners are accountable for effectiveness of service delivery. Using a systematic approach to address concerns is important, including establishing baseline data on children's performance that can be monitored weekly through functional activities (Frolek Clark & Miller, 1996). Qualitative data offer information but are difficult to use for decision making (eligibility for services, baseline, effectiveness of interventions, progress toward outcomes or goals).

For practitioners working under IDEA, these data provide information about eligibility, effectiveness of services, need for discontinuation or ongoing programming, and need for extended-year services (Part B).

REFERENCES

American Occupational Therapy Association. (2010). Standards of practice for occupational therapy. *American Journal of Occupational Therapy, 64*(6, Suppl.), S106–S111. https://doi.org/10.5014/ajot.2010.64S106

American Occupational Therapy Association. (2015). Standards of practice for occupational therapy. *American Journal of Occupational Therapy, 69*(Suppl. 3), 6913410057. https://doi.org/10.5014/ajot.2015.696S06

American Occupational Therapy Association. (2018). Guidelines for documentation of occupational therapy. *American Journal of Occupational Therapy, 72*(Suppl. 2), 7212410010. https://doi.org/10.5014/ajot.2018.72S203

American Occupational Therapy Association. (2020). Occupational therapy practice framework: Domain and process (4th ed.). *American Journal of Occupational Therapy, 74*(Suppl. 2), 7412410010. https://doi.org/10.5014/ajot.2020.74S2001

Every Student Succeeds Act of 2015, Pub. L. 114-95, 20 U.S.C. §§ 6301.

Fawcett, L., & Strickland, R. (1998). Accountability and competence: Occupational therapy practitioner perceptions. *American Journal of Occupational Therapy, 52*, 737–743. https://doi.org/10.5014/ajot.52.9.737

Frolek Clark, G. (2019). Best practices in school occupational therapy documentation and data collection. In G. Frolek Clark, J. Rioux, & B. Chandler (Eds.), *Best practices for occupational therapy in schools* (2nd ed., pp. 373–383). AOTA Press.

Frolek Clark, G., & Handley-Moore, D. (2017). *Best practices for documenting occupational therapy services in schools.* AOTA Press.

Frolek Clark, G., & Miller, L. (1996). Providing effective occupational therapy services: Data-based decision making in school-based practices. *American Journal of Occupational Therapy, 50*, 701–708. https://doi.org/10.5014/ajot.50.9.701

Individuals With Disabilities Education Improvement Act of 2004, Pub. L. 108-446, 20 U.S.C. §§ 1400–1482.

Law, M., Baptiste, S., Carswell, A., McColl, M., Polatajko, H., & Pollock, N. (2019). *Canadian Occupational Performance Measure* (5th ed., rev.). COPM, Inc.

Losardo, A., & Notari-Syverson, A. (2011). *Alternative approaches to assessing young children* (2nd ed.). Brookes.

Ottenbacher, K., & Cusick, A. (1990). Goal attainment scaling as a method of clinical service evaluation. *American Journal of Occupational Therapy, 44*, 519–525. https://doi.org/10.5014/ajot.44.6.519

U.S. Department of Education. (n.d.). *Every Student Succeeds Act: Accountability, state plans, and data reporting: Summary of final regulations.* https://www2.ed.gov/policy/elsec/leg/essa/essafactsheet170103.pdf

Best Practices in the Use of Assistive Technology to Enhance Participation

Judith Schoonover, MEd, OTR/L, ATP, FAOTA

7

KEY TERMS AND CONCEPTS

- Assistive technology
- Augmentative and alternative communication
- Interdisciplinary approach
- Let's Participate! Project
- Student, Environments, Tasks, and Tools
- Switch
- Technology Related Assistance for Individuals With Disabilities Act of 1988
- Universal design
- Universal Design for Learning

A solid foundation and understanding of AT is a first step in what for most children with disabilities is a lifelong journey. Technology will grow and change as they do but may always be a part of their life. (Simon Technology Center, 2015, p. 2)

OVERVIEW

Childhood experiences directly influence independence, attitudes, and success in adulthood. The learning that takes place in the early months and years through meaningful interaction with people and objects in natural settings and during everyday activities and routines is critical to later understanding and development. The level of participation young children enjoy is dependent on their ability to access their environment, participate, and become engaged.

For young children with disabilities who encounter barriers to accessing their natural environments, *assistive technology* (AT) can provide a gateway to communication, self-help, mobility, exploration, play, and learning. Examples of AT equipment are as varied as the children, contexts, and needs they support but may include simple adaptations to typical toys and materials, positioning supports, mobility aids, specialized utensils, communication devices, switches, and computers and tablets. These tools can help young children acquire important developmental skills and provide compensatory experiences.

Modifications to the environment, activities, materials, and instructional practices; accommodations; and individualized and specific AT help young children practice cause and effect and early choice making, fine motor and visual–motor skills, and self-help. Assistive devices and services can influence the growth and development of infants and young children with disabilities, thereby providing opportunities to learn and interact with the environment in ways that might not otherwise be possible and allowing participation in family, school, and community activities.

Research suggests that AT is underused with children ages birth to 5 years, yet it can significantly affect them, along with their caregivers (Trivette et al., 2012). National reports have consistently reported that fewer than 10% of children ages 3–5 years served under the Individuals With Disabilities Education Improvement Act of 2004 (IDEA; P. L. 108-446) Part B received AT services in 2015 (U.S. Department of Education, 2015). AT for young children may look different than it does for older children, youths, and adults and should support ongoing development and learning during everyday roles and routines (Mistrett, 2018). It is used primarily in the child's natural environments to support participation in daily activities and may be "do it yourself" (DIY) or highly specialized.

Gilormini et al. (2017) discussed various myths about AT and young children. See Exhibit 7.1.

Most important, there are no prerequisites for AT. Although children may require specific skills to benefit from certain interventions or devices, no child is too young or has too many disabling conditions to be considered. AT is need based rather than related to a specific disability and can compensate for missed milestones. More than one device may be required, depending on the context and environment in which it is used.

Federal Laws Supporting Assistive Technology

The *Technology Related Assistance for Individuals With Disabilities Act of 1988* (Tech Act; P. L. 105-394) first described an AT *device* as "any item, piece of equipment, or product system, whether acquired commercially off the shelf, modified, or customized, that is used to increase, maintain, or improve functional capabilities of individuals with disabilities." This broad definition can be interpreted

---

EXHIBIT 7.1.   Myths Regarding Assistive Technology and Young Children

Common myths about AT and young children:
- A child must be "old enough" to benefit from AT.
- AT must be powered: wired, electronic, or digital.
- AT is an alternative to what other children use.
- AT must be selected by a specialist.
- AT is only appropriate for children with low-incidence disabilities.
- AT can keep children from developing as fully as possible.
- AT is expensive and designed for children with disabilities.

Gilormini et al. (2017) refuted each of these myths with research and websites.

Note. AT = assistive technology.

---

to range from homemade interventions created from easily found materials, Velcro, and adapted toys to complex and costly devices such as computers, powered mobility, communication systems, and more. The Tech Act described the training and support to choose and use AT as "any service that directly assists an individual with a disability in selection, acquisition or use of an assistive technology device."

Early intervention and preschool

IDEA (2004) used the same definition of *AT* as the Tech Act. The final regulations also state that "related services" do not include surgically implanted medical devices. Considering AT in the individualized family service plan (IFSP) or individualized educational program (IEP) is a legal requirement as part of IDEA, and AT devices and services must be made available to children with a disability if required during the evaluation process or as part of the IFSP or IEP. Although this consideration is mandated, there is no specific information on how this deliberation is to be conducted.

Infants and toddlers eligible for early intervention should receive services to assist family members and to enhance learning and development through everyday learning opportunities. Each child's unique needs are considered, including AT, when devices and services are necessary to increase, maintain, or improve the child's functional capabilities in terms of physical, communication, cognitive, social–emotional, or adaptive development. Any AT should be provided, as much as possible, in natural environments (e.g., home, preschool, community settings) as part of the IFSP and reviewed at least every 6 months. The Every Student Succeeds Act of 2015 (ESSA; P. L. 114-95), as it relates to early childhood, enables school districts to improve early learning for all children, including those with disabilities. Nonregulatory ESSA early learning guidance from the U.S. Department of Education (2016) notes that funding can be used

to increase preschool teachers' competencies in instructing children with disabilities; ensuring that appropriate accommodations are in place, such as AT, so that children can access the curriculum or participate in assessments; implementing schoolwide models of positive interventions and supports to promote healthy social, emotional, and behavioral development; and supporting the universal design of the environment or instructional materials. (p. 20)

ESSENTIAL CONSIDERATIONS

Occupational therapy interventions for infants and young children include the use of activities, education and training, application of universal design principles, recommendations pertaining to changes to the environment or activity to support the child's ability to engage in identified occupations, and use of AT (American Occupational Therapy Association [AOTA], 2020). AT is considered a specialty area, yet occupational therapy practitioners incorporate environmental modification and specialized tools, including basic or "low-tech" AT items (e.g., utensils with built-up handles) and complex or "high-tech" AT devices (e.g., custom seating and mobility systems, adapted computer access, environmental control units), in their interventions to enable caregiving and participation of young children with disabilities. (*Note. Occupational therapy practitioner* refers to both occupational therapists and occupational therapy assistants.)

Use of AT includes assessment, selection, provision, and education and training. Currently there is no legislation requiring specific credentials for individuals providing AT services; however, certificate programs and advanced degrees in AT are offered by a growing number of universities, and online self-study series are available through various organizations. The Rehabilitation Engineering and Assistive Technology Society of North America (RESNA) has provided one mechanism for verifying a minimum level of competence for individuals acting as AT providers through an examination process that provides credentialing for persons working as AT professionals.

The *2020 Occupational Therapy Code of Ethics* (AOTA, 2020a) is based on the principles of beneficence, nonmaleficence, autonomy, justice, veracity, and fidelity and states that practitioners are responsible for taking "steps (e.g., professional development, research, supervision, training) to ensure proficiency, use careful judgment, and weigh potential for harm when generally recognized standards do not exist in emerging technology or areas of practice" (p. 8). Although the use of AT continues to rise, inequality of access in terms of AT deployment remains (Greenfield & Musolino, 2012).

Awareness of available tools, products, and modifications is essential for practitioners to responsibly suggest interventions and participate in training in the use of selected tools as part of a team. It is important for occupational therapy practitioners to educate themselves regarding current trends in AT (AOTA, 2016) as well as recognize and document the adaptations and strategies they implement every day as AT. Cook (2009) discussed that the process of selecting AT should include identifying potential consequences of the use of the tool. Finding a balance between the positive and potentially less than satisfactory outcomes can directly affect the use or nonuse of AT.

It is essential that decision makers take into account the child and family, the context in which a potential solution will be used, and the impact of incorporating the tool into roles and routines as part of the process of implementing AT devices and services. Occupational therapy practitioners should empower children and their families to be strong advocates for their needs to give them their best chance for success. Consumers of AT should know their rights, including considering the need for AT and the benefits of such devices and services to get on the road to a successful, independent, and meaningful life.

BEST PRACTICES

Historically, occupational therapy practitioners have a documented expertise in fabricating or incorporating tools as a way to enable or enhance occupational performance (AOTA, 2016). Introducing assistive devices and services as early as possible while coaching those who are directly involved with the child can facilitate engagement in developmentally appropriate experiences and can create exciting opportunities for children to explore, interact with, and function in their environments; however, salient factors need to be considered. The following section discusses critical considerations in determining the need for AT to promote access and enhance occupational performance in early childhood.

Apply Universal Design Concepts in Environments

Occupational therapy practitioners should be familiar with the concept of *universal design,* the idea of simplifying life for everyone by making products, communications, and the built environment more usable by as many people as possible at little or no extra cost (Center for Universal Design, 1997). With universal design, many features traditionally associated with AT are currently embedded in products such as toys and tablets, resulting in items that are easier to grip, hold, manipulate, visualize, figure out, or use in more than one way, providing accessibility to a wider range of users while decreasing the stigma connected with specialized devices.

Universal Design for Learning (UDL) is an educational initiative for the reform of the learning environment, expanded from the universal design movement in architecture. The Center for Applied Special Technology (2019) applied the concept of universal design in the physical environment to a framework proposing change in the way students are taught, with a focus on providing curricula to support student diversity. UDL assumes that students with diverse skills and needs are active participants in learning and that the goals, curriculum, instructional materials, and assessments need to anticipate and address this diversity through alternatives, options, and adaptations. Like the flexible design of occupational therapy services, UDL principles call for providing multiple means of engagement, representation, and action and expression.

To create accessible learning opportunities for learners, early childhood teams should consider the design of the environment, incorporate a range of teaching strategies, and provide multiple ways to demonstrate knowledge and skills while considering individual needs and preferences in the context of content, process, and products (Dinnebeil et al., 2013). This practice is practical and least restrictive, and it considers existing resources and supports rather than immediately introducing complex tools and devices that might be difficult to learn or embed in natural contexts or that might conflict with family expectations or cultural norms.

The *Let's Participate! Project* (https://www.letsparticipate.org/), a model demonstration project funded by the Office of Special Education Programs, was designed to help IDEA Part C early intervention and Part B preschool programs use AT effectively with infants, toddlers, and young children with disabilities, allowing them to participate more fully in everyday activities. This site provides practical ideas for adaptations; checklists to review the physical, social, and temporal environments where learning takes place; and suggestions for simple modifications to improve access for all. There are also checklists for group programs that provide examples of easily found or adapted items and methods to support a child's movement, communication, use of materials, and participation behavior.

Determine the Need for Assistive Technology

Although universal design methodologies can meet the needs of most young children, when a more specific need is determined for a child with a disability, AT must be considered. In addition to the initial evaluation, ongoing assessment and intervention are required.

Because of rapidly occurring changes in the dynamic interplay among the child, the activities, the tools, and the contexts that make up the essence of participation in early childhood, evaluation of strengths and needs is an ongoing process rather than a one-time event. Successful consideration, evaluation, and implementation of AT begins with individualized and contextual assessments leading to the identification of appropriate devices and services. AT solutions continue to evolve and diversify, as does the skill set required to relate more complex aspects of technology and person–environment factors in the decision-making process supporting an *interdisciplinary approach* (AOTA, 2016), where the combined knowlege of various team members, including educators, related service providers, and administrators, is used to work toward a common goal.

Individuals contributing to the evaluation process might include parents and family members; teachers, principal, or program director; occupational, physical, and speech–language therapists; a professional with specialized knowledge of the AT available to support the child in the areas identified by the team; medical professionals; a rehabilitation engineer (a specialist in customizing a device); and a social worker, service coordinator, or case manager. The evaluation might be completed by individuals who will also provide the intervention (e.g., fitting and training the device) or by a team that has been formed or contracted with specifically for the purpose of completing AT assessments. If vendors or separate teams are responsible for evaluation and intervention, they ideally collaborate with those working with the child on an ongoing basis to make decisions and recommendations.

Use collaborative decision-making tools

Because of the highly individualized nature of AT, there is not a standardized AT protocol, although assessment tools and models to guide AT consideration, assessment, decision making, and service delivery have been developed by multiple disciplines. The **Student, Environments, Tasks, and Tools** (SETT) framework is one of the best known interdisciplinary collaborative tools used for considering the need for AT in schools (Zabala, 2005, 2010). Individuals familiar with the student describe the student's distinct strengths and needs, examine their customary environments to determine obstacles or potential supports and alternatives, and consider what the student wants or needs to do in order to successfully participate. This deliberate discussion provides a "road map" to help teams recognize barriers to student performance and identify the particular features or items that can be used to overcome those barriers.

Consistent with the type of information that occupational therapy practitioners gather as part of an occupational profile and occupational performance analysis (AOTA, 2020) and applicable to a variety of settings, application of the SETT framework should result in student-centered, environmentally specific, and task-focused tool systems to support participation. Zabala and Mistrett (2011) suggested early childhood teams can also use the SETT framework to ask themselves what the child needs to do, what is preventing them from "doing it," and their current interests and abilities.

Teams should then review the child's daily environments (e.g., home, day care, playground) and discuss who else is in those environments, what equipment and materials are available, and what resources exist for the caregivers. For young children, *tasks* are their typical routines and activities. Examining the critical elements of the routines can lead to possible modifications to how they are accomplished, what outcomes identify successful completion, and effective tools and strategies.

In their book *Assistive Technology for Young Children: Creating Inclusive Learning Environments,* Sadao and Robinson (2010) provided printable forms, including "Functional Evaluation for Early Technology," and examples for evaluating AT needs, determining what AT to choose, and creating individualized "toolkits." The Simon Technology Center's Technology to Improve Kids' Educational Success Project has developed easy-to-use documents to help IFSP and IEP teams consider the use of AT for children ages birth to 5 years. These documents include

- The *AT Consideration Flowchart,* designed to function as a visual planning guide of the possible outcomes of consideration;
- The *Child-Centered AT Plan,* developed to help teams focus on the desired outcome of the interventions; and
- The *Expanded Child-Centered AT Plan,* which goes into greater depth pertaining to any current AT use, areas of need, and AT trials; identifies any training needs and device or system set-up and maintenance; determines a back-up plan; assigns AT roles; provides documentation; and more.

Provide assistive technology for self-care routines

AT for caregiving and self-care influences the ability of infants and young children to participate in feeding, bathing, personal hygiene, and dressing routines. Collaboratively,

occupational therapy practitioners discuss the child's daily routines, strengths, and needs in the contexts of family, culture, and community with parents, hospital teams, caregivers, and early childhood special educators to consider how AT can help the child to engage in the desired activity. For example, the occupational therapist evaluates positioning supports and feeding and hygiene equipment to allow children to participate more fully in ADLs.

From simple adaptations, such as the use of rolled towels to help a child sit in a typical high chair, a bathtub insert to aid in bathing and allow water play, or dishes secured with nonskid shelf liner, to more complex positioning and mobility devices, occupational therapy practitioners have an instrumental role in coaching caregivers, working directly with them in activities and routines. This level of support can contribute to caregivers' feelings of competence in using adaptation and AT (Kling et al., 2010). When providers and caregivers work together to use AT, caregivers report feeling competent, particularly in identifying solutions for facilitating their children's involvement in activities and routines and in using a continuum of tools to do so.

Provide assistive technology for play

Play and exploration is a primary occupation of childhood and acts as a foundation for the development of fine motor, gross motor, perceptual, social, and cognitive skills. It is important to consider the attributes of toys and how to best match them with the child's needs and interests; the indoor and outdoor opportunities for play; and the child's developmental level, family lifestyle, siblings, and friends.

Exploration allows children to develop new skills and learn more about the world around them. However, not all children are able to move by themselves. "Children with mobility limitations have been shown to also demonstrate limitations in cognition and attention, spatial awareness, visual perception and postural responses, and social and emotional development. In the realm of spatial awareness, children are reported to lack object permanence and are not appropriately wary of heights" (Center on Technology and Disability, 2012, p. 1). Children who are unable to actively explore their environment and learn the consequences of their actions run the risk of becoming passive, which can lead to additional delays in motor skills, self-determination, and learning (Wehmeyer, 2002). Interventions include using typical, adapted, or specialized toys; self-care; and mobility equipment. Often, the foundation for other AT begins with equipment and strategies used for positioning, seating, and mobility. These interventions can be used to improve body stability and provide proximal trunk and head support needed for viewing and accessing the environment.

Identify Power Mobility Needs

Numerous research studies have been conducted relating to the use of power mobility with infants and young children. Founded by Dr. Cole Galloway at the University of Delaware, Go Baby Go is a national, community-based research, design, and outreach program providing customized battery-operated, adapted ride-on toy vehicles for young children with disabilities. AOTA has sponsored training and build events at annual conferences since 2015. The cars are adapted to be operated with either commercially manufactured or DIY switches. A *switch* is an input–output device that can be used by individuals with limited mobility to operate various AT, switch-adapted toys, environmental controls, computer software, and more through a specific action such as pressure. Switches can include additional sensory feedback such as lights, sounds, or vibration and be customized and used with different access points. For example, a switch placed behind a child operating a Go Baby Go car could be activated by the child sitting up straight and pressing against the switch with their back. Inserts are fabricated and customized on the basis of the child's needs using easily found materials, such as PVC pipe, foam, pool noodles, and Styrofoam paddleboards. In RESNA's *Position on the Application of Power Mobility Devices for Pediatric Users,* Rosen et al. (2017) concluded that

> early utilization of powered mobility for children with mobility limitations enhances independence, improves development in multiple areas, and enables children to grow to become productive and integrated members of society. Ideally, mobility should be effortless and provide children with the opportunity to attend to and fulfill all daily tasks as typically expected from their non-disabled peers. Age, limited vision or cognitive deficits, difficulty accessing controls, parental concerns, and the ability to utilize other means of mobility for very short distances should not, in and of themselves, eliminate the child as a candidate for powered mobility. (p. 13)

Adapt Materials for Child's Use

Many toys can be easily adapted or purchased off the shelf for use by children with differences in the way they move, see, hear, comprehend, or communicate. These include puzzles with knobs or magnets, motion toys with big button switches, push or ride-on toys with wheels wrapped in Velcro for stability, and game pieces with handles. Using universally designed toys, adaptive equipment, and specific AT (e.g., switches); creating new ways to play; and using the setting are all ways to make play accessible at home, in the community, or while hospitalized. Mainstream and specialized technology, such as smart devices, tablets, software applications, and computers, can engage young children and support motor, social, cognitive, and communication skills. Development in these skills provides a wide array of cause and effect, entertainment, emergent literacy, and educational choices. These devices can circumvent motor difficulties, provide opportunity for choice making, and offer an engaging interface with multisensory stimuli and feedback.

Emergent literacy and play experiences can be provided though e-books and simple games and activities that the child can control with a computer mouse, switch, or touch interface. *Emergent literacy* is the normal process by which a child develops an understanding of language and print through naturally occurring contact with books and print in context. Children who are read to, explore books, and are exposed to print throughout the home and community in the form of packaging, on signs, and in stores begin to relate the symbols they see to words. When children scribble and their marks are commented upon, they understand their marks can have meaning.

Caution must be used to ensure that electronic devices do not replace the opportunity to be a participant rather than an audience and that children are exposed as much as possible to the typical childhood experience children enjoy and learn from.

Consider Communication Needs

As stated by the National Joint Committee for the Communications of Persons With Severe Disabilities (Brady et al., 2016),

> all people with a disability of any extent or severity have a basic right to affect, through communication, the conditions of their existence. Beyond this general right, a number of specific communication rights should be ensured in all daily interactions and interventions involving persons who have severe disabilities. (p. 123)

AOTA is a stakeholder on this committee, which recognizes the essential role communication plays in occupation throughout the lifespan and how occupational therapy practitioners contribute to ensuring that all individuals have access to a means of communicating.

Augmentative and alternative communication (AAC) systems provide expressive and receptive language support for children experiencing communication difficulties. AAC can be used to make existing speech and language more effective, or take the place of verbal speech. An AAC system might include communicative behaviors and speech as well as mobile apps, speech-generating devices, and eye-gaze systems. Unaided AAC systems include the communicator's facial expressions, vocalizations, gestures, and sign language. Aided AAC systems require the use of a tool or device such as pictures, words, or a speech-generating device to supplement or replace speech. The right tools can help in the development of language and emerging literacy skills; enhance participation in all settings; facilitate friendships; and promote meaningful exchanges with family members, caregivers, and people in the greater community (Cook & Polgar, 2015).

Communication devices can be as simple as visuals (e.g., photos, icons, line drawings, symbols) or more complex, such as a voice output device that produces an auditory message when activated directly, through a switch, or by eye gaze. Systems often used by young children include pictures, homemade binders or books of picture symbols, recorded speech devices, tablet speech applications, and dynamic-screen speech-generating devices (Chazin et al., 2016). Visual supports can help young children understand where to find things and where they belong, when things will happen, what to do and when to do it, how to interact with others, and how to communicate thoughts and choices. They can be used by both the child for whom they are intended and the child's communication partners. The Visual Supports Checklist (Bennett-Armistead et al., 2016) can assist teams in reviewing the child's environment and determining whether needed interventions are in place.

Determining the best communication system to use, training and implementation of the system, and data collection are shared responsibilities. With an ever-increasing range of AAC systems and diversity among those requiring communication support, there is a greater need than ever before for interdisciplinary teams with expertise in speech and language skills, literacy skills, human–computer interface, visual–cognitive processing, motor performance, and instructional design (Light & McNaughton, 2014). Various members of the team bring different perspectives and skills: The child and caregivers have the best knowledge of daily communication needs and routine, teachers have knowledge related to emergent literacy and instruction, speech–language pathologists are experts in language development, and occupational and physical therapists provide services related to positioning and physically operating the AAC system.

Occupational therapy practitioners can provide valuable information pertaining to the child's visual perception, motor skills, and sensory regulation and make suggestions for transporting and setting the device so that it is accessible. For AT to be successful, it is important to facilitate, educate, and encourage use of the device throughout the day. In addition to addressing perception, muscle control, mobility, and seating in relation to the chosen system, occupational therapy practitioners should be familiar with the selected system and model its use, not only expecting the child to use it but using it themselves to interact with the child.

Consider Need for Switches

For some infants and young children with disabilities, their mobility, communication, or emergent literacy and play begin with the use of one or more switches. Switches can be used to teach cause and effect, provide opportunity for control, or communicate. Connecting switches to simple battery-operated devices or more complex technologies, such as tablets, computers, communication devices, and environmental control units, provides opportunities for access and participation that might not otherwise be possible because of the child's physical limitations. Any part of the body can be used to activate a switch, and activation can occur with various contact methods, such as pushing, pulling, light touch, or deep pressure, depending on the child's abilities and the switch chosen.

Switches come in many shapes and sizes and can be homemade, customized with tools such as 3-D printers, or purchased commercially. Off-the-shelf battery-operated toys can be switch-adapted with online instructions and materials from a hardware store. With their skills in assessment and task analysis, occupational therapy practitioners are ideal collaborators in determining the impact of motor, sensory, and cognitive abilities on operating a switch. Best practices use these findings to match with specific features of a switch to help determine the type of switch that might work best and how it should be positioned. Positioning the switch and device may require the use of mounts to put each object in the optimal position for access. Mounts can be fabricated from easily found materials (e.g., nonskid shelf liner, suction cups, Velcro, PVC pipe, C-clamps) or can be purchased.

Consider Funding Sources

The local education agency or early intervention programs may fund AT or allow families to borrow equipment on the basis of team decisions. Sources of funding may also include private insurance, medical assistance, lending libraries, AT reuse programs, micro-loans, DIY, and service organizations. Implementation of the device requires careful consideration of how and where it will be used and how success is measured. Training the child, family, caregiver, and team members is essential to prevent disuse.

Contribute to Ongoing Research Needs

Research on AT services and outcomes is limited. Despite the benefits of AT and AT services for infants and young children, AT remains underdocumented, underused, and inconsistently integrated in the context of daily activities and routines in natural environments. Long et al. (2007) reported that training for occupational therapy practitioners working with children who need AT devices or services has not kept pace with the explosion of new, more sophisticated AT devices now available. A survey of occupational therapy practitioners indicated they felt they had inadequate training in policies governing AT services and the organization and function of the service system and that they desired accessible and affordable training in the areas of funding of technology and services; collaborating with families and other service providers; and accessing reliable, knowledgeable vendors.

Because of the ever-changing nature of this field, the complexity of the devices, and the need for individualized decisions, it is difficult to build a large evidence base in this area of practice that is consistent with the constantly shifting features and volume of available technology; however, there are certain aspects of AT effectiveness that remain constant. For example, there seems to be a strong correlation between acceptance and use of AT and training methods by practitioners or parents (Dunst et al., 2011, 2013; Kling et al., 2010). Other barriers to increased usage of AT with young children include funding issues, lack of knowledge of the potential of AT, and insufficient lending libraries or AT device loan support (Sadao & Robinson, 2010).

According to Kling et al. (2010), information and training from early intervention providers increases both caregiver competence and successful use of AT as a solution to circumvent barriers in their children's activities and routines. Increased information and training also contribute to providers' competence and effectiveness in adequately supporting caregivers (Kling et al., 2010). Therefore, it is essential for occupational therapy practitioners working with infants and young children to be aware of available technologies and be competent in training and coaching caregivers in the use of needed interventions. To help teams determine whether they are providing best practices, leaders in AT have helped establish guidance in determining and maintaining best practices in AT. The Quality Indicators of Assistive Technology (QIAT) matrices can be found on https://qiat.org/. Subscribing to the QIAT email list also provides practitioners with a forum in which to post questions and discuss all aspects of AT.

SUMMARY

Occupational therapy practitioners collaborate with service providers, family members, and caregivers to promote a child's development in physical, communication, cognitive, adaptive, and social–emotional domains, planning and implementing strategies that promote participation in meaningful occupations by developing opportunities to establish, restore, or maintain skills. AT is one of many tools occupational therapy practitioners use to promote or substitute for the acquisition of developmental skills and engagement in activities that are purposeful and satisfying. AT can serve as a door opener and provide access for all who encounter barriers in their natural environments, paving over the gap between potential and participation with possibilities. For young children with disabilities and their families, AT redefines possibilities and opportunities, saying, "Yes, you can!" and establishes a foundation for future successes.

Technically, there are no prerequisites or age requirements for AT consideration. The early introduction and judicious use of AT can provide children with disabilities from birth through age 5 years and their caregivers with access to natural learning opportunities for child-centered movement, play, communication, and self-care experiences paralleling those of typically developing children. Best practice dictates that services to children with disabilities be closely tied to the natural context; thus, the need for understanding the attributes, tasks, and tools necessary to facilitate successful participation increases.

AT services include collaboration for evaluating the needs of the child and family, selecting and acquiring appropriate devices, training the family and other caregivers, and monitoring the use of the device. Occupational therapy practitioners can and should advocate for universal design and environmental modifications that remove barriers in homes, schools, and communities to ensure access to supportive community services, including transportation, personal care, health care, education, and play, and to facilitate engagement in natural environments. By holistically considering the hopes and dreams of the child, the family, and caregivers as well as attending to the natural context of early childhood, occupational therapy practitioners can guide the selection of appropriate AT devices and services to support play, ADLs, education, and social participation.

RESOURCES

- **Able Play:** https://ableplay.wordpress.com
  Toy rating system and website associated with the National Lekotek Center that provides comprehensive information on toys for children with special needs to help parents and others make the best decisions when purchasing products
- **Center for Applied Special Technology:** www.cast.org
  Works to expand learning opportunities for all individuals through research and development of universal design for learning
- **Center on Technology and Disability:** www.ctdinstitute.org
  Online library of resources on AT and disabilities
- **Center for Parent Information and Resources:** www.parentcenterhub.org
  Information for parent centers on serving families with disabilities

- **Let's Participate! Project:** www.letsparticipate.org
  Model demonstration project designed to assist IDEA Part C and Part B preschool programs in implementing and sustaining promising practices in the effective use of AT by infants, toddlers, and preschool children with disabilities
- **PACER Center's Simon Technology Center publications:** www.pacer.org/stc/publications.asp
  Resources that help families learn about AT:
  - EZ AT: https://www.pacer.org/stc/pubs/STC-16.pdf
  - EZ AT 2: https://www.pacer.org/stc/pubs/EZ-AT-book-2011-final.pdf
- **PEAT's (Physical Environment and Assistive Tools) Suite:** www.dec-sped.org/peats-suite
  Planning materials to assist service providers to make decisions about how to plan or change the physical environment so it is more accessible to a child and to use assistive tools connecting demands of daily routines and activities with a child's ability to meet adult expectations of successful participation
- **Quality Indicators for Assistive Technology Services:** www.qiat.org
  Network that supports teachers, other professionals, and parents in evaluating AT service delivery
- **Technology to Improve Kids' Educational Success:** www.pacer.org/stc/tikes
  Began as a 5-year model demonstration project designed to improve outcomes for children with disabilities ages birth to 5 years by helping parents and providers understand how AT can help. Originally funded by the U.S. Department of Education, Office of Special Education Programs; now a project of PACER Center.
- **Visual Supports Checklist:** https://ccids.umaine.edu/resource/visual-supports-checklist-pdf/
  Based on a review of current literature, practical knowledge, and reported experiences from early childhood educators on the topic of visual supports

REFERENCES

American Occupational Therapy Association. (2016). Assistive technology and occupational performance. *American Journal of Occupational Therapy, 70,* 7012410030. https://doi.org/10.5014/ajot.2016.706S02

American Occupational Therapy Association. (2020a). 2020 occupational therapy code of ethics. *American Journal of Occupational Therapy, 74*(Suppl. 3), 7413410005. https://doi.org/10.5014/ajot.2020.74S3006

American Occupational Therapy Association. (2020b). Occupational therapy practice framework: Domain and process (4th ed.). *American Journal of Occupational Therapy, 74*(Suppl. 2), 7412410010. https://doi.org/10.5014/ajot.2020.74S2001

Bennett-Armistead, S., Blagojevic, B., Neal, E., & Taylor, B. (2016). *Visual Supports Checklist.* University of Maine. https://ccids.umaine.edu/resource/visual-supports-checklist-pdf/

Brady, N. C., Bruce, S., Goldman, A., Erickson, K., Mineo, B., Ogletree, B. T., . . . Wilkinson, K. (2016). Communication services and supports for individuals with severe disabilities: Guidance for assessment and intervention. *American Journal on Intellectual and Developmental Disabilities, 121,* 121–138. https://doi.org/10.1352/1944-7558-121.2.121

Center for Applied Special Technology. (2019). *About CAST.* http://www.cast.org/about#.X0Udf9xKh6o

Center on Technology and Disability. (2012). *Powered mobility for young children.* https://www.ctdinstitute.org/library/2014-10-22/powered-mobility-infants-and-toddlers

Center for Universal Design. (1997). *The principles of universal design.* https://projects.ncsu.edu/ncsu/design/cud/about_ud/udprinciplestext.htm

Chazin, K. T., Quinn, E. D., & Ledford, J. R. (2016). *Augmentative and alternative communication (AAC).* http://ebip.vkcsites.org/augmentative-and-alternative-communication

Cook, A. M. (2009). Ethical issues related to the use/non-use of assistive technologies. *Developmental Disabilities Bulletin, 37*(1), 127–152. https://files.eric.ed.gov/fulltext/EJ920692.pdf

Cook, A. M., & Polgar, J. M. (Eds.). (2015). *Assistive technologies: Principles and practice* (4th ed.). Elsevier Mosby.

Dinnebeil, L., Boat, M., & Bae, Y. (2013). Integrating principles of universal design into the early childhood curriculum. *Dimensions in Early Childhood, 41,* 3–13. https://www.collaborative.org/sites/default/files/Dimensions_Vol41_1_Dinnebeil.pdf

Dunst, C., Trivette, C., Hamby, D., & Simkus, A. (2013). Systematic review of studies promoting the use of assistive technology devices by young children with disabilities. *Tots N Tech Research Brief, 5*(1). https://files.eric.ed.gov/fulltext/ED565254.pdf

Dunst, C. J., Trivette, C. M., Meter, D., & Hamby, D. W. (2011). Influences of contrasting types of training on practitioners' and parents' use of assistive technology and adaptations with infants, toddlers and preschoolers with disabilities. *Tots N Tech Research Brief, 3*(1). https://files.eric.ed.gov/fulltext/ED565255.pdf

Every Student Succeeds Act of 2015, Pub. L. No. 114-95, 20 U.S.C. §§ 6301.

Gilormini, B., Milbourne, S., & Mistrett. (2017). *Assistive technology use with young children: Myths and mythbusters!* (Let's Participate! FHI360). https://inclusioninstitute.fpg.unc.edu/sites/inclusioninstitute.fpg.unc.edu/files/handouts/ATMythsandMythbusters.docx.pdf

Greenfield, P., & Musolino, G. (2012). Technology in rehabilitation: Ethical and curricular implications for physical therapist education. *Journal of Physical Therapy Education, 26*(2), 81–90. https://journals.lww.com/jopte/Abstract/2012/01000/Technology_in_Rehabilitation__Ethical_and.12.aspx

Individuals With Disabilities Education Improvement Act of 2004, Pub. L. 108-446, 20 U.S.C. §§ 1400–1482.

Kling, A., Campbell, P. H., & Wilcox, J. (2010). Young children with physical disabilities: Caregiver perspectives about assistive technology. *Infants and Young Children, 23,* 169–183. https://doi.org/10.1097/IYC.0b013e3181e1a873

Light, J., & McNaughton, D. (2014). Communicative competence for individuals who require augmentative and alternative communication: A new definition for a new era of communication? *Augmentative and Alternative Communication, 30,* 1–18. https://doi.org/10.3109/07434618.2014.885080

Long, T. M., Woolverton, M., Perry, D. F., & Thomas, M. J. (2007). Training needs of pediatric occupational therapists in assistive technology. *American Journal of Occupational Therapy, 61,* 345–354. https://doi.org/10.5014/ajot.61.3.345

Mistrett, S. G. (2018). *Let's Participate! Using assistive technology with young children with disabilities* [PowerPoint]. http://eiplp.org/wp-content/uploads/2015/10/Lets-Participate-ICC-June-2017-.pdf

Rosen, L., Plummer, T., Sabet, A., Lange, M. L., & Livingstone, R. (2017). *RESNA's position on the application of power mobility devices for pediatric users.* https://doi.org/10.1080/10400435.2017.1415575

Sadao, K. C., & Robinson, N. B. (2010). *Assistive technology for young children: Creating inclusive learning environments.* Baltimore: Brookes.

Simon Technology Center. (2015). *Technology to Improve Kids' Educational Success (TIKES).* PACER Center.

Technology Related Assistance for Individuals With Disabilities Act of 1988, Pub. L. 105-394, 29 U.S.C. §§ 3001.

Trivette, C. M., Dunst, C. J., Hamby, D. W., & Meter, D. (2012). Relationship between early childhood practitioner beliefs and the adoption of innovative and recommended practices. *Tots N Tech Research Brief, 6*(1), 1–12. http://tnt.asu.edu/files/TotsN-Tech_ResearchBrief_v6_n1_2012.pdf

U.S. Department of Education. (2015). *37th annual report to Congress on the implementation of the Individuals With Education Disabilities Act, Parts B and C.* 2015. https://www2.ed.gov/about/reports/annual/osep/2015/parts-b-c/index.html

U.S. Department of Education. (2016). *Non-regulatory guidance: Early learning in the Every Student Succeeds Act: Expanding opportunities to support our youngest learners.* https://www2.ed.gov/policy/elsec/leg/essa/essaelguidance10202016.pdf

Wehmeyer, M. L. (2002). Promoting the self-determination of students with severe disabilities. *ERIC Digest.* https://files.eric.ed.gov/fulltext/ED470522.pdf

Zabala, J. (2005). *Using the SETT framework to level the learning field for students with disabilities.* http://www.joyzabala.com/uploads/Zabala_SETT_Leveling_the_Learning_Field.pdf

Zabala, J. (2010). *The SETT framework: Straight from the horse's mouth* [PowerPoint]. www.joyzabala.com/uploads/CA_Kananaskis__SETT_Horses_Mouth.pdf

Zabala, J., & Mistrett, S. (2011). Applying the SETT framework to early childhood. www.teachingei.org/technology/documents/4.1%20SETT%20for%20Early%20Childhood.pdf

Best Practices in Supporting Family Partnerships

8

Anna Wallisch, PhD, OTR/L, and Lauren M. Little, PhD, OTR/L

KEY TERMS AND CONCEPTS

- Client-centered care
- Collaborative goals
- Context
- Cultural competency
- Cultural reciprocity
- Ecological systems theory
- Ecology of Human Performance
- Family capacity building
- Family-centered care
- Family partnerships
- Family routines
- Parent storytelling
- Participatory practice
- Relational practice
- Resource-based interventions
- Siblings
- Strengths-based practice

OVERVIEW

Occupational therapy practitioners work with families and caregivers to create goals and intervention plans that are meaningful to children's and families' everyday lives. (*Note. Occupational therapy practitioner* refers to both occupational therapists and occupational therapy assistants.) They understand that family partnerships are important in early childhood settings and work to build these in their work settings. This chapter discusses the concept and history of family partnerships in occupational therapy practice, theories that inform family partnerships in therapy, essential elements of family partnerships, and strategies to create positive family partnerships.

ESSENTIAL CONSIDERATIONS

The importance of *family-centered care* (i.e., when family priorities guide practice) in early childhood is well established (Hanna & Rodger, 2002; Sumsion & Law, 2006). Within family-centered care, occupational therapy practitioners must be intentional in creating and maintaining partnerships with family members.

What Are Family Partnerships?

Family partnerships refers to the relationship between the occupational therapy practitioner and families. Family partnerships are driven by two components: *relational practice* (e.g., respect, active listening) and *participatory practice* (i.e., family is engaged in the goal setting, intervention, and evaluation process; An et al., 2018). When occupational therapy practitioners engage in relational practice, they are building a relationship with a family that is built on trust and shared values around the activities of therapy for the child. Through this relationship building, practitioners

and families develop a belief that they both are involved in all aspects of therapy, including evaluation, intervention, and goal setting. When the partners engage in participatory practice, they are actively problem solving and collaborating to set goals and identify ideas for intervention.

Positive partnerships are considered by parents (Wallisch et al., 2019) and service providers as an active ingredient of effective interventions, yet research suggests family-centered practice is perceived as challenging to implement (Dickens et al., 2011). For example, one study found that approximately 50% of parents were not involved during early intervention (EI) sessions (Dunst et al., 2014). This is troublesome because family-centered practice is associated with less delayed care, fewer unmet service needs, a reduction in out-of-pocket costs, greater parent optimism about their child's future, increased parent self-efficacy, increased family functioning, and greater access to care (Guralnick, 2017; Kuhlthau et al., 2011; Kuo et al., 2011).

Family partnerships mean that occupational therapy practitioners collaborate with family to understand the goals and everyday routines that are most meaningful to them (e.g., need to find a job, need assistance with bathing their toddler). In family partnerships, the practitioner works with the family to build their capacity to identify and implement strategies to increase their child's participation in everyday activities. In the rest of this chapter, the term *parent* is used to refer to the primary caregivers of the child, and the word *sibling* is used to refer to a child's brothers and sisters, although the parent and siblings may not be the child's biological parent or siblings.

How Have Practice Models Changed Over Time to Address Family Partnerships?

Historical models of therapy in early childhood settings focused primarily on the child as separate from the child's participation in family routines (Bazyk, 1989; Rosenbaum et al., 1998). In an "expert model," the occupational therapy practitioner is the expert, and parents are expected to follow directions (e.g., home program) provided by the practitioner. Using this model often results in noncompliance, largely because parents do not share the value of the prescribed activities or understand how the activities relate to their everyday lives.

As practice models have evolved, occupational therapy practitioners have come to value parents as authentic partners in the therapy process and follow best practice principles that consider parents' attitudes, beliefs, and goals as vital components of intervention (Hanft, 1988). The *Occupational Therapy Practice Framework: Domain and Process* (4th ed.; American Occupational Therapy Association [AOTA], 2020) highlights the importance of a **client-centered care,** defined as an "approach to service that incorporates respect for an partnership with clients as active participants in the therapy process" (Boyt Schell et al., 2014, p. 1230). In the case of children, parents were viewed as an integral part of the client-centered approach. Early childhood professional organizations also developed documents to move practice toward a family-centered approach. See Chapter 2, "Influences From Early Childhood Professional Organizations and Technical Assistance Centers," for more information.

What Theoretical Perspectives Inform Family Partnerships?

There has been extensive work within and beyond occupational therapy to understand how theory may best inform family-centered care. Two theories are described next, both of which have shaped early childhood practices.

Ecological systems theory

Bronfenbrenner's (1977) **ecological systems theory** began a transformation of how scholars and practitioners understood child development and EI. Previous methods of understanding children's development occurred outside of the children's everyday environments and activities; Bronfenbrenner (1977) challenged researchers and practitioners to embed interventions and science in the everyday contexts of children. This foundational theory is driven by the necessity to analyze the child's reciprocal interactions among multiple layers of their environment.

In particular, occupational therapy practitioners cannot understand child behavior unless they understand the environmental features surrounding a child (Bronfenbrenner, 1977). The ecological theory depicts five environments (i.e., microsystems, mesosystems, exosystems, macrosystems, chronosystems) that directly and indirectly influence a child. Families are an important piece of all environmental systems (e.g., interactions with children, culture, community, routines), so it is crucial that practitioners partner with families to support the environmental features surrounding a child's development.

Ecology of Human Performance

The **Ecology of Human Performance** (EHP) provides an ecological perspective to occupational therapy intervention and is based on Bronfenbrenner's (1977) theory (Dunn et al., 1994). EHP contains four primary constructs: (1) *person* (i.e., sensorimotor, cognitive, and psychosocial abilities as well as personal interests, values, and experiences), (2) *task* (i.e., a distinct set of behaviors necessary to reach a goal), (3) *context* (i.e., temporal, social, physical, cultural environments), and (4) *performance* (i.e., a person's engagement in tasks within a context). These constructs interact with each other, and one cannot understand them without analyzing the contextual features surrounding a person, because each new context provides new opportunities, demands, supports, and barriers to performance.

EHP provides concrete ways intervention strategies may align with contextual or person factors, including

- Establish and restore,
- Alter,
- Adapt and modify,
- Prevent, and
- Create (Dean et al., 2019).

Establish and restore is the only intervention strategy that focuses on changing person factors, but it recognizes that occupational therapy practitioners need to account for context, because this affects an individual's performance. **Context**, or the physical, social, temporal, cultural, and virtual aspects of the environment (Dunn et al., 1994), is critical to family-centered care, and using the natural environments of families is necessary for intervention development. As practitioners recognize the unique everyday contexts of families, interventions are more applicable and more likely implemented by families. See Table 8.1 for specific examples of intervention strategies within each EHP concept.

BEST PRACTICES

Occupational therapy practitioners have a knowledge base in child development, environmental modifications, and strategies to increase children's occupations (e.g., dressing, play, eating, social interactions) and performance skills (e.g., fine motor, social communication). The family has specific knowledge about their child, their daily routines, and strengths and barriers in their environment. Partnering with families is essential to family-centered practice and is central to recommended practices and legislation in the United States (e.g., Individuals With Disabilities Education Improvement Act of 2004; P. L. 108-446). The Division of Early Childhood's (DEC; 2014) *Recommended Practices in Early Intervention/Early Childhood Special Education 2014* highlights the importance of collaborating with families and offers strategies to do so, and AOTA (2017, 2020) also recognizes partnering with families as essential to practice.

Implement Family-Centered Practices

Family-centered practice means including families in all aspects of service delivery, using interventions that are respectful and based on individual family needs (DEC, 2014). This allows the family to guide the occupational therapy session, and results in building strong partnerships with families. Merely briefing a parent on what was accomplished in a session or just including families in creating goals is simply not enough to embody true family-centered

TABLE 8.1. Ecology of Human Performance Interventions and Examples

EHP INTERVENTION	COMMON LANGUAGE	INTERVENTION FOCUS	EARLY INTERVENTION EXAMPLE
Establish and restore	Learn something new every day	Person[a]	When parents begin potty training their child, the occupational therapy practitioner may assist them in establishing a new, consistent toileting routine with their child. However, the therapist must consider how this new routine will be embedded in current family routines.
Alter	Find a better place	Context	An occupational therapy practitioner helps a parent decide on a toddler-friendly park. Together, the therapist and family select a park that typically has toddlers (for social interaction opportunities) and that has a playground structure that is lower to the ground, with fewer steps, to make it easier to climb.
Adapt	Make it easier to do	Task and context	The occupational therapy practitioner provides bowls with a suction cup on the bottom to prevent the bowl from moving when the child uses a spoon. With a simple change of bowl (context), it becomes easier for the child to scoop food from the bowl.
Prevent	Think ahead	Person, context, task	Parents may provide pictures or visuals to prepare their child for a new activity they will transition to.
Create	Make it work for everyone	Person, context, task	Placing child toys on lower shelves allows all children easier access to independently select toys during free play in a preschool classroom.

[a]Must consider context for the intervention.
Note. EHP = ecology of human performance.
Source. Adapted from Dean et al. (2019).

practice. In using this practice, the idea is not to shift all responsibilities to parents but to actively support, collaborate with, and engage parents during the intervention process (King & Chiarello, 2014). Across various intervention settings (EI, early childhood, health care), services should be provided with families, not parallel to families.

Partner with siblings

Much of the research on family partnerships has focused on parents, but occupational therapy practitioners have unique opportunities to partner with siblings. Research suggests *siblings* (i.e., brothers and sisters) of children with disabilities often play multiple roles, including teacher, friend, helper, and caregiver, that support the development of children with disabilities (Stoneman et al., 1989). Additionally, siblings are often motivated to develop a sibling relationship, because such relationships often provide a long-lasting source of support (Brody, 2004). When children have family members who positively perceive disabilities and possess greater knowledge about disabilities, siblings also have more positive perceptions and experiences (Petalas et al., 2009).

Rather than providing siblings with home-based programs or "homework" to complete, occupational therapy practitioners can view siblings as integral partners in the therapy process to understand their goals, hopes, and dreams for their sibling with a disability. Family partnerships may be extended to all family members, which may increase intervention efficacy. Overall, siblings are a lifelong support, whereas parents are often with their children for fewer years; this means it is critical for practitioners to support positive relationships between siblings early.

Embed interventions in family routines

When occupational therapy practitioners focus on engagement and participation in daily life skills in the family routine, they enhance the child's occupational performance and role in the family (AOTA, 2020). **Family routines,** or the regularly occurring and observable patterns of a family's daily life (Denham, 2002), are an essential aspect of the context surrounding a child's development and incorporate the cultural values and community in which a child is situated (Weisner, 2002). The contexts of families provide the developmental pathways for children and a structure for numerous learning opportunities (Weisner, 2002). When a practitioner understands the typical routines of a family, they gain insight into the values, goals, resources, and activities of the family in various contexts (Weisner et al., 2005). Daily routines provide the structure for the reciprocal interactions that occur between parents and children (e.g., conversing at mealtime, reading a bedtime story, playing at the park), and warm, responsive parent–child interactions support children's cognitive, language, and social development (Guralnick, 2017; Spagnola & Fiese, 2007).

When intervention is embedded in a family's typical progression of daily activities and in naturally occurring occupations, intervention efficacy increases (AOTA, 2020; Bernheimer & Weisner, 2007). When interventions are viewed as separate from families' daily routines, parents are less likely to implement strategies to address children's skills and participation. For example, if a parent wants a child to be more independent in dressing, they should use strategies at the natural times during a day when dressing occurs. Occupational therapy practitioners must listen to and collaborate with parents to problem solve about when strategies may be used during the day, because every family's routines look different and interventions must be relevant to family life.

Cultivate cultural competence and reciprocity

The cultural contexts surrounding a child are paramount to family-centered practices. Different cultural contexts afford distinct routines, beliefs, roles, values, daily activities, communities, opportunities, and parenting ideologies. *Cultural competency* means acknowledging the importance of culture, cross-cultural relations, and the dynamics that result from cultural differences; expanding cultural knowledge; and adapting services to fit cultural needs (Betancourt et al., 2003).

A more contemporary term, *cultural reciprocity,* refers to the efforts by early childhood personnel to understand the families' cultural beliefs to promote healthy development among young children (Zero to Three, 2016). Cultural reciprocity is the process of becoming aware of and understanding subtle values in our professional beliefs and practice so that we can explain them to families from culturally and linguistically diverse backgrounds who might not share these same values. By clarifying to ourselves why we recommend a particular practice to a family, we become aware of our entrenched cultural values and begin to recognize that our assumptions about what is the "right" practice may not be universal (Kalyanpur & Harry, 2012).

In one study of occupational therapists' views of cultural competence and reciprocity strategies, they reported
- Using strategies to learn about a family's culture,
- Using cultural knowledge to adapt interventions and promote cultural inclusion,
- Becoming aware of their own cultural beliefs, and
- Using family-centered practices to build rapport and respect with families (Wray & Mortenson, 2010).

Occupational therapy practitioners should recognize their cultural contexts and beliefs as well as the cultural contexts of families; otherwise, they risk losing a parent's respect as well as failing to provide services relevant to a family's culture.

Build Family Capacity

Family capacity building refers to affording parents opportunities to strengthen their existing strategies and knowledge to promote new parenting skills and self-efficacy (DEC, 2014). Building family capacity is especially important because intervention outcomes are partially dependent on parent characteristics (Osborne et al., 2008). According to family systems models, capacity-building interventions entail three core constructs:
1. Parent concerns and priorities,
2. Family strengths, and
3. Family resources and supports (Dunst et al., 2014).

Using a family capacity model is associated with increased parent self-efficacy and parent well-being, which is linked to better parent–child interactions and child outcomes (Trivette et al., 2010). In the sections following,

each of the core components of building family capacity is discussed.

Listen to parent concerns

The American Academy of Pediatrics (2014) recommends listening to parent concerns as an effective strategy to identify children with disabilities earlier. Gathering the occupational profile during evaluation provides the occupational therapist with information about the child's health and development, family concerns and priorities, and occupation and environmental strengths and barriers (AOTA, 2020).

During intervention, occupational therapy practitioners should actively listen to parents' priorities and concerns. Understanding parent concerns, resources, and top priorities lays the foundation for family-centered goal setting. Parent concerns not only provide the opportunity for goal development and insight into intervention areas relevant to families but also provide a quick opportunity to screen children's occupations rather than testing each area. Given that early identification is linked to earlier access to services and that EI is crucial for the developmental trajectories of children with disabilities (Dawson, 2008), practitioners may support parents to seek diagnostic evaluations. Listening closely and collaborating with parents is a powerful tool for linking families to vital services.

Use a strengths-based approach

Central to family-centered practice and family capacity building is capitalizing on family strengths to guide intervention. This idea stems from positive psychology and social work practices and is recognized as a best practice in EI by AOTA (2017) and the DEC (2014). There are five core components to *strengths-based practice:*
1. Respect (i.e., valuing peoples' rights and dignity)
2. Teamwork (i.e., collaborating with families)
3. Sharing (i.e., building a family's knowledge and power to make decisions)
4. Social justice (i.e., equality, acceptance, and social determination)
5. Transparency (i.e., openly communicating all information; Carlson et al., 2010).

These constructs dovetail with the aforementioned principles of family-centered practices.

Although a strengths-based approach is necessary to partner with families, this ideology is often not integrated into care. When researchers analyzed professional documentation of children with disabilities, results suggested that clinicians typically used deficit-based language more than neutral or strengths-based language (Braun et al., 2017). When practitioners use strengths-based language during assessment procedures, children have significantly better outcomes, and parent satisfaction significantly increases (Cox, 2006). Even multidisciplinary team members' perceptions change when documentation uses strengths-based language, as opposed to deficit-based language (Donovan & Nickerson, 2007).

The language occupational therapy practitioners use to describe children with disabilities not only changes the

TABLE 8.2.   Make the Switch to Strengths-Based Language

DEFICIT-BASED STATEMENT	STRENGTHS-BASED STATEMENT
Jonas is aggressive and bites his peers during classroom activities.	Jonas uses biting to communicate with his peers.
Delilah cannot use a spoon and a fork to eat.	Delilah uses her hands to eat.
Stephen lacks eye contact when communicating.	Stephen looks at his toys when communicating.
Veronica lacks the fine motor coordination to tie her shoes.	Veronica puts her shoes on, and her mom ties her shoes.

way others perceive the child but may also influence parent perceptions. In particular, the language used to explain a diagnosis to parents is often related to how parents later describe the deficits of their child (Karst & Van Hecke, 2012). In turn, the type of language parents use is related to parent well-being, child functioning, and the types of treatments families select (Shyu et al., 2010). When practitioners use a strengths-based approach, parents are more likely to positively perceive their child, use positive statements, and increase their affection with their child (Steiner, 2011). The words practitioners use to describe children are malleable and, when framed to incorporate the child's strengths, have a powerful impact on child and family function (see Table 8.2).

Identify family resources and supports

The contexts surrounding families provide various resources, supports, and barriers to child development. Although it is critical to acknowledge parents as experts during intervention sessions, occupational therapy practitioners may also support families when they request information about available resources (e.g., preschools, transportation, community activities, assistance with understanding individualized education programs [IEPs] or individualized family service plans [IFSPs]). *Resource-based interventions,* designed to increase family capacity, consist of

- Identifying parent priorities and what resources are needed,
- Determining current access to resources, and
- Reflecting on how effective the resource is (Rush & Sheldon, 2011).

Family resources may indirectly affect a child and intervention effectiveness. For example, research suggests that adequate resources for mothers are associated with maternal health as well as the amount of time, energy, and investment available to a mother when she implements an intervention with her child (Dunst et al., 1988). Furthermore, when parents have social support, this often acts as a protective factor and reduces parent-related stress (Guralnick, 2017). By collaborating with parents, occupational therapy practitioners may assist them in identifying the available resources and supports they have and devise a plan to access resources to fill in gaps.

One way to identify available resources is the use of a narrative approach, or *parent storytelling.* This provides an understanding of a parent's experiences with their child and helps maintain parent–therapist collaboration (Hanna & Rodger, 2002). Practitioners may elicit storytelling related

to a parent's vision of their child's future, current child performance, resources currently available, needed resources, and meaningful family activities. A narrative approach not only supports a parent–therapist collaboration but also provides a starting point to develop goals and intervention strategies.

Identify Family-Centered Goals

A common challenge in implementing family-centered practice is ensuring goals reflect the family's areas of concern (King & Chiarello, 2014; Leiter, 2004). In a family-centered approach, therapists collaborate with parents and use the parents' priorities to guide goal setting (Hanna & Rodger, 2002). Research supports that these *collaborative goals* are linked to goal achievement, increased parent motivation and competency, and improved child outcomes (King & Chiarello, 2014; Øien et al., 2010).

Incorporating components of family-centered practice (i.e., family routines, strengths, concerns, resources, culture) aligns with and supports the development of family-driven goals. Furthermore, using a narrative approach may also support parent–therapist collaboration to understand a child's current performance and how parents would like to see their child progress. This allows the therapist and parent to measure progress over time and make small steps toward a larger goal. Overall, goal setting is considered one of the most important components linked to the effectiveness of family partnerships.

Case Examples 8.1–8.4 illustrate how occupational therapy practitioners may use evidence-based strategies to develop family partnerships in an EI, preschool, outpatient clinic, and telehealth practice setting.

SUMMARY

Partnering with families is essential to family-centered practice. By respecting family values, actively listening to concerns, capitalizing on the child's strengths, and engaging parents in all aspects of service delivery, occupational therapy practitioners may develop successful partnerships with families. Although family-centered practice is challenging to implement and requires practitioners to put family priorities before their expert opinions, practitioners must be charged with providing evidence-based practice during the critical years of child development. This way, practitioners may develop more effective partnerships and practices and, most of all, considerably affect the lives of children and families.

CASE EXAMPLE 8.1. ALEX: EARLY INTERVENTION (HOME)

Background: Alex, age 2 years, has a diagnosis of autism spectrum disorder and receives EI services in his home. Spanish is the family's primary language.

Preparation: Before visiting the home, the occupational therapist and translator meet to discuss ways to be culturally responsive to the family during the visit. The translator states it is important to accept a drink or food offered by the family.

Home Visit: The therapist begins the evaluation by using a routines-based interview to learn about the family routines. The parents are asked to share Alex's strengths and interests during each routine. They state he loves to pick out and organize his clothes. He also loves dogs, playing with his sister, using the computer, and bath time. After learning about the family routines and Alex's strengths, the occupational therapist asks the family about their concerns. Because Alex eats only five foods, his parents are concerned about his nutrition and that they must make him a meal separate from what the rest of their family is eating.

Observation: After obtaining the family's approval, the therapist arrives at dinnertime to observe Alex. The family invites the therapist to join the meal, which she accepts to be culturally responsive. The occupational therapist observes that Alex eats with his fingers and wanders throughout the kitchen during mealtime.

The therapist asks the parents, "What would a dream mealtime routine look like for you and your family?" Although the parents indicate they would love to see everyone eating the same meal at the table, they would be happy with Alex just trying new foods at this time. Thinking about Alex's strengths, the therapist asks the family, "How could we use his strength in picking out his clothing for picking out foods he might try?" The parents decide they will have Alex assist in organizing foods that "go together" for the meal.

CASE EXAMPLE 8.2. EMILY: PRESCHOOL

Background: Emily is a 3-year-old girl who is diagnosed with mild cerebral palsy and attends a Head Start preschool. She previously received EI services at home and was recently referred for an occupational therapy evaluation to support her participation in her classroom.

Evaluation: The occupational therapist starts by observing Emily during regular classroom routines and collaborating with her parents and teachers on priorities, needs, interests, and strengths to gather the occupational profile. When completing the observation, the therapist notices that Emily is often happy and excited when around her peers; however, when circle time begins, she is often crying. The occupational therapist schedules a meeting with Emily's teacher and her parents. Her teacher indicates that Emily is usually very happy during the day and loves mealtime, playing outside, and playing with musical instruments but cries during circle time, which disrupts the activity for the other children.

The therapist asks Emily's parents, "In what other situations has Emily become upset that are similar to circle time?" Her mom shares that Emily became upset during story time at the library when she was sitting on the floor. They learned that she was able to enjoy the story when supported by sitting in a chair with armrests; otherwise, she focuses too much on coordinating muscles to sit and becomes upset that she is missing the story. The therapist recognizes that collaborating with Emily's parents provided insight that Emily's challenges during circle time were not behavior related but motor related. Parents are crucial members of the child's team and have critical knowledge to share.

CASE EXAMPLE 8.3. MARIA: OUTPATIENT CLINIC

Background: Maria, age 5 years, is outgoing, is interested in jewelry, and loves playing games on her tablet. She lives with her mother, father, grandmother, and three older typically developing siblings. While attending her preschool program, she receives occupational therapy services once a week to address fine motor and behavior regulation related to her diagnosis of Down syndrome.

Health care visit: The occupational therapist in a health care setting conducts a structured assessment and shares the results with the family. Maria has many strengths but struggles with self-care activities, such as dressing herself, because of delays in motor and adaptive skills. Maria's parents share that Maria's teacher wants to start working on self-dressing with pants during toileting and coat for recess.

The occupational therapist notices the parents continue to refer to goals from Maria's IEP rather than stating their concerns and priorities for Maria. Shifting her method of questioning, the therapist asks them to describe a typical day for their family. Their discussion of the morning routine is vague, so the therapists states, "It sounds like you have a great team at school to address some of Maria's skills; what are Maria's strengths? What is she really good at?" Maria's parents share that Maria chooses a piece of jewelry to wear and often selects her elastic bracelets every morning.

The therapist asks the parents how they could use Maria's strength in picking out bracelets and other jewelry to help her with putting on her clothes. The parents feel that Maria's motivation for dressing would increase if she were given the opportunity to pick her clothes out independently. Because she manages most elastic accessories well, they will start with pants that have elastic waistbands and stretchy shirts.

CASE EXAMPLE 8.4. DANIEL: EARLY INTERVENTION TELEHEALTH

Background: Daniel is 34 months old and receives EI services for a developmental delay. In particular, he shows difficulties with fine motor skills as well as expressive and receptive language. Daniel lives with his mother, grandmother, and grandfather in a rural area and receives intervention sessions with an occupational therapist through telehealth.

Intervention: The occupational therapist uses a coaching model with Daniel's mother during the sessions, which are based on the IFSP outcomes. Daniel's mother identifies toileting as very important because she thinks that independence is critical for Daniel's upcoming transition to a preschool setting. She is concerned about classroom staff having to change Daniel's diapers.

To facilitate a family partnership, the occupational therapist focuses on the occupation of toileting. She listens to Daniel's mother's concerns about toilet training and knows that this is what best practice looks like— valuing the parents' concerns as well as offering coaching and guidance. Using her professional reasoning skills and task analysis skills, the occupational therapist asks questions about Daniel's current behaviors around toilet training. Specific questions include, "How can we use what Daniel is really good at to get him interested in the potty?" "When you taught him a new skill in the past, what worked best for him?" and, "What do you think is the best way to begin the toilet training process?" The occupational therapist capitalizes on Daniel's mother's eagerness to have him toilet trained as well as her understanding of what is most motivating for her son.

Through coaching, Daniel's mother and therapist realize that Daniel learns best when provided clear modeling, with each step in the activity broken down. He also is motivated by anything related to Elmo. The therapist provides some suggestions about an Elmo toilet training app that Daniel's mother could use to model the steps in toilet training, and then they problem solve together on ways Daniel could practice and build upon each step.

REFERENCES

American Academy of Pediatrics. (2014). AAP publications reaffirmed or retired. *Pediatrics, 134*(5), e1520. https://doi.org/10.1542/peds.2014-2679

American Occupational Therapy Association. (2017). Guidelines for occupational therapy services in early intervention and schools. *American Journal of Occupational Therapy, 71,* 7112410010. https://doi.org/10.5014/ajot.2017.716S01

American Occupational Therapy Association. (2020). Occupational therapy practice framework: Domain and process (4th ed.). *American Journal of Occupational Therapy, 74*(Suppl. 2), 7412410010. https://doi.org/10.5014/ajot.2020.74S2001

An, M., Palisano, R. J., Yi, C. H., Chiarello, L. A., Dunst, C. J., & Gracely, E. J. (2018). Effects of a collaborative intervention process on parent–therapist interaction: A randomized controlled trial. *Physical & Occupational Therapy in Pediatrics, 39,* 259–275. https://doi.org/10.1080/01942638.2018.1496965

Bazyk, S. (1989). Changes in attitudes and beliefs regarding parent participation and home programs: An update. *American Journal of Occupational Therapy, 43,* 723–728. https://doi.org/10.5014/ajot.43.11.723

Bernheimer, L. P., & Weisner, T. S. (2007). "Let me just tell you what I do all day…": The family story at the center of intervention research and practice. *Infants & Young Children, 20,* 192–201. https://doi.org/10.1097/01.IYC.0000277751.62819.9b

Betancourt, J. R., Green, A. R., Carrillo, J. E., & Ananeh-Firempong, O. (2003). Defining cultural competence: A practical framework for addressing racial/ethnic disparities in health and health care. *Public Health Reports, 118,* 293–302. https://doi.org/10.1093/phr/118.4.293

Boyt Schell, B. A., Gillen, G., & Scaffa, M. (2014). Glossary. In B. A. Boyt Schell, G. Gillen, & M. Scaffa (Eds.), *Willard and Spackman's occupational therapy* (12th ed., pp. 1229–1243). Lippincott Williams & Wilkins.

Braun, M. J., Dunn, W., & Tomchek, S. D. (2017). A pilot study on professional documentation: Do we write from a strengths perspective? *American Journal of Speech–Language Pathology, 26,* 972–981. https://doi.org/10.1044/2017_AJSLP-16-0117

Brody, G. H. (2004). Siblings' direct and indirect contributions to child development. *Current Directions in Psychological Science, 13,* 124–126. https://doi.org/10.1111/j.0963-7214.2004.00289.x

Bronfenbrenner, U. (1977). Toward an experimental ecology of human development. *American Psychologist, 32,* 513–531. https://doi.org/10.1037/0003-066X.32.7.513

Carlson, G., Armitstead, C., Rodger, S., & Liddle, G. (2010). Parents' experiences of the provision of community-based family support and therapy services utilizing the strengths approach and natural learning environments. *Journal of Applied Research in Intellectual Disabilities, 23,* 560–572. https://doi.org/10.1111/j.1468-3148.2010.00562.x

Cox, K. F. (2006). Investigating the impact of strength-based assessment on youth with emotional or behavioral disorders. *Journal of Child and Family Studies, 15,* 278–292. https://doi.org/10.1007/s10826-006-9021-5

Dawson, G. (2008). Early behavioral intervention, brain plasticity, and the prevention of autism spectrum disorder. *Development and Psychopathology, 20,* 775–803. https://doi.org/10.1017/S0954579408000370

Dean, E. E., Wallisch, A., & Dunn, W. (2019). Adaptation as a transaction with the environment: Perspectives from the Ecology of Human Performance model. In L. C. Grajo & A. K. Boissele (Eds.), *Adaptation through occupation: Multidimensional perspectives* (pp. 141–155). Slack.

Denham, S. A. (2002). Family routines: A structural perspective for viewing family health. *Advances in Nursing Science, 24*(4), 60–74. https://doi.org/10.1097/00012272-200206000-00010

Dickens, K., Matthews, L. R., & Thompson, J. (2011). Parent and service providers' perceptions regarding the delivery of family-centered paediatric rehabilitation services in a children's hospital. *Child: Care, Health and Development, 37,* 64–73. https://doi.org/10.1111/j.1365-2214.2010.01125.x

Division for Early Childhood. (2014). *DEC recommended practices in early intervention/early childhood special education 2014.* http://www.dec-sped.org/recommendedpractices

Donovan, S. A., & Nickerson, A. B. (2007). Strength-based versus traditional social–emotional reports: Impact on multidisciplinary team members' perceptions. *Behavioral Disorders, 32,* 228–237. https://doi.org/10.1177/019874290703200401

Dunn, W., Brown, C., & McGuigan, A. (1994). The ecology of human performance: A framework for considering the effect of context. *American Journal of Occupational Therapy, 48,* 595-607. https://doi.org/10.5014/ajot.48.7.595

Dunst, C. J., Bruder, M. B., & Espe-Sherwindt, M. (2014). Family capacity-building in early childhood intervention: Do context and setting matter? *School Community Journal, 24*(1), 37–48. http://www.puckett.org/family-capacity-building-eco-context-setting.pdf

Dunst, C. J., Leet, H. E., & Trivette, C. M. (1988). Family resources, personal well-being, and early intervention. *Journal of Special Education, 22,* 108–116. https://doi.org/10.1177/002246698802200112

Guralnick, M. J. (2017). Early intervention for children with intellectual disabilities: An update. *Journal of Applied Research in Intellectual Disabilities, 30,* 211–229. https://doi.org/10.1111/jar.12233

Hanft, B. (1988). The changing environment in early intervention services: Implications for practice. *American Journal of Occupational Therapy, 42,* 724–731. https://doi.org/10.5014/ajot.42.11.724

Hanna, K., & Rodger, S. (2002). Towards family-centred practice in paediatric occupational therapy: A review of the literature on parent–therapist collaboration. *Australian Occupational Therapy Journal, 49,* 14–24. https://doi.org/10.1046/j.0045-0766.2001.00273.x

Individuals With Disabilities Education Improvement Act of 2004, Pub. L. 108-446, 20 U.S.C. §§ 1400–1482.

Kalyanpur, M., & Harry, B. (2012). *Cultural reciprocity in special education: Building family–professional relationships.* Brookes Publishing.

Karst, J. S., & Van Hecke, A. (2012). Parent and family impact of autism spectrum disorders: A review and proposed model for intervention evaluation. *Clinical Child and Family Psychology Review, 15,* 247–277. https://doi.org/10.1007/s10567-012-0119-6

King, G., & Chiarello, L. (2014). Family-centered care for children with cerebral palsy: Conceptual and practical considerations to advance care and practice. *Journal of Child Neurology, 29,* 1046–1054. https://doi.org/10.1177/0883073814533009

Kuhlthau, K., Bloom, S., Van Cleave, J., Knapp, A. A., Romm, D., Klatka, K., . . . Perrin, J. M. (2011). Evidence for family-centered care for children with special health care needs: A systematic review. *Academic Pediatrics, 11,* 136–143. https://doi.org/10.1016/j.acap.2010.12.014

Kuo, D. Z., Mac Bird, T., & Tilford, J. M. (2011). Associations of family-centered care with health care outcomes for children with special health care needs. *Maternal and Child Health Journal, 15,* 794–805. https://doi.org/10.1007/s10995-010-0648-x

Leiter, V. (2004). Dilemmas in sharing care: Maternal provision of professionally driven therapy for children with disabilities. *Social Science & Medicine, 58,* 837–849. https://doi.org/10.1016/S0277-9536(03)00258-2

Øien, I., Fallang, B., & Østensjø, S. (2010). Goal-setting in paediatric rehabilitation: Perceptions of parents and professional. *Child: Care, Health and Development, 36,* 558–565. https://doi.org/10.1111/j.1365-2214.2009.01038.x

Osborne, L. A., McHugh, L., Saunders, J., & Reed, P. (2008). Parenting stress reduces the effectiveness of early teaching interventions for autistic spectrum disorders. *Journal of Autism and Developmental Disorders, 38,* 1092–1103. https://doi.org/10.1007/s10803-007-0497-7

Petalas, M. A., Hastings, R. P., Nash, S., Dowey, A., & Reilly, D. (2009). "I like that he always shows who he is": The perceptions and experiences of siblings with a brother with autism spectrum disorder. *International Journal of Disability, Development and Education, 56,* 381–399. https://doi.org/10.1080/10349120903306715

Rosenbaum, P., King, S., Law, M., King, G., & Evans, J. (1998). Family-centred service: A conceptual framework and research review. *Physical and Occupational Therapy in Pediatrics, 18,* 1–20. https://doi.org/10.1080/J006v18n01_01

Rush, D. D., & Sheldon, M. L. (2011). *The early childhood coaching handbook.* Brookes Publishing.

Shyu, Y. L., Tsai, J., & Tsai, W. (2010). Explaining and selecting treatments for autism: Parental explanatory models in Taiwan. *Journal of Autism and Developmental Disorders, 40,* 1323–1331. https://doi.org/10.1007/s10803-010-0991-1

Spagnola, M., & Fiese, B. H. (2007). Family routines and rituals: A context for development in the lives of young children. *Infants & Young Children, 20,* 284–299. https://doi.org/10.1097/01.IYC.0000290352.32170.5a

Steiner, A. M. (2011). A strength-based approach to parent education for children with autism. *Journal of Positive Behavior Interventions, 13,* 178–190. https://doi.org/10.1177/1098300710384134

Stoneman, Z., Brody, G. H., Davis, C. H., & Crapps, J. M. (1989). Role relations between children who are mentally retarded and their older siblings: Observations in three in-home contexts. *Research in Developmental Disabilities, 10,* 61–76. https://doi.org/10.1016/0891-4222(89)90029-2

Sumsion, T., & Law, M. (2006). A review of evidence on the conceptual elements informing client-centred practice. *Canadian Journal of Occupational Therapy, 73*(3), 153–162. https://doi.org/10.1177/000841740607300303

Trivette, C. M., Dunst, C. J., & Hamby, D. W. (2010). Influences of family-systems intervention practices on parent–child interactions and child development. *Topics in Early Childhood Special Education, 30,* 3–19. https://doi.org/10.1177/0271121410364250

Wallisch, A., Little, L., Pope, E., & Dunn, W. (2019). Parent perspectives of an occupational therapy telehealth intervention. *International Journal of Telerehabilitation, 11*(1), 15–22. https://doi.org/10.5195/ijt.2019.6274

Weisner, T. S. (2002). Ecocultural understanding of children's developmental pathways. *Human Development, 45,* 275–281. https://doi.org/10.1159/000064989

Weisner, T. S., Matheson, C., Coots, J., & Bernheimer, L. P. (2005). Sustainability of daily routines as a family outcome. In A. E. Maynard & M. I. Martini (Eds.), *Learning in cultural context: Family, peers, and school* (pp. 41–73). Springer.

Wray, E. L., & Mortenson, P. A. (2011). Cultural competence in occupational therapists working in early intervention therapy programs. *Canadian Journal of Occupational Therapy, 78,* 180–186. https://doi.org/10.2182/cjot.2011.78.3.6

ZERO TO THREE. (2016). *What is cultural reciprocity?* https://www.zerotothree.org/resources/1577-what-is-cultural-reciprocity

Best Practices in Collaborating With Community, School, and Health Care Partners

9

Lea Ann Lowery, OTD, OTR/L

KEY TERMS AND CONCEPTS

- Advocacy
- Coaching
- Collaborative approach
- Communication logs
- Community partnering
- Data-driven decision making
- Interdisciplinary standardized care plans
- Intraprofessional collaboration
- Resolve conflict
- Self-evaluation
- Telehealth
- Transdisciplinary model
- Tuckman's Model

OVERVIEW

As members of various health care and education teams, occupational therapy practitioners are strong advocates of collaboration (e.g., teaming, networks, consortiums, partnerships, alliances). (*Note. Occupational therapy practitioner* refers to both occupational therapists and occupational therapy assistants.) A *collaborative approach* is defined as "orientation in which the occupational therapy practitioner and client work in the spirit of egalitarianism and mutual participation. Collaboration involves encouraging clients to describe their therapeutic concerns, identify their own goals, and contribute to decisions regarding therapeutic interventions" (Boyt Schell et al., 2014, as cited in American Occupational Therapy Association [AOTA], 2020, p. 84). Regardless of the language used, collaboration in pediatric occupational therapy practice begins with a relationship with and between children and families.

Collaborative effort can lead to achievement of goals that would not otherwise be attainable by individual effort alone (Gajda, 2004). High-quality collaboration requires professionals to understand the role of other agencies and systems, how services are provided, referral mechanisms, and the strengths and limitations of respective agencies or systems (Dunn, 2011).

Factors that influence collaboration include the location of services, goals and objectives, funding, and policy-related expectations. Most important, collaboration requires an understanding of the various stakeholders and their vision for the relationship. Collaborative practice should occur throughout the trajectory of care, including the child and family level, the inter- and intra-agency levels, with community stakeholders, and at the system and policy level. The literature from community-based practice and research provides a valuable framework for thinking about collaboration (see Table 9.1).

ESSENTIAL CONSIDERATIONS

Key elements of collaboration include shared goals and vision for the future, an awareness of team members, clarification of goals and expectations, and leadership and structure for the group to operate (D'Amour et al., 2008). This section discusses inter- and intra-agency collaborations between occupational therapy practitioners and important stakeholders.

Collaboration Within Settings

Inpatient health care

Infants and young children who are hospitalized are often experiencing serious illness and require the support of numerous health care providers. Families may experience greater stress, feelings of loss of control over decision making, and decreased self-confidence in understanding their child's needs during hospitalizations. It is essential for health care providers in hospital settings to be in tune with signs of caregiver stress and identify specific strategies that support families over the course of the hospitalization and after discharge.

Collaboration with families at the hospital level should include the use of language that is clear and easy to understand and should occur at intervals that allow processing. Rather than asking families, "Do you have any questions?" ask, "What questions do you have?" or, "What information that we've discussed would you like to talk over further?" Partnering with families during a child's hospitalization should include support for mental health and wellness, including adequate rest.

Occupational therapy practitioners may also experience increased stress when working in health care settings, because visits may be brief and coordination of care more complex. To increase collaboration in hospital settings,

---

TABLE 9.1. Conceptual Framework for Collaboration and Examples of Collaborative Practice

CATEGORY	EXAMPLES OF COLLABORATION AND POTENTIAL OUTCOMES
Child and family	Collaboration with families and other caregivers to identify priorities for care and goals for the future. The use of specific approaches, such as coaching, can be a collaborative intervention.
Organizational	Organizations benefit from education and consultation to increase understanding of the respective roles of providers and to enhance service delivery.
Community	Partnering with communities can lead to increased access and sense of belonging for children and families. The use of consultation and approaches such as environmental adaptation are important collaborative approaches for community settings and can promote health and wellness.
Public policy	Advocacy through stakeholders such as legislators can lead to policy changes, such as legal mandates for insurance coverage for therapy services.
Systems	The use of data-driven assessment and quality indicators can lead to important systems change and better outcomes for children and families.

Source. Adapted from (Scaffa, 2019).

team members may need to use more structured methods of communication. Strategies such as the use of case conferences and opportunities to engage in "rounds" (bedside team conferencing in hospital settings) can increase opportunities for collaboration among team members (Fewster-Thuente & Velsor-Friedrich, 2008).

Another model that has shown effectiveness is the use of *interdisciplinary standardized care plans,* which create a framework for team members to have an established approach for select populations they more frequently encounter, therefore increasing provider knowledge of expected care and offering a timeline of service delivery (Fewster-Thuente & Velsor-Friedrich, 2008). For teams that do not have prescribed intervention plans or organized opportunities to meet, identifying a team leader, such as floor nurses or social workers, who can function as the hub of the team and relay information from the physician to other providers and the family can increase a sense of coordination around care of children and their families in hospital settings.

Outpatient health care

The environmental and organizational structure of outpatient facilities creates many opportunities for collaborative practice. Frequently, health care providers in outpatient settings function in multi- or interdisciplinary teams. Outpatient settings often feature large gyms and open treatment spaces that create more natural interactions for team members to work together through approaches such as cotreatment or, at a minimum, within proximity of each other. Working in proximity can lead to a greater understanding of other team members' treatment goals and facilitate coordinated intervention planning.

Outpatient settings frequently use specialty teams that focus on select populations or intervention approaches to offer integrated expertise as a part of the diagnostic or intervention process. For example, health care settings such as hospitals and outpatient facilities often use specialty teams in areas (e.g., feeding, technology, mobility devices) or on the basis of specific conditions (e.g., cerebral palsy, autism spectrum disorder, muscular disorders). Within

these organized teams, opportunities for collaboration are high because of the structure of appointments, assessment methods, and designated times for debriefing and planning.

Specialty clinics frequently operate within a hierarchy with a clear team leader, such as the physician. Communication often occurs among team members and directly to the team leaders. Parents and children can benefit from this more streamlined and focused approach to care.

Preschool setting

Occupational therapy practitioners in preschool settings have opportunities to provide both direct and consultative services with other personnel, including teachers and paraprofessionals, in a more multi- or interdisciplinary approach. As members of the educational team, occupational therapy practitioners engage in collaboration when developing the individualized education program goals, including implementating strategies and monitoring progress. Shared decisions through the development of curriculum and implementation of classroom-wide educational opportunities provide rich opportunities for collaboration between teachers and occupational therapy practitioners. In community-based preschools, practitioners can collaborate with teachers and paraprofessionals to increase environmental access and to provide consultation regarding strategies to support children with diverse developmental needs.

Although collaboration in community- and education-based preschools can and should include family input, the ability to interact regularly with parents can pose significant challenges. Collaboration in these settings requires more deliberate efforts to share information and discuss approaches to ensure generalization to the home. The use of communication notebooks and regular opportunities for parent–teacher–provider conferences can increase the consistency of interactions.

Home setting

Early intervention (EI) has a greater focus on the child and family relationship. EI is based on a *transdisciplinary model,* which requires strong coordination among team members and effective partnerships to empower decision making and create a sense of competency for caregivers. Incorporating extended family members and important persons in the life of the child is an essential component of collaboration in EI settings that can lead to greater generalization of intervention approaches.

The use of *coaching* is an example of a collaborative intervention approach that can lead to enhanced feelings of competence among caregivers (Rush et al., 2003). Coaching is an evidence-based approach based on adult learning principles that utilizes a collaborative exchange among practitioner, families, and other providers. The primary focus of coaching is a guided facilitation process with an emphasis on the receiver developing ideas, testing theories, and problem solving with support from the "coach" (Friedman et al., 2012). Transdisciplinary approaches can provide families with a more streamlined delivery of services. Challenges to collaboration in a transdisciplinary model include role blurring and a decreased sense of autonomy (King et al., 2009).

Intraprofessional Collaboration Between Occupational Therapy Practitioners in Different Practice Settings

All occupational therapy services focus on enhancing the person's health, well-being, and ability to engage in their occupations (American Occupational Therapy Association [AOTA], 2020); however, the environment, payer and funding sources, and various laws affect how services are delivered (see Table 9.2). For example, in the home, the occupational therapy practitioner focuses on the family's needs and priorities, whereas in hospitals, the practitioner may focus on specific performance skills. A shift to addressing contexts and environment often characterizes the relationship of occupational therapy providers when working at the community level.

Intraprofessional collaboration consists of cooperation among team members who are from the same discipline but who serve the child in different practice settings. The benefit of intraprofessional collaboration is that each provider offers a unique perspective on the care of the whole child, which leads to more well-rounded programming. Conversely, when not well coordinated, intraprofessional collaboration can result in confusion for the families if there is disagreement among providers about priority of care, potential duplication of services, and increased time and use of resources on the part of the families.

For intraprofessional collaboration to be successful, occupational therapy practitioners must devote time to understanding the policies, laws, and funding associated with unique settings (Table 9.2). A strong understanding of the values and priority of care of the family is essential. Practitioners should seek opportunities to communicate through coordinated meetings or phone calls. Occupational therapy practitioners should consider privacy differences between settings when engaged in intraprofessional collaboration. The Health Insurance Portability and Accountability Act of 1996 (P. L. 104-191) and Family Educational

TABLE 9.2. Similarities and Differences Between Work Settings Influence Collaboration

TOPIC	HOME: EARLY INTERVENTION (AGE BIRTH–3 YEARS)	PRESCHOOLS (AGE 3–5 YEARS)	HEALTH CARE (AGE BIRTH–5 YEARS)
How child and family are viewed	Child, family as team member and partner	Student–learner, family as critical team member and partner	Patient, client, family partner
Determination of need for services	IFSP team (occupational therapist is a member)	IEP team (occupational therapist is a member)	Occupational therapist, occupational therapist and family, occupational therapist and physician (depending on payer source)
Legal delivery of services (in addition to state professional license)	IDEA Part C: Child- and family-centered goals, natural environment, medical necessity for billing Medicaid	IDEA Part B: Least restrictive environment, free and appropriate education, medical necessity for billing Medicaid	Follow payer requirements, medical necessity for billing Medicaid
Documentation and privacy	IFSP, FERPA, occupational therapy intervention plan, AOTA (2018a) *Guidelines for Documentation of Occupational Therapy*	IEP, FERPA, occupational therapy intervention plan, AOTA (2018a) *Guidelines for Documentation of Occupational Therapy*	Occupational therapy treatment plan (plan of care), HIPAA regulations, AOTA (2018a) *Guidelines for Documentation of Occupational Therapy*
Payment	Federal, state, and local funds; Medicaid; private insurance	Federal, state, and local funds; Medicaid; private insurance	Private insurance, Medicaid, private pay, contracts (with EI, local education agency)

Note. AOTA = American Occupational Therapy Association; EI = early intervention; FERPA = Family Educational Rights and Privacy Act of 1974; HIPAA = Health Insurance Portability and Accountability Act of 1996; IDEA = Individuals With Disabilities Education Improvement Act of 2004; IEP = individualized education program; IFSP = individualized family service plan.

Rights and Privacy Act of 1974 (P. L. 93-380) regulations both ensure the privacy of consumers, but they have distinct differences that practitioners must understand and adhere to when working across and between settings.

Interprofessional Collaboration: Occupational Therapy Practitioners and Other Professionals

Occupational therapy practitioners frequently interact with professionals such as physicians, equipment vendors, care coordinators, and other therapists. One of the greatest threats to effective collaboration between professionals, including those from different professional backgrounds, is the lack of opportunity to regularly communicate about shared visions for the child and family. With increasing demands on practitioners to deliver high-quality services in the most efficient method possible, opportunities to speak by phone or coordinate a meeting may be limited or challenging at best. Ways to improve communication among providers from different settings include reducing jargon in documentation and establishing regular meeting times. Respecting and adhering to family priorities can guide decision making about priority of services, frequency of visits, and best approaches.

Communication strategies that can assist with collaboration among providers and with the family include the use of *communication logs,* records used to track communication among providers. In hospital settings, specific communication strategies, such as Situation–Background–Assessment–Recommendation (Institute of Medicine, n.d.; see Exhibit 9.1), have been developed to ensure that communication between providers is clear and delivered in a consistent manner, which is particularly important in settings such as acute care, where interprofessional collaboration can be challenging.

Other practice settings, such as specialty clinics, often have more formal processes for communication. For example, when occupational therapists are evaluating and making recommendations for devices such as augmentative communication devices or adaptive seating, strong collaboration among families, therapists, and vendors is essential to ensure recommendations meet the needs of the child.

When collaborating with physicians, occupational therapy practitioners may choose to use strategies such as attending appointments with families or providing written updates for families to share during medical appointments. Specialty physicians, such as physiatrists and developmental pediatricians, often rely on the input of practitioners when making decisions about the health care plan, such as potential surgeries, recommendations for equipment, and referral to other providers. Follow-up with physicians is important after medical procedures and implementation of specific intervention approaches to ensure that the child is progressing well.

Collaboration at the community level

Collaboration at the community level provides occupational therapy practitioners an opportunity to engage with stakeholders to improve accessibility and the health and wellness of children and families. *Communities* typically refers to localities but can also include groups with a common interest (Green et al., 2001). **Community partnering** involves the coming together of many individuals, agencies, and organizations and can include both the public and the private sectors. The beauty of collaboration at the community level is that like-minded groups and individuals share expertise and a vision (see Exhibit 9.2). The benefit to children and families can include an increased sense of acceptance and engagement in the communities in which they live. At the child level, increased sense of competence and social acceptance can occur when communities are inclusive.

Collaboration at the community level frequently involves addressing the context and environment to support occupational engagement. This can include consultation and education with stakeholders, such as community recreation settings, child care centers, and churches. For example, collaboration of occupational therapy practitioners with parks and recreation departments can lead to accessible play spaces and increased engagement of all children. Similarly, community providers such as dance, gymnastics, and swimming instructors can benefit from alliances with practitioners to support children with diverse developmental needs.

Occupational therapy practitioners also can partner with businesses. Information on environmental features such as lighting, door width to accommodate wheelchairs, and adaptive strollers and seating space is an important way to enhance accessibility and ease of care in the community. Of great importance to many families is accessibility of bathroom changing spaces that offer privacy and ability to lay down a larger child with greater physical needs. More common in recent years is the availability of sensory-friendly events, which make going to movies, zoos, and other community-based activities more child and family friendly. Churches and other places of worship can also benefit from consultation and support from practitioners to enhance opportunities for participation (Carter et al., 2016).

EXHIBIT 9.1.	Situation–Background–Assessment– Recommendation Manualized Communication Strategy

Situation: Provide concise overview of the situation
Background: Share relevant information and history
Assessment: Explicit findings, summary of evaluation
Recommendation: Recommended plan

EXHIBIT 9.2.	Benefits of Community Partnerships

Community partnerships
- Provide more freedom and opportunity for creativity and collaboration outside of traditional roles,
- Bring greater awareness of respective stakeholders and their expertise,
- Allow shared responsibility and collaboration so larger projects can to come to fruition, and
- Can reduce duplication of services and maximize limited resources.

Source. Adapted from Green et al., 2001.

Collaboration at the policy level

Collaboration at the state or national level can promote long-term change and improvements for the health and well-being of children and families. One example is representation of occupational therapy on boards and governing bodies at the local, state, regional, and national levels. Advocacy at these levels requires that practitioners be well versed in existing policies and other regulatory aspects, such as accreditation, organizational structure, political dynamics, and fiscal management.

Advocacy can come in the form of political involvement, ranging from running for an office or seat to working with advocacy groups or lobbyists who are promoting legislation important for practice. For example, state mandates regarding insurance coverage for children with autism spectrum disorder as well as other developmental disabilities have led to important changes in access to care for many children who were not previously eligible for therapy coverage by private insurance. Occupational therapy practitioners can work with legislators through Hill Day and other events that create opportunities to share important information about occupational therapy and promote legislative change on behalf of consumers.

BEST PRACTICES

Collaboration requires leadership skills, such as strong verbal and written communication, respect for other stakeholders, and an understanding of the respective systems in which partners work. There are many theories and frameworks that enhance occupational therapy practitioners' understanding of collaboration. Early literature on organizational change often references *Tuckman's Model,* which is known for its 4-stage sequence: (1) form, (2) storm, (3) norm, and (4) perform (Gajda, 2004). In Tuckman's Model, collaborative relationships must evolve through stages that include getting to know each other, experiencing challenges and conflict between group members, learning to work cooperatively, and evolving into a well-functioning unit.

More contemporary models have expanded to include group identification of a sense of purpose (i.e., vision), strategies and tasks required of team members, leadership and decision making, and communication. Collaboration may be limited to low levels of interaction, such as networking, or may include more unified and formal processes with high-level interaction (Gajda, 2004). Regardless of the frequency, proximity, or level of interaction, collaboration requires that each partner evaluate their unique contribution and work toward a shared goal of improved outcomes for children and families. Other critical elements for effective collaboration include establishing priorities of partnerships (form), developing relationships (form), using data to inform decision making (norm), engaging in self-assessment (norm), resolving conflicts (storm), and developing innovations for best practice (perform).

Identify Priorities of Care

Allocation of resources can be a threat to the delivery of services in both educational and health care settings. Specific examples can include long wait lists for diagnostic and therapy services, high caseloads, limitations on number of allowed therapy visits by reimbursement models, and geographic access to services and supports. Limited access to services can lead to increased stress for families and missed opportunities to maximize outcomes for children (Kolehmainen et al., 2012). When teams form, collaborators may benefit from developing a framework of care that identifies a best fit for delivery of services. Identifying key outcomes, such as frequency, duration, and cessation of services, can facilitate improved understanding of services for providers as well as families and maximize resources (Bailes et al., 2008).

Develop Relationships and Partnerships

No effective partnership has ever existed without positive feelings of regard for individuals and groups that work together. Teams that function best devote time to creating relationships and trust. During the *forming* stage, creating opportunities for formal meetings when possible, understanding the perspectives of other collaborators, and being willing to listen are essential components. Similarly, during the early stages of relationship development, partners may focus less on accomplishing specific tasks and instead identify a shared goal or vision. When possible, relationships among providers, agencies, and groups can be strengthened through opportunities to interact outside of work-related activities. Partnerships that will have high-frequency interactions and a need for strong collaborative relationships may benefit from formal team development activities.

Use Data to Guide Decision Making and Evaluate Effectiveness

In evaluations of the effect of programming, the identification and use of effective procedures can assist with defining outcomes and determining when revision is needed. Important considerations include how partnerships will be strengthened through collaboration, what level of collaboration is needed, and how client outcomes can be evaluated. Other considerations, such as the group composition and structure and the tasks and environments where collaboration occurs, provide a framework for *data-driven decision making* (Gaboury et al., 2009), a process that analyzes patterns and information gleaned from data to make decisions. Data collection can take many forms and is highly dependent on the goals of the group.

More formal processes of assessment can include structured observation of specific procedures and processes to ensure consistency, checklists, and the development of measurable objectives and outcomes. Other methods for collaborative relationships may include active reflection using questions to explore expectations, outcomes, and potential changes to intervention and education plans (Rush et al., 2003). Evaluating outcomes at the occupational therapy practitioner or family level can include satisfaction surveys or the use of qualitative data, such as focus groups. Measures such as goal attainment scaling can be used to systematically evaluate positive or negative changes in outcomes (Turner-Stokes, 2009). Evaluation of collaborative relationships between providers and agencies can occur through systematic review of referrals to other providers, satisfaction surveys, and examination of intake procedures.

Conduct Self-Evaluation

Self-evaluation, the appraisal of one's own performance, is an essential step in evaluation of collaborative partnerships and requires a careful examination of one's own values and beliefs. How do our own values drive decision making? What is our own understanding (or lack of) of the roles of other group and team members? What previous interactions have we experienced that may color our point of view?

Occupational therapy practitioners should use several strategies to support self-assessment, such as cultural competence training to increase understanding of family beliefs and decision making, when caring for children. Developing knowledge regarding health and education systems can promote practitioners' understanding of the unique contributions of collaborative partners. Seeking educational opportunities that enhance leadership skills and effective communication strategies can provide important tools for self-assessment.

Resolve Conflicts

Even with the best of intentions, collaboration can be hard, and conflict is inevitable. For partnerships to be successful, all members must work to achieve a climate that allows sharing ideas, beliefs, and concerns. The ability to *resolve conflict* is essential for successful group functioning and the well-being of members. Conflicts, whether passive or overt, typically take shape in the form of behaviors such as power plays, blaming, withholding information, and other passive–aggressive acts. In particular, conflict typically consists of challenges at the task, relationship, and process levels (Behfar, 2008). The nature and structure of groups may give rise to greater incidences of specific types of conflict. Groups or partnerships that are in proximity and have regular opportunities to work together and interact both formally and informally typically experience fewer conflicts.

Role blurring is another common area of conflict (Suter et al., 2009). Team structure and role clarification may be less well defined, which can lead to feelings of confusion or

---

EXHIBIT 9.3.   Tips for Supporting Communication in Collaborative Practice

- Plan for regular meeting times.
- Encourage opportunities to interact in social situations and activities not directly related to client care.
- Spend time learning more about the background and training of other team members to increase a sense of value among all.
- Create mentoring opportunities between team members from different disciplines to increase understanding of different roles and responsibilities among team members.
- Encourage dialogue and openness to diverse opinions.
- Identify the priorities of the group members, and strive to keep a focus on meeting the objectives.
- Schedule opportunities for team-building experiences, and allow adequate time for reflection.
- Develop a clear orientation process for new members.
- Understand differences between practice settings, including reimbursement, documentation requirements, and organizational structure.

---

frustration. For example, the primary service provider (PSP) approach selects one member of the team to serve as the primary contact for the family. Although this is typically a person who knows the family best or is based on the child's current needs (e.g., feeding, mobility), some teams use one discipline as the PSP for the children, thus causing frustration for the family or team members who have limited access.

To address conflict, teams should consider the use of specific strategies, such as discussing or debating ideas, working to reach a consensus or compromise, and voting. They may develop a set of rules, such as algorithms that can guide decision making and reduce conflict, that are specific to the type of conflict (Behfar, 2008). Encouraging opportunities for sharing of different points of view is an important step for creating healthy relationships among team members. Exhibit 9.3 provides tips for communication in collaborative practice.

Use Technology to Promote Collaboration

The nature of health and education systems demands that occupational therapy practitioners be highly efficient and cost-effective in the delivery of care and necessitate the use of innovative practices. *Telehealth* is "the application of evaluation, consultative, preventive, and therapeutic services delivered through information and communication technology" (AOTA, 2018b, p. 1). Services are cost-effective and potentially allow access among practitioners, children, families, and preschool staff in areas that experience personnel challenges, especially in rural areas (Cason, 2011).

Potential benefits of telehealth include ability for families to access services in a timely manner, access to practitioners with expertise in specific areas of practice, opportunities to provide consultation to families to enhance outcomes, and opportunities for collaboration among team members who might not ordinarily meet or work side by side. Telehealth can provide opportunities for professionals to interact with each other in more convenient ways, including team meetings and professional development.

However, occupational therapy practitioners face challenges when using innovative approaches such as telehealth, and the use of "netiquette" ground rules can ensure a more positive experience for all participants (see Appendix J "Occupational Therapy Telehealth Practices in Early Childhood"). Examples of netiquette rules for telehealth delivery include finding an environment that is free from other distractions, such as a television or other background sounds; creating a clear agenda and time frame for the meeting; and designating a leader for facilitation of the discussion. Other considerations for technology-based service delivery and teaming include confidentiality, technology connections and requirements, sound and image quality, equipment accessibility, and comfort of providers and recipients of services (Cason, 2011). Access to high-speed internet can be limited for families residing in more rural areas. Practitioners must understand reimbursement and state practice guidelines before implementing telehealth methods.

SUMMARY

Collaboration is an essential component of high-quality programming for children and families that is often unique to the setting and team. Positive outcomes, such as increased efficiency, sense of competency, and belonging among members, can occur with effective collaboration. However, collaboration is not always easy, and each member must contribute to the development of shared goals, demonstrate respect for all stakeholders, commit to the reduction of conflict, and use effective communication strategies. Occupational therapy practitioners should also identify resources that support their understanding and knowledge of collaborative practice.

Understanding specific aspects of practice settings as well as payer requirements, documentation, handling of records, and overall goals for the child and family is essential. Collaboration requires occupational therapy practitioners to adopt a big-picture approach to delivery of services. Effective collaboration at the community level requires important communication skills that focus first and foremost on listening to key stakeholders while developing goals and a sense of cohesion related to program development or improvement of existing services. Systems collaboration requires a great understanding of organizational structure, policy, and legal aspects of agencies and organization. When practitioners collaborate at the systems level, they provide opportunity to create far-reaching policy and positive changes to services for consumers. Applying basic leadership strategies, such as establishing clear lines of communication, identifying mutual goals, delegating tasks, and recognizing and supporting the respective roles and strengths of partners, can lead to more effective service delivery and enhanced systems of care.

Telehealth is an innovative approach for service delivery regardless of proximity and is a method for reducing stress on families accessing care while affording an opportunity for various team members to collaborate. Continued exploration regarding management of confidentiality, reimbursement for services, and user comfort is needed for this new frontier of health care delivery and collaborative practice.

RESOURCES

- **Association of University Centers on Disability's Leadership Education in Neurodevelopmental Disabilities programs:** https://www.aucd.org/template/page.cfm?id=473
- **Institute for Healthcare Improvement:** http://www.ihi.org/about/Pages/default.aspx
- **Interprofessional Education Collaborative:** https://www.ipecollaborative.org/
- **National Center for Interprofessional Practice and Education:** https://nexusipe.org/
- **World Health Organization's** *Framework for Action on Interprofessional Education and Collaborative Practice:* https://www.who.int/hrh/resources/framework_action/en/

REFERENCES

American Occupational Therapy Association. (2018a). Guidelines for documentation of occupational therapy. *American Journal of Occupational Therapy, 72*(Suppl. 2), 7212410010. https://doi.org/10.5014/ajot.2018.72S203

American Occupational Therapy Association. (2018b). Telehealth in occupational therapy. *American Journal of Occupational Therapy, 72*(Suppl. 2), 7212410059. https://doi.org/10.5014/ajot.2018.72S219

American Occupational Therapy Association. (2020). Occupational therapy practice framework: Domain and process (4th ed.). *American Journal of Occupational Therapy, 74*(Suppl. 2), 7412410010. https://doi.org/10.5014/ajot.2020.74S2001

Bailes, A. F., Reder, R., & Burch, C. (2008). Development of guidelines for determining frequency of therapy services in a pediatric medical setting. *Pediatric Physical Therapy, 20,* 194–198. https://doi.org/10.1097/PEP.0b013e3181728a7b

Behfar, K. J. (2008). The critical role of conflict resolution in teams: A close look at the links between conflict type, conflict management strategies, and team outcomes. *Journal of Applied Psychology, 93,* 170–188. https://doi.org/10.1037/0021-9010.93.1.170

Boyt Schell, B. A., Gillen, G., & Scaffa, M. (2014). Glossary. In B. A. Boyt Schell, G. Gillen, & M. Scaffa (Eds.), *Willard and Spackman's occupational therapy* (12th ed., pp. 1229–1243). Lippincott Williams & Wilkins.

Carter, E. W., Boehm, T. L., Annandale, N. H., & Taylor, C. E. (2016). Supporting congregational inclusion for children and youth with disabilities and their families. *Exceptional Children, 82,* 372–389. https://doi.org/10.1177/0014402915598773

Cason, J. (2011). Telerehabilitation: An adjunct service delivery model for early intervention services. *International Journal of Telerehabilitation, 3*(1), 19–28. https://doi.org/10.5195/IJT.2011.6071

D'Amour, D., Goulet, L., Labadie, J. F., Martin-Rodriguez, L. S., & Pineault, R. (2008). A model and typology of collaboration between professionals in healthcare organizations. *BMC Health Services Research, 8,* 188. https://doi.org/10.1186/1472-6963-8-188

Dunn, W. (2011). *Best practice occupational therapy for children and families in community settings* (2nd ed.). Slack.

Family Educational Rights and Privacy Act of 1974, Pub. L. 93-380, 20 U.S.C. § 1232g; 34 CFR Part 99.

Fewster-Thuente, M. N., & Velsor-Friedrich, B. (2008). Interdisciplinary collaboration for healthcare professionals. *Nursing Administration Quarterly, 32,* 40–48. https://doi.org/10.1097/01.NAQ.0000305946.31193.61

Friedman, M., Woods, J., & Salisbury, C. (2012). Caregiver coaching strategies for early intervention providers. Moving toward operational definitions. *Infants and Young Children, 25,* 62–82. https://doi.org/10.1097/IYC.0b013e31823d8f12

Gaboury, I., Bjjold, M., Boon, H., & Moher, D. (2009). Interprofessional collaboration within Canadian integrative healthcare clinics: Key components. *Social Science & Medicine, 69,* 707–715. https://doi.org/10.1016/j.socscimed.2009.05.048

Gajda, R. (2004). Utilizing collaboration theory to evaluate strategic alliances. *American Journal of Evaluation, 25*(1), 65–77. https://doi.org/10.1177/109821400402500105

Green, L., Daniel, M., & Novick, L. (2001). Partnerships and coalitions for community-based research. *Public Health Reports, 116*(Suppl. 1), 20–31. https://doi.org/10.1093/phr/116.S1.20

Health Insurance Portability and Accountability Act of 1996 (HIPAA), Pub. L. 104-191, 42 U.S.C. § 300gg, 29 U.S.C §§ 1181–1183, and 42 U.S.C. §§ 1320d–1320d9.

Individuals With Disabilities Education Improvement Act of 2004, Pub. L. 108-446, 20 U.S.C. §§ 1400–1482.

Institute of Medicine. (n.d.). *SBAR tool: Situation–background–assessment–recommendation.* http://www.ihi.org/resources/Pages/Tools/SBARToolkit.aspx

King, G., Strachan, D., Tucker, M., Duwyn, B., Desserud, S., & Shillington, M. (2009). The application of a transdisciplinary model for early intervention services. *Infants and Young Children, 22,* 211–223. https://doi.org/10.1097/IYC.0b013e3181abe1c3

Kolehmainen, N., MacLennan, G., Ternent, L., Duncan, E. A., Duncan, E. M., Ryan, S. B., . . . Francis, J. J. (2012). Using shared goal setting to improve access and equity: A mixed methods study of the Good Goals intervention in children's occupational therapy. *Implementation Science, 7,* 76. https://doi.org/10.1186/1748-5908-7-76

Rush, D., Sheldon, M., & Hanft, B. (2003). Coaching families and colleagues: A process for collaboration in natural settings. *Infants and Young Children, 16,* 33–47.

Scaffa, M. E. (2019). Occupational therapy interventions for groups, communities and populations. In B. Boyt Schell & G. Gillen (Eds.), *Willard and Spackman's occupational therapy* (13th ed., pp. 436–447). Wolters Kluwer.

Suter, E., Arndt, J., Arthur, N., Parbosingh, J., Taylor, E., & Deutschlander, S. (2009). Role understanding and effective communication as core competencies for collaborative practice. *Journal of Interprofessional Care, 23,* 41–51. https://doi.org/10.1080/13561820802338579

Turner-Stokes, L. (2009). Goal attainment scaling (GAS) in rehabilitation: A practical guide. *Clinical Rehabilitation, 23,* 362–370. https://doi.org/10.1177/0269215508101742

Best Practices in Early Childhood Transitions

Joanne Jackson Foss, PhD, OTR, FAOTA, and Christine T. Myers, PhD, OTR/L

10

KEY TERMS AND CONCEPTS

- Coaching
- Family-centered approaches
- Individuals With Disabilities Education Improvement Act of 2004
- Infant mental health
- Late referral
- Modeling
- Natural environments
- Transition plan
- Transition supports
- Transitions

OVERVIEW

Young children participate in a variety of short-term and long-term changes within the first 5 years of life, such as coming home from the hospital after birth, beginning center-based care, and entering preschool (PS) and kindergarten. These changes, termed *transitions,* "refer to the events, activities, and processes associated with key changes between environments or programs during the early childhood years and the practices that support the adjustment of the child and family to the new setting" (Division for Early Childhood, 2014, p. 16). Children and their families may feel stress and uncertainty during these transitions; however, this stress may be much greater if the child has special needs (Waters & Friesen, 2019). Not only do transitions signal a change of environment and context, but the additional needs of a child with a disability may require extra time and energy to ensure the process unfolds without problems (Rosenkoetter et al., 2009).

Occupational therapy practitioners have the knowledge and skills to support children and families who wish to make a smooth transition between environments and programs (Myers et al., 2011; Podvey & Myers, 2015). (*Note. Occupational therapy practitioner* refers to both occupational therapists and occupational therapy assistants.) Training in family-centered practices, an understanding of how to use activity analysis for successful outcomes in the natural environment, and a background in interprofessional practice make occupational therapy an important addition to early childhood transition teams. Practitioner involvement in transition planning and the adjustment to the new environment may improve the child's and family's outcomes through coaching, adaptation, modifications, and collaboration with other team members.

This chapter describes the roles of occupational therapy practitioners working in early childhood transitions, the policies that direct transitions in public schools and early intervention (EI) programs, and the best practices for supporting positive transitions and optimizing transition outcomes for children ages birth to 5 years and their families.

ESSENTIAL CONSIDERATIONS

Early Childhood Transitions Under IDEA

In 2017, more than 300,000 infants and toddlers exited EI services (U.S. Department of Education, Office of Special Education Programs, 2016). Many of these children transitioned to local PS programs, with approximately 130,000 students eligible for special education in PS. The *Individuals With Disabilities Education Improvement Act of 2004* (IDEA; P. L. 108-446) has provisions related to early childhood transitions. Various possibilities are discussed next.

Transitions from hospital to Part C

Infants and children younger than age 3 years may be referred for Part C EI while still in the hospital if they have an established risk or anticipated developmental delays (each state determines its own eligibility criteria). In this case, the neonatal intensive care unit (NICU) team may contact the EI team before the transition to home, with services beginning after hospital discharge. This transition is guided by IDEA Part C federal and state regulations that determine family and child needs through a comprehensive, multidisciplinary evaluation (IDEA, 2004). *Transition supports* for the family, such as instruction in child development and preschool readiness, may also be provided through state and local agencies not affiliated with EI, such as early childhood home visiting programs funded by Medicaid (Johnson, 2019).

Transitions from IDEA Part C to Part B

When children with disabilities transition to PS, they may do so from an EI program (Part C of IDEA) or without having had previous services. For a child who has been receiving EI services, the team develops a ***transition plan*** (i.e., a written plan of activities and services needed to provide a smooth transition from early intervention to preschool) as part of the child's individualized family service plan (IFSP), not less than 90 days and not more than 9 months before the child's third birthday. If the team members suspect the child has an educational disability that falls under Part B of IDEA, they will share their concerns with the parent and contact the local educational agency (LEA) to refer the child for an evaluation to determine eligibility for special education services. The parent must give written consent before the evaluation. Occupational therapy practitioners who provided EI services share their information with the preschool team, which may include the occupational therapist working in the PS, to assist with the eligibility determination and intervention planning.

Transitions from home or community to IDEA Part B

For children who transition to PS without previous enrollment in EI, the process to determine eligibility for special education and related services begins with a parent's consent for evaluation. The occupational therapists working in the PS may be asked to complete evaluations to assist the team in determining eligibility. See Figure 10.1 for an overview of the transition timeline for children transitioning from Part C to Part B services.

Transitions near 3rd birthday

If a child is referred to EI as they approach age 3 years, specific guidelines provide guidance to LEAs. A ***late referral*** is one that comes 135 days or fewer before a child's third birthday, and the process is similar to that for children who are already receiving EI services except that the initial IFSP meeting and transition planning conference may be combined (Diefendorf & Lucas, 2010). For children referred 90–45 days before turning age 3 years, a transition plan is not required; however, the initial IFSP must include transition planning.

For children referred fewer than 45 days before turning age 3 years, an initial evaluation by the EI program and a transition planning conference are not required. In this

---

FIGURE 10.1. Early childhood transition timeline for SPP/APR indicators C-8A, 8B, 8C, B-11, and B-12 for Part C children determined to be eligible at least 90 days prior to their third birthday.

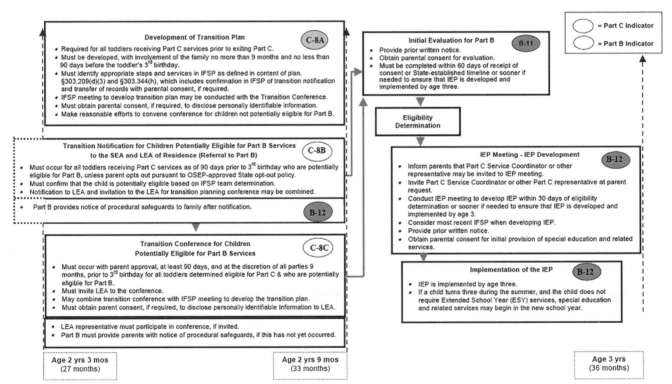

Developed by NECTAC in collaboration with the Early Childhood Transition Workgroup of the RRCP General Supervision Priority Team and the Office of Special Education Programs (OSEP), September, 2012

Note. APR = annual performance report; IEP = individualized education program; IFSP = individualized family service plan; LEA = local education agency; OSEP = Office of Special Education Programs; SEA = state education agency; SPP = state performance plan.

Source. Reprinted from "Early Childhood Transition Timeline for SPP/APR Indicators C-8A, 8B, 8C, B-11 and B-12" by the Early Childhood Technical Assistance Center, 2012, https://ectacenter.org/~pdfs/topics/transition/timeline_flowchart_APR_indicators_09-12_OSEP_approved.pdf. Developed by NECTAC in collaboration with the Early Childhood Transition Workgroup of the RRCP General Supervision Priority Team and the Office of Special Education Programs (OSEP).

case, the EI program may provide parents with information about Part B 619 PS program and may refer the child to the LEA, if the parent consents. Occupational therapy practitioners may participate in the IFSP meetings, transition planning, and eligibility determination for late referrals.

Transitions from preschool to kindergarten

Transition to kindergarten should emphasize school readiness and a positive adjustment to school. Children may be transitioning without PS experience, from PS with or without an individualized education program (IEP), or with concerns that may require an IEP. Though IDEA provides limited guidance for children transitioning to kindergarten, the IEP team should discuss strategies for a smooth transition for children with IEPs. If the child has concerns that may require special education and related services, the child will need an evaluation to determine eligibility. Children transitioning from Head Start to kindergarten receive continuity of services through coordination between educational and social agencies (Improving Head Start for School Readiness Act of 2007; P. L. 110-134).

Office of Special Education Programs Indicators and Outcomes

The U.S. Department of Education's Office of Special Education Programs receives an annual report from states with data from Part C and Part B programs to monitor compliance with IDEA. Two specific indicators relate to transition from EI (Part C of IDEA) to PS services:

- C-8 (Early Childhood Transition): Percentage of all children exiting Part C who received timely transition planning to support their transition to PS and other appropriate community services by their 3rd birthday, including
  - An IFSP with transition steps and services;
  - Notification to state and local education agencies, if the child potentially is eligible for Part B; and
  - Transition conference, if the child potentially is eligible for Part B (IDEA, 2004, 1416[a][3][B] and 1442).
- B-12 (Early Childhood Transition): Percentage of children referred by Part C before age 3 years who are found eligible for Part B and who have an IEP developed and implemented by their 3rd birthday (IDEA, 2004, 1416[a][3][B]).

Occupational therapists working in EI and PS support local programs to meet the requirements of these indicators by providing timely evaluations, participating in transition planning, and assisting with determining eligibility for services.

Two Part B indicators relate to PS to kindergarten transitions:

- B-7 (Preschool Outcomes): Percentage of preschool children with IEPs who demonstrate improved
  - Positive social–emotional skills (including social relationships),
  - Acquisition and use of knowledge and skills (including early language and communication and early literacy), and
  - Use of appropriate behaviors to meet their needs.

- B-8 (Parent Involvement): Percentage of parents with a child receiving special education services who report that schools facilitated parent involvement as a means of improving services and results for children with disabilities.

These indicators relate to school readiness for preschoolers receiving special education services and transitioning to kindergarten. Children who have appropriate social–emotional skills and who are able to communicate and make their needs known are more likely to adjust to kindergarten (Mann et al., 2016; Quirk et al., 2017). Parent involvement in transition activities may lead to better adjustment outcomes in kindergarten (Kang et al., 2017).

Each state collects data on a state-identified measurable result (SIMR) for Part B and for Part C and reports results based on an annual performance report indicator. Occupational therapy practitioners may have a role in supporting states to meet their SIMR. For example, in Florida, the Part C SIMR is to increase the percentage of infants and toddlers who exit EI with an increased rate of growth in positive social–emotional skills. As discussed above, appropriate social–emotional skills improve children's adjustment to a new school environment. Occupational therapy practitioners who address social–emotional skills with young children are supporting their ability to adjust to PS (Myers & Podvey, 2019).

BEST PRACTICES

The unique perspective of occupational therapy practitioners can be particularly valuable for transition planning. Research suggests that transitions can prove especially challenging for children with disabilities and their families (Podvey et al., 2010; Waters & Friesen, 2019). Occupational therapy practitioners understand the personal and social environments and the contextual factors of participation and can help children and families adjust to changes in expectations, routines, and social environments. The federal laws that influence best practices in early childhood transitions promote three concepts of intervention: family-centered services, natural environments, and transition planning.

Support Family-Centered Services

A comprehensive understanding of early social, emotional, and behavioral development can help improve the outcomes of families and children affected by less than optimal environments and experiences. The following sections address developmental considerations, effects of stress on families, family-centered approaches, and capacity building.

Developmental considerations in early childhood

The field of **infant mental health** (IMH) emerged in the late 1970s. This perspective acknowledges that all domains of development are interdependent and supported by the dynamics of the young child's environment. Therefore, optimal development is dependent on a safe environment with supportive social interactions (Center on the Developing Child, Harvard University, 2010). The complex interactions of biological development and environmental and social contexts facilitate the development of the emotional regulation and social functioning necessary for competence in relationships, learning, and eventual adult life roles (Podvey & Myers, 2015). EI services can minimize developmental delay and enhance the capacity of the family to adjust to the inevitable transitions that will occur as the child ages (American Occupational Therapy Association [AOTA], 2017).

Research supports the importance of early caregiver and child relationships as the context for brain organization (Center on the Developing Child, Harvard University, 2010). Appropriate brain organization supports social-emotional capacities and cognitive, language, and physical development. IMH research has concluded that the optimal and most cost-effective time for interventions supporting children and their families or caregivers is in early childhood (Center on the Developing Child, Harvard University, 2016). The occupations of infants and toddlers develop through play, learning, and social interactions with family and caregivers. Early learning provides the foundation for later learning. The ability of the parents and family to assist the child to engage in the occupations that promote mastery, competency, and identity is critical.

Effects of stress on early childhood

Experiences in infancy and early childhood shape development and brain function (Center on the Developing Child, Harvard University, 2010). The period between birth and age 5 years is critical for the development of significant brain maturity; social–emotional capacities; and cognitive, language, and physical skills needed for long-term mental health (Center on the Developing Child, Harvard University, 2016). During this sensitive time, brain organization is highly receptive to both positive and negative experiences. Infants and young children need high levels of warm, sensitive, and responsive caregiving. Parents struggling with stress or with mental health issues of their own may find it difficult to consistently respond with the warmth and support that lay the foundation for secure attachments and trust in relationships (Grady, 2016).

EI services that promote the family's capacity to meet their child's needs can prevent long-term issues and promote favorable outcomes. Research supports that earlier interventions are more effective than later interventions to try to reverse the developmental and behavioral issues created by stressful experiences in infancy and early childhood (Center on the Developing Child, Harvard University, 2016).

Family-centered approach

A 2013 review of EI studies revealed that interventions that facilitated family participation and training resulted in positive outcomes (Kingsley & Mailloux, 2013). To promote a young child's preparation for academics and participation in ADLs through optimal development, parent–child relationships are the focus of intervention. Family-centered, relationship-based services facilitate the family's capacity to care for and support the critical development of the young child. The family is the main social unit, the first teachers, and experts in the care and capacities of their child (Muhlenhaupt et al., 2019). Therefore, enhancing the parents' competence can prevent developmental disability and lead to more favorable long-term outcomes (Ferretti & Bub, 2017).

Family-centered approaches include *coaching,* which fosters the development of strategies and skills through problem solving, practice, and feedback, and *modeling,* which fosters the development of behaviors and skills through imitation and observation (Holloway & Chandler, 2010). These approaches provide training in the child's natural environment (see Table 10.1). The occupational therapy practitioner can model strategies or behaviors that the parents can add to their repertoire of actions. Parents learn new skills to promote their child's learning during everyday family routines and interactions. Colyvas et al. (2010) found that parents seemed to learn behavior strategies best when the strategies were explicitly modeled and the parents were given the chance to practice in the presence of the occupational therapy practitioner.

The coaching approach centers on the parent and occupational therapy practitioner team. As a team, the parent and the practitioners can collaboratively work through environmental issues that are affecting the family's capacity to adjust and support the child. Although the parent is the learner, the child can benefit from new strategies and skills that assist the family to adapt routines and encourage

TABLE 10.1.   Family-Centered Approaches and Examples

FAMILY-CENTERED APPROACH AND DEFINITION	APPLICATION EXAMPLES
Modeling: Family-centered approach that fosters the development of behaviors and skills through imitation and observation	▪ Hospital: Recognizing stressors and adapting behavioral interactions for family ▪ EI: Encouraging parent–child social interactions during routines (e.g., diapering, feeding) ▪ PS: Helping family incorporate practice of PS routines (e.g., washing hands, eating lunch in a group). ▪ Kindergarten: Using motivating strategies to increase attention span and persistence
Coaching: Family-centered approach that fosters the development of strategies and skills through problem solving, practice, and feedback	▪ Hospital: Recognizing barriers and adapting context and environments ▪ EI: Recognizing sources of family stress and problem-solving strategies for improvement (e.g., sleep routine, feeding behaviors) ▪ PS: Building skills to communicate with school personnel and advocate for the child ▪ Kindergarten: Incorporating academic skills (e.g., reading, math) in family activities

Note. EI = early intervention; PS = preschool.

positive experiences (Case-Smith, 2013). Overall, parents report positive perceptions of family-centered and routines-based intervention (Kingsley & Mailloux, 2013).

Building capacity

Part C of IDEA focuses on building the family's capacity to support their child through the transition process. When working with families and young children using family-centered approaches, professionals must establish a strong collaborative relationship with the family. Family-centered approaches build the family's confidence and capacity to meet the needs of their child. In family-centered approaches, the occupational therapy practitioner works to build a strong relationship with the family (Muhlenhaupt et al., 2019). Through this relationship, parents gain confidence in their ability to focus on the steps needed to support their child with life events, including the inevitable transitions of childhood. Intervention goals should strive to help the parent gain more confidence with new skills and strategies to add to their repertoire of skills.

Emphasize Childhood Occupations and Routines in Early Childhood

Successful transitions support the child's engagement in the natural occupations and routines that serve as a foundation for adaptation to challenging contextual demands of the future.

Natural environments

Natural environments are the home and community settings that are typical for the child's same-age peers without disabilities (IDEA, 2004). Services provided in natural settings offer opportunities for families to implement strategies in the environments where they will be used or to practice new skills in a familiar environment during the child's routine before the changes brought on by transitions occur (AOTA, 2017).

Preparing for future transitions

A child's first transition is typically from the hospital to their home environment. Although most transitions occur naturally as a child develops, they also occur because of changes in programs or facilities, the child's age, the child's disability status, or family needs or location. Changes in environment or service provisions can be stressful for the child and family. Children and caregivers leave behind familiar environments and often the professionals familiar with their child. Early family-centered collaboration and planning can facilitate a smoother transition process, ensuring continuity in the child's engagement and participation (Fain & Eason, 2016).

Family-centered approaches can encourage participation in pretransition planning. Parents should receive guidance to collaborate with new personnel and visit new environments. As the child and family prepare for transition to new services, parents should feel more confident in their capacity to advocate for their child and have the skills to assist their child to adjust to the changes.

Support Transitions Across Settings

Early childhood interventions that include collaboration and planning with families can equip children with the skills and support they need for successful transitions. The following section addresses supports needed for fluid transitions across settings in the early childhood years.

Hospital to home and community

Some children may spend an extended period of time in a NICU setting, where they receive specialized care by a team of medical professionals designed specifically for medically challenged newborns. This intensive level of care is most often funded by medical insurance or Medicaid. The care of newborns in this medical environment, although lifesaving, also emphasizes individualized developmental care. Interventions to encourage the development of newborn occupations (e.g., feeding, sleeping, adjusting to environmental stimuli) are provided, and participation by families is supported while they adjust to the critical needs of the infant (AOTA, 2018).

Family-centered approaches inherent in developmental care encourage optimal development and parent–child attachment and bonding. In general, interventions for infants born before 37 weeks gestational age that address the parent–child relationship as well as developmental skills have promise in improving cognitive and motor outcomes during infancy and seem to have a positive influence on cognitive outcomes into PS (Dusing et al., 2018; Frolek Clark & Kingsley, 2020; Spittle et al., 2015).

Communication is an important aspect of the transition process for children and families transitioning from the NICU to home (Early Childhood Technical Assistance Center, 2018b). Occupational therapy practitioners should be prepared to answer questions about community resources and use reflective listening skills as caregivers and family members discuss their concerns. Practitioners may need to initiate the gathering of information from families, including asking the family to share their priorities and goals for their child, identifying any particular supports the family may need when they go home, and inquiring how the family perceives the role that EI may have in supporting their child and the family after the transition.

Children may also experience medical conditions or accidents that result in hospitalizations. In anticipation of discharge from hospital-based settings, families receive training and guidance for the child's medical needs (Breneol et al., 2017). While focusing on these needs, occupational therapy practitioners can provide a perspective that emphasizes skills needed for optimal growth and development. Collaborating closely with the family before discharge fosters a successful transition by identifying potential issues and barriers (AOTA, 2018). On discharge, children and families may receive referrals to determine eligibility for IDEA EI or early childhood programs or outpatient occupational therapy, along with follow-up medically based services. Occupational therapy practitioners work to build a strong collaborative relationship with the family, assisting them with their priorities and the skills they need to meet the needs of their child in their family context (AOTA, 2017).

Home to community settings

EI services are provided for infants and toddlers with developmental delays and for children who may be at risk for developmental delay (on the basis of each state's eligibility guidelines). Because young children learn best in the context of their own home and community, EI services are family centered and delivered in the child's natural environments (Muhlenhaupt et al., 2019).

EI service providers anticipate and guide transition planning to community-based settings, such as center- and home-based child care and private and public PS programs. When the child is transitioning to new environments, discussing the expectations of the new environment with the caregiver, visiting the new environment with the child and family, and assisting the staff in the new environment to plan for the individualized needs of the child may be beneficial. Often, occupational therapy practitioners provide EI services at the child's care center, which allows interventions that support the child's engagement in the routines of the center through environmental adaptations and modifications and staff coaching. Continuity of practitioners in child care and PS may improve the transition to PS; thus, it is preferable for practitioners to be consistent over time in early care and EI (McMullen et al., 2016).

Early intervention to preschool

Children typically enter community-based PS settings with services that promote school readiness, language, preliteracy, and math skills. When needed, children who are age 3 years may be eligible for Head Start or special education and related services at their PS. Unlike the family-centered approach with one-on-one coaching of caregivers in the natural environment, PS programs use a student-centered approach with less family involvement. Occupational therapy practitioners can help prepare families for these differences through pretransition discussions and descriptions of what to expect once their child enters PS. Practitioners can also answer questions about programs offered in the LEA if they are knowledgeable about the local service system.

The Division for Early Childhood (2014) provides two recommended practices for early childhood transitions:

1. *TR1:* Practitioners in the sending and receiving programs exchange information before, during, and after transition about practices most likely to support the child's successful adjustment and positive outcomes.
2. *TR2:* Practitioners use a variety of planned and timely strategies with the child and family before, during, and after the transition to support successful adjustment and positive outcomes for both the child and the family.

Occupational therapy practitioners have a role in supporting both of these practices. They may attend transition planning meetings, where their expertise in activity analysis, as well as insights on the child's engagement in participation, can help the team develop individualized support strategies. Likewise, practitioners should plan to attend IFSP and IEP meetings that include transition planning activities to provide their knowledge and recommendations. EI providers should offer their evaluations and recommendations to the next setting before the first day of school.

Because occupational therapy practitioners have a distinct expertise in understanding the relationship among person, occupation, and environment, they should actively contribute to the decision-making process in advocating for the least restrictive environment and inclusion. Practitioners should undertake a leadership role on IFSP and IEP teams to provide a justifiable rationale for an inclusive learning environment as well as for removing context-related barriers.

Occupational therapy practitioners can also support parents by encouraging them to identify questions they may have about the transition process and by encouraging parents to share those questions at transition meetings (Early Childhood Technical Assistance Center, 2018a). If the practitioner is able to visit the new classroom with the child and family before the transition, they will be able to provide suggestions for adapting and modifying the classroom environment; help the PS team make plans for transportation; and identify any potential concerns associated with the child's engagement, such as lunchtime in the cafeteria (Myers, 2006; Rous et al., 2007).

The relationship between the caregiver and the providers across all environments is crucial to a successful transition with positive child adjustment (Rosenkoetter et al., 2009). In locations where the occupational therapy practitioners work in both the EI and the PS programs, transition may be smoother for the family. Otherwise, the practitioner in the PS setting will contact the child's parents before the transition to initiate building a relationship.

If caseload assignments are not known until after the start of the school year, the occupational therapy practitioner should prioritize children who have recently transitioned to PS, because their need for occupational therapy services may be increased by the adjustment to the new setting. The school practitioner should work with the parents, teacher, and others on the special education team to support the child's engagement and participation in school activities. Assisting with environmental modifications, behavioral approaches, task adaptation, and assistive technology may help to improve the adjustment period and the child–teacher relationship. Ultimately, this may support positive outcomes in PS (Rous, 2008).

Preschool to kindergarten

Pretransition preparation in anticipation of changes in home routine, setting requirements, and family and child roles provides an important foundation for successful early school experiences (Gomez, 2016). PS settings emphasize school-readiness skills to prepare children for school. Academic and social expectations of kindergarten-age children have increased with a government focus on student performance and accountability. Occupational therapy practitioners provide critical assistance in identifying barriers to the child's participation and adjustment to the expectations of kindergarten.

According to Myers and Podvey (2019), the transition practices and strategies for the occupational therapy practitioner working in PS should center on improving child participation by

- Addressing the needs of the child before they transition to kindergarten by being aware of the expectations of kindergarten and making recommendations for

- adaptations and modifications to the environment and classroom materials;
- Helping the child learn skills needed for kindergarten through development of both environment-specific skills (e.g., hanging a backpack in a cubby) and executive functioning skills (e.g., self-regulation, problem solving);
- Supporting families through frequent communication about the transition, explaining parents' rights and the eligibility processes of programs, and encouraging visits to the new school and classroom; and
- Engaging in interprofessional communication with team members during transition planning meetings and IEP meetings.

SUMMARY

Many transitions occur during the early years for children and families. For children with disabilities, stress with change is typical; however, stress may be decreased through planning and active involvement from all team members. Occupational therapy practitioners have a distinct contribution to the team through their understanding of how occupational performance is influenced by changes in the environment and how child and family preparation can improve transition outcomes.

By using family-centered approaches that build capacity in natural environments, occupational therapy practitioners in EI programs help to prepare children and families for transitions to child care and PS programs. Practitioners in PS can promote a child's adjustment to the new classroom and school environment through activity analysis, adaptation, and modification. Practitioners in both EI and PS can decrease the stress of transition and enhance successful transitions by working with children and families to develop skills needed for the new environment, collaborating with team members, and communicating intentionally with caregivers to build a strong, supportive relationship.

REFERENCES

American Occupational Therapy Association. (2017). Guidelines for occupational therapy services in early intervention and schools. *American Journal of Occupational Therapy, 71*(Suppl. 2), 7106160010. https://doi.org/10.5014/ajot.2017.716S01

American Occupational Therapy Association. (2018). Occupational therapy's role in the neonatal intensive care unit. *American Journal of Occupational Therapy, 72*, 7212410060. https://doi.org/10.5014/ajot.2018.72S204

Breneol, S., Belliveau, J., Cassidy, C., & Curran, J. A. (2017). Strategies to support transitions from hospital to home for children with medical complexity: A scoping review. *International Journal of Nursing Studies, 72*, 91–104. https://doi.org/10.1016/j.ijnurstu.2017.04.011

Case-Smith, J. (2013). Systematic review of interventions to promote social–emotional development in young children with or at risk for disability. *American Journal of Occupational Therapy, 67*, 395–404. https://doi.org/10.5014/ajot.2013.004713

Center on the Developing Child, Harvard University. (2010). *The foundations of life long health are built in early childhood.* https://46y5eh11fhgw3ve3ytpwxt9r-wpengine.netdna-ssl.com/wp-content/uploads/2010/05/Foundations-of-Lifelong-Health.pdf

Center on the Developing Child, Harvard University. (2016). *From best practices to breakthrough impacts: A science-based approach to building a more promising future for young children and families.* https://46y5eh11fhgw3ve3ytpwxt9r-wpengine.netdna-ssl.com/wp-content/uploads/2016/05/From_Best_Practices_to_Breakthrough_Impacts-4.pdf

Colyvas, J., Sawyer, B., & Campbell, P. (2010). Identifying strategies early intervention occupational therapists use to teach caregivers. *American Journal of Occupational Therapy, 64*, 776–785. https://doi.org/10.5014/ajot.2010.09044

Diefendorf, M., & Lucas, A. (2010). *Federal IDEA Part C & Part B transition requirements for late referrals to IDEA Part C.* https://fpg.unc.edu/node/8952

Division for Early Childhood. (2014). *DEC recommended practices in early intervention/early childhood special education 2014.* https://www.dec-sped.org/dec-recommended-practices

Dusing, S. C., Tripathi, T., Marcinowski, E. C., Thacker, L. R., Brown, L. F., & Hendricks-Muñoz, K. D. (2018). Supporting play exploration and early developmental intervention versus usual care to enhance development outcomes during the transition from the neonatal intensive care unit to home: A pilot randomized controlled trial. *BMC Pediatrics, 18*, 46. https://doi.org/10.1186/s12887-018-1011-4

Early Childhood Technical Assistance Center. (2018a). *Practitioner practice guide: Transition from early intervention to preschool special education services.* https://ectacenter.org/pdfs/decrp/PGP_TRN2_eitopreschool_2018.pdf

Early Childhood Technical Assistance Center. (2018b). *Practitioner practice guide: Transition from hospital to home.* https://ectacenter.org/~pdfs/decrp/PGP_TRN1_hospitalto-home_2018.pdf

Fain, A., & Eason, D. (2016). Collaborating for seamless transitions from early childhood education into elementary schools in Tulsa, Oklahoma. *Voices in Urban Education, 43*, 15–21. https://files.eric.ed.gov/fulltext/EJ1101327.pdf

Ferretti, L., & Bub, K. (2017). Family routines and school readiness during the transitions to kindergarten. *Early Childhood Education and Development, 28*, 59–77. https://doi.org/10.1080/10409289.2016.1195671

Frolek Clark, G., & Kingsley, K. (2020). Occupational therapy practice guidelines for early childhood: Birth–5 years. *American Journal of Occupational Therapy, 74*, 7403397010. https://doi.org/10.5014/ajot.2020.743001

Gomez, R. (2016). Sustaining the benefits of early childhood education experiences: A research overview. *Voices in Urban Education, 43*, 5–14. https://files.eric.ed.gov/fulltext/EJ1101330.pdf

Grady, M. (2016). Supporting early education transitions: Alignment, collaboration, and community engagement. *Voices in Urban Education, 43*, 2–4. https://files.eric.ed.gov/fulltext/EJ1101420.pdf

Holloway, E., & Chandler, B. (2010). Family-centered practice: It's all about relationships. In B. Chandler (Ed.), *Early childhood: Services for children birth to five* (pp. 131–178). AOTA Press.

Improving Head Start for School Readiness Act of 2007, Pub. L. 110-134, 42 U.S.C.§ 9801 *et seq.*

Individuals With Disabilities Education Improvement Act of 2004, Pub. L. 108-446, 20 U.S.C.§ 1400–1482.

Johnson, K. (2019). *Medicaid financing for home visiting: The state of states' approaches.* https://ccf.georgetown.edu/wp-content/uploads/2019/01/Medicaid-and-Home-Visiting.pdf

Kang, J., Horn, E. M., & Palmer, S. (2017). Influences of family involvement in kindergarten transition activities on children's early school adjustment. *Early Childhood Education Journal, 45,* 789–800. https://doi.org/10.1007/s10643-016-0828-4

Kingsley, K., & Mailloux, Z. (2013). Evidence for the effectiveness of different service delivery models in early intervention services. *American Journal of Occupational Therapy, 67,* 431–436. https://doi.org/10.5014/ajot.2013.006171

Mann, T. D., Humd, A. M., Hesson-McInnis, M. S., & Roman, Z. J. (2016). Pathways to school readiness: Executive functioning predicts academic and social–emotional aspects of school readiness. *Mind, Brain and Education, 11,* 21–31. https://doi.org/10.1111/mbe.12134

McMullen, M. B., Yun, N. R., Mihai, A., & Kim, H. (2016). Experiences of parents and professionals in well-established continuity of care infant toddler programs. *Early Education and Development, 27,* 190–220. https://doi.org/10.1080/10409289.2016.1102016

Muhlenhaupt, M., de Sam Lazaro, S., Fabrizi, S., Schelkind, S., & Owens, A. (2019). Interprofessional core competencies to enhance occupational therapy services in early childhood settings. *OT Practice, 24*(3), 12–16. https://pdfs.semanticscholar.org/9695/0411eb6ee60592c294bc0098f8ef1a876412.pdf?_ga=2.205944080.2076357162.1598543529-940277187.1598543529

Myers, C. T. (2006). Exploring occupational therapy and transitions for young children with special needs. *Physical and Occupational Therapy in Pediatrics, 62,* 212–220. https://doi.org/10.1080/J006v26n03_06

Myers, C. T., & Podvey, M. (2019). Best practices in transition planning for preschoolers. In G. Frolek-Clark, J. E. Rioux, & B. E. Chandler (Eds.), *Best practices for occupational therapy in schools* (2nd ed., pp. 235–243). AOTA Press.

Myers, C. T., Schneck, C. M., Effgen, S. K., McCormick, K. M., & Shasby, S. B. (2011). Factors associated with therapists' involvement in children's transition to preschool. *American Journal of Occupational Therapy, 65,* 86–94. https://doi.org/10.5014/ajot.2011.09060

Podvey, M. C., Hinojosa, J., & Koenig, K. (2010). The transition experience to pre-school for six families with children with disabilities. *Occupational Therapy International, 17,* 177–187. https://doi.org/10.1002/oti.298

Podvey, M. C., & Myers, C. T. (2015). Early childhood transitions. In M. Orentlicher, R. Gibson, & S. Schefkind (Eds.), *Transitions across the lifespan* (pp. 51–80). AOTA Press.

Quirk, M., Dowdy, E., Goldstein, A., & Carnazzo, K. (2017). School readiness as a longitudinal predictor of social–emotional and reading performance across the elementary grades. *Assessment for Effective Instruction, 42,* 248–253. https://doi.org/10.1177/1534508417719680

Rosenkoetter, S., Schroeder, C., Rous, B., Hains, A., Shaw, J., & McCormick, K. (2009). *A review of research in early childhood transition: Child and family studies* (Technical Report No. 5). University of Kentucky, Human Development Institute, National Early Childhood Transition Center.

Rous, B. (2008). *Recommended transition practices for young children and families: Results from a national validation survey* (Technical Report No. 3). University of Kentucky, Human Development Institute, National Early Childhood Transition Center.

Rous, B., Myers, C., & Stricklin, S. (2007). Strategies for supporting transitions of young children with special needs and their families. *Journal of Early Intervention, 30,* 1–18. https://doi.org/10.1177/105381510703000102

Spittle, A., Orton, J., Anderson, P. J., Boyd, R., & Doyle, L. W. (2015). Early developmental intervention programmes provided post hospital discharge to prevent motor and cognitive impairment in preterm infants. *Cochrane Database of Systematic Reviews, 2015,* CD005495. https://doi.org/10.1002/14651858.CD005495.pub4

U.S. Department of Education, Office of Special Education Programs. (2016). *IDEA Section 618 data products: State level data files: 2016–2017 Part C exiting.* https://www2.ed.gov/programs/osepidea/618-data/state-level-data-files/index.html#ccc

Waters, C. L., & Friesen, A. (2019). Parent experiences of raising a young child with multiple disabilities: The transition to preschool. *Research and Practice for Persons With Severe Disabilities, 44,* 20–36. https://doi.org/10.1177/1540796919826229

Section II.

Knowledge Essential to Early Development

11

Brain Development in the Early Years

Stefanie C. Bodison, OTD, OTR/L

KEY TERMS AND CONCEPTS

- Associational systems
- Auditory receptors
- Autonomic nervous system
- Central nervous system
- Cognition
- Emotions
- Extreme stress
- Fear circuitry
- Fetal alcohol spectrum disorder
- Interoception
- Maternal nutrition
- Motor commands
- Motor systems
- Multisensory interactions
- Myelination
- Nasal chemoreceptors
- Neural circuits
- Neurodevelopment
- Neurodevelopmental perspective
- Neurons
- Neuroplasticity
- Parasympathetic responses
- Peripheral nervous system
- Proprioceptors
- Pruning
- Selective attention
- Sensory systems
- Somatosensory system
- Sympathetic nervous system responses
- Tactile receptors
- Taste receptors
- Toxicant
- Vestibular receptors
- Visual receptors

OVERVIEW

Occupational therapy practitioners possess specialized knowledge and skills to appreciate the complex interplay between person and environmental factors, and their impact on the development of childhood occupations (Case-Smith, 2013; Lane & Bundy, 2011; Law et al., 1996). (*Note. Occupational therapy practitioner* refers to both occupational therapists and occupational therapy assistants.) A broad understanding of neurodevelopment is foundational to support practitioners' ability to accurately assess the person-related factors driving and supporting social and environmental interactions.

Neurodevelopment, or neural development, "refers to the [biological] processes that generate, shape, and reshape the nervous system" ("Development of the nervous system," n.d.) from conception throughout the life course. Occupational therapy practitioners must integrate concepts from neuroscience, including genetics, anatomy, and systems physiology, to develop a "coherent understanding of brain structure and function" (Purves et al., 2012, p. 1). Practitioners must then use this knowledge to inform their analysis of the ways participation in childhood occupations might be affected.

From a *neurodevelopmental perspective* (i.e., involving the development of the nervous system), the trajectory of brain growth is well understood (Bodison et al., in press). As the scientific methods to document brain processes have evolved over time, occupational therapy practitioners' comprehension of the relationship between these neurodevelopmental processes and observable behaviors has become more refined (Casey et al., 2005; Lebel & Beaulieu, 2009; Luna et al., 2010; Squeglia et al., 2013). In practice, practitioners are rightly focused on supporting the development of skills to improve participation, but it is critical that they recognize the need to first understand, then potentially improve, the underlying neurodevelopmental processes that subserve the skills in which they are interested. Therefore, the purpose of this chapter is to provide an overview of structural and functional brain development in neurotypical and neurodiverse populations to support the clinical reasoning of practitioners working with children from ages birth to 5 years.

ESSENTIAL CONSIDERATIONS

Occupational therapy practitioners play a vital role in supporting the development of the foundational sensory, motor, emotional, social, attentional, and cognitive abilities that undergird childhood occupations. By first reflecting on the ways the brain develops in utero, practitioners are equipped to assess the relationship between individual person factors and prenatal insults that are likely to affect the development of functional skills and behaviors in early life. Additionally, the selection of theories and frames of reference to guide practice should be informed by the practitioner's understanding of brain development throughout the early years and the ways insults to this neurodevelopmental process can influence the child's interactions in the environment and with other people.

https://doi.org/10.7139/2021.978-1-56900-610-8.011

Current neuroscience theories suggest that neural systems are interrelated in the following ways:

Sensory systems represent information about the state of the organism and its environment; *motor systems* organize and generate actions; and *associational systems* link the sensory and motor components of the nervous system, providing the basis for "higher order" brain functions such as perception, attention, cognition, emotions, language, and rational thinking. (Purves et al., 2012, p. 1, bold and italics added)

For occupational therapy practitioners working with young children, an important concept to internalize centers on understanding that one neural system does not control or oversee the functions of the other; rather, these neural systems work collaboratively with one another to support the development of the child's complex social and environmental interactions.

Core Concepts of Neurodevelopment

Neurodevelopment begins at embryogenesis (i.e., embryonic development after fertilization; Purves et al., 2012) and is a result of gene expression. Multiple regulatory processes influence the expression and quantity of specific genes (Purves et al., 2012), but, essentially, neurodevelopment proceeds in a generally predictable way. *Neurons* are the building blocks of the nervous system and transmit all data throughout the entire nervous system. Neurons do not act in isolation; instead, they are organized into specific *neural circuits* that process distinct types of information (Purves et al., 2012).

These neural circuits are broadly organized within the peripheral nervous system (PNS) and central nervous system (CNS). The *PNS* includes the sensory receptors and sensory neurons that take relevant information about the body and the environment into the brain, as well as the motor system that sends signals from the brain to the muscles and organs, allowing interaction in the world (Purves et al., 2012). The *CNS* consists of the spinal cord and the brain, where processing and integration of all neural information occurs.

In utero, as the brain and spinal cord form, there is generation, proliferation, and migration of neurons that ultimately form the mature neural networks that undergird neurotypical processes (Gazzaniga et al., 2014). Throughout neurodevelopment, in utero and during the first years of life, there is continued *myelination* (i.e., formation of myelin around the axon) and *pruning* (i.e., process of eliminating extra neurons, synapses, and axons within the brain and nervous system) of neurons as the child interacts in the world, which assists the brain in developing refined, specific neural networks (Ayres, 2005; Kandel et al., 2013). Current theories in the neuroscience community, supported by research with both child and adult populations, assert that the human brain has the capacity to reorganize neural networks when there is damage (Kandel et al., 2013). This concept, known as *neuroplasticity,* is an underlying theoretical principle that has informed and will continue to enhance the development of rehabilitation interventions provided by occupational therapy practitioners working with young children.

Brain development in utero

The core neurodevelopmental processes described above begin in utero. For occupational therapy practitioners working with young children, the most important thing to consider about brain development in utero is that there are critical periods when specific neural structures are formed, and this development can be influenced by genetic factors or exposure to toxicants.

Most sensory structures are fully developed at birth, but their complex functional development continues during the first weeks and months of life. For most neural structures of the brain, the developmental trajectory represented for the sensory systems here occurs similarly. At birth, all of the major brain structures are present, but their individual capacity and complex interconnectedness continue to develop, with ongoing cellular growth and pruning processes, as the infant (and, later, the young child) interacts with the environment and the people surrounding them.

Impact of maternal nutrition and extreme stress on brain development in utero

There is a growing body of research linking poor *maternal nutrition* and extreme stress to changes in neurodevelopmental outcomes. Morrison and Regnault (2016) noted that "poor maternal nutritional intake after the periconceptional period during pregnancy can negatively impact fetal genetic growth trajectory and can result in fetal growth restriction" (p. 1). As early as 22 days after conception, the neural plates are forming the neural tube (which becomes the brain and spinal cord). Division of the cells within the neural tube, which occurs 7 weeks after conception, creates nerve cells and glial cells. Axon and dendrite growth and the formation of synapses occur next. Research has shown that these processes, which lead to brain development, are susceptive to extreme maternal stress and nutrient deficiencies, including severe acute malnutrition, chronic undernutrition, iron deficiency, and iodine deficiency (Prado & Dewey, 2014).

Depending on when the malnutrition or *extreme stress* (e.g., abuse, financial concerns, housing insecurity) occurs during pregnancy, these may cause ineffective transport of nutrients and oxygen to the fetus through the placenta, resulting in low birthweight (Zhang et al., 2015), increased risk of cardiovascular disease because of the effects of protein restriction (Zohdi et al., 2015), and influences on the development of other organs. Higher systolic blood pressure in childhood may be linked to poor maternal diet (Blumfield et al., 2015).

Brain recovery or neural plasticity is influenced by the timing and degree of the deprivation as well as the child's environment and experience (Prado & Dewey, 2014). Although there are not yet specific practice guidelines or policies influencing referrals to occupational therapy practitioners for developmental assessment, young children whose mothers were malnourished or experienced extremely stressful conditions while pregnant may have delays in motor or cognitive development that could alter their ability to participate fully in childhood occupations.

Prenatal exposure to toxicants

A *toxicant* is "a poison that is made by humans or that is put into the environment by human activities" ("Toxicant," n.d., para. 1). Although all human development can be negatively affected by exposure to toxicants, prenatal exposure to toxicants in utero is especially damaging to the developing brain. Anything experienced by the maternal respiratory, circulatory, or digestive systems influences the developing fetus. There are multiple ways toxicant exposures can be categorized, but, generally speaking, environmental toxicants include lead, pesticides, and other air pollutants; inhaled toxicants include cigarettes, marijuana, and other psychoactive substances that can be smoked; ingestible toxicants include some drugs prescribed for medicinal purposes, alcohol, and illicit drugs; and injectable toxicants include pharmacological agents used for medical purposes and psychoactive illicit drugs.

In the United States, the Centers for Disease Control and Prevention [CDC] and other national agencies have worked intensely to educate the general public about the effects of inhaled, ingestible, and injectable toxicants on the developing fetus (CDC, 2019). Presently, multiple research efforts are underway to study the effects of environmental toxicants on the developing brain (Lebel et al., 2008), which may significantly influence national policies about exposure to environmental toxicants.

When working with young children who may have experienced prenatal exposure to toxicants, occupational therapy practitioners should consider the type and amount of toxicant exposure experienced and when the exposure occurred during prenatal development (if known). Often, the amount or timing of the exposure is unknown, but, as previously described, there are critical periods of brain development that could be influenced differently depending on the type of toxicant exposure and when the exposure occurred. Regardless, practitioners should be prepared to assess any of the neurodevelopmental areas described in this section, because they all could be negatively influenced by prenatal toxicant exposure.

One common condition resulting from prenatal alcohol exposure is *fetal alcohol spectrum disorder* (FASD). Current research indicates that the neurodevelopment issues experienced by children with FASD include problems with emotion regulation, poor inhibition, difficulty with working memory, and delayed fine and gross motor abilities (Doney et al., 2014; Jirikowic, Kartin, & Olson, 2008; Jirikowic, Olson, & Kartin, 2008). For more information, see Chapter 39, "Best Practices Supporting Families of Children With Prenatal Substance Exposure and Postnatal Trauma."

Development of the Autonomic Nervous System

The *autonomic nervous system* (ANS) is composed of the sympathetic and parasympathetic branches, which work synergistically to control the neural and hormonal regulation of homeostatic functions (Gazzaniga et al., 2014). Generally speaking, *sympathetic nervous system responses* have an arousing effect on the visceral structures of the body (e.g., heart, lungs, gastrointestinal tract), whereas *parasympathetic responses* have a calming effect on the same visceral structures.

In neurotypical children and adults, the ANS has the capacity to stimulate the sympathetic branch when necessary while automatically balancing out this autonomic response with the activation of the parasympathetic branch. The brain structures most responsible for activating the ANS include the thalamus, limbic system, and hypothalamus (Kandel et al., 2013). It is important for occupational therapy practitioners to remember that the functions of the ANS occur automatically, outside of conscious control. As is highlighted throughout this chapter, the ANS is likely to be influenced by or involved in sensory processing, emotion regulation, attentional processes, and cognitive processes, so practitioners should consider each of these when they suspect that a young child's ANS is overactive.

Development of the Sensory Systems and Sensory Processing

Humans are constantly bombarded by sensory data that the brain processes and integrates to aid in the development of attentional processes, emotion regulation, perception, and action (Ayres, 2005; Bremner et al., 2012). At present, the medical and scientific communities have identified and explicated the structure and function of the sensory systems: tactile, proprioceptive, vestibular, visual, auditory, gustatory, and olfactory. Each sensory system consists of specialized receptors designed to detect and transform data from the body and environment into electrical signals interpretable by the brain (Bremner et al., 2012; Kandel et al., 2013). Each receptor is connected to specialized sensory neurons that transmit the sensory data to the CNS, where they are processed and integrated in both unimodal (one type of sensory information) and multimodal ways in specific areas of the brain (Bremner et al., 2012; Kandel et al., 2013). Leading scientific inquiry about sensory processing theorizes that the senses provide complementary information about the body and the environment for humans to form a comprehensive understanding of the world and their place in it (Ayres, 2005; Bremner et al., 2012).

When working with young children, occupational therapy practitioners must have a basic understanding of the structure and function of the sensory systems, the primary areas in the brain where the sensory information is processed and integrated, and the functions influenced by the incoming sensory experiences. Generally speaking, all sensory information except olfaction passes through the brainstem and interacts with the reticular activating and limbic systems, with the potential to contribute to the emotion regulation, alerting, and arousing functions of the nervous system as well as basic motor functions, such as breathing and postural responses. These facts are not repeated for each of the specific sensory systems as they are reviewed in this section, but it is important for practitioners to keep in mind that the processing of sensory experiences could significantly affect the child's arousal and ANS responses. The review provided below is not meant to be exhaustive, and only major brain structures and functions are highlighted.

Tactile system

Tactile receptors are located all over every inch of skin and inside the mouth. There are many types of tactile receptors that are designed to detect temperature, pain, light touch, deep touch, vibration, and movement across the skin. The primary areas in the brain where tactile information is processed and integrated include the thalamus, limbic system, somatosensory cortex, posterior parietal cortex, and association areas.

The information detected by the tactile receptors keeps the child safe from noxious or harmful stimuli and helps them understand the intensity, quality, and nature of what they are touching. Functionally, the tactile system contributes to the young child's ability to develop an accurate body schema, motor planning, in-hand manipulation and fine motor abilities, and oral motor skills (Ayres, 2005; Bremner et al., 2012). Additionally, varying types of touch can have either an alerting or a calming effect on the child's nervous system, and touch is often closely associated with emotional connectivity with others (Ayres, 2005; Gazzaniga et al., 2014).

Proprioceptive system

Proprioceptors are located in the muscles, tendons, and joints and include the muscle spindle and Golgi tendon organ. These receptors are designed to detect the change in the tension–length relationship of the muscle belly, muscle isometric contractions, and tendon stretch that occurs when the muscle is near end range. In the brain, the primary areas where proprioceptive input is processed and integrated include the cerebellum, thalamus, somatosensory cortex, posterior parietal cortex, and association areas, which perform the integration. Functionally, the proprioceptors provide information about the force exerted by the muscles of the body, joint position sense, limb movement, and the co-contraction of muscles during weight-bearing and weight-shifting activities (Ayres, 2005; Kandel et al., 2013).

Vestibular system

Vestibular receptors are located inside the interior auditory canal of each ear. Otoliths detect gravity in the saccule, whereas linear horizontal movement is detected in the utricle. The three semicircular canals within each ear are oriented in three planes of motion and are stimulated when the head undergoes any type of angular movement. Vestibular information travels along cranial nerve VIII into the brainstem, where it is processed and integrated in the vestibular nuclei, the vestibulocerebellum, and the posterior parietal cortex.

Functionally, the vestibular system contributes to the young child's ability to automatically and consciously dissociate head and eye movements, develop postural and balance reactions, coordinate the two sides of the body, and develop a three-dimensional spatial reference that will allow them to effectively navigate the environment (Gazzaniga et al., 2014). Additionally, varying types of vestibular input can have either an alerting or a calming effect on the child's nervous system. In particular, slow, linear, rhythmic vestibular input is calming, whereas fast, dysrhythmic movement is alerting (Ayres, 2005).

Visual system

Visual receptors are housed inside the eyes and include the rods and cones, which detect light and color. The primary brain areas responsible for processing and integrating visual information include the primary visual cortex, occipital cortex, posterior parietal lobe, superior temporal sulcus, and anterior inferior temporal cortex. The functions of the visual system include seeing what and where something is, developing a perception of what is being seen, and honing depth and visual topographical skills to aid in navigating the environment (Kandel et al., 2013).

Auditory system

Auditory receptors are located inside the cochlea, which is housed in the internal auditory canal. The auditory system transforms sound waves into electrical signals that travel along cranial nerve VIII into the brainstem. The brain areas that process and integrate auditory information include the thalamus, left temporal cortex, inferior parietal lobe, left inferior frontal cortex, and left insular cortex (Kandel et al., 2013). Functionally, the auditory system supports the development of the young child's expressive and receptive language abilities and assists in the perception of environmental auditory stimuli to support navigation (Kandel et al., 2013; Purves et al., 2012).

Gustatory system

The gustatory or **taste receptors** are located in the tongue and are systematically organized to detect sour, bitter, salty, and sweet sensations (Gazzaniga et al., 2014). The brain areas that process and integrate taste sensations include the thalamus and the limbic system. Functionally, the gustatory system contributes to the perception of taste and the strong emotional connections humans make to these tastes and various foods (Gazzaniga et al., 2014).

Olfactory system

The olfactory system includes **nasal chemoreceptors** in the olfactory bulb that have a direct connection to the limbic system in the brain. The limbic system is one of the phylogenetically oldest structures in the brain and helps the nervous system learn what is safe versus unsafe. One of the major functions of the olfactory system is to immediately develop the mother–infant bond that begins with first contact (Ayres, 2005; Gazzaniga et al., 2014). Additionally, the olfactory system supports the perception of taste and helps the young child identify foods and other people in the environment (Gazzaniga et al., 2014) through smell.

Multisensory integration

Many of the sensory systems work closely together in complementary ways. In fact, the structure and functions of the tactile and proprioceptive systems are often combined and called the **somatosensory system.** Although it is outside the scope of this chapter to detail the most commonly understood and studied **multisensory interactions,** many of people's daily functions are influenced by visual and auditory associations; tactile, proprioceptive, and vestibular interactions; and olfactory and gustatory combinations. Young children are multisensory beings living in a complex world, and their brain devotes the first months of life to making sense of the unimodal and multimodal sensory data to build a foundation on which higher level, more complex perceptual and motor skills can be built (Ayres, 2005; Bremner et al., 2012).

Interoception

Interoception allows the individual to perceive internal bodily states, such as their heartbeat, intestinal discomfort, and the urge to go to the bathroom (Critchley, 2009; Gazzaniga et al., 2014; Pollatos et al., 2007). The area of the brain thought to support interoception is the insular cortex, where it is hypothesized that all visceral and somatic input is integrated to form a representation of the individual's internal state of the body (Craig, 2009; Gazzaniga et al., 2014). Research by Critchley (2009) hypothesized a close connection among interoception, the activation of the insular cortex, and the processing of emotions. In particular, this research suggested that the ability to accurately identify one's own emotions is directly tied to one's ability to perceive internal bodily states. Although the mechanisms of interoception are not yet fully understood, occupational therapy practitioners should consider the role poor interoception may play for children who have difficulty toileting or otherwise relying on internal states to know when and when not to eat.

Motor Development

The *motor commands* that guide action originate in the frontal lobe, in the premotor and supplementary motor cortices. Once the motor commands have been generated, they are simultaneously transmitted to the primary motor cortex, basal ganglia, and cerebellum (Kandel et al., 2013). Through a variety of interactions in these subcortical structures, the motor commands are sent to the motor neurons and, ultimately, muscles of the body, through spinal connections. Specific muscle movement occurs when the motor commands from the brain stimulate the skeletal muscles in organized ways.

When there is damage to any of the aforementioned motor centers, muscle control is likely to be disordered. For example, research across various clinical populations has illuminated that damage to the cerebellum can produce ataxic or dysrhythmic motor movements (Schmahmann, 2004), and irregular functioning in the basal ganglia can cause excessive tonal responses, such as spasticity and dystonia (Neychev et al., 2008; Vitek et al., 1999).

When working with young children who have problems with motor control, occupational therapy practitioners must be able to apply professional reasoning to understand how the known or suspected underlying neurodevelopmental issue is associated with the functional behaviors observed. Only when practitioners are able to accurately theorize connections between brain centers and motor responses will they be able to select the best assessments and interventions to guide therapeutic interactions and improve function. For example, for a child with cerebral palsy who experiences spasticity when moving, the practitioner should reason that the problems with motor control are likely a result of disordered processes in the basal ganglia and cerebellum and therefore not related to poor

sensory processing. When they conceptualize in this way on the basis of a comprehensive understanding of neuroscience, the practitioner should professionally reason that the best assessment and intervention choices for this child are grounded in motor learning theories rather than sensory integration theory.

Development of Selective Attention

Selective attention is the ability to prioritize and cognitively focus on relevant inputs, thoughts, and actions while ignoring irrelevant or distracting ones (Gazzaniga et al., 2014). *Arousal,* in contrast, refers to the global physiological state of the organism and can be described as a continuum from asleep to hyperaroused (as in a fear state; Gazzaniga et al., 2014). Researchers have theorized that individuals can maintain selective attention in spite of their arousal state, but the ease at which they can most productively attend is influenced by the state of arousal (Gazzaniga et al., 2014). The brain centers that are involved in attentional processes include the pulvinar of the thalamus, superior colliculus, temporal–parietal junction, posterior parietal lobe, superior prefrontal lobe, and ventral prefrontal lobe (Gazzaniga et al., 2014; Kandel et al., 2013).

Recent research has illuminated that several conditions affecting selective attention (e.g., attention-deficit disorder, both inattentive and hyperactive types) are likely a result of neurochemical differences in the aforementioned brain attentional networks. Research of this nature assists occupational therapy practitioners in recognizing when neurodevelopmental processes affecting participation might or might not be significantly altered through occupational therapy intervention directed at improving underlying neural networks. In fact, when the practitioner reasons that the attentional problem is related to disordered neurochemical processes rather than sensory processing, the assessment and intervention approaches might be based on the use of cognitive or educational strategies rather than sensory integration theory.

Development of Emotions

Emotions are defined as "valanced responses [pleasure–displeasure] to external stimuli and/or internal mental representations that . . . [consist of] . . . a physiologic reaction to a stimulus, a behavioral response, and a feeling" (Gazzaniga et al., 2014, p. 427). Although it is clear to scientists that multiple neural circuits are involved in processing emotions, the thalamus, limbic system, hypothalamus, orbitofrontal cortex, and corpus callosum likely play major roles (Gazzaniga et al., 2014). Emotional stimuli, which come from either external events or memories, are "highly relevant for the well-being and survival" (Gazzaniga et al., 2014, p. 428) of the individual and therefore can influence the development of higher order functions, such as cognition and implicit (i.e., hidden) or explicit (i.e., known) learning processes.

During development, as the child interacts with the environment and the individuals in it and, for example, experiences a dangerous encounter, their brain associates a physiologic response (increased ANS response) with a flight-or-fight reaction and feelings of fear. Similar processes occur when the emotional stimulus is one of pleasure.

Over time, the child learns to consciously manage or self-regulate their emotional responses in socially acceptable ways, depending on the stimulus and context.

With this global understanding of how the brain develops emotions, occupational therapy practitioners are better able to professionally reason potential underlying causes for the emotional disturbances sometimes experienced by young children. This should broaden practitioners' perspective and keep them from assuming that a child with negative emotions or poor self-regulation is purposefully seeking to be "naughty."

Foundations of Cognitive Development

In the neuroscience community, *cognition* "refers to the ability to attend to external stimuli or internal motivations; to identify the significance of such stimuli; and to make appropriate responses" (Purves et al., 2012, p. 587). This definition, although broad, helps occupational therapy practitioners working with children from age birth–5 years conceptualize the various units of skills that are needed as a foundation to cognitive development. For example, before infants can identify the significance of external stimuli, they must first learn about the sensory characteristics of the external stimuli, relate the external stimuli to themselves, recognize that they can act on the stimuli (cause and effect), and, ultimately, remember that their actions have value and meaning.

The primary brain structures that assist in developing these cognitive processes include the association areas of the cortex, which receive and integrate information from the sensory and motor cortices, the thalamus, and the brainstem (Gazzaniga et al., 2014; Kandel et al., 2013). Given the involvement of these various neurodevelopmental structures, it should be clear to occupational therapy practitioners that very young children are essentially developing the foundation for cognition through the enhancement of the sensory and motor systems. Only through interaction with the environment and the people in it can children develop their own perceptual abilities and recognize that their physical actions can influence things around them. Practitioners working with young children are integral in supporting the neurodevelopment of sensory and motor functions that serve as the foundation for high-order cognitive and executive functions (e.g., learning, prereading, prewriting).

BEST PRACTICES

Various factors can significantly alter the developing brain and influence the child's developmental trajectory. Some neurodevelopmental conditions are congenital; others are acquired over the young child's life. It is important that occupational therapy practitioners have a clear understanding of how the brain might be altered by the various neurodevelopmental conditions, because each could influence the theoretical model and frames of reference the practitioner chooses to assess the child's abilities and design an intervention.

As is now well understood and valued, developing children's abilities are a product of both their neurological makeup and the social and environmental interactions experienced over time. Although neurodevelopment often proceeds in a predictable way, variations in structure and function of the brain can influence social and environmental interactions. The purpose of the following section is to help occupational therapy practitioners consider the ways behaviors might be differently shaped by specific types of neurodiverse brain development.

The development of the brain is influenced by many factors, including a child's relationships, experiences, and environment. The first 8 years of a child's life build a foundation for future health and development. The cumulative impact of early experiences, both positive and negative, on a child's development can be profound (Robinson et al., 2017). See Chapter 29, "Best Practices in Supporting Learning and Early Literacy Skills (Cognitive Skills)," for additional evidence-based interventions to enhance cognitive development, including learning and executive functioning.

Identify Families and Children With Needs and Make Appropriate Referrals

Occupational therapy practitioners work with many children and caregivers. Understanding the family's resources is as critical as identifying their priorities and concerns. For example, if a parent has lost their job and the family is unable to make home payments, they may end up homeless. Referring them to appropriate agencies is essential to the health of the family.

Collaborate Across Systems to Support Brain Development

Although the health care, social services, and education systems that serve young children and their families provide opportunities to support responsive relationships and environments that support brain development, efforts by these systems are often fragmented. Integrating relationship-based prevention and intervention services for children early in life, when the brain is developing most rapidly, can optimize developmental trajectories (Robinson et al., 2017).

Support Cutting-Edge Science to Enhance Healthy Development

In 2016, the Center on the Developing Child at Harvard University published a paper based on insights from cutting-edge science to support healthy development among vulnerable children. These concepts are discussed in more detail in this section.

Build responsible relationships and positive experiences in environments

"Experiences affect the nature and quality of the brain's developing architecture by influencing which circuits are reinforced and which are pruned due to lack of use" (Center of the Developing Child, Harvard University, 2016, p. 8). These experiences can turn genes on and off (e.g., well-functioning immune system). Without responsible interaction from caregivers, the child's developing brain may weaken (Center on the Developing Child, Harvard University, 2016).

To create positive relationships, decrease the risk of obesity, and increase the quality of evening sleep, the American Academy of Pediatrics (AAP; 2018) recommends that children younger than 2 years avoid digital media, other than video chatting, and that children ages 2–5 years watch only 1 hour of high-quality children's programming daily. Interaction between the child and caregiver during the screen time builds positive relationships rather than decreasing development in the long run (AAP, 2018).

Occupational therapy practitioners can assist in positive experiences among the family, caregivers, and child. For example, after constant morning sickness and lethargy during a high-risk pregnancy, a mother gave birth to three children who had various medical conditions, one severe enough to require in-home nursing service. During the home visit, the occupational therapy practitioner observed that the mother did not interact with any of her children but sat in a chair staring outside, while a respite worker and a home nurse cared for the children. Every week, the practitioner came to work with the children and specifically focused on engaging the mother during the session by giving positive feedback and requesting assistance (e.g., hold one child). Soon the mother was meeting the practitioner at the door to describe new skills she was seeing during her interactions with her children.

Decrease adversity and stressors

Environments with supportive adults may block children's stress-response systems to prevent stress hormones and keep biological functions in check. However, children experiencing child abuse or neglect, violence, extreme poverty, family turmoil, and other hardships or trauma can become hyperresponsive to adversity, and these experiences are associated with increased physical and mental health issues (Center on the Developing Child, Harvard University, 2016). This *fear circuitry* in the brain activates the fight-or-flight response, increases the chance of perceiving and focusing attention on potential threats, and may lead to a low sense of self-efficacy. Findings indicate that "deprivation, neglect, or emotional abuse . . . can cause more harm to a young child's development, with effects including subsequent cognitive delays, impairments in executive functioning, and increased risk of a wide range of health problems over a lifetime" (Center on the Developing Child, Harvard University, 2016, p. 7). Occupational therapy practitioners can support and model nurturing, capacity-building experiences for caregivers, which will enhance a child's positive outcomes.

Promote positive relationships to build children's resilience

Developing new skills or behaviors early, before brain circuits have been wired, is important. Research also supports that having at least one stable and responsible relationship with an adult, no matter the hardship the child has experienced, helps children develop the ability to respond to adversity and thrive (Center on the Developing Child, Harvard University, 2016; Dicker & Gordon, 2004). Occupational therapy practitioners work closely with children and their caregivers. Promoting family strengths and positive relationships is necessary to support positive lifetime outcomes.

Support a set of core life skills for adults

Research indicates that adults' core life skills include their self-regulation and executive functions. Results from poor core life skills may include poor planning, focus, self-control, awareness, and flexibility (Center on the Developing Child, Harvard University, 2016). By creating more positive environments and providing coaching or training in specific self-regulation or executive functions, occupational therapy practitioners assist adults in developing and using these skills, which may relieve some of the key stressors. For example, a parent who is overwhelmed with managing their child with attention deficit hyperactivity disorder may benefit from calming strategies, assistance in setting up a waking routine to decrease the stress of getting to preschool on time, and strategies for reinforcing positive behavior.

SUMMARY

Best practice requires that occupational therapy practitioners who work with young children have a comprehensive understanding of brain development and consider how varying conditions might alter developmental trajectories. This knowledge will influence the selection of theories and frames of reference practitioners use to guide assessment and intervention procedures. By infusing their practice with knowledge about the underlying neurodevelopmental processes that support participation in childhood occupations, occupational therapy practitioners will be best prepared to significantly, positively affect young children's development.

RESOURCES

- ◾ *Brain Facts: A Primer on the Brain and Nervous System:* https://www.brainfacts.org/the-brain-facts-book
  A free, downloadable resource describing brain structure and function
- ◾ **Centers for Disease Control and Prevention:** https://www.cdc.gov/ncbddd/childdevelopment/early-brain-development.html
  Information on early brain development and health
- ◾ **Center on the Developing Child, Harvard University:** https://developingchild.harvard.edu/resources/inbrief-applying-the-science-of-child-development-in-child-welfare-systems/
  Information on child development
- ◾ **ZERO TO THREE:** https://www.zerotothree.org/espanol/brain-development
  Information on brain development

REFERENCES

American Academy of Pediatrics. (2018). *Children and media tips from the American Academy of Pediatrics.* https://www.aap.org/en-us/advocacy-and-policy/aap-health-initiatives/Pages/Media-and-Children.aspx

Ayres, A. J. (2005). *Sensory integration and the child.* Western Psychological Services.

Blumfield, M., Nowson, C., Hure, A., Smith, R., Simpson, S., Raubenheimer, D., . . . Collins, C. (2015). Lower protein-to-carbohydrate ratio in maternal diet is associated with higher childhood systolic blood pressure up to age four years. *Nutrients, 7,* 3078–3093. https://doi.org/10.3390/nu7053078

Bodison, S. C., Colby, J., & Sowell, E. R. (in press). Structural brain development: Birth through adolescence. In J. Rubenstein & P. Rakic (Eds.), *Neural circuit and cognitive development* (Vol 2). Elsevier.

Bremner, A. J., Lewkowicz, D. J., & Spence, C. (2012). The multisensory approach to development. In A. Bremner, D. Lwekowicz, & C. Spence (Eds.), *Multisensory development* (pp. 1–26). Oxford University Press.

Case-Smith, J. (2013). Development of childhood occupations. In J. Case-Smith & J. C. O'Brien (Eds.), *Occupational therapy for children* (pp. 56–83). Mosby.

Casey, B. J., Tottenham, N., Liston, C., & Durston, S. (2005). Imaging the developing brain: What have we learned about cognitive development? *Trends in Cognitive Sciences, 9,* 104–110. https://doi.org/10.1016/j.tics.2005.01.011

Center on the Developing Child, Harvard University. (2016). *Applying the science of child development in child welfare systems.* https://developingchild.harvard.edu/resources/child-welfare-systems/

Centers for Disease Control and Prevention. (2019, July 24). *Substance use during pregnancy.* https://www.cdc.gov/reproductivehealth/maternalinfanthealth/substance-abuse/substance-abuse-during-pregnancy.htm

Craig, A. D. (2009). How do you feel—now? The anterior insula and human awareness. *Nature Reviews Neuroscience, 10,* 59–70. 10.1038/nrn2555

Critchley, D. H. (2009). Psychophysiology of neural, cognitive, and affective integration: fMRI and autonomic indicants. *International Journal of Psychophysiology, 73,* 88–94. https://doi.org/10.1016/j.ijpsycho.2009.01.012

Development of the nervous system. (n.d.). In *Wikipedia.* https://en.wikipedia.org/wiki/Development_of_the_nervous_system

Dicker, S., & Gordon, E. (2004). *Ensuring the healthy development of infants in foster care: A guide for judges, advocates and child welfare professionals.* ZERO TO THREE Policy Center.

Doney, R., Lucas, B. R., Jones, T., Howat, P., Sauer, K., & Elliott, E. J. (2014). Fine motor skills in children with prenatal alcohol exposure or fetal alcohol spectrum disorder. *Journal of Developmental & Behavioral Pediatrics, 35,* 598–609. https://doi.org/10.1097/DBP.0000000000000107

Gazzaniga, M. S., Ivry, R. B., & Mangun, G. R. (2014). *Cognitive neuroscience: The biology of the mind.* Norton.

Jirikowic, T., Kartin, D., & Olson, H. C. (2008). Children with fetal alcohol spectrum disorders: A descriptive profile of adaptive function. *Canadian Journal of Occupational Therapy, 75,* 238–248. https://doi.org/10.1177/000841740807500411

Jirikowic, T., Olson, H. C., & Kartin, D. (2008). Sensory processing, school performance, and adaptive behavior of young school-age children with fetal alcohol spectrum disorders. *Physical & Occupational Therapy in Pediatrics, 28,* 117–136. https://doi.org/10.1080/01942630802031800

Kandel, E. R., Schwartz, J. H., Jessell, T. M., Siegelbaum, S. A., & Hudspeth, A. J. (2013). *Principles of neural science* (5th ed.). McGraw-Hill.

Lane, S. J., & Bundy, A. C. (2011). *Kids can be kids: A childhood occupations approach.* F.A. Davis.

Law, M., Cooper, B., Strong, S., Stewart, D., Rigby, P., & Letts, L. (1996). The Person–Environment–Occupation Model: A transactive approach to occupational performance. *Canadian Journal of Occupational Therapy, 63,* 9–23. https://doi.org/10.1177/000841749606300103

Lebel, C., & Beaulieu, C. (2009). Lateralization of the arcuate fasciculus from childhood to adulthood and its relation to cognitive abilities in children. *Human Brain Mapping, 30,* 3563–3573. https://doi.org/10.1002/hbm.20779

Lebel, C., Rasmussen, C., Wyper, K., Walker, L., Andrew, G., Yager, J., & Beaulieu, C. (2008). Brain diffusion abnormalities in children with fetal alcohol spectrum disorder. *Alcoholism: Clinical and Experimental Research, 32,* 1732–1740. https://doi.org/10.1111/j.1530-0277.2008.00750.x

Luna, B., Padmanabhan, A., & O'Hearn, K. (2010). What has fMRI told us about the development of cognitive control through adolescence? *Brain and Cognition, 72,* 101–113. https://doi.org/10.1016/j.bandc.2009.08.005

Morrison, J., & Regnault, T. (2016). Nutrition in pregnancy: Optimising maternal diet and fetal adaptations to altered nutrient supply. *Nutrients, 8,* 342. https://doi.org/10.3390/nu8060342

Neychev, V. K., Fan, X., Mitev, V. I., Hess, E. J., & Jinnah, H. A. (2008). The basal ganglia and cerebellum interact in the expression of dystonic movement. *Brain, 131,* 2499–2509. https://doi.org/10.1093/brain/awn168

Pollatos, O., Gramann, K., & Schandry, R. (2007). Neural systems connecting interoceptive awareness and feelings. *Human Brain Mapping, 28,* 9–18. https://doi.org/10.1002/hbm.20258

Prado, E., & Dewey, K. (2014). Nutrition and brain development in early life. *Nutrition Reviews, 72,* 267–284. https://doi.org/10.1111/nure.12102

Purves, D., Augustine, G. J., Fitzpatrick, D., Hall, W. C., LaMantia, A., & White, L. E. (2012). *Neuroscience* (5th ed.). Sinauer.

Robinson, L., Bitsko, R., Thompson, R., Dworkin, P., McCabe, M., Peacock, G., & Thorpe, P. (2017). CDC grand rounds: Addressing health disparities in early childhood. *Morbidity and Mortality Weekly Report, 66,* 769–772. https://doi.org/10.15585/mmwr.mm6629a1

Schmahmann, J. D. (2004). Disorders of the cerebellum: Ataxia, dysmetria of thought, and the cerebellar cognitive affective syndrome. *Journal of Neuropsychiatry and Clinical Neurosciences, 16,* 367–378. https://doi.org/10.1176/jnp.16.3.367

Squeglia, L. M., Jacobus, J., Sorg, S. F., Jernigan, T. L., & Tapert, S. F. (2013). Early adolescent cortical thinning is related to better neuropsychological performance. *Journal of the International Neuropsychological Society, 19,* 962–970. https://doi.org/10.1017/S1355617713000878

Toxicant. (n.d.). In *National Cancer Institute Dictionary of Cancer Terms.* https://www.cancer.gov/publications/dictionaries/cancer-terms/def/toxicant

Vitek, J. L., Chockkan, V., Zhang, J. Y., Kaneoke, Y., Evatt, M., DeLong, M. R., . . . Bakay, R. A. (1999). Neuronal activity in the basal ganglia in patients with generalized dystonia and hemiballismus. *Annals of Neurology, 46,* 22–35. https://doi.org/10.1002/1531-8249(199907)46:1<22::aid-ana6>3.0.co;2-z

Zhang, S., Regnault, T., Barker, P., Botting, K., McMillen, I., McMillan, C., . . . Morrison, J. (2015). Placental adaptations in growth restriction. *Nutrients, 7,* 360–389. https://doi.org/10.3390/nu7010360

Zohdi, V., Lim, K., Pearson, J., & Black, M. (2015). Developmental programming of cardiovascular disease following intrauterine growth restriction: Findings utilising a rat model of maternal protein restriction. *Nutrients, 7,* 119–152. https://doi.org/10.3390/nu7010119

Early Childhood Mental Health

Kris Pizur-Barnekow, PhD, OTR/L, IMH–E®, and Stephan Viehweg, LCSW, ACSW, IMH–E®, CYC-P

12

KEY TERMS AND CONCEPTS

- Adverse childhood experiences
- Co-occupational engagement
- Distal relationships
- Early childhood mental health
- Healthy working alliance
- Intentional Relationship Model
- Learn the Signs. Act Early. campaign
- PAUSE method
- Perinatal posttraumatic stress disorder
- Postpartum depression
- Proximal relationships
- Reflective practices
- Relationship
- Relationship-centered practices
- Substance use disorder
- Therapeutic use of self

OVERVIEW

Mental health is at the heart of occupational therapy practice and is historically rooted in the foundational years of the profession's development (Kielhofner & Burke, 1977). During the early 1900s, humanistic moral treatment was developed in response to the inhumane treatment of people with mental illness in asylums (Kielhofner & Burke, 1977). More recently, the American Occupational Therapy Association's (AOTA's) *Occupational Therapy Practice Guidelines for Mental Health Promotion, Prevention, and Intervention for Children and Youth* (Bazyk & Arbesman, 2013) outlined occupational therapy's role in early childhood mental health. Although this area of practice is becoming more widely accepted, addressing complexities of families and meeting families where they are require knowledge, skills, and professional behaviors that embrace relationship-centered and reflective practices.

Early Childhood Mental Health Development

Relationship-centered practices (i.e., using a relationship with parents to effect change) and *reflective practices* (i.e., using reflection to improve thinking and enhance skills) are key in the prevention of early childhood mental health disorders and the promotion of early childhood mental health (Tomlin & Viehweg, 2016). *Early childhood mental health,* or the developing capacity of children ages birth–5 years to explore the environment, cope with routine daily stressors, express emotions, and develop relationships and learn, affects many developmental domains (ZERO TO THREE, 2020). Young children who possess the ability to develop physically, cognitively, and socially so that they can cope during difficult events or times are considered mentally healthy (Centers for Disease Control and Prevention [CDC], 2019a).

In early childhood, children's mental health develops through nurturing and responsive relationships (ZERO TO THREE, 2020), and occupational therapy practitioners play an important role in promoting healthy relationships through the lens of co-occupational engagement. (*Note. Occupational therapy practitioner* refers to both occupational therapists and occupational therapy assistants.) Early childhood mental health is an area of practice that consists of assessment and intervention in social–emotional domains of development and includes understanding relationships and co-occupational interactions between the caregiver and child, caregiver and practitioner, and practitioner and child.

Although scholars in occupational science conceptualize co-occupation differently (Pickens & Pizur-Barnekow, 2009; Pierce, 2003; Zemke & Clark, 1996), many have agreed that co-occupations are highly interactive. Healthy *co-occupational engagement* occurs when two or more people participate in meaningful pursuits, and it is an essential consideration during early childhood. A young child only exists in relation to a caregiver (Winnicott, 1960) suggesting that wherever one finds a baby, there is a caregiver, and without care, there would be no infant. That is, a child without co-occupational engagement would cease to exist. When co-occupational engagement between a child and a caregiver is characterized by a lack of responsivity and nurturing, the child's social–emotional, cognitive, and physical development are at risk.

Children at Risk for Mental Health Concerns

Children with impaired or delayed social–emotional skills may also have a concomitant mental health condition. The prevalence of mental health conditions in young children underscores the need for qualified occupational therapy practitioners who are passionate about this work. Cree et al. (2018) estimated that one in six children ages 2–8 years in the United States has a developmental, behavioral, or mental health disorder. Adverse childhood experiences (ACEs) account for neurobiological changes (alterations in brain chemistry) that subsequently affect behavioral and mental health. Such challenges result in preschool (PS) expulsion and increased suspension rates (Zeng et al., 2019). On the basis of survey data from the 2016 National Survey of Children's Health dataset, an estimated 174,309 preschoolers (2.0%) and 17,248 (0.2%) older children were expelled annually (Zeng et al., 2019). Suspensions and expulsions may exacerbate mental health issues and increase the likelihood of occupational deprivation.

In addition to ACEs, other factors, such as person and environment factors, contribute to mental health conditions in early childhood (Ghandour et al., 2018). Among children ages 2–8 years, boys are more likely than girls to have a behavioral, mental, or developmental disorder (Cree et al., 2018). More than one in five children living below 100% of the federal poverty level have a behavioral, mental, or developmental disorder. In addition, socioeconomic status is related to access to treatment (Cree et al., 2018). The estimated annual cost of childhood mental health disorders is a staggering $247 billion (CDC, 2019a).

Role of Occupational Therapy in Early Childhood Mental Health

Occupational therapy practitioners are uniquely trained to engage children and families in healthy co-occupations that promote early childhood mental health and development across multiple settings and contexts, including home, early care and learning settings, and PS environments. These settings are considered natural environments as outlined in the Individuals With Disabilities Education Improvement Act of 2004 (IDEA; P. L. 108-446), Part C. Part C describes service delivery for infants and toddlers (ages birth–3 years) at risk for or diagnosed with a disability; Part B provides guidance on service delivery for children with disabilities ages 3–5 years. In addition, practitioners working in health care also promote mental health and development with children and families.

Regardless of the practice setting or the co-occupation addressed, relationships are key to successful early childhood mental health interventions and the prevention of childhood mental health disorders or conditions. In early intervention (EI) practice, relationships are formed through coaching activities and embedded interventions (Salisbury et al., 2018). In early care and learning environments or PS settings, occupational therapy practitioners support social participation with peers while working closely with the teacher and educational staff to promote healthy co-occupational participation and age-appropriate social–emotional skills.

This chapter describes the role that relationships play in early childhood mental health practice and social–emotional development. Evidence from neuroscience is presented to support the need for a mental health approach in EI and early childhood practice settings. In addition, this chapter links the evidence to occupational therapy practices to support children in independent occupations through engagement in healthy co-occupations. Best practices in home visiting and routines-based interventions are presented as tools to assist occupational therapy practitioners in this area of practice.

ESSENTIAL CONSIDERATIONS

In both EI and PS settings, young children achieve optimal social–emotional developmental milestones through the relationships they have with their primary caregivers (e.g., parents, foster parents, early care and learning professionals and teachers). The CDC's (2019b) *Learn the Signs. Act Early. campaign* (CDC, 2019b) promotes developmental monitoring in all domains of development, including social–emotional development. Occupational therapy practitioners practicing in EI and PS settings may use the CDC's resources to help family members and early care and learning professionals identify when a child is demonstrating red flags for poor social–emotional development.

After completion of developmental monitoring and screening for social–emotional development, the occupational therapist considers the role of relationships in the child's development. Healthy relationships are contextualized through co-occupational engagement and characterized by warm, responsive, and nurturing care (Ainsworth, 1967). Although warm, responsive nurturing is at the core of healthy social–emotional development in early childhood, it is important to remember that young children with disabilities may respond to nurturing and responsive care differently than their typically developing peers (Wolke et al., 2013). The differences in responsiveness of children with disabilities may lead to challenges with attachment, bonding, co-regulation, and social participation (Wolke et al., 2013). Occupational therapy practitioners use their knowledge about body structures and functions and co-occupational and occupational engagement to optimize attachment, bonding, co-regulation, self-regulation, social participation, and relationships (AOTA, 2020).

Relationships

A *relationship* is defined as a state of being connected ("Relationship," 2019), and during early childhood, this connection develops through social participation and co-occupational engagement (Pizur-Barnekow, 2019). From an occupational therapy perspective, the state of being connected through engagement in co-occupation forms children's identities, develops their competence, and adds meaning and value to their lives (AOTA, 2014; Pizur-Barnekow, 2019).

Proximal and distal relationships

In early childhood mental health practice, relationships exist in proximal and distal forms. *Proximal relationships* include therapist–parent/caregiver and parent/caregiver–child relationships. *Distal relationships* are the connections that exist between the family and the larger community (Bronfenbrenner, 1989). When considering child development, it is important to recognize that both proximal and distal relationships are key to organizing all domains of development (National Scientific Council on the Developing Child, 2005/2014).

Proximal relationships between children and primary caregivers serve as a foundational regulator for children's behavior, emotion, cognition, and physiology (Barnekow & Kraemer, 2005). The infant brain develops rapidly, with more than a million neural connections formed every second (National Scientific Council on the Developing Child, 2020). In young children, the ability to self-regulate, learn, be motivated, and achieve in school is strongly associated with nurturing and responsive caregiving (McClelland & Tominey, 2014; National Scientific Council on the Developing Child, 2005/2014). Conversely, persistent and toxic stress resulting from unhealthy relationships can adversely affect the brain's structure, function, and architecture over the life course.

Primary caregiving relationships during early childhood are extremely important and contribute to distal relationships that develop over the lifespan. Both are critical in helping children navigate challenges, manage stress, and develop an adaptive coping style that leads to successful participation later in life (National Scientific Council on the Developing Child, 2005/2014). Occupational therapy practitioners are well suited to support parents and caregivers while building their capacity through a **healthy working alliance**, which refers to the collaborative relationship between the parent or caregiver and the provider (Bordin, 1979). A healthy and productive working alliance enhances family–caregiver engagement in social participation occupations. When practitioners and caregivers engage in a healthy working alliance, practitioners recognize the importance of validating caregivers' feelings and responding with inquiry and empathy (Fialka, 1997). Parents may not expect professionals to alleviate or erase their concerns. Rather, parents appreciate acknowledgment of their feelings and support in challenging situations (Fialka, 1997).

Factors influencing relationships

This chapter will focus later on practical ways to promote relationships with children and their caregivers as a meaningful way to achieve intervention goals. However, many factors influence productive working alliances and attachment relationships, both positively and negatively. Among these factors are perinatal mood disorders; postpartum depression; substance use disorder; and ACEs, including trauma and neglect. Table 12.1 provides the definitions, symptoms, and prevalence of these conditions.

Regardless of the factors that influence healthy relationships and attachment, occupational therapy practitioners

TABLE 12.1. **Factors Influencing Relationships**

DISORDER	SYMPTOMS	PREVALENCE OR OCCURRENCE
Perinatal mood disorders: **postpartum depression** (PPD)	Persistent symptoms of PPD may start before birth and continue through the first year of the infant's life. Symptoms include mood swings, difficulty bonding with the child, changes in appetite and sleep, fatigue, loss of interest, difficulty with concentration, and thoughts of harming self or baby (Mayo Clinic, 2020).	On average, 1 in 9 women in the United States will experience PPD, and the likelihood of experiencing PPD varies by race/ethnicity, age, education, birth complications, exposure to stressful life events, and marital status. PPD is more common in women who have a history of depression or financial difficulty (Ko et al., 2017).
Perinatal mood disorders: **perinatal posttraumatic stress disorder** (PTSD)	Perinatal PTSD occurs when a mother or father believes or witnesses that the baby's or mother's life is in danger (Simkin, 2017). Symptoms include intrusive memories, avoidance and numbing, and hyperarousal. These symptoms generally occur between conception and 6 months postpartum and affect the relationship between parents and their infant, resulting in impaired bonding and poorer child cognitive outcomes (Vignato et al., 2017).	Perinatal PTSD affects 9% of women in the United States, and as many as 18% are at risk (Beck et al., 2011; Grekin & O'Hara, 2014).
Substance use disorder (SUD)	Symptoms of SUD vary and are dependent on the substance that is being used. From an occupational therapy perspective, a hallmark behavior associated with SUD is that people continue to use substances even though use interrupts their participation in everyday life, including their ability to perform IADLs such as caregiving (Plach & Stoffel, 2019).	According to the National Survey on Drug Use and Health, 66% of all Americans ages 12 years or older reported using alcohol, and 17.8% reported using illicit drugs in the year before the survey (Center for Behavioral Health Statistics and Quality, 2016).
Adverse childhood experiences (ACEs)	ACEs include all types of traumatic experience, including neglect and abuse, that occur to children and youth ages birth–18 years (CDC, 2019a). ACEs may lead to risky behavior (e.g., alcoholism and drug abuse, encounters with the legal or justice system), chronic conditions (e.g., depression, cardiovascular disease, cancer), and early death.	Two-thirds of the ACE study sample ($N = 17,337$) reported at least 1 ACE, and more than 1 in 5 reported 3 or more ACEs (CDC, 2019a).

Note. CDC = Centers for Disease Control and Prevention; IADLs = instrumental activities of daily living.

use the *therapeutic use of self* to develop collaborative relationships with family members and professional caregivers (AOTA, 2020). In early childhood practice settings, practitioners draw on narrative and professional reasoning to provide family-centered care and interventions that build capacity within an empathic framework (AOTA, 2020). Practitioners who implement a therapeutic use of self approach foster open communication while recognizing the emotional aspects of the people they serve. In turn, the therapeutic use of self enhances social participation at both proximal and distal levels (AOTA, 2020).

BEST PRACTICES

Significant interventions and supports exist to help professionals consider best practice guidelines and competencies across a variety of disciplines in the early childhood field. In early education settings, a multitiered system of supports addresses challenging behaviors through prevention and data-driven interventions (Sugai & Horner, 2009). When children's behaviors are disruptive, occupational therapy practitioners may refer to a behavioral specialist who can develop a plan that includes positive behavioral supports. When addressing trauma in school-age children, practitioners collaborate with teachers to identify strengths and increase resiliency. When children feel secure, they should subsequently begin to self-regulate (Whiting, 2018). Engagement in early co-occupational experiences such as play and social participation are key when serving children in early childhood school settings (Whiting, 2018).

In EI settings, referral to a behavioral specialist may enhance child outcomes. Working with children and their families in their various settings and situations requires listening and collaboration. Working with children inherently means including their parents and caregivers. Each child and family is different, and families have different cultural norms and values and individual experiences that can complicate partnerships and intervention. Occupational therapy practitioners may be hesitant to explore relationships with children and their parents as part of their work for fear of practicing outside of their skill set. Certainly, when children and their caregivers exhibit serious and challenging behaviors, referral to a qualified mental health provider is warranted. Practitioners may also want to collect parent-friendly handouts on topics such as typical sleep patterns, nutrition in babies and toddlers, behavior management, and the like for those occasions when families are in crisis and need something immediate to help them navigate a challenging situation. However, in the longer term, greater progress can be gained in the therapeutic process when the practitioner pays attention to the relationships. This section discusses two tools that practitioners can use as well as a case example to integrate this information.

Consider the PAUSE Method

Tomlin and Viehweg (2016) offered a problem-solving tool called the *PAUSE method* to support professionals in considering all of the perspectives involved in creating and implementing treatment approaches with young children and their families. The intent of this framework is to better understand and maximize relationship opportunities in this work.

This problem-solving model is represented by the acronym *PAUSE*, which serves as a reminder to slow down and consider the relationship aspect of the work. The five components of the model are:
1. *Perceive;* observe and listen
2. *Ask* questions to learn more about what is happening
3. *Understand* each participant's experience or viewpoint
4. *Strategize;* select and take action
5. *Evaluate* the outcomes using reflective processes (Tomlin & Viehweg, 2016).

These components are likely to be familiar to occupational therapy practitioners who use problem-solving models and reflective practice. A key component of the PAUSE framework is consideration of the relational aspects of each participant, including the child. To better understand this model, consider Case Example 12.1, which includes a more detailed discussion of each PAUSE component.

CASE EXAMPLE 12.1. JOSHUA: USING THE PAUSE METHOD

Joshua, a 2-year-old boy, was referred for occupational therapy services to address the EI team's concerns about his delays in development, including language and adaptation. After reading about reflective practice skills, Liz, the occupational therapist, has become more aware of her connection with families. She has worked hard to develop a relationship with Joshua's parents, Phil and Katrina, who seem loving and are consistent with attendance at sessions but often lack follow-through with home recommendations and activities discussed during their visits. She has noticed that Phil and Katrina seem to struggle with managing Joshua's behaviors and regulating their own reactions to Joshua's actions. They have also talked about ways to engage Joshua during mealtime with nutritious foods and discussion while eating. Liz realizes that she feels frustrated with the family, yet she wants to be helpful. She arrives for the regularly scheduled session prepared to continue working on the activities they discussed at the last home visit.

Perceive
The first component, *perceiving,* or observing and listening, takes skill and practice. In early childhood practice, providers recognize that listening includes paying attention to both what is said and how it is said (Weatherston, 2000). When providers pause and reflect, they can also consider what is not said (Tomlin & Viehweg, 2016).

(Continued)

CASE EXAMPLE 12.1. JOSHUA: USING THE PAUSE METHOD *(Cont.)*

What can Liz discover by intentionally listening to and observing this child and family?

Imagine that when Liz arrives at 4:00 p.m. for her home visit with the family, she encounters one of these scenarios:

- Joshua is asleep and Katrina goes to wake him up: Liz perceives that this is an ongoing issue and wonders why a regular naptime continues to be a challenge, especially when she contacts the family the day before an appointment to confirm the appointment time.
- Phil has just arrived with fast-food sandwiches and fries for everyone: Liz perceives that although they have talked about ways to use mealtime to address developmental goals, Phil continues to seemingly misunderstand and disrupt the progress made.
- Joshua is having a tantrum with Katrina, who seems frustrated that he will not pick up his toys. He has just thrown his blocks, hitting Katrina in the face: Liz perceives that Katrina must not have been successful with the behavior management strategies they talked about during the last session and is still arguing with the toddler.

Ask questions

Liz wants to be more open to knowing more about her clients' experiences to inform her perceptions before she makes any judgment or changes her plans. By considering each person's perspective, Liz is likely to have additional questions as she wonders about each participant's views and experiences. The second component of the framework, *ask*, reminds Liz that gathering additional information can help inform a productive and successful intervention plan.

Beyond listening, observing, and gathering information, it is important to ask the right questions (Heffron & Murch, 2010). Using open questions and statements in a supportive way can lead to occupational therapy practitioners learning a great deal from families. Initial questions can lead to additional inquiries to more deeply understand the child's and family's experience (Green & Palfrey, 2000). What might Liz ask Phil and Katrina, based on her observations and perceptions? What would be helpful to know about their life situation, past experiences, and plans for the future? Consider possible questions Liz might ask for each of the potential scenarios described earlier:

- Liz might ask, "Is Joshua taking a nap now?" If Katrina says yes, she might explore when he went to sleep, whether he is feeling well, how he slept the night before, and so forth. Knowing more about why he is sleeping at the time of the appointment could be useful as Liz begins to understand more about the current situation and what course of action she might suggest.
- Liz might ask the family whether the sandwiches are to use in the session to work on feeding issues. She

might reflect with the family on how their mealtime activities worked over the past week in relation to the goals they discussed.

- Liz might use open-ended statements to learn more about the current situation, such as "Wow, Joshua seems upset today. What happened before I arrived?" Or she might observe, "You seem pretty frustrated with Joshua's behavior. Tell me more." She might invite more conversation about the block throwing by reflecting, "He hit you with one of the blocks and that made you mad. What happened before he got upset and threw them?"

Understand

With additional information, Liz can begin to more deeply *understand* what is happening from the perspectives of Joshua and his parents, as well as her own. Knowing more about Phil's and Katrina's experiences can provide insights about strategies and approaches to provide useful interventions. Considering the child's experience and perspective can be insightful, and better understanding the parents' perspective and needs are key pieces of helping them to develop skills (Bernstein & Edwards, 2012). Moreover, considering how the child perceives the family's experience can provide crucial insight for appropriate, potential therapy approaches. Young children cannot speak for themselves; therefore, providers are reminded to ask, "What about the child?" to ensure attention to the needs of the identified client (Weatherston, 2001, 2005). Liz may gain insights in each of the possible scenarios:

- Katrina shares that Joshua has not been sleeping very well this past week. Liz might therefore modify her expectations and plans for the session. She could explore Joshua's recent sleep history to learn more about his patterns and any recent changes to the family's schedule that might be affecting his sleep. She might suggest they let Joshua sleep and discuss the past week before waking him because he might wake up naturally; they can use that time to talk about Katrina's frustrations and challenges.
- Liz may better understand the late lunch after learning that Phil's work schedule changed, and he really wants to have time to share a meal with Joshua because they have talked about ways to work on developmental milestones during mealtimes. This understanding may influence how they plan for today and future sessions.
- Understanding how Joshua might feel and react when his parents get upset at his behaviors could provide some insight into how hard it is for him to calm down when those around him are actually encouraging him to escalate his behaviors. Wondering aloud with Joshua's parents, Liz might say something such as "It might be hard for Joshua to be calm when others around him are upset" and "I wonder if Joshua knows

(Continued)

CASE EXAMPLE 12.1. JOSHUA: USING THE PAUSE METHOD *(Cont.)*

how to calm down. Maybe we could talk about ways to help him learn how to do that."

Strategize

With deeper appreciation for each team member's perspective, including the child's, the occupational therapy practitioner can engage the family in creating *strategies* to address the identified concerns. Liz can use this knowledge in discussing with Phil and Katrina how to address their expressed concerns and identify ideas and actions that are doable for them and will have the most impact on addressing their concerns.

Evaluate

While developing strategies, Liz can ask Phil and Katrina how they will know when goals have been accomplished while also setting a timeline to check in and *evaluate* progress. Responding to the insights gained while using the PAUSE framework can provide invaluable assistance to Liz in supporting the family as needed while maintaining her focus on therapeutic activities to address the goals in their plan. Liz can use her insights as she

partners with the family to strategize and evaluate progress in each of the scenarios:

- Because Joshua seems to be having new sleep challenges, Liz might offer to talk with Katrina and Phil about exploring resources to help them better manage sleep routines. Liz might also share a handout about typical sleep patterns to help them in their understanding of Joshua's needs for sleep and potential routines that can accommodate their family schedule.
- Liz can acknowledge the value of family time, Phil's desire to connect with his son, and how mealtime can be used to support developmental outcomes. She could offer to explore some activities the family might consider that include healthy food options for Joshua to try and ways to maximize mealtime as a learning experience.
- Liz might discuss inviting another team member with expertise in behavior management to assess Joshua and offer suggestions. With Katrina's and Phil's agreement, she could ask the service coordinator to help make the referral. Liz might offer a handout about typical behavior with suggestions for ways to respond effectively to Joshua's challenging behaviors.

Consider the Intentional Relationship Model

In addition to the PAUSE framework (Tomlin & Viehweg, 2016), the ***Intentional Relationship Model*** (IRM; Taylor, 2008) may assist occupational therapy practitioners with professional reasoning as they serve children and families. The IRM model provides a framework for the therapeutic use of self. As suggested by the model's name, therapeutic relationships are intentional or deliberate (Taylor, 2008). When practitioners use IRM as a lens to view relationships, they understand that the therapeutic relationship is key to occupational (Taylor, 2008) and co-occupational performance. Intentional or deliberate therapeutic relationships serve as the foundation of a healthy working alliance that may benefit the child and family. In interactions with parents and early childhood professionals, IRM provides a framework that considers enduring and situational characteristics of the relationship partner that may contribute to interpersonal events. Interpersonal events, or challenges to relationships, are unavoidable, and when they are not addressed, the therapeutic relationship may be at risk. Consequently, the potential exists for an interpersonal event to negatively affect occupational (Taylor, 2008) and co-occupational performance.

Occupational therapy practitioners possess interpersonal skills, therapeutic styles, and a capacity for professional reasoning to enhance therapeutic relationships (Taylor, 2008). These skills and styles contribute to preferred mode use. Taylor (2008) identified six modes commonly used in therapeutic relationships: (1) advocating, (2) collaborating, (3) empathizing, (4) encouraging, (5) instructing, and (6) problem solving. The key to effective

therapeutic relationships is to practice with mindful empathy, be flexible in mode use, and be family centered when applying IRM in practice (Taylor, 2008). Practitioners can also combine IRM and reflective supervision to enhance and strengthen therapeutic relationships.

Reflective supervision

Returning to the case example, Liz may experience an interpersonal dilemma when she encounters challenging family situations that she feels go beyond her role and expertise. Liz may want to discuss her feelings of frustration and worry with a reflective supervisor or consultant. Having a regularly scheduled time to talk about challenging situations can provide insight for practitioners and help guide plans for future sessions. This approach, often referred to as *reflective supervision* or *reflective consultation* (Heller & Gilkerson, 2009), allows providers to explore their own personal reactions to child and family situations, clarify boundaries, establish and maintain work–life balance, and stay energized by this type of work and avoid burnout. Recognizing that everyone who works with young children and families is vulnerable to their own reactions and related feelings may be helpful.

After meeting with her reflective supervisor, Liz might think about the mode she used during interactions with Katrina and Phil. Through reflective supervision, Liz may decide to try a problem-solving approach and ask Katrina and Phil to identify potential solutions to address the issues they have identified. By paying attention to the relationship dilemma, Liz may better understand Katrina's and Phil's perspectives, which may lead to enhanced co-occupational engagement.

Check in with the family

Occupational therapy practitioners enhance the likelihood of progress and success when they attend to their relationship with the child and caregivers. Checking in with the family on arrival to talk about how life has been between home visits provides an opportunity to evaluate progress and goals while discovering where challenges with selected activities and interventions may exist. When caregivers feel comfortable with their EI provider, they are more likely to share when they have questions or doubts about suggested strategies and activities. Including caregivers in the hands-on work during the session allows them to try out the activity, ask questions, and get useful input from the occupational therapy practitioner. At the end of the session, establishing a plan for what will happen before the next appointment can be an effective way to establish evaluation criteria to know when progress occurs.

Providing early childhood occupational therapy services in the home setting can be both rewarding and challenging. Occupational therapy practitioners naturally consider relationship as part of their work. Pausing to pay attention to emerging issues, learning about and understanding these issues from each person's perspective, and creating strategies in partnership with the family can greatly enhance the quality of the relationship as well as the success of the intervention and developmental goals. In addition, achieving success in reaching treatment goals can lead to more satisfaction with the work.

SUMMARY

Attending to relationships is natural for occupational therapy practitioners. Using the PAUSE framework (Tomlin & Viehweg, 2016) and the IRM (Taylor, 2008) while building the skills needed to focus on relationships can enhance therapeutic outcomes. When practitioners recognize mental health concerns among children and their families, they can use their connections to link the family to additional services to address concerns and needs that go beyond occupations. The partnership or working alliance among the practitioner, parents, and caregivers is equally as important as the services provided to the child.

In addition, engaging in reflective practices characterized by collaboration, reflection, and consistency with a reflective supervisor develops a partnership that enhances professional growth and strengthens practice. Practice in early childhood mental health is enhanced by interprofessional working relationships in which the role of each profession is valued and team communication is timely and respectful (Interprofessional Education Collaborative, 2016). Resources obtained through statewide early childhood mental health endorsement programs and early childhood mental health alliances and associations enhance knowledge and skills in this practice area.

Weatherston and Fitzgerald (2018, para. 8) offered some key elements to remember in promoting and assuring positive early childhood mental health, noting that each of these elements includes a focus on relationship:

- "Healthy relationships with stable, nurturing caregivers" are an essential aspect of healthy social–emotional development.

- "Strong and supported parents" and caregivers "are seen as *mediators of change* as they enter into sensitive, responsive, and nurturing relationships with their infants and young children."
- "Reduction of child poverty through focus on two-generational or relational strategies that reduce the social and emotional risks of infancy and stresses of early parenthood and address the wellbeing of infants, very young children, caregiving families, and communities" may assure positive early childhood mental health.
- "A well-prepared, high quality," interprofessional "work force that is relationship driven" increases the likelihood of optimal care.

Interdisciplinary partnerships focusing on early childhood mental health while contributing occupational therapy's therapeutic skills focused on co-occupations can go a long way in ensuring children grow and develop to their fullest potential.

RESOURCES AND ACTIVITIES

- Think about a challenging scenario from your own experience, and consider how this model might help you approach your work in a different way.
- Learn more about early childhood mental health through your state's infant mental health alliance or association or related organization.
- Explore the benefits of reflective consultation or supervision by visiting ZERO TO THREE's website (https://www.zerotothree.org) and seek opportunities to access it.
- Discover ways to connect families to other families in your community (look for your state's Family to Family Health Information Center, Parent to Parent program, and Parent Training Information Center resources).
- Search the Internet for the variety of learning opportunities available using such keywords as *social–emotional development, infant mental health, early childhood mental health, reflective practice, reflective supervision/consultation, parallel process,* and *trauma informed.*
- Provide families with evidence-based information to learn more about early childhood development through resources such as the CDC's free *Learn the Signs. Act Early.* campaign (https://www.cdc.gov/actearly).
- Identify useful, family-friendly, and evidence-based handouts for families that provide information about behavior management, sleep, nutrition, biting, anxiety, tantrums, aggression, and so forth by looking at trusted websites or books such as *Tackling the Tough Stuff: A Home Visitor's Guide to Supporting Families at Risk* (Tomlin & Viehweg, 2016).
- Explore AOTA resources about trauma-informed care at https://www.aota.org/~/media/Corporate/Files/Publications/CE-Articles/CE-article-May-2019-Trauma.pdf.
- Check out a research synthesis on infant mental health and early care and education providers at http://csefel.vanderbilt.edu/documents/rs_infant_mental_health.pdf.

REFERENCES

Ainsworth, M. D. S. (1967). *Infancy in Uganda: Infant care and the growth of love.* Johns Hopkins University Press.

American Occupational Therapy Association. (2020). Occupational therapy practice framework: Domain and process (4th ed.). *American Journal of Occupational Therapy, 74*(Suppl. 2), 7412410010. https://doi.org/10.5014/ajot.2020.74S2001

Barnekow, K. A., & Kraemer, G. W. (2005). The psychobiological theory of attachment: A viable frame of reference for early intervention providers. *Physical and Occupational Therapy in Pediatrics, 25,* 3–15. https://doi.org/10.1080/J006v25n01_02

Bazyk, S., & Arbesman, M. (2013). *Occupational therapy practice guidelines for mental health promotion, prevention, and intervention for children and youth.* AOTA Press.

Beck, C. T., Gable, R. K., Sakala, C., & Declercq, E. R. (2011). Posttraumatic stress disorder in new mothers: Results from a two-stage U.S. national survey. *Birth, 38,* 216–227. https://doi.org/10.1111/j.1523-536X.2011.00475.x

Bernstein, V. J., & Edwards, R. C. (2012). Supporting early childhood practitioners through relationship-based, reflective supervision. *NHSA Dialog, 15,* 286–301. https://doi.org/10.1080/15240754.2012.694495

Bordin, E. S. (1979). The generalizability of the psychoanalytic concept of the working alliance. *Psychotherapy: Research, Theory, and Practice, 16,* 252–260. https://doi.org/10.1037/h0085885

Bronfenbrenner, U. (1989). Ecological systems theory. In R. Vasta (Ed.), *Annals of child development* (pp. 187–249). JAI Press.

Center for Behavioral Health Statistics and Quality. (2016). *2015 National Survey on Drug Use and Health: Detailed tables.* Substance Abuse and Mental Health Services Administration.

Centers for Disease Control and Prevention. (2019a). *Data and statistics on children's mental health.* https://www.cdc.gov/childrensmentalhealth/data.html

Centers for Disease Control and Prevention. (2019b). *Learn the signs. Act early.* https://www.cdc.gov/ncbddd/actearly/index.html

Cree, R. A., Bitsko, R. H., Robinson, L. R., Holbrook, J. R., Danielson, M. L., Smith, D. S., & Peacock, G. (2018). Health care, family, and community factors associated with mental, behavioral, and developmental disorders and poverty among children aged 2–8 years—United States, 2016. *MMWR, 67,* 1377–1383. https://doi.org/10.15585/mmwr.mm6750a1

Fialka, J. (1997). *It matters: Lessons from my son.* Huntington Woods, MI: Author.

Ghandour, R. M., Sherman, L. J., Vladutiu, C. J., Ali, M. M., Lynch, S. E., Bitsko, R. H., & Blumberg, S. J. (2018). Prevalence and treatment of depression, anxiety, and conduct problems in U.S. children. *Journal of Pediatrics, 206,* 256–267.e3. https://doi.org/10.1016/j.jpeds.2018.09.021

Green, M., & Palfrey, J. (2000). *Bright futures: Guidelines for health supervision of infants, children, and adolescents* (2nd ed.). American Academy of Pediatrics.

Grekin, R., & O'Hara, M. W. (2014). Prevalence and risk factors of post-partum posttraumatic stress disorder: A meta-analysis. *Clinical Psychology Review, 34,* 389–401. https://doi.org/10.1016/j.cpr.2014.05.003

Heffron, M. C., & Murch, T. (2010). *Reflective supervision and leadership in infant and early childhood programs.* ZERO TO THREE.

Heller, S., & Gilkerson, L. (Eds.). (2009). *A practical guide to reflective supervision.* ZERO TO THREE.

Individuals With Disabilities Education Improvement Act of 2004, Pub. L. 108-446, 20 U.S.C. §§ 1400–1482.

Interprofessional Education Collaborative. (2016). *Core competencies for interprofessional collaborative practice: 2016 update.* Interprofessional Education Collaborative.

Kielhofner, G., & Burke, J. P. (1977). Occupational therapy after 60 years: An account of changing identity and knowledge. *American Journal of Occupational Therapy, 31,* 675–689.

Ko, J. Y., Rockhill, K. M., Tong, V. T., Morrow, B., & Farr, S. L. (2017). Trends in postpartum depressive symptoms—27 states, 2004, 2008, and 2012. *MMWR, 66,* 153–158. https://doi.org/10.15585/mmwr.mm6606a1

Mayo Clinic. (2020). *Postpartum depression.* https://www.mayoclinic.org/diseases-conditions/postpartum-depression/symptoms-causes/syc-20376617

McClelland, M. M., & Tominey, S. L. (2014). The development of self-regulation and executive function in young children. *ZERO TO THREE, 35*(2), 2–8.

National Scientific Council on the Developing Child. (2020, May 9). *Brain architecture.* https://developingchild.harvard.edu/science/key-concepts/brain-architecture/

National Scientific Council on the Developing Child. (2014). *Excessive stress disrupts the architecture of the developing brain* (Working Paper 3, updated ed.). Cambridge, MA: Author. (Original work published 2005). http://developingchild.harvard.edu/wp-content/uploads/2005/05/Stress_Disrupts_Architecture_Developing_Brain-1.pdf

Pickens, N. D., & Pizur-Barnekow, K. (2009). Co-occupation: Extending the dialogue. *Journal of Occupational Science, 16*(3), 151–156. https://doi.org/10.1080/14427591.2009.9686656

Pierce, D. (2003). *Occupation by design: Building therapeutic power.* Philadelphia, PA: F. A. Davis.

Pizur-Barnekow, K. (2019). Early intervention: A practice setting for infant mental health. In C. Brown, V. C. Stoffel, & J. Muñoz (Eds.), *Occupational therapy in mental health: A vision for participation* (2nd ed., pp. 573–584). F. A. Davis.

Plach, H., & Stoffel, V. C. (2019). Substance abuse and co-occurring disorders. In C. Brown, V. C. Stoffel & J. P. Muñoz (Eds.), *Occupational therapy in mental health: A vision for participation* (2nd ed., pp. 238–249). F. A. Davis.

Relationship. (2019). In *Merriam-Webster dictionary.* https://www.merriam-webster.com/dictionary/relationship

Salisbury, C., Woods, J., Snyder, P., Moddelmog, K., Mawdsley, H., Romano, M., & Windsor, K. (2018). Caregiver and provider experiences with coaching and embedded interventions. *Topics in Early Childhood and Special Education, 38,* 17–29. https://doi.org/10.1177/0271121417708036

Simkin, P. (2017). *Birth trauma: Definition and statistics.* http://pattch.org/resource-guide/traumatic-births-and-ptsd-definition-and-statistics/

Sugai, G., & Horner, R. J. (2009). Responsiveness-to-intervention and school-wide positive behavior supports: Integration of multi-tiered system approaches. *Exceptionality, 17,* 223–237. https://doi.org/10.1080/09362830903235375

Taylor, R. (2008). *The intentional relationship: Occupational therapy and use of self.* F. A. Davis.

Tomlin, A., & Viehweg, S. (2016). *Tackling the tough stuff: A home visitor's guide to supporting families at risk.* Paul H. Brookes.

Vignato, J., Georges, J. M., Bush, R. A., & Connelly, C. D. (2017). Post-traumatic stress disorder in the perinatal period: A concept analysis. *Journal of Clinical Nursing, 26,* 3859–3868. https://doi.org/10.1111/jocn.13800

Weatherston, D. (2000). The infant mental health specialist. *ZERO TO THREE, 21,* 3–10.

Weatherston, D. (2001). Infant mental health: A review of the relevant literature. *Psychoanalytic Social Work, 8*(1), 39–69. https://doi.org/10.1300/J032v08n01_04

Weatherston, D. (2005). Returning the treasure to babies: An introduction to infant mental health service and training. In K. M. Finello (Ed.), *The handbook of training and practice in infant and preschool mental health* (pp. 3–30). Jossey-Bass.

Weatherston, D., & Fitzgerald, H. E. (2018). Public policy and infant mental health. https://perspectives.waimh.org/2018/08/21/public-policy-and-infant-mental-health/

Whiting, C. C. (2018). Trauma and the role of the school-based occupational therapist. *Journal of Occupational Therapy, Schools, and Early Intervention, 11,* 291–301. https://doi.org/10.1080/19411243.2018.1438327

Winnicott, D. W. (1960). The theory of the parent–infant relationship. *International Journal of Psycho-Analysis, 41,* 585–595.

Wolke, D., Eryigit-Madzwamuse, S., & Gutbrod, T. (2013). Very preterm/very low birthweight infants' attachment: Infant and maternal characteristics. *Archives of Disease in Childhood: Fetal and Neonatal Edition, 99,* F70–F75. 10.1136/archdischild-2013-303788

Zemke, R., & Clark, F. (1996). *Occupational science: The evolving discipline.* F. A. Davis.

Zeng, S., Corr, C. P., O'Grady, C., & Guan, Y. (2019). Adverse childhood experiences and preschool suspension expulsion: A population study. *Child Abuse & Neglect, 97,* 104149. https://doi.org/10.1016/j.chiabu.2019.104149

ZERO TO THREE. (2020). *Infant and early childhood mental health.* https://www.zerotothree.org/early-development/infant-and-early-childhood-mental-health

Understanding Early Literacy Development

Stephanie Parks, PhD, OT/L, and Gloria Frolek Clark, PhD, OTR/L, BCP, FAOTA

KEY TERMS AND CONCEPTS

- Alphabet knowledge
- Concepts of print
- Dual language learners
- Early literacy development
- Early literacy learning
- Emergent literacy development
- Executive functioning skills
- Handwriting tasks
- Literacy skills
- Oral language
- Phonological awareness
- Phonological memory
- Preliteracy development
- Print knowledge
- Rapid naming of letters and digits
- Rapid naming of objects and colors
- Reading readiness
- Visual processing
- Writing name

OVERVIEW

Currently, the U.S. education system places a strong emphasis on literacy development to ensure that all children learn to read (Neuman & Cunningham, 2009). If children do not develop strong reading comprehension by third grade, their chances of graduating from high school or going to college are greatly diminished (Duncan & Murnane, 2011). However, 65% of America's fourth graders are not reading at a proficient level (Annie E. Casey Foundation, 2014). Because success in reading is dependent on early and emergent literacy skills (National Institute for Literacy, 2008), occupational therapy practitioners working in early intervention, child care, preschool, and health care settings are increasingly focused on literacy skills (Frolek Clark, 2016). (*Note. Occupational therapy practitioner* refers to both occupational therapists and occupational therapy assistants.)

Early Literacy Skills and Reading Difficulties

Children develop early *literacy skills* (i.e., reading, writing, listening, speaking) through exposure to early language and literacy experiences. These foundational skills for reading and writing begin at birth and are refined during early childhood as children learn to identify letters and sounds and understand basic concepts of print.

For young children with sensory, physical, or cognitive challenges, opportunities for early literacy learning are limited. Barriers such as limited verbal abilities, difficulty holding books independently and turning pages, and limited vision may prevent active participation in early literacy activities. Occupational therapy practitioners can provide adaptations and strategies to mediate limitations and remove barriers for these children (Stauter et al., 2017).

Literacy and Behavioral Difficulties

A child who enters school without early literacy skills not only may struggle academically but also may have behavioral difficulties at school (Halonen et al., 2006). As the child falls behind peers, the long-term effects of poor literacy skills increase. Such effects include dropping out of school, participating in antisocial activities, and achieving poorly in educational and occupational areas (Bennett et al., 2003; Maughan et al., 1985).

Roughly 58%–96% of children with developmental disabilities and delays entering kindergarten do not demonstrate skills needed for transition to kindergarten (Lloyd et al., 2009). When assessed in fourth grade, 62% of these children were reading below academic standards. The children with developmental disabilities or delays who were at the highest risk for poor outcomes (e.g., low academic performance, low educational attainment, early criminal activities) included those with behavioral and social difficulties (Trout et al., 2003). For children with developmental disability, there is a direct correlation between deficits in critical reading skills and the severity of their behavioral and social problems (Trout et al., 2006). These children do not show gains in reading skills as readily as children with disabilities but no behavioral problems (Anderson et al., 2001). Providing intervention during early childhood to enhance early literacy skills is critical.

Connections between behavior and reading ability have been found among typically developing children as well as those with developmental disabilities (Anderson et al., 2001; Gray et al., 2014; King et al., 2016; Morgan et al., 2008). Gray and colleagues (2014) found that a developmental trajectory of toddlers' externalizing behaviors—in particular, inattention—predicted their second-grade reading outcomes.

Literacy: Handwriting Concerns

With the increasing demands of writing for kindergarteners, a predictor of their performance is their ability to complete **handwriting tasks** (e.g., using marker to attempt to print name) in preschool (Fogo, 2008). Significant correlations exist between ability to identify letter names and handwriting skills among preschoolers and early kindergarteners (Bus et al., 2001; Frolek Clark & Luze, 2014; Molfese et al., 2006).

One of the earliest writing skills is writing alphabet letters. Research has found children master writing capital (i.e., uppercase) letters before lowercase, even when instruction is provided simultaneously for both (Adams, 1990; Frolek Clark & Luze, 2014; Ritchey, 2008). Capital letters are the same height and easy to identify.

Students who have difficulty with letter names, letter sounds, and phonemic awareness struggle with reading and writing skills (Berninger et al., 2006; Fischel et al., 2007; Frolek Clark & Luze, 2014). Research has linked poor handwriting among elementary students to poor visual–motor skills (Cornhill & Case-Smith, 1996; Graham et al., 2006; Weintraub & Graham, 2000), fine motor skills (Cornhill & Case-Smith, 1996; Exner, 2005), and in-hand manipulation (e.g., fine motor dexterity; Breslin & Exner, 1999; Cornhill & Case-Smith, 1996).

The best single predictor of the length and quality of children's written work in Grades 1–6 is automatic letter writing (Graham et al., 1997). In 2014, Frolek Clark and Luze found significant positive correlations between writing scores (writing non-sequential alphabet letters from dictation and writing first and last name) and reading scores among kindergarteners—in particular, knowing letter sounds, naming letters, and knowing phonemes. There was also a positive and significant correlation among writing, reading, fine motor skills (in-hand dexterity), and visual–motor integration. The best predictors of a child's ability to write the alphabet letters included the ability to write their first and last name, whether they knew initial sounds of letters, and their age (Frolek Clark & Luze, 2014). The best predictors of a child's ability to write their name (first and last) were age, ability to write the alphabet from dictation, and scores on the Beery Visual–Motor Integration Test and Beery Motor Coordination subtest (Beery & Beery, 2006; Frolek Clark & Luze, 2014).

Occupational Therapy Role

Occupational therapy practitioners support participation in life through engaging in occupations (American Occupational Therapy Association, 2020). Literacy activities such as reading, writing, listening, and speaking are meaningful occupations that are essential to children's performance at home, in the community, and in preschools and are within the domain of occupational therapy (Frolek Clark, 2016).

ESSENTIAL CONSIDERATIONS

Occupational therapy practitioners working in early childhood settings must understand the research supporting early literacy and incorporate these concepts into their evaluations and intervention for children and their families. Early identification of children with cognitive, motor, and behavioral issues can promote essential interventions.

Predictors of Literacy Achievement

In response to the growing interest in research-based practices, the National Early Literacy Panel (NELP) was formed and conducted a meta-analysis of more than 500 empirical studies of early literacy development (National Institute for Literacy, 2008). The goal of this panel was to determine which instructional practices promoted the development of children's early literacy skills and were precursors of later literacy achievement. Six variables representing early literacy skills had moderate to large predictive relations with later measures of literacy (even when IQ and socioeconomic status [SES] were considered; see the first six variables in Table 13.1). Although they were moderately correlated with at least one measure of literacy achievement, the five additional skills listed at the end of Table 13.1 did not maintain predictive power when other variables were added or were not yet evaluated by the researchers.

Since the NELP publication, more recent studies have continued to confirm the research synthesis findings. Research findings indicate that **executive functioning skills** (e.g., working memory, inhibition, cognitive flexibility) predict math and reading ability among prekindergarteners and kindergarteners (Blair, 2016). Without efficient early literacy skills, kindergartners struggle to read at grade level; if they are still struggling by third grade, they are more likely to drop out of high school than their peers (Hernandez, 2012).

Stages of Literacy

There are three phases or stages of **early literacy learning** (Dunst et al., 2006). Like development in other domains, these developing literacy skills are not linear, discrete, or independent. Rather, the skills in these stages are overlapping and interrelated.

1. **Preliteracy development**
   - Prelanguage and early nonverbal communication and social skills acquired before language onset that form the foundation for language acquisition and emergent literacy skills (ages birth–15 months)
2. **Emergent literacy development**
   - Language onset and vocabulary development (ages 12–20 months)
   - Language growth and emergent literacy development as the foundation for the process of future literacy-related abilities (ages 24–42 months)
3. **Early literacy development**
   - Acquisition and mastery of the fundamentals of reading, writing, and other literacy-related skills (ages 36–48 months)
   - Conventional literacy, including the actual skills used for reading and writing (i.e., decoding, oral reading, fluency, demonstrating comprehension, generating written sentences or paragraphs, spelling; ages 48–60 months).

Influence of Home Environment

In the mid-1990s, researchers Hart and Risley (1995) conducted a seminal study referred to as the *30 Million Word*

TABLE 13.1. Skills That Predict Literacy Achievement

LITERACY SKILLS	DEFINITION
Alphabet knowledge	Knowing the names and sounds of letters
Phonological awareness	The ability to detect, manipulate, or analyze the auditory aspects of spoken language independent of meaning
Rapid naming of letters and digits	The ability to name a sequence of random letters and digits, rapidly
Rapid naming of objects and colors	The ability to name a sequence of repeating random sets of pictures of objects or colors
Writing name	The ability to write one's own name
Phonological memory	The ability to remember spoken information for a short period of time
Concepts of print	Knowledge of print conventions (e.g., left–right, front–back) and concepts (e.g., book cover, author)
Print knowledge	Skill reflecting a combination of elements of alphabet knowledge, concepts about print, and early decoding
Reading readiness	Combination of alphabet knowledge, concepts of print, vocabulary, memory, and phonological awareness
Oral language	The ability to produce or comprehend spoken language
Visual processing	The ability to match or discriminate visually presented symbols

Source. Definitions from National Institute for Literacy (2008).

Gap, which has influenced the way educators, parents, and policymakers think about language development and the importance of talking to very young children, especially those living in poverty. Researchers audio recorded hours of verbal language in the homes of 45 participant families once a month over 2.5 years. Families were sorted or classified by SES into *high* (professional), *middle* (working class) and *low/welfare* (poverty) groups. The researchers extrapolated the results and concluded that in 4 years, an average child in a professional family would hear almost 45 million words, an average child in a working-class family would hear 26 million words, and an average child from a family living in poverty would hear only 13 million words. Thus, the gap between high-SES families and low-SES families was 30 million words. The authors found a correlation between word exposure and the rate of vocabulary acquisition of the child participants (Walker et al., 1994) and posited that the word gap could partially explain the achievement gap (e.g., school readiness, literacy) the country is currently experiencing related to SES, race, and persistent disparity.

Although Hart and Risley's study (1992) and their book, *Meaningful Differences in the Everyday Experience of Young American Children* (1995), came out decades ago, controversy surrounding this research still exists. Replication studies (e.g., Sperry et al., 2019) suggest that a more accurate gap is approximately 4 million, as opposed to 30 million. Scholars have also raised criticisms of the study, including the small sample size (only 45 families), methodology, lack of investigation regarding the quality of language heard, and potentially being racially discriminatory (Adair et al., 2017; Cartmill, 2016).

Although the results and conclusions of 30 Million Word Gap should be interpreted with healthy caution, scholars in early childhood generally agree on the positive impact the study has had in increasing public awareness and policy on the importance of intervention for families with infants, toddlers, and young children. Several 30 Million Word Gap–funded initiatives were launched across communities and continue to target lower SES families through home visiting interventions.

Dual Language Learners

In 2015, *dual language learners* (DLLs), learners who acquire two or more languages simultaneously, composed 29% of Head Start enrollment nationally, with 25% coming from Spanish-speaking families (Baker & Páez, 2018). Experts and educators suggest that there are many benefits to raising a bilingual child, including ability to communicate with family members, increased employment options in adulthood, and adaptability to new and culturally diverse environments. Research has also shown that bilingual children perform higher on tests involving multitasking, creative thinking, and problem solving (Bialystok et al., 2012).

Research shows that DLLs can benefit significantly from high-quality early childhood education by learning language skills in both their home language and English, as well as literacy skills that promote school readiness (Castro et al., 2011). Preschool practitioners in high-quality programs should make strategic decisions about how and when to incorporate home languages in materials and books to promote early literacy practices. Additional effective curriculum adaptations and modifications helpful for DLLs include using visual supports (e.g., pictures as labels and environmental print in both languages, as well as color coding).

BEST PRACTICES

This section provides information about specific strategies to promote and provide early literacy through formal and informal learning opportunities and a literacy-rich environment.

Promote Literacy and Learning

Occupational therapy practitioners have a critical role in promoting, supporting, and implementing literacy activities (e.g., reading, writing, speaking, listening) across all early childhood settings.

Advocate for literacy-rich environments

Early literacy includes conversations, books, stories, and print (ZERO TO THREE, 2003). Evans et al. (2014) found that having any books in the home had a statistically significant positive impact on a child's test scores in 42 nations, even after controlling for family wealth, occupations, and educational level. In addition to having books in the environment, caregivers should talk to the child. Huttenlocher and colleagues (1991) found that children whose mothers spoke to them had almost 300 more words by age 2 years than children whose mothers rarely spoke to them. Occupational therapy practitioners should collaborate with families, family literacy organizations, community libraries, child care centers, and preschools to educate and promote the importance of literacy-rich environments for all children, especially those with low SES.

Promote informal early literacy learning opportunities

Starting at a few weeks of age, parents can enhance their child's literacy and academic performance by reading to them. Raikes and colleagues (2006) found that regularly reading to a child promotes greater language comprehension, increased vocabulary, and higher cognitive skills, as compared with peers. A child whose family read to them at least 3 times a week was almost twice as likely to score in the top 25% in reading, as compared with peers (Denton & West, 2002). In a study of parents who asked questions and talked with their child during reading, DeTemple (2001) found that children whose parents paused to engage in conversation were able to ask more questions, talked more, and engaged more in conversation. Parents in impoverished regions who read to their toddlers for 6 weeks were found to make statistically significant improvements in their child's attention and comprehension (Cooper et al., 2014).

Support formal early literacy learning opportunities

Many preschools provide formal literacy opportunities for children, including those with special needs. Yet many teachers focus on reading skills but are not prepared to teach handwriting (Graham et al., 2008). Occupational therapy practitioners in early childhood settings often support educational teams in choosing evidence-based curricula and instruction.

Preschoolers with special needs. As stated previously, preschoolers with developmental disabilities or delays are at risk for not being prepared to transition to kindergarten. The Kids in Transition to School (KITS) program, a short-term intervention, was provided during the summer before children's kindergarten year (Pears et al., 2016). This program focused on school readiness skills (e.g., early literacy, social, self-regulation) and parent groups to increase parental awareness of school readiness and involvement. Research indicates that the children receiving

the KITS intervention had an increase in early literacy skills (e.g., phonemic awareness, letter knowledge, understanding of print concepts) and success in kindergarten. In another study, preschoolers ages 3–6 years with Down syndrome who were provided with a 45-week program of phonological awareness, word analysis, sight word training, and shared book reading demonstrated a statistically significant improvement in letter name identification, letter sound identification, and identification of sight words (Colozzo et al., 2016).

Preschoolers at risk for literacy delays because of low socioeconomic status. Occupational therapy practitioners should support formal instruction using evidence-based curricula. A 2-year multisite study with large sample sizes using the Get Ready intervention (which is designed to enhance parent–child interactions and academics) in Head Start found the treatment group's scores in writing, reading, and oral language had made statistically significant increases, as compared with the control group (Sheridan et al., 2011).

Another multisite study with a large sample size found that children who used Head Start's Research-Based Developmentally Informed program, an emergent literacy curriculum, demonstrated statistically significant positive changes in learning engagement and attention compared with the control group (Nix et al., 2013). Several studies using the Read It Again prekindergarten program, which focused on phonological awareness and print knowledge, found statistically significant increases in literacy (e.g., alphabet knowledge, print knowledge, rhyme; Hilbert & Eis, 2013; Justice et al., 2010; Schryer et al., 2015).

General education preschoolers at risk for learning difficulties. Across the United States, states are providing interventions for at-risk preschoolers using multitiered systems of support. A multisite study with a large sample of at-risk 4-year-olds provided explicit Tier II interventions to enhance reading skills. After 9 weeks of 30-minute lessons twice a week focused on developmentally appropriate activities (e.g., letter names and sounds) in small groups, the researchers found statistically significant improvements in reading scores (Bailet et al., 2013).

Another study compared preschoolers who received Tier I supports or Tier II supplemental instruction with a control group. Results indicated the experimental group had statistically significant increases in letter names, letter sounds, and print knowledge (Lonigan & Phillips, 2015). Four-year-old children who received 3 months of instruction using the Handwriting Without Tears—Get Set for School program three times a week for 20 minutes each session made statistically significant improvement on prewriting (name, copying shapes), kindergarten readiness, and fine motor skills (Lust & Donica, 2011).

Adaptations and assistive technology for literacy

Occupational therapy practitioners also play a significant role in supporting access to books and literacy materials for all young children, including those with disabilities. For example, strategies and adaptations may include

- Interactive book reading activities using props from the story to increase and maintain engagement,
- Adapting writing tools for functional grasp,
- Visual supports to increase understanding of written communication and increase functional communication and symbolic representation, and
- Adaptations to promote engagement and independence to hold books and turn pages (e.g., large plastic paperclips on pages, books stabilized and mounted on an easel vertically).

Children with and without disabilities may use technology such as tablets, computers, and smart devices to engage in literacy activities for short periods. Technology can provide children with motor or language difficulties with opportunities to engage in literacy activities. For example, using a switch may enable a child to learn cause and effect. For more information on literacy and assistive technology, see Chapter 7, "Best Practices in the Use of Assistive Technology to Enhance Participation," and Chapter 29, "Best Practices in Supporting Learning and Early Literacy Skills (Cognitive Skills)."

SUMMARY

Development of literacy skills during early childhood significantly affects children's academic performance and life skills. Occupational therapy practitioenrs collaborate with families, educators, and other groups to enhance literacy skills among young children. Practitioners have the knowledge and skills to enhance literacy through interventions, modifications, environmental adaptations, and assistive technology. Interventions should use evidence-based resources to enhance children's skills in reading, writing, speaking, and listening.

Occupational therapy practitioners working with young children and their families have many resources available. The list and links in the Resources section include early organizations, national centers, and early literacy resources for practitioners in early childhood settings.

RESOURCES

- **American Occupational Therapy Association** (includes a literacy community on practice, journal articles, practice section with toolkits, fact sheets, and more): https://www.aota.org/
- **American Speech–Language–Hearing Association:** www.asha.org/public/speech/emergent-literacy/
- **Center for Early Literacy Learning:** http://www.earlyliteracylearning.org/
- **Kansas Inservice Training System's Virtual Kit:** Learning to Read: Early Literacy Birth to Five http://kskits.dept.ku.edu/ta/virtualKits/learningToReadEarlyLiteracy0to5.shtml
- **National Association for the Education of Young Children:** https://naeyc.org/resources/topics/literacy
- **National Center on Quality Teaching and Learning (Office of Head Start):** https://eclkc.ohs.acf.hhs.gov/
- **Paths to Literacy for Students Who Are Blind or Visually Impaired:** https://www.pathstoliteracy.org/
- **ZERO TO THREE:** https://www.zerotothree.org/early-learning/early-literacy

REFERENCES

Adair, J. K., Colegrove, K. S. S., & McManus, M. E. (2017). How the word gap argument negatively impacts young children of Latinx immigrants' conceptualizations of learning. *Harvard Educational Review, 87*(3), 309–334. https://doi.org/10.17763/1943-5045-87.3.309

Adams, M. (1990). *Beginning to read: Thinking and learning about print.* MIT Press.

American Occupational Therapy Association. (2020). Occupational therapy practice framework: Domain and process (4th ed.). *American Journal of Occupational Therapy, 74*(Suppl. 2), 7412410010. https://doi.org/10.5014/ajot.2020.74S2001

Anderson, J. A., Kutash, K., & Duchnowski, A. J. (2001). A comparison of the academic progress of students with EBD and students with LD. *Journal of Emotional and Behavioral Disorders, 9,* 106–115. https://doi.org/10.1177/106342660100900205

Annie E. Casey Foundation. (2014). *Early reading proficiency in the United States: A KIDS COUNT data snapshot.* https://www.aecf.org/resources/early-reading-proficiency-in-the-united-states/

Bailet, L. L., Repper, K., Murphy, S., Piasta, S., & Zettler-Greeley, C. (2013). Emergent literacy intervention for prekindergartners at risk for reading failure: Years 2 and 3 of a multiyear study. *Journal of Learning Disabilities, 46,* 133–153. https://doi.org/10.1177/0022219411407925

Baker, M., & Páez, M. (2018). *The language of the classroom: Dual language learners in Head Start, public pre-K, and private preschool programs.* Migration Policy Institute.

Beery, K., & Beery, N. (2006). *Beery™ VMI: Administration, scoring and teaching manual* (5th ed.). NCS Pearson, Inc.

Bennett, K. J., Brown, K. S., Boyle, M., Racine, Y., & Offord, D. (2003). Does low reading achievement at school entry cause conduct problems? *Social Science and Medicine, 56,* 2443–2448. https://doi.org/10.1016/S0277-9536(02)00247-2

Berninger, V., Abbott, R., Jones, J., Wolf, B., Gould, L., Anderson-Youngstrom, M., . . . Apel, K. (2006). Early development of language by hand: Composing reading, listening, and speaking connections; three letter-writing modes; and fast mapping in spelling. *Developmental Neuropsychology, 29*(1), 61–92. https://doi.org/10.1207/s15326942dn2901_5

Bialystok, E., Craik, F. I., & Luk, G. (2012). Bilingualism: Consequences for mind and brain. *Trends in Cognitive Sciences, 16,* 240–250. https://doi.org/10.1016/j.tics.2012.03.001

Blair, C. (2016). Executive function and early childhood education. *Current Opinion in Behavioral Sciences, 10,* 102–107. https://doi.org/10.1016/j.cobeha.2016.05.009

Breslin, D., & Exner, C. (1999). Construct validity of the in-hand manipulation test: A discriminant analysis with children without disability and children with spastic diplegia. *American Journal of Occupational Therapy, 53,* 381–386. https://doi.org/10.5014/ajot.53.4.381

Bus, A., Both-de Vries, A., de Jong, M., Sulzby, E., de Jong, W., & de Jong, E. (2001). *Conceptualizations underlying prereaders' story writing* (CIERA Report No. 2-015). University of Michigan, School of Education, Center for Improvement of Early Reading Achievement.

Castro, D., Espinosa, L., & Paez, M. (2011). Defining and measuring quality in early childhood practices that promote dual language learners' development and learning. In M. Zaslow, I. Martinez-Beck, K. Tout, & T. Halle (Eds.), *Quality measurement in early childhood settings* (pp. 257–280). Brookes.

Cartmill, E. A. (2016). Mind the gap: Assessing and addressing the word gap in early education. *Policy Insights from the Behavioral and Brain Sciences, 3*(2), 185–193. https://doi.org/10.1177/2372732216657565

Colozzo, P., McKeil, L., Petersen, J. M., & Szabo, A. (2016). An early literacy program for young children with Down syndrome: Changes observed over one year. *Journal of Policy and Practice in Intellectual Disabilities, 13,* 102–110. https://doi.org/10.1111/jppi.12160

Cooper, P. J., Vally, Z., Cooper, H., Radford, T., Sharples, A., Tomlinson, M., & Murray, L. (2014). Promoting mother–infant book sharing and infant attention and language development in an impoverished South African population: A pilot study. *Early Childhood Education Journal, 42,* 143–152. https://doi.org/10.1007/s10643-013-0591-8

Cornhill, H., & Case-Smith, J. (1996). Factors that relate to good and poor handwriting. *American Journal of Occupational Therapy, 50,* 732–739. https://doi.org/10.5014/ajot.50.9.732

Denton, K., & West, J. (2002). *Children's reading and math achievement in kindergarten and first grade* (NCES Report No. 2002-125). National Center for Education Statistics.

DeTemple, J. M. (2001). Parents and children reading books together. In D. Dickinson & P. Tabor (Eds.) *Beginning literacy with language* (pp. 31–52). Brookes.

Duncan, G. J., & Murnane, R. J. (Eds.). (2011). *Whither opportunity? Rising inequality, schools, and children's life chances.* Russell Sage.

Dunst, C. J., Trivette, C. M., Masiello, T., Roper, N., & Robyak, A. (2006). Framework for developing evidence based early literacy learning practices. *CELLpapers, 1*(1), 1–12. http://www.earlyliteracylearning.org/cellpapers/cellpapers_v1_n1.pdf

Evans, M., Kelley, J., & Sikora, J. (2014). Scholarly culture and academic performance in 42 nations. *Social Forces, 92,* 1573–1605. https://doi.org/10.1093/sf/sou030

Exner, C. (2005). Development of hand skills. In J. Case-Smith (Ed.), *Occupational therapy for children* (5th ed., pp. 304–355). Mosby.

Fischel, J., Bracken, S., Fuchs-Eisenberg, A., Spira, E., Katz, S., & Shaller, G. (2007). Evaluation of curricular approaches to enhance preschool early literacy skills. *Journal of Literacy Research, 39,* 471–501. https://doi.org/10.1080/10862960701675333

Fogo, J. (2008). *Writing in preschool.* Unpublished doctoral dissertation, Purdue University, West Lafayette, IN.

Frolek Clark, G. (2016). The occupations of literacy: Occupational therapy's role. *Journal of Occupational Therapy, Schools, and Early Intervention, 9*(1), 27–37. https://doi.org/10.1080/19411243.2016.1152835

Frolek Clark, G., & Luze, G. (2014). Predicting handwriting performance in kindergarteners using reading, fine-motor, and visual–motor measures. *Journal of Occupational Therapy, Schools, & Early Intervention, 7*(1), 29–44. https://doi.org/10.1080/19411243.2014.898470

Graham, S., Berninger, V., Abbott, R., Abbott, S., & Whitaker, D. (1997). The role of mechanics in composing of elementary school students: A new methodological approach. *Journal of Educational Psychology, 89*(1), 170–182. https://doi.org/10.1037/0022-0663.89.1.170

Graham, S., Harris, K., Mason, L., Fink-Chorzempa, B., Moran, S., & Saddler, B. (2008). How do primary grade teachers teach handwriting? A national survey. *Reading and Writing, 21,* 49–60. https://doi.org/10.1007/s11145-007-9064-z

Graham, S., Struck, M., Santoro, J., & Berninger, V. (2006). Dimensions of good and poor handwriting legibility in first and second graders: Motor programs, visual–spatial arrangement, and letter formation parameter setting. *Developmental Neuropsychology, 29,* 43–60. https://doi.org/10.1207/s15326942dn2901_4

Gray, S. A. O., Carter, A. S., Briggs-Gowan, M. J., Jones, S.M., & Wagmiller, R. L. (2014). Growth trajectories of early aggression, overactivity, and inattention: Relations to second-grade reading. *Developmental Psychology, 50,* 2255–2263. https://doi.org/10.1037/a0037367

Halonen, A., Aunola, K., Ahonen, T., & Nurmi, J. E. (2006). The role of learning to read in the development of problem behaviour: A cross-lagged longitudinal study. *British Journal of Educational Psychology, 76,* 517–534. https://doi.org/10.1348/000709905X51590

Hart, B., & Risley, T. (1992). American parenting of language-learning children: Persisting differences in family–child interactions observed in natural home environments. *Developmental Psychology, 28,* 1096–1105. https://doi.org/10.1037/0012-1649.6.1096

Hart, B., & Risley, T. R. (1995). *Meaningful differences in the everyday experience of young American children.* Brookes.

Hernandez, D. (2012). *Double jeopardy: How third-grade reading skills and poverty influence high school graduation.* https://www.aecf.org/resources/double-jeopardy/

Hilbert, D. D., & Eis, S. D. (2013). Early intervention for emergent literacy development in a collaborative community pre-kindergarten. *Early Childhood Education Journal, 42,* 105–113. https://doi.org/10.1007/s10643-013-0588-3

Huttenlocher, J., Haight, W., Bryk, A., Seltzer, M., & Lyons, T. (1991). Early vocabulary growth: Relation to language input and gender. *Developmental Psychology, 27,* 236–248. https://doi.org/10.1037/0012-1649.27.2.236

Justice, L. M., McGinty, A. S., Cabell, S. Q., Kilday, C. R., Knighton, K., & Huffman, G. (2010). Language and literacy curriculum supplement for preschoolers who are academically at risk: A feasibility study. *Language Speech & Hearing Services in Schools, 41,* 161–178. https://doi.org/10.1044/0161-1461(2009/08-0058)

King, K. R., Lembke, E. S., & Reinke, W. M. (2016). Using latent class analysis to identify academic and behavioral risk status in elementary students. *School Psychology Quarterly, 31*(1), 43–57. https://doi.org/10.1037/spq0000111

Lloyd, J. E. V., Irwin, L. G., & Hertzman, C. (2009). Kindergarten school readiness and fourth-grade literacy and numeracy outcomes of children with special needs: A population-based study. *Educational Psychology, 29,* 583–602. https://doi.org/10.1080/01443410903165391

Lonigan, C. J., & Phillips, B. M. (2015). Supplemental material for response to instruction in preschool: Results of two randomized studies with children at significant risk of reading difficulties. *Journal of Educational Psychology, 108,* 114–129. https://doi.org/10.1037/edu0000054.supp

Lust, C. A., & Donica, D. K. (2011). Effectiveness of a handwriting readiness program in Head Start: A two-group controlled trial.

American Journal of Occupational Therapy, 65, 560–568. https://doi.org/10.5014/ajot.2011.000612

Maughan, B., Gray, G., & Rutter, M. (1985). Reading retardation and antisocial behaviour: A follow-up into employment. *Journal of Child Psychology and Psychiatry, 26,* 741–758. https://doi.org/10.1111/j.1469-7610.1985.tb00588.x

Molfese, V., Beswick, J., Molnar, A., & Jacobi-Vessels, J. (2006). Alphabetic skills in preschool: A preliminary study of letter naming and letter writing. *Developmental Neuropsychology, 29,* 5–19. https://doi.org/10.1207/s15326942dn2901_2

Morgan, P. L., Farkas, G., Tufis, P. A., & Sperling, R. A. (2008). Are reading and behavior problems risk factors for each other? *Journal of Learning Disabilities, 41,* 417–436. https://doi.org/10.1177/0022219408321123

National Institute for Literacy. (2008). *Developing early literacy: Report of the National Early Literacy Panel.* Washington, DC: Author.

Neuman, S. B., & Cunningham, L. (2009). The impact of professional development and coaching on early language and literacy instructional practices. *American Educational Research Journal, 46,* 532–566. https://doi.org/10.3102/0002831208328088

Nix, R. L., Bierman, K. L., Domitrovich, C. E., & Gill, S. (2013). Promoting children's social–emotional skills in preschool can enhance academic and behavioral functioning in kindergarten: Findings from Head Start REDI. *Early Education and Development, 24,* 1000–1019. https://doi.org/10.1080/10409289.2013.825565

Pears, K. C., Kim, H. K., Fisher, P. A., & Yoerger, K. (2016). Increasing pre-kindergarten early literacy skills in children with developmental disabilities and delays. *Journal of School Psychology, 57,* 15–27. https://doi.org/10.1016/j.jsp.2016.05.004

Raikes, H., Pan, B. A., Luze, G., Tamis-LeMonda, C. S., Brooks-Gun, J., Constantine, J., . . . Rodrigues, E. T. (2006). Mother–child book reading in low-income families: Correlates and outcomes during the first three years of life. *Child Development, 77,* 924–953. https://doi.org/10.1111/j.1467-8624.2006.00911.x

Ritchey, K. (2008). The building blocks of writing: Learning to write letters and spell words. *Reading & Writing, 21,* 27–47. https://doi.org/10.1007/s11145-007-9063-0

Schryer, E., Sloat, E., & Letourneau, N. (2015). Effects of an animated book reading intervention on emergent literacy skill development: An early pilot study. *Journal of Early Intervention, 37,* 155–171. https://doi.org/10.1177/1053815115598842

Sheridan, S. M., Knoche, L. L., Kupzyk, K. A., Edwards, C. P., & Marvin, C. A. (2011). A randomized trial examining the effects of parent engagement on early language and literacy: The Getting Ready intervention. *Journal of School Psychology, 49,* 361–383. https://doi.org/10.1016/j.jsp.2011.03.001

Sperry, D. E., Sperry, L. L., & Miller, P. J. (2019). Reexamining the verbal environments of children from different socioeconomic backgrounds. *Child Development, 90,* 1303–1318. https://doi.org/10.1111/cdev.13072

Stauter, D. W., Myers, S. R., & Classen, A. I. (2017). Literacy instruction for young children with severe speech and physical impairments: A systematic review. *Journal of Occupational Therapy, Schools, & Early Intervention, 10,* 389–407. https://doi.org/10.1080/19411243.2017.1359132

Trout, A. L., Epstein, M. H., Nelson, R., Synhorst, L., & Hurley, K. D. (2006). Profiles of children served in early intervention programs for behavioral disorders: Early literacy and behavioral characteristics. *Topics in Early Childhood Special Education, 26,* 206–218. https://doi.org/10.1177/02711214060260040201

Trout, A. L., Nordness, P. D., Pierce, C. D., & Epstein, M. H. (2003). Research on the academic status of children with emotional and behavioral disorders: A review of the literature from 1961 to 2000. *Journal of Emotional and Behavioral Disorders, 11*(4), 198–210. https://doi.org/10.1177/10634266030110040201

Walker, D., Greenwood, C., Hart, B., & Carta, J. (1994). Prediction of school outcomes based on early language production and socioeconomic factors. *Child Development, 65,* 606–621. https://doi.org/10.1111/j.1467-8624.1994.tb00771.x

Weintraub, N., & Graham, S. (2000). The contribution of gender, orthographic, finger function, and visual–motor processes to the prediction of handwriting status. *Occupational Therapy Journal of Research, 20,* 121–141. https://doi.org/10.1177/153944920002000203

ZERO TO THREE. (2003). *Early literacy.* https://www.zerotothree.org/espanol/early-literacy

Section III.

Considerations for Early Intervention: IDEA Part C

Understanding Part C: Early Intervention Law and the Individualized Family Service Plan (IFSP) Process

14

Anne Lucas, MS, OTR/L

KEY TERMS AND CONCEPTS

- Child Find
- Comprehensive system of personnel development
- Developmental delay
- Lead agency
- Monitoring activities
- Natural environments
- Part C of the Individuals With Disabilities Education Improvement Act of 2004
- Procedural safeguards
- Service coordinator
- System of payment
- Team

OVERVIEW

As an outgrowth of the Education for All Handicapped Children Act of 1975 (P. L. 94-142), the early intervention federal grant program was established by Congress in 1986 as P. L. 99-457. This program is now ***Part C of the Individuals With Disabilities Education Improvement Act of 2004*** (IDEA; P. L. 108-446). It was established to address "an urgent and substantial need" to enhance the development of infants and toddlers with disabilities; reduce educational costs by minimizing the need for special education; maximize independent living; enhance the capacity of families to meet their child's needs; and identify, evaluate, and meet the needs of all children, particularly underserved populations (IDEA, §1431[a]).

Before the enactment of the early intervention federal grant program in 1986, states provided services to different populations of infants and toddlers with disabilities through various agencies (Spiker et al., 2000). As a result, this program was designed to assist states to coordinate existing interagency, multidisciplinary early intervention services and implement coordinated, statewide systems of services for infants and toddlers with disabilities, ages birth to 3 years years and their families (IDEA, §303.1). Although participation in the Part C of IDEA early intervention (EI) program is voluntary, states must ensure that appropriate EI services are available to all eligible infants and toddlers and their families if they chose to participate (IDEA, §303.101). According to the Early Childhood Technical Assistance (ECTA) Center (n.d.-a), all states and territories currently participate in the Part C program.

Occupational therapy is one of 17 EI services identified in Part C of IDEA (§303.13) and is considered a primary EI service under Part C, while under Part B, occupational therapy is a related service. Occupational therapy is required to be offered by both Part B and Part C. Because the provision of high-quality EI services is dependent on the knowledge and skills of EI personnel (Kasprzak et al., 2019), it is incumbent that occupational therapy practitioners understand the requirements of Part C and the processes and practices used in implementing these requirements. (*Note. Occupational therapy practitioner* refers to both occupational therapists and occupational therapy assistants.) The American Occupational Therapy Association (AOTA; 2017) *Guidelines for Occupational Therapy Services in Early Intervention and Schools* indicate that occupational therapy practitioners need to be "knowledgeable about systems that influence practice," "procedures and practices of the early intervention system," and the "principles of family centered practice" used in providing EI services (p. 5). This chapter provides an overview of the Part C requirements, how states implement these requirements, and how these requirements translate into occupational therapy practice.

ESSENTIAL CONSIDERATIONS

According to the ECTA Center (2015), "building and sustaining high-quality early intervention . . . systems is a complex and ongoing process for states" (p. 1). Not only do states need to comply with Part C of IDEA requirements, but they must ensure their EI system infrastructure (e.g., funding, policies and procedures, oversight and accountability, workforce development, program standards, data system) is of high quality to support service providers in implementing evidence-based practices that result in positive outcomes for infants and toddlers with disabilities and their families. How each state designs its EI system to meet Part C requirements is influenced by a multitude of factors such as existing state requirements; which agencies provided EI services before the 1986 EI program; and state politics, priorities, and funding (Greer et al., 2007; Spiker et al., 2000). As a result, EI program structures and service delivery systems vary across states, and these variations are likely to influence eligibility for EI services, as well as the quality of the services provided. In states with local control and local decision-making authority, there is also variation within the state in the design of local EI systems and how services are delivered (Spiker et al., 2000). While each state program may look different, they are all required to adhere to a minimum set of services and activities; states may go above and beyond, which will be influenced by these factors.

Lead Agency Designation

States are required to have a **lead agency** designated by the governor to administer, supervise, and monitor programs and activities; identify and coordinate all available resources; establish financial responsibilities of agencies to pay for EI services; resolve disputes; and ensure that EI services are delivered pending resolution of disputes (IDEA, §303.120). Multiple states (e.g., Vermont) have co-lead agencies, but IDEA clearly states that each state system must have a single line of responsibility. The type of lead agency designated by most states is a health agency; some states designate "other" agency (i.e., pertaining to developmental disabilities, human services, early learning agencies, and co-lead agencies), and slightly fewer states have an education lead agency (ECTA Center, 2016).

Contracts and Interagency Agreements

State lead agencies are required to enter into contractual or other written arrangements with entities for the delivery of EI services (IDEA, §303.121). Many states contract with local providers (individuals, public agencies, or private businesses) for the provision of all EI services for eligible children, from child referral through transition in a specific catchment area. Some states contract with agencies for activities, from child referral to the development of the initial individualized family service plan (IFSP), and also contract with other providers and agencies to deliver services once the IFSP is developed. Several other states have different service arrangements (IDEA Infant & Toddler Coordinators Association, 2018a).

Supervision and Monitoring

Each state lead agency is responsible for monitoring programs and activities to ensure compliance with Part C requirements (IDEA, §303.120[a][2]). States' **monitoring activities** are required to focus primarily on improving results for children and families and ensuring that programs are compliant with Part C requirements (IDEA, §303.700[b]). These activities include monitoring EI program performance on the state performance plan (SPP) and annual performance report (APR) indicators (i.e., delivery of timely services, delivery of services in natural environments, child and family outcomes, Child Find, completion of evaluation and assessment in 45 days, completion of timely transition activities including a transition plan, transition notification, and transition conference; IDEA, §303.700[d]; U.S. Department of Education, 2018a). When monitoring, states must identify noncompliance and ensure correction of the noncompliance within 1 year of identification (IDEA, §303,700[e]). States can use a variety of methods to conduct monitoring, including but not limited to, desk audits, onsite visits, record reviews, and self-assessments (ECTA Center, 2015).

Financial Requirements

To ensure an effective and responsive EI system of services and supports, states must have an adequate and stable funding base, which includes coordinating and accessing available federal, state, and local resources (ECTA Center, n.d.-b). Part C of IDEA (§303.501) requires states to use federal Part C funds to pay for direct services as identified on the IFSP, including frequency, intensity, and duration, only if no other funding sources are available to pay for these services.

IDEA (§303.501) allows states to establish a **system of payment** policy that defines whether public and private insurance is used to pay for any EI services and whether families incur a cost for services; IDEA is specific that it is a "Payor of Last Resort," meaning that funds provided by Part C may not be used to pay for services that "otherwise would have been paid for by another public or private source." Family costs may include a fee for services based on a family's ability to pay (e.g., a sliding fee scale) or cost participation associated with the use of public or private insurance (e.g., co-payments, deductibles, premiums). The policy must also clarify that family fees will not be charged for Child Find activities, evaluation and assessment, service coordination, development and review of the IFSP, and administration of procedural safeguards. Parents must consent before the use of public or private insurance to pay for IFSP services and when there is an increase in frequency, length, duration, or intensity of services when using private insurance. If the parent does not provide consent, services must still be provided (IDEA, §303.520). If the state opts to charge family fees, the fees must be based on the state's definition of ability to pay (IDEA, §303.521).

Overall, states have discretion regarding which fund sources to use. Almost all states (47) access Medicaid to pay for EI services (IDEA Infant & Toddler Coordinators Association, 2017). In many states, Medicaid accepts the IFSP as the prior authorization document. Approximately half of states (27) access private insurance; fewer states (17) implement family fees (e.g., annual fees, monthly fees, copayments; IDEA Infant & Toddler Coordinators Association, 2018b). Because funding sources used to pay for services vary, occupational therapy practitioners should become familiar with their state's system of payment policies and other state-specific financial processes.

Personnel Standards and Personnel Development System

To provide high-quality EI services, states must ensure "knowledgeable, skilled, competent, and highly qualified personnel and that sufficient numbers of these personnel are available in the state to meet service needs" (ECTA Center, 2015, p. 25). Part C of IDEA (§303.118) requires states to establish a **comprehensive system of personnel development,** including training and technical assistance for EI personnel on evidence-based practices and legal requirements. Personnel standards must also be in place for all disciplines that provide EI services to ensure that qualified personnel are working in EI (IDEA, §303.119). These standards should be consistent with standards established by national professional organizations (e.g., Council for Exceptional Children [CEC], American Speech-Language-Hearing

Association, AOTA) and with state criteria for certification, licensure, credentialing, and endorsement (Kasprzak et al., 2019). In addition to requiring all EI personnel, including occupational therapy practitioners, to meet state personnel standards, some states require EI certification through participation in state certification training (Early Childhood Personnel Center, n.d.).

Definition of *Developmental Delay*

Each state is required by IDEA (§303.111) to include a rigorous definition of **developmental delay** to appropriately identify infants and toddlers with disabilities who are eligible for Part C EI services. The definition must describe the procedures used to measure a child's development and the level of developmental delay that constitutes a delay in one or more of the following areas of development: cognitive, physical including vision and hearing, communication, social or emotional, and adaptive. States must also identify conditions that have a high probability of resulting in developmental delay. At state discretion, children at risk for developmental delay may be included in the eligibility definition (IDEA, §303.21).

States' definitions of developmental delay range between restrictive (e.g., 50% delay in one or more domains, two standard deviations in one domain) and broad (e.g., at risk, any delay, 25% delay in one or more domains). Many states' definitions fall in between these parameters (e.g., 25% in two or more domains, 30% delay in one or more domains, or 1.5 standard deviations in one domain; IDEA Infant & Toddler Coordinators Association, 2018c). The ECTA Center's compilation of each state's eligibility definitions of developmental delay (see https://ectacenter.org/~pdfs/topics/earlyid/partc_elig_table.pdf) is a helpful resource.

Part C Option: Flexibility to Serve Children Beyond Age 3 Years and Birth Mandate

Part C of IDEA regulations permits states to provide EI services under Part C from age 3 years until the beginning of the school year or until the child enters, or is eligible to enter, kindergarten or elementary school. If a state chooses to extend EI services, it must be a joint policy decision between the Part C lead agency and the state education agency and include an educational component that promotes school readiness (i.e., preliteracy, language, and numeracy skills; IDEA, §303.211). Two states currently have elected to serve children beyond the age of 3 years under this Part C option. One state provides early intervention services for children until age 4 years, and the other state serves children until the beginning of the school year after the child's fourth birthday (J. Barrett-Zitkus, U.S. Department of Education, personal communication, May 6, 2019).

States may also enact a state law or birth mandate that permits children younger than age 3 years to be served under free appropriate public education according to Part B of IDEA or to use Part B funds for providing early intervention services. If a state enacts a birth mandate, both Part B and Part C of IDEA requirements must be met, and fees cannot be charged to parents for these services (IDEA, §303.521[c]). There are five birth mandate states. All five

have an education lead agency (one has a co-lead) and had birth mandates in place before the initiation of Part C (Michigan Association of Administrators of Special Education, 2014).

Public Awareness and Child Find

A public awareness system must be in place to disseminate information on the availability of EI services; how to refer a child under the age of 3 years for an evaluation or EI services; and the state's central directory of services, resources, and experts in the state (IDEA, §303.301). Each state must also have a comprehensive **Child Find** system, which identifies, locates, and evaluates all infants and toddlers with disabilities who are eligible for EI services, including those who reside on an Indian reservation or are homeless, in foster care, or a ward of the state. The system must be coordinated with other Child Find efforts, including but not limited to, Part B of IDEA, the Maternal and Child Health Bureau, Head Start, the Child Welfare Agency, and the Early Hearing Detection and Intervention Program (IDEA, §303.302).

Service Coordination

Part C of IDEA requires each infant or toddler with a disability and their family to be provided with one service coordinator (e.g., case manager) to serve as the single point of contact for the team and assist parents in accessing services and resources. The **service coordinator** coordinates evaluations, facilitates IFSP meetings, informs families of their rights and procedural safeguards, coordinates funding, coordinates and monitors services, and facilitates transition (IDEA, §303.34). Service coordinators may be "dedicated," meaning that service coordination is their only role, or may have "blended" roles. In a blended model, a service coordinator would be assigned from any one of the professionals on the EI team, including occupational therapy practitioners, who provide EI services (Raver & Childress, 2014). States more frequently use a dedicated model of service coordination than a blended model or a combination of both (IDEA Infant & Toddler Coordinators Association, 2019).

Screening, Evaluation, and Assessment

Part C of IDEA (§303.310) requires that screening (if adopted), evaluation, and assessment, as well as the initial IFSP meeting, be conducted within 45 days of referral unless the parent is unavailable as a result of exceptional family circumstances. States have the option of including screening to determine whether a child is suspected of having a disability before initial evaluation and assessment. The parents must provide consent for screening, and if at any time the parent requests evaluation and assessment, they must be provided (IDEA, §303.320). According to an informal review of states' policies and procedures by the ECTA Center in April 2019, 39% of states incorporate screening as an option in their referral and intake process.

A timely, comprehensive, multidisciplinary evaluation and assessment must be conducted by qualified personnel to determine a child's eligibility in accordance with the state's definition of developmental delay and to assess the unique strengths and needs of the child to determine appropriate services. A child's medical and other records may be used to establish eligibility without conducting an evaluation of the child. Assessment of the child includes reviewing results of the evaluation, observing the child, and determining needs in each developmental area. A family assessment, which is voluntary, is conducted to assess the family's resources, priorities, and concerns and to determine the supports and services necessary to enhance the family's capacity to meet the developmental needs of

FIGURE 14.1.   The early intervention and individualized family service plan process.

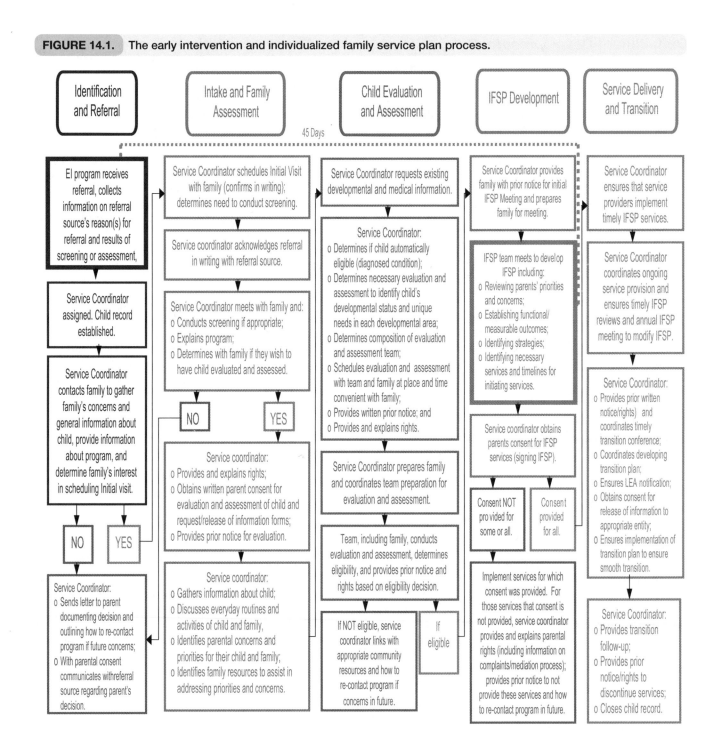

Lucas, Hurth & Shaw, NECTAC 2006. Adapted from Solutions Consulting Group, LLC with permission   *Note: Programs differ in who is assigned to each responsibility. Service coordinator could be other service provider.

Source. Reprinted from *The Early Intervention/IFSP Process,* by ECTA Center, 2006, retrieved from https://ectacenter.org/~pdfs/topics/families/ifsp_process_chart .pdf. Reprinted with permission.

the child. Informed clinical opinion must be used in conducting the evaluation and assessment and may be used to establish a child's eligibility without negating the results of the evaluation instrument (IDEA, §303.321). See Figure 14.1 for an overview of the process.

Child and Family Outcome Measurement

The U.S. Department of Education (2018a) require states to collect child and family outcome data and to report annually on state performance compared to the target in their SPP and APR. For family outcomes, states report on "the percent of families who report that early intervention services have helped their family: 1) know their rights; 2) effectively communicate their child's needs; and 3) help their children develop and learn" (p. 5). States use a family survey to collect these data (ECTA Center, n.d.-c).

States also report data on child outcomes, including "the percent of infants and toddlers with IFSPs who demonstrate improved: (1) Positive social-emotional skills (including social relationships); (2) Acquisition and use of knowledge and skills (including early language/communication); (3) Use of appropriate behavior to meet needs" (U.S. Department of Education, 2018a, p. 3). Most states use the Child Outcomes Summary (COS) to measure the three child outcomes. The COS summarizes multiple assessment tools, including information from the family, and compares this summary of the child's functioning to age expectations. A small number of states use only a publisher's tool (e.g., Battelle Developmental Inventory, 2nd ed.; Newborg, 2005) to measure child outcomes (ECTA Center, 2018). Regardless of the approach, all states collect child outcomes data at entry and at exit from Part C and then compare entry and exit data for children who have received services for at least 6 months to determine the child's progress while receiving EI services (U.S. Department of Education, 2018a).

States also use child and family outcomes data for program improvement. Almost all states use one or more child or family outcome as the focus of their state systemic improvement plan, an indicator used in the SPP and APR (U.S. Department of Education, 2018b).

IFSP Development, Review, and Evaluation

For each eligible infant and toddler and their family, an IFSP must be collaboratively developed by a team. The team includes the child's family, advocates, service coordinator, people involved in conducting the evaluation and assessment, and as appropriate, service providers who will be providing services (e.g., developmental specialist, service coordinator, speech pathologist, occupational therapist, physical therapist; IDEA, §303.343). Part C of IDEA (§303.344) requires specific content in the IFSP, including but not limited to

- The child's present levels of development across all domains;
- The parent's resources, priorities, and concerns;
- Outcomes or results to be achieved;
- EI services (including frequency, intensity, and duration of services; natural environment; payment arrangements; and so forth);
- Other services;

- The service coordinator; and
- A transition plan with steps and services.

An IFSP review must be conducted at least once every 6 months, and an annual IFSP meeting must be held within 365 days of the initial IFSP to evaluate and revise the IFSP as needed. Information from current evaluations and ongoing assessments, including family priorities, concerns, and resources, are used by the team to make decisions about needed IFSP changes (e.g., outcomes, service types, service frequency and intensity; IDEA, §303.342).

Service Delivery

Part C of IDEA requires EI services be provided under public supervision, regardless of the payment source. Parental consent must be obtained before initiation of IFSP services. Services, including frequency, intensity, and duration (including start date), and the setting of the service must be provided in accordance with the IFSP and must be initiated in a timely manner (IDEA, §303.13). Many states define timely services as services initiated within 30 days of the parent's signature on the IFSP (U.S. Department of Education, 2012).

EI services are also required to be based on scientifically based research (IDEA, §303.112). In other words, the selection of services and interventions must be based on available evidence of their efficacy or effectiveness in improving results as reflected in research, data, and collective knowledge and input of professionals and families (ECTA Center, n.d.-d). States frequently use evidence-based practices per established service delivery models that focus on specific practices such as coaching (Coaching in Natural Learning Environments; North Carolina Early Intervention Infant-Toddler Program, 2019), routines-based intervention (Routines-based Early Intervention [The RAM Group, 2015] and Family Guided Routines Based Intervention [2020]), and positive behavioral intervention and support (Pyramid Model [National Center for Pyramid Model Innovations, n.d.). States also use the CEC's Division of Early Childhood Recommended Practices (2014) in the areas of leadership, assessment, environment, family, instruction, interaction, teaming and collaboration, and transition (U.S. Department of Education, 2018b).

Procedural Safeguards

Under Part C of IDEA (§§303.400–303.449), ***procedural safeguards*** protect the rights of parents and infants and toddlers with disabilities and include mechanisms for the resolution of disputes. Procedural safeguards requirements and dispute resolution procedures must be shared with and explained to parents. Parents and children have the right to such safeguards as a timely evaluation and assessment, timely EI services, the ability to accept or refuse (through written consent) screening, evaluation and assessment, EI services, use of public or private insurance (if applicable), and the confidentiality of child or family personally identifiable information. The ECTA Center has a resource that describes which procedural safeguards must be provided at specific times in the IFSP process, from referral through transition (see flow chart for procedural safeguards at https://bit.ly/31GqX1z).

Transition

When a child is ready to exit the Part C EI program, every effort must be made to ensure that children and families experience a smooth transition. Part C of IDEA (§303.209) requires

- A timely transition plan to be developed in the IFSP for children exiting Part C,
- A timely transition notification to be provided to the local education agency where the child resides and to the state education agency for toddlers potentially eligible for Part B of IDEA (unless the state allows parents to opt out of the notification), and
- A timely transition conference to be convened with the receiving agency, with approval of the family.

At age 3 years, children more frequently transition to preschool special education under Part B of IDEA than to other programs such as Head Start, child care, and so forth (U.S. Department of Education, 2018c).

BEST PRACTICES

Understanding the requirements of Part C of IDEA, the intent of the law, and variation in how states implement the law is complex. What is more challenging is using the decades of available evidence on what constitutes effective EI services under Part C and implementing practices that result in improved child and family outcomes (Bruder, 2010; Hebbeler et al., 2012).

Provide Service in Natural Environments

Natural environments are settings that are typical for a same-age child without a disability and may include the home or community settings such as the library, the park, or child care (IDEA, §303.26). Research supports that children learn best while interested and engaged in naturally occurring learning opportunities that are embedded in everyday activities and routines of their family (Shelden & Rush, 2001, as cited in Lucas et al., 2014). Families spend the most time with their children and have the greatest impact on their children's development (Bruder, 2010; Raver & Childress, 2014). In addition, McWilliam (2012) contends that what happens between intervention sessions is central for enhancing the child's learning, independence, and participation in family and community life.

In 2008, this evidence was used by the Workgroup on Principles and Practice in Natural Environments (WPPNE) to develop consensus documents outlining the mission and key principles (WPPNE, 2008a) as well as agreed-upon practices for providing early intervention services in natural environments (WPPNE, 2008b). WPPNE (2008a) defined the mission as using "Part C early intervention [to build] upon and [provide] supports and resources to assist family members and caregivers to enhance children's learning and development through everyday learning opportunities" (p. 2).

Occupational therapy's focus on promoting participation through engagement in occupations clearly aligns with Part C of IDEA's focus on providing EI in the context of a family's everyday routines and activities (AOTA, 2017; Minard, 2018). Occupational therapy enhances the family's capacity by supporting families in problem-solving challenging activities that are important and meaningful, such as rest, sleep, mealtime, play, and social development, and in making adaptations to support their child's functional skills, engagement, and participation (AOTA, 2017). A resource that reflects the alignment between occupational therapy literature and the key principles of early intervention is *Key Principles of Early Intervention and Effective Practices: A Crosswalk With Statements From Discipline Specific Literature* (see https://ectacenter.org/topics/eiservices/natenv_position.asp).

Although variations in states' EI systems can affect the roles and responsibilities of occupational therapy practitioners across states (AOTA, 2017), there are best practices that all practitioners can use throughout the IFSP process, from referral through transition. These practices support dynamic and individualized interactions with families and reflect the context, culture, values, and beliefs of the child and family (AOTA, 2017).

Provide Family Service Coordination

Occupational therapists are well qualified to function as service coordinators (AOTA, 2010, 2014), especially in states that use a blended model of service coordination. According to AOTA (2010), occupational therapists' "holistic, science-driven, evidence-based approach" can be used in carrying out the functions of service coordinator (p. 1). As service coordinators, occupational therapists use leadership practices to coordinate evaluation and assessments and IFSP meetings; promote collaborative decision making and problem solving with the team; coordinate with community partners to support the family in accessing needed supports and resources; and foster a strengths-based, capacity-building partnership with the child's family (AOTA, 2017).

Conduct Screening, Evaluation, and Assessment

In conducting screening, evaluation, and assessment, occupational therapists administer appropriate instruments, use observation, and apply clinical reasoning (AOTA, 2014a, 2017). Ideally, evaluation and assessment of the child should be conducted in settings where the child typically participates and in the context of naturally occurring routines and activities to best identify the child's strengths and needs related to functional performance (WPPNE, 2008b).

Identifying the child's skills in each developmental domain is important, but it is most critical to assess the child's performance across domains and settings to determine how these skills affect the child's engagement in occupation and participation in family routines. Barriers and facilitators of engagement and participation are identified (AOTA, 2017, 2020; Campbell, n.d., as cited in Lucas et al., 2014). Although occupational therapy practitioners focus on the whole child, they uniquely contribute to the team's assessment of the child's strengths and needs regarding "adaptive development, adaptive behavior, and play and sensory, motor, and postural development" (AOTA, 2017, p. 6).

The assessment team, including the occupational therapist, gathers information from the child's family on what is working and what is challenging in everyday routines and activities; the strategies they have tried and found successful or not; the child and family's interests, including what they would like their child and their family to be able to do; the supports and resources they have access to or would like to access; and their priorities for their child and family (AOTA, 2017; WPPNE, 2008b). For more details about evaluation and assessment, see Chapter 15, "Best Practices in Early Intervention Screening and Evaluation."

Complete Child Outcome Measurement

According to the ECTA Center (n.d.-e), the three global child outcomes measured for accountability and program improvement describe a child's appropriate application of behaviors, knowledge, and skills in a meaningful way for successful participation and engagement in everyday occupations at home and in the community. When using the COS, occupational therapists can uniquely contribute to the team process by sharing assessment information on the child's functional performance in occupations, helping the team synthesize assessment information, and using their knowledge of typical development to jointly rate the child's performance in the three outcomes compared with age-expected behavior (James et al., 2016).

Develop and Review the IFSP

In developing or reviewing the IFSP, occupational therapy practitioners actively participate in the IFSP team, which includes the family. The team reviews child evaluation and assessment and family assessment information to identify or modify child and family IFSP outcomes to address the individualized needs and preferences of the child and the family (AOTA, 2017; Lucas et al., 2014). According to Bruder (2010), IFSP outcomes should "cross disciplines and agency boundaries" (p. 344). Lucas and colleagues (2014) contended that outcomes should not be discipline specific but rather describe the child's participation in naturally occurring routines and activities and promote skill development across multiple domains so that any IFSP team member can address them.

Child IFSP outcomes should enhance the child's learning, engagement, and participation (child as learner and actor); be important and meaningful to the family; expand settings in which the child can be competent; and build on the child's interests. Similarly, IFSP family outcomes should enhance the capacity of the family to support their child's development and participation (family as learner and actor) and support the family in accessing community resources and supports (Lucas et al., 2014). Criteria for developing and rating high-quality and functional IFSP outcomes have been identified by the ECTA Center (see https://ectacenter.org/~pdfs/pubs/rating-ifsp.pdf).

When determining the services needed to meet child and family outcomes, the IFSP team should choose a primary service provider based on the individual needs of the child and family (AOTA, 2014). In selecting the primary service provider, the team considers the desired outcomes and practitioner expertise and matches them with the child

and family, practitioner availability, and geography (Shelden & Rush, 2007; Woodruff & McGonigel, 1988, as cited in Boyer & Thompson, 2014). According to AOTA (2014, p. 1), "Occupational therapists are ideally suited to function as primary service providers, as determined by the IFSP team" as long as other services are provided by team members as needed and the services provided by the primary provider are not outside the scope of practice or one's license or certification. Shelden and Rush (2007) saw the primary service provider as a mobilizer and mediator of resources to support the child and family.

In determining frequency and intensity of services, Infant Toddler Connection of Virginia (2018) considered whether the service is new or ongoing, the degree to which the relationship between the provider and the child and family is established, the parents' or caregivers' level of understanding and capacity to embed learning opportunities into everyday activities, and the urgency of the outcome to be achieved. Any of these factors may warrant more frequent services for a limited period with a gradual reduction of frequency over time. Caldwell and colleagues (2018) contended that "frequent contact with a therapist may be an important component to maintain a newly established routine" (p. 6).

The team considers the home and community settings where the child and family typically participate or would like to participate when determining the natural environments where services will be provided. A service can be delivered in multiple settings such as in the home, at a child care center, or on the playground, depending on child and family needs. If the IFSP team determines that the outcomes cannot be met in natural settings, a justification must be developed that describes how the services provided in specialized settings will be generalized into everyday routines and activities and designates a timeline for returning the services to natural settings (WPPNE, 2008b).

Provide Services in the Context of a Team

Early intervention services, as identified on the IFSP, are provided in the context of the *team,* including the family. Team composition is usually flexible based on the individual needs of each child and family (Raver & Childress, 2014). However, a core team with representatives across key disciplines (e.g., occupational therapy, speech-language pathology, physical therapy, early childhood education) that accesses other professionals as needed can be used to serve children in a specific geographic area (Shelden & Rush, 2007). Regardless of structure, the team meets frequently to share knowledge and expertise, promote a collective understanding of the child and family's evolving strengths and needs, build team and family capacity, problem solve challenges, and monitor progress (AOTA, 2017; Boyer & Thompson, 2014; Shelden & Rush, 2007).

In preparation for service delivery, the occupational therapy practitioner develops occupation-based goals and interventions that align with the IFSP outcomes and the settings where the interventions will occur (AOTA, 2017). Each visit focuses on building family capacity to attend and respond to their child's interests and abilities in everyday activities to promote the child's development and learning as well as to identify or obtain needed resources and supports (McWilliam, 2012; Shelden & Rush, 2007).

The visit begins with a conversation with the family focusing on what has occurred since the previous visit, including any significant family events, what is working and challenging, what the family has tried, and the outcomes and strategies they would like to focus on during the visit (WPPNE, 2008b). Each visit is individualized to meet the family where they are, taking into consideration changing child and family circumstances and characteristics (McWilliam, 2012; Raver & Childress, 2014). All interactions with the family need to reflect that families have strengths and capabilities and are the primary change agents for their child's learning and development (McCollum & Yates, 2017; McWilliam, 2012).

Modifications, adaptations, and assistive technology are used as needed by occupational therapy practitioners to enhance children's development, level of engagement in activities, and functional participation in family and community life (AOTA, 2017). Observation, modeling, teaching, coaching, prompting, joint problem solving, and joining the ongoing interactions of the family and child are also used throughout visits to support the family in making established routines more responsive to the child's needs (Raver & Childress, 2014; WPPNE, 2008b).

Supporting the family and caregiver as the primary interactor with the child during each visit and providing multiple opportunities for them to practice the intervention strategies discussed or modeled are critical (McCollum & Yates, 2017; Raver & Childress, 2014). Before each visit ends, the occupational therapy practitioner and family jointly decide next steps and identify needs for team member support (e.g., consultation, information sharing, co-visit; WPPNE, 2008b). Throughout service delivery, the changing needs of children and families, data on the effectiveness of interventions, and progress toward outcomes should drive the interventions and be used to identify potential changes needed to IFSP outcomes and services through an IFSP review (AOTA, 2017).

Support Transition From Early Intervention

Occupational therapy practitioners can assist in supporting children and families exiting Part C to preschool special education or other community services (AOTA, 2017). Myers and colleagues (2011) stated that "occupational therapists' knowledge of activity analysis and environmental adaptation makes them valuable team members who have the skills to anticipate possible problems in the next environment and work in partnership with families and other professionals to identify solutions before the transition" (p. 87).

Myers and colleagues (2011) emphasized the importance of involving parents in transition planning and establishing collaborative communication between the sending and receiving agencies to support a seamless transition and minimize parental stress and anxiety caused by changing environments. Occupational therapy practitioners can support the family in advocating for their child's needs, attend transition meetings, assist in developing the individualized education program if the child is transitioning to preschool special education under Part B of IDEA, and consult with the receiving therapist and program staff. More information about transition is included in Chapter 10, "Best Practices in Early Childhood Transitions."

SUMMARY

Part C of IDEA is a complex law that outlines specific requirements that states must meet in implementing EI services for infants and toddlers with disabilities and their families. It provides flexibility in how states implement these requirements. This flexibility leads to variation in states' design of their EI systems that can affect the quality of services delivered to children and families. It can also affect the roles and responsibilities of occupational therapy practitioners. Overall, a high-quality system infrastructure is essential to support service providers in effectively implementing evidence-based practices that result in improved outcomes for infants and toddlers with disabilities and their families.

Based on available evidence that suggests that children learn best when interested and engaged in naturally occurring everyday activities and routines, EI services focus on building the family's capacity to use everyday activities to enhance their child's development and support participation in family and community life. This use of everyday activities to promote engagement, participation, and learning aligns well with occupational therapy practices as outlined in the *Occupational Therapy Practice Framework: Domain and Process* (4th ed.; AOTA, 2020). Occupational therapy, a core service in EI, brings expertise to the team decision-making process and helps ensure that appropriate services and supports are in place to address each child and family's unique strengths and needs. Many sources agree that families and caregivers have the greatest influence on children's learning and development; therefore, what happens between intervention visits is most critical for learning.

REFERENCES

American Occupational Therapy Association. (2014). *AOTA practice advisory on the primary provider approach in early intervention.* https://www.aota.org/~/media/Corporate/Files/Practice/Children/Browse/EI/Role-of-OT_1/Early-Intervention-FAQ.pdf

American Occupational Therapy Association. (2017). Guidelines for occupational therapy services in early intervention and schools. *American Journal of Occupational Therapy, 71*(Suppl. 2), 7112410010. https://doi.org/10.5014/ajot.2017.716S01

American Occupational Therapy Association. (2020). Occupational therapy practice framework: Domain and process (4th ed.). *American Journal of Occupational Therapy, 74*(Suppl. 2), 7412410010. https://doi.org/10.5014/ajot.2020.74S2001

Bruder, M. B. (2010). Early childhood intervention: A promise to children and families for their future. *Exceptional Children, 76,* 339–355. https://doi.org/10.1177/001440291007600306

Boyer, V. E., & Thompson, S. D. (2014). Transdisciplinary model and early intervention: Building collaborative relationships. *Young Exceptional Children, 17*(3), 19–32. https://doi.org/10.1177/1096250613493446

Caldwell, A. R., Skidmore, E. R., Raina, K. D., Rogers, J. C., Terhorst, L., Danford, C. A., & Bendixen, R. M. (2018). Behavioral activation approach to parent training: Feasibility of promoting routines of exploration and play during mealtime (Mealtime PREP). *American Journal of Occupational Therapy, 72,* 7206205030. https://doi.org/10.5014/ajot.2018.028365

Council for Exceptional Children, Division for Early Childhood. (2014). *DEC recommended practices in early intervention/early childhood special education 2014.* https://www.dec-sped.org/dec-recommended-practices

Early Childhood Personnel Center. (n.d.). *Database of state personnel standards.* https://ecpcta.org/

Early Childhood Technical Assistance Center. (2006). *The early intervention/IFSP process.* https://ectacenter.org/~pdfs/topics/families/ifsp_process_chart.pdf

Early Childhood Technical Assistance Center. (2015). *A System Framework for Building High-Quality Early Intervention and Preschool Special Education Programs.* https://ectacenter.org/~pdfs/pubs/ecta-system_framework.pdf

Early Childhood Technical Assistance Center. (2016). *Part C lead agencies.* https://ectacenter.org/partc/ptclead.asp

Early Childhood Technical Assistance Center. (2018). *State approaches to child outcomes measurement Part C APR Indicator 3: FFY 2016 (2016–2017).* https://ectacenter.org/~pdfs/eco/map_partC32018.pdf

Early Childhood Technical Assistance Center. (n.d.-a). *Part C of IDEA.* https://ectacenter.org/partc/partc.asp

Early Childhood Technical Assistance Center. (n.d.-b). *Finance.* https://ectacenter.org/topics/finance/finance.asp

Early Childhood Technical Assistance Center. (n.d.-c). *Family outcomes.* https://ectacenter.org/eco/pages/familyoutcomes.asp

Early Childhood Technical Assistance Center. (n.d.-d). *Evidence-based practices.* https://ectacenter.org/topics/evbased/evbased.asp

Early Childhood Technical Assistance Center. (n.d.-e). *Outcomes FAQ.* https://ectacenter.org/eco/pages/faqs.asp

Education for All Handicapped Children Act of 1975, Pub. L. 94-142, reauthorized as the Individuals With Disabilities Education Improvement Act, codified at 20 U.S.C. §§ 1400–1482.

Family Guided Routines Based Intervention. (2020). *FGRBI for providers.* http://fgrbi.com/providers

Greer, M., Taylor, A., & Mackey Andrews, S. D. (2007). *A framework for developing and sustaining a Part C finance system* (NECTAC notes No. 23). The University of North Carolina, FPG Child Development Institute, National Early Childhood Technical Assistance Center.

Hebbeler, K., Spiker, D., & Kahn, L. (2012). Individuals With Disabilities Education Act's early childhood programs: Powerful vision and pesky details. *Topics in Early Childhood Special Education, 31,* 199–207. https://doi.org/10.1177/0271121411429077

IDEA Infant & Toddler Coordinators Association. (2017). *ITCA finance survey.* https://www.ideainfanttoddler.org/pdf/2016-ITCA-Finance-Survey.pdf

IDEA Infant & Toddler Coordinators Association. (2018a). *ITCA annual survey: State challenges and responses.* https://www.ideainfanttoddler.org/pdf/2018-ITCA-State-Challenges-Report.pdf

IDEA Infant & Toddler Coordinators Association. (2018b). *2018 ITCA finance survey: Use of public and private insurance and family fees.* https://www.ideainfanttoddler.org/pdf/Finance-Survey-Report-Pt-2-public-private-insurance-family-fees.pdf

IDEA Infant & Toddler Coordinators Association. (2018c). *Percentage of all children under the age of one receiving services by eligibility (single day count 10/1/–12/1/2017).* https://www.ideainfanttoddler.org/pdf/2017-Child-Count-Data-Charts.pdf

IDEA Infant & Toddler Coordinators Association. (2019). *ITCA service coordination survey report.* https://www.ideainfanttoddler.org/pdf/2019-Service-Coordination-Survey-Reports.pdf

Individuals With Disabilities Education Improvement Act of 2004, Pub. L. 108-446, 20 U.S.C. § 1400 et seq C.F.R. (2004).

Infant Toddler Connection of Virginia. (2018). *Practice manual, Chapter 7: IFSP development.* http://www.infantva.org/documents/PracticeManual-Chapter7,9.18Final.pdf

James, L. W., Stoffel, A., Schefkind, S., & Khetani, M. (2016). Occupational therapy in the child outcome summary process in early intervention and preschool. *OT Practice, 21*(5), 13–16. https://ectacenter.org/~pdfs/meetings/ecidea16/OT-Brief.pdf

Kasprzak, C., Hebbeler, K., Spiker, D., McCullough, K., Lucas, A., Walsh, S., . . . Bruder, M. B. (2019). A state system framework for high-quality early intervention and early childhood special education. *Topics in Early Childhood Special Education.* 97–109, https://doi.org/10.1177/0271121419831766

Lucas, A., Gillaspy, K., & Peters, M. (2014). *Developing high quality, functional IFSP outcomes and IEP goals training package.* https://ectacenter.org/knowledgepath/ifspoutcomes-iepgoals/ifspoutcomes-iepgoals.asp

McCollum, J. A., & Yates, T. (2017). *PIWI: The evidence base.* https://eiclearinghouse.org/wp-content/uploads/2018/06/1aEvidence-Supporting-PIWI-Model.pdf

McWilliam, R. A. (2012). Implementing and preparing for home visits. *Topics in Early Childhood Special Education, 31,* 224–231. https://doi.org/10.1177/0271121411426488

Michigan Association of Administrators of Special Education. (2014). *Comparing early childhood systems: IDEA early intervention systems in the birth mandate states.* http://maase.pbworks.com/w/file/fetch/96292569/MAASE%20Birth%20Mandate%20States%20Report%20FINAL%2005.20.14.pdf

Minard, C. (2018). The underutilization of occupational therapy in transdisciplinary early intervention services. *Journal of Occupational Therapy, Schools, and Early Intervention, 11*(1), 15–20. https://doi.org/10.1080/19411243.2017.1408441

Myers, C. T., Schneck, C. M., Effgen, S. K., McCormick, K. M., & Shasby, S. B. (2011). Factors associated with therapists' involvement in children's transition to preschool. *American Journal of Occupational Therapy, 65,* 86–94. https://doi.org/10.5014/ajot.2011.09060

National Center for Pyramid Model Innovations. (n.d.). *Pyramid Model overview.* https://challengingbehavior.cbcs.usf.edu

Newborg, J. (2005). *Battelle Developmental Inventory* (2nd ed.). Riverside.

North Carolina Early Intervention Infant-Toddler Program. (2019). *The earlier you know, the better they'll grow.* https://beearly.nc.gov/data/files/pdf/provider/NCITP_Coaching%20_NLEP_Toolkit_09272019.pdf

The RAM Group. (2015). *Routines-Based Model.* https://robin-mcwilliam3.wixsite.com/ram-group/content1

Raver, S., & Childress, D. (2014). Collaboration and teamwork with families and professionals. In S. A. Raver & D. C. Childress (Eds.), *Family centered early intervention: Supporting infants and toddlers in natural environments* (pp. 31–52). Paul H. Brookes.

Shelden, M. L., & Rush, D. D. (2007). Characteristics of a primary coach approach to teaming in early childhood programs.

CASEinPoint, 3(1), 1–8. https://fipp.org/static/media/uploads/caseinpoint/caseinpoint_vol3_no1.pdf

Spiker, D., Hebbeler, K., Wagner, M., Cameto, R., & McKenna, P. (2000). A framework for describing variations in state early intervention systems. *Topics in Early Childhood Special Education, 20,* 195–207. https://doi.org/10.1177/027112140002000401

Workgroup on Principles and Practices in Natural Environments, Office of Special Education Programs Technical Assistance Community of Practice: Part C Settings. (2008a). *Agreed upon mission and key principles for providing early intervention services in natural environments.* https://ectacenter.org/~pdfs/topics/families/Finalmissionandprinciples3_11_08.pdf

Workgroup on Principles and Practices in Natural Environments, Office of Special Education Programs Technical Assistance Community of Practice: Part C Settings. (2008b). *Agreed upon practices for providing early intervention services in natural environments.* https://ectacenter.org/~pdfs/topics/families/AgreedUponPractices_FinalDraft2_01_08.pdf

U.S. Department of Education. (2012). *Part C SPP/APR 2012 indicator analyses - (FFY 2010).* https://ectacenter.org/~pdfs/partc/part-c_sppapr_12.pdf

U.S. Department of Education. (2018a). *Part C state performance plan/annual performance report (Part C SPP/APR)* Part C 2019 measurement table. https://osep.grads360.org/#communities/pdc/documents/17410

U.S. Department of Education. (2018b). *Part C state performance plan/annual performance report 2018 indicator analyses.* https://osep.grads360.org/#communities/pdc/documents/17332

U.S. Department of Education. (2018c). *40th Annual report to Congress on the implementation of the Individuals With Disabilities Education Act.* https://www2.ed.gov/about/reports/annual/osep/2018/parts-b-c/index.html

Best Practices in Early Intervention Screening and Evaluation

15

Beth Elenko, PhD, OTR/L, BCP, CLA

KEY TERMS AND CONCEPTS

- Assessment
- Authentic assessment
- Child Find
- Child Outcome Summary Form
- Criterion-referenced assessments
- Developmental delay
- Eligibility criteria
- Evaluation
- Family-centered practices
- Family-directed assessment
- Family service coordinators
- Individualized family service plan
- Informed clinical opinion
- Multidisciplinary evaluation and assessment
- Norm-referenced assessments
- Occupations
- Occupational profile
- Referral sources
- Routines-based interview
- Screening

OVERVIEW

Screening and evaluation in Part C of the Individuals With Disabilities Education Improvement Act of 2004 (IDEA; P. L. 108-446) for early intervention (EI) are critical processes to identify young children's and family's strengths and needs. The information gleaned provides administrators, service providers, and families with a fundamental understanding of a child's developmental needs, progress, and status and how well they are learning, as well as determines necessary provision of needed services. The evaluation process is often the family's first encounter with the special education process and occupational therapy. The outcome of this first impression may have powerful significance for the future of that family and the trajectory that follows. This chapter explores the screening and evaluation process for EI services specific to the role of occupational therapy practitioners. (*Note. Occupational therapy practitioner* refers to both occupational therapists and occupational therapy assistants.)

The term *screening* refers to processes used to identify potential developmental issues of young children that may need more in-depth evaluation. The term *evaluation* refers to the comprehensive process of gathering necessary data to determine the young child's eligibility for services under IDEA. The term *assessment* refers to the specific tests, standardized tools, and authentic observations that are part of the evaluation process (American Occupational Therapy Association [AOTA], 2015). Other disciplines may use the terms *evaluation* and *assessment* interchangeably, which may cause confusion to families and providers.

Laws and Regulations Regarding the Evaluation Process in Early Intervention

AOTA provides guidelines and resources that occupational therapy practitioners must follow during service delivery. Examples include the *Occupational Therapy Practice Framework: Domain and Process* (4th ed.; *OTPF*; AOTA, 2020) and *Standards of Practice for Occupational Therapy* (AOTA, 2015). *Practitioners must adhere to licensure laws established by the state regulatory board or risk losing the ability to practice in that state.*

There are federal laws, such as the IDEA, Early Head Start (Improving Head Start for School Readiness Act of 2007; P. L. 110-134), and the Child Abuse Prevention and Treatment Act (1974; P. L. 93-247), that authorize funding to states and that practitioners must follow. Although Part C of IDEA is voluntary, all states that participate must comply with the regulations, such as providing a timely, comprehensive, ***multidisciplinary evaluation and assessment*** conducted by qualified personnel (e.g., service coordinator, special instructor, nurse, discipline-specific therapists) to determine a child's eligibility.

In addition, state agencies establish regulations that must be followed. For instance, each state identifies a lead agency, its evaluation process, and eligibility criteria. Occupational therapy practitioners must be aware of all of these federal and state evaluation and eligibility regulations and understand their state's Part C system (AOTA, 2017). See Chapter 14, "Understanding Part C: Early Intervention Law and the Individualized Family Service Plan (IFSP) Process," for more information on EI law, eligibility determination, and the individualized family service plan (IFSP) process.

Occupational Therapy Role

Under Part C, occupational therapy practitioners have multiple roles (AOTA, 2017). These are discussed briefly here and at more length in the Best Practices section.

Family service coordinator

Occupational therapy practitioners may serve as *family service coordinators,* the single contact for the team and family. This role requires coordinating evaluations and assessments; facilitating and participating in the development, review, and evaluation of the IFSP; and providing access to services and resources for the family. A critical role of the family service coordinator is to help families navigate the Part C EI process, from initial evaluation through transition to preschool or child care.

Member of multidisciplinary team to determine eligibility

The comprehensive multidisciplinary evaluation to determine eligibility must involve at least two professionals. The occupational therapist may serve as a member of the multidisciplinary team and conduct assessments of the five required developmental domains to determine whether the child meets the state's eligibility for EI services.

Occupational therapy evaluator to determine need for services and plan interventions

Another role for occupational therapists is conducting an occupational therapy evaluation focused on more specific skills (e.g., observe feeding to determine strengths and needs) for intervention planning purposes. The occupational therapist reports the findings and recommendations to the IFSP team.

ESSENTIAL CONSIDERATIONS

State Eligibility Criteria for Part C Services

Each state determines their *eligibility criteria,* the specific standards needed in order to receive EI services. For eligibility, each state's policy identifies a rigorous definition of *developmental delay* and includes established physical and mental conditions that will most likely lead to a delay. The definition of developmental delay must include the procedures to measure the child's development in all of the following areas: cognitive, physical (including vision and hearing), communication, social or emotional, and adaptive. Many states define *developmental delay* using standardized assessments (e.g., 25% delay or 1.5 standard deviation below the mean in two or more domains).

Based on the state's criteria, some children who are at risk for developmental delay may be determined eligible for Part C EI services if the conditions have a high probability of resulting in developmental delay (e.g., Down syndrome). IFSP teams often use children's medical records to establish eligibility without conducting an evaluation of the child (but an assessment of the child's needs in each of the five developmental areas must be conducted; IDEA, § 303.321).

Another method for determining eligibility is on the basis of *informed clinical opinion,* use of qualitative and quantitative information to assist in forming a determination regarding difficult-to-measure aspects of current developmental status and the potential need for EI (IDEA, § 303.321[a][3][ii]). Informed clinical opinion is warranted especially when conventional standardized tests are unable to provide reliable or appropriate methods to measure delays in certain populations (Bagnato et al., 2008; Macy et al., 2016; Shackelford, 2002). The occupational therapist must substantiate the use of clinical opinion to help lead agencies understand the conditions. These areas need a description of the young child's performance and function (e.g., inability to suck from a bottle), and how this affects the child's health and development (e.g., poor growth and weight gain) rather than a score. Variables that affect informed clinical opinion may include the young child's life experiences, quality of movement, and play, and the occupational therapy practitioner's professional judgment. Occupational therapists have professional experience that is valued and supported by federal regulations (Bagnato et al., 2008; Office of Special Education Programs [OSEP], 2011; Shackelford, 2002).

Part C child evaluation and assessment terminology and guidelines

IDEA uses the terms *evaluation* and *assessment* for very specific processes. *Evaluation* is used to determine the child's initial and continued eligibility (IDEA, § 303.321[a][1]). *Assessment* means ongoing procedures to identify the child's unique strengths and needs and the EI services appropriate to meet those needs (IDEA, § 303.321[a][2][ii]). IDEA requires that all evaluations and assessments of the child and family are conducted by qualified individuals in a nondiscriminatory manner and are selected and administered without racial or cultural discrimination. No single procedure is used to determine a child's eligibility. IDEA Part C requires that evaluation of the child must include

- Administering an evaluation instrument;
- Obtaining the child's history (e.g., family interview);
- Identifying the child's level of functioning in each developmental area (cognitive; physical, including vision and hearing; communication; social or emotional; adaptive);
- Reviewing information from other sources (e.g., health care workers, family members); and
- Reviewing medical, education, or other records.

Family-directed assessment

The *family-directed assessment* is a voluntary process of interviewing family members to identify their concerns, priorities, and resources. This assessment must be conducted by qualified personnel. In addition, the family helps identify the supports and services needed to enhance their capacity to meet the developmental needs of their child.

Occupational therapists play a significant role under Part C to identify families' concerns, priorities, and resources during the evaluation, gathering relevant data to address functional needs of the young child and synthesize information with the family to identify possible outcomes and needs for services (AOTA, 2017).

Culturally and linguistically appropriate evaluation practice

Families have their own unique culture, language, and routines that occupational therapists need to pay attention to during the evaluation process. By doing this, they can determine the true picture of the young child's and family's functioning and therefore meet their needs most optimally (OSEP, 2011). Each family brings developmental beliefs and traditions that are reflected in their child-rearing strategies. Families have their own cultures and styles of routines, and assumptions should not be made during evaluation.

Families engage in occupations and routines differently. For example, mealtimes can include different types of foods, times, locations, people who are present, and ways young children are fed or feed themselves. Soliciting information about cultural expectations is critical to understanding the young child's level of functioning and validates families' concerns with sensitivity to family values, needs, language, and culture. The occupational therapist's ability to consider the young child's and family's cultural and linguistic preferences helps to limit bias and promote effective collaboration and communication with families (AOTA, 2017; de Sam Lazaro, 2017; Hansen & Lynch, 2004; Lynch & Hansen, 2004; Macy et al., 2016).

Evaluation Should be Family-Centered

Regardless of the lead agency, rules, and regulations of the state, one consistent principle found across early childhood and EI is the emphasis on family-centered practices. *Family-centered practices* involve a set of beliefs, principles, and values for supporting and strengthening the capacity of families to promote and enhance their child's devlopment (Dunst, 2002). Therefore, engaging the family as active participants in the EI process is critical. Families become part of the evaluation process from the initial contact in hopes of building the family's capacities. Research indicates that using family-centered practices during the assessment process yields increased satisfaction and family well-being (Dunst et al., 2006). See Exhibit 15.1 for salient features of family-centered practices.

Occupational therapy practitioners can use many strategies to promote collaboration and partnerships between the family and team. They can begin with talking to families and gathering information about their observations to include in the evaluation. Asking families about their daily routines and how their child functions within those routines assists in completing a better picture of the child and family.

The Division for Early Childhood's (DEC; 2014) *Recommended Practices* emphasizes the family's essential partnership in the evaluation process in the child's natural environments (e.g., home, child care, church, park). DEC's *Recommended Practices* call for an integrated and individualized evaluation that includes the family's concerns; the young child's functional participation in everyday routines, interests, materials, and play partners; and a shared partnership between professionals and families to enhance teaching and learning. In other words, the evaluation process should be family centered, authentic, developmentally appropriate, culturally and linguistically responsive, and multidimensional. The concepts of family-centered practices in natural environments and authentic assessment practices are discussed in the following section. See Chapter 8, "Best Practices in Supporting Family Partnerships," for more information on supporting family-centered practices and family partnerships.

Authentic Assessment Practices

When determining eligibility and planning for services, EI evaluators may use authentic assessment of the young child in their natural environments. *Authentic assessment* is a term "used to describe data collected through the evaluation process that is actually produced as part of the child's natural routine and activities" (Frolek Clark, 2010, p. 147). Authentic assessment is also known as *play-based assessment* or *functional assessment*.

The authentic assessment may involve conducting an ecological evaluation of the child and caregivers in their everyday routines and contexts. Of equal importance is understanding the routines of daily life in natural environments, including the unique strengths and needs of the child and family. Authentic contextual observation creates opportunities to evaluate the infant or toddler's physical, sensory, emotional, and adaptive abilities as well as the interactions among caregivers, siblings, and peers during daily routines. Therefore, the occupational therapist observes the young child and family in their natural environments to identify areas of strengths and challenges in their everyday contexts. Natural environments are critical in the evaluation process because "infants and toddlers learn best through everyday experiences and interactions with familiar people in familiar contexts" (Workgroup on Principles and Practices in Natural Environments, OSEP TA Community of Practice: Part C Settings, 2008, p. 1).

Observations should be scheduled when routine activities are occurring, with those caregivers who are usually part of that routine. Therefore, observation may occur on one visit or over time. Often, observations over time help to create a more holistic picture of the young child and family to prevent assumptions practitioners might make from a one-time "snapshot." Because young children's performance is varied at different times and across different contexts with different caregivers, multiple observations ensure a true representation of the young child's functioning.

EXHIBIT 15.1.	Salient Features of Family-Centered Practice

Respect for:
- The family as the expert on the child
- The family as the ultimate decision maker for the child and family
- The family as the constant in the child's life
- The family's choice in level of participation in evaluation and intervention
- The family's priorities and concerns as the driver for outcomes
- The family's cultural beliefs and values.

Source. Adapted from Baird & Peterson (1997).

Another critical aspect of authentic assessment involves using materials and equipment found in the young child's home or community, as opposed to professionals bringing their tabletop testing materials to assess young children. The materials should resemble real-life conditions needed for the young child to engage in the activity (Bagnato & Macy, 2010; Macy et al., 2016).

BEST PRACTICES

The *OTPF* (AOTA, 2020) provides guidance on occupational therapy evaluation, including the development of the occupational profile and analysis of occupational performance. The following section describes occupational therapists' role in children's evaluation and assessment to determine eligibility as the best practices of an occupational therapy evaluation in EI to identify the child's strengths and needs for services. IDEA Part C requires that screening (if adopted), evaluation and assessment, and the initial IFSP meeting be conducted within 45 days of referral unless the parent is unavailable because of exceptional family circumstances.

Referral

States are required to identify, locate, and evaluate infants and toddlers with disabilities as early as possible. This is often referred to the state's **Child Find** system, designed to ensure ongoing efforts are in place to raise awareness about EI services. Primary **referral sources** for EI often include hospitals, physicians, child care programs, local education agencies and schools, homeless family shelters, domestic violence shelters and agencies, and families themselves. Referral of specific at-risk infants and toddlers who require a referral may include substantiated cases of child abuse or neglect or children affected by illegal substance abuse (e.g., prenatal drug exposure; IDEA, § 303.303).

Screening

IDEA allows the lead agency to adopt screening procedures to determine whether children are suspected of having a disability. Screening must be carried out by or under the supervision of the lead agency or the EI provider. Parental notice must be provided and consent must be obtained. During the screening process, if the parent requests and consents to an evaluation, the child must be evaluated, even if the child is not suspected of having a disability (IDEA, 2004, § 303.320). Approximately 40% of states have an option for screening.

Conduct a Child Evaluation and Child and Family Assessment: Determine Eligibility and Identify Strengths and Needs

A timely, comprehensive, multidisciplinary evaluation and assessment must be conducted by qualified personnel to determine a child's eligibility for EI services in accordance with the state's definition of developmental delay or disability. IDEA defines *multidisciplinary* as "two or more separate disciplines or professions" (IDEA, 2004, § 303.24). Parental consent is required before the child may evaluated. The

occupational therapist may be one of the professionals who conducts an evaluation of the child's developmental in five areas (i.e., cognitive development; physical development, including vision and hearing; communication development; social–emotional development; and adaptive development) to determine eligibility. A single assessment tool cannot be the only method or procedure by which eligibility is determined. Record review, observation, and interviews of the family and child care providers may also be useful in determining the child's performance and needs.

The evaluation may be conducted in a play-based arena style, which involves one person who has contact with the child while other team members support the facilitator by documenting data, providing cues or missed items, and so forth. Another method is to divide the five developmental areas between the professionals, so that one is observing while the other person is working directly with the child. Engaging the family during the evaluation process is important. Examples of active roles for the family include interpreting their child's behavior, participating in the assessment, and validating the assessment and results.

The occupational therapist, as service coordinator or along with the service coordinator, may conduct the family-directed assessment of the family's concerns, resources, and priorities. This information provides a basis for identifying appropriate family outcomes and determining EI services needed to meet these outcomes.

Conduct an Occupational Therapy Evaluation: Determine Programming Needs

When an occupational therapy evaluation has been determined to be necessary, the occupational therapist conducts the evaluation to provide information to the team regarding the child's strengths and needs and to determine the need for occupational therapy services.

Develop an occupational profile

An essential component of occupational therapy evaluation is developing the **occupational profile,** a summary of the child's history and experiences, daily living skills, interests, values, and needs. Occupational therapists gather this information through interviews with the family and caregivers to identify their priorities and concerns for the child.

To gather data to understand the child's occupational performance, the occupational therapist should speak with as many people as possible who are involved in the child's daily routine, including parents, grandparents, babysitters, siblings, teachers, and child care providers. Interview strategies often work best to explore the young child's daily routines and to determine how they function within these routines. If available, other documents to examine may include records and reports from hospitals, doctors, or other EI professionals. A thorough birth and developmental history is also important to understand how the child has progressed thus far. This history is gathered through interviewing the parent or caregiver on information such as pregnancy issues, gestational date of birth, delivery options, prematurity, as applicable, and is necessary to gain a complete picture of the child's birth. A brief discussion of developmental milestones that the child has achieved thus far also helps paint a picture of where the child is in terms of developmental domains. If applicable, medical history may be necessary if the child has had other medical issues unrelated to their birth.

Use routines-based interview strategies. One method that can assist in gathering the occupational profile of the strengths and needs during the child's occupational performance is a ***routines-based interview,*** which is an effective tool to gather information across different settings and contexts and is highly useful in developing the occupational profile (Jennings et al., 2012; McWilliam, 2010; McWilliam et al., 2009). Asking about the daily routines of families helps to develop a relationship with the family or caregivers; obtain a full description of the young child's functioning in their daily activities; and plan and create a list of functional child and family concerns, priorities, resources, and outcomes (AOTA, 2017; McWilliam, 2010; McWilliam et al., 2009).

Occupational therapy practitioners can initiate the routines-based interview by simply asking what a typical day is like for the family, with the purpose of understanding areas where the family needs assistance. How does the family feel about engaging in their daily routines? Which routines are sources of difficulty with their child and may need further evaluation and intervention? This is a valuable opportunity for the family to share how they engage in routines and for the practitioner to identify where they can provide guidance and coaching strategies.

Analyze occupational performance

In addition to completing an occupational profile, occupational therapists use their uniquely qualified skills to evaluate developmental skills of young children with suspected delay or disability in natural environments to analyze ***occupations,*** such as self-care (eating, dressing, hygiene), play, learning, leisure, rest and sleep, and social participation (AOTA, 2014). The occupational therapist may evaluate performance skills (e.g., motor, process, social interaction), performance patterns (e.g., habits, routines, rituals, roles), and client factors (e.g., body functions, body structures) in the child's and family's context and environment (e.g., physical, social, temporal, cultural). Assessment for planning intervention usually encompasses more in-depth observations.

Use assessment tools appropriately. Occupational therapists should consider the purpose of the tool needed. Do they need to determine whether there is a problem (e.g., interview, screening tool), determine with the multidisciplinary team whether the child is eligible (tool that measures all five developmental areas), determine child and family needs (interviews or tools to identify the child's strengths and needs for programming), or determine whether the outcome was successful (ongoing data collection; Frolek Clark, 2010)? The answers to these questions should guide which tools are chosen.

Traditionally, standardized assessments, both criterion- and norm-referenced, were commonly used to determine a young child's level of developmental functioning.

Although they are useful, ***norm-referenced assessments*** compare young children with their peers and give statistical information to quantify their level of developmental function. ***Criterion-referenced assessments*** show a range of skills that a young child may be able to perform. Both require specific controlled, preset standard conditions designed to determine the child's level of functioning. Occupational therapists have many options to assess the domains specific to occupational therapy (Macy et al., 2015; Mulligan, 2014).

Occupational therapists should consider occupation-based strategies and tools to measure the functioning of the child in the environment. Depending on the areas of concern, these may include formal observations, play scales, and feeding checklists. For measurement of performance skills (e.g., motor, sensory), tools that include a parental interview are helpful, because there are limitations to standardized assessment tools used with young children. Often, infants and toddlers are not be able to perform the tasks or follow the instructions provided to them that are often required by norm-referenced, standardized tests. Another limitation is that the statistical nature and interpretation of results may not be understood by families and teachers. In addition, families are often not included in the administration-standardized, norm-referenced tests, which contradicts family-centered principles (Bagnato et al., 2010; de Sam Lazaro, 2017; Macy et al., 2015).

Some assessment tools may not be culturally sensitive and change as the norms change, which makes them challenging for the early childhood population (de Sam Lazaro, 2017). Many practitioners feel criterion-referenced tests are a better measure and parallel the ideals of authentic assessment (Macy et al., 2015, 2016). Reviewing tools for their purpose, authenticity, and realism will be critical going forward in the early childhood field so that measurement is more than just an administrative task meeting criteria but one that matches the early childhood principles occupational therapy practitioners aspire to (Bagnato et al., 2010).

Although the field of early childhood is moving toward more authentic evaluations, Part C lead agencies may still require providers to use conventional quantitative assessment and scoring results to determine eligibility. Table 15.1 includes common examples of methods and assessment tools used by occupational therapists and other members of EI evaluation teams. See also Appendix F, "Examples of Assessments for Early Childhood (Birth to 5 Years)."

Develop Individualized Family Service Plan

The data gathered by the team are written into a comprehensive report that establishes a perspective of the young child's functioning to determine eligibility. Information gathered through interviews, observations, and assessments serves as the context for the development of the IFSP. Evaluation team members should communicate effectively so that families understand evaluation results in a jargon-free, culturally and linguistically appropriate manner. See Appendix G, "Sample Early Intervention Team Report."

If the child is eligible, information gathered through interviews, observations, and assessments serves as the context for the development of the IFSP. The ***IFSP*** is a legal document identifying the child's and family's needs,

TABLE 15.1.   Examples of Assessment Tools Used in Early Intervention

PURPOSE	METHOD OR TOOL	DESCRIPTION	AGE RANGE
Screening	Ages & Stages Questionnaires® (3rd ed.; Squires et al., 2009)	Includes communication, gross motor, fine motor, problem solving, and personal–social areas	1–66 months
	Ages & Stages Questionnaires®: Social–Emotional (2nd ed.; Squires et al., 2015)	Includes social–emotional development	1–72 months
	Edinburgh Postnatal Depression Scale (Cox et al., 1987)	Screening tool for postpartum depression	Pregnant women or women who have recently given birth
Parent interviews	Asset-Based Context Matrix (Wilson & Mott, 2006)	A contextually based assessment protocol for parents and caregivers of young children and families	Birth–3 years
	Routines-Based Interview and observations (McWilliam et al., 2009)	Interviews and observations of child and family across natural environments	Birth–3 years
	Measurement of Engagement, Independence, and Social Relationships (MEISR™) manual: Research edition. (McWilliam, & Younggren, 2019)	This instrument has been designed to develop a profile of functional behaviors of a child from ages birth to 3 years, in home routines completed by parent or caregiver	Birth–3 years
Measures to determine eligibility (5 major domains)	Assessment, Evaluation, and Programming System for Infants and Children® (2nd ed.; Bricker et al., 2020)	Includes fine motor, gross motor, cognitive, adaptive, social–communication, and social skills. The assessment encompasses preacademic content areas, such as preliteracy, numeracy, and prewriting.	Birth–6 years
	Battelle Developmental Inventory (3rd ed.; Newborg, 2020)	Includes adaptive, personal–social, communication, motor, and cognitive skills	Birth–7 years, 11 months
	Bayley Scales of Infant and Toddler Development® (4th ed.; Bayley & Aylward, 2019)	Includes cognitive, language, motor, and social–emotional skills and adaptive behavior	1–42 months
	Brigance Inventory of Early Development–III (Brigance & French, 2013)	Includes physical, language, academic and cognitive, and self-help and social–emotional skills	Birth–7 years
	Developmental Assessment of Young Children (2nd ed.; Voress & Maddox, 2013)	Includes cognition, communication, social–emotional development, physical development, and adaptive behavior	Birth to 5 years, 11 months
Other commonly used tools	Alberta Infant Motor Scales (Piper & Darrah, 1994)	Norm-referenced test to assess motor maturation	Birth–18 months
	Early Learning Accomplishment Profile (Glover et al., 2002)	Criterion-referenced tool that includes gross motor, fine motor, prewriting, cognitive, language, and social–emotional areas	Birth–3 years
	Hawaii Early Learning Profile (Warshaw, 2000)	Criterion-referenced tool that includes cognitive, language, gross motor, fine motor, social–emotional, and self-help areas	Birth–3 years
	Miller Function and Participation Scales (Miller, 2006)	Assessment of a child's developmental performance related to home and school environment	2–7 years, 11 months
	Pediatric Evaluation of Developmental Inventory (PEDI). (Haley et al., 1992)	Norm-referenced observation of self-care, mobility, and social function to measure both capability and performance.	6 months–7 years
	Peabody Developmental Motor Scales (PDMS-2) (Folio & Fewell, 2000)	Norm- and criterion-referenced early childhood motor development program that assesses gross and fine motor skills. The assessment is composed of six subtests that measure interrelated motor abilities that develop early in life. PDMS-3 is currently being standardized.	Birth–5 years
	Sensory Profile™ 2 (Dunn, 2014)	A standardized tool to evaluate a child's sensory processing patterns in the context of home, school, and community-based activities	Birth–14 years, 11 months
	Revised Knox Preschool Play Scale (Knox, 2008)	Includes play behavior in four dimensions: space management, material management, pretense and symbolic play, and participation	Birth–6 years

services, and outcomes. Practitioners should build a partnership with the family to enhance capacity building as parents become advocates for their children. For more detailed information on IFSP development and intervention, see Chapter 16, "Best Practices in Intervention Under Part C."

Report Early Childhood Outcomes

EI programs document success in meeting program goals and outcomes and effective intervention for accountability purposes through the ***Child Outcome Summary Form*** (COSF) developed by the Early Childhood Technical Assistance Center (ECTA, 2018). This form is not an assessment; rather, it is a summary of multiple assessment tools and information from the family that compares this child's current functioning with age-expected performance. The COSF and companion tools (e.g., Early Childhood Outcomes Decision Tree) assist the team to score the child's functioning at entry and exit of EI services. States and local programs are making child and family outcome measurements more efficient and more effective by integrating those processes within the IFSP implementation.

The following three outcomes inform the initial evaluation process and what is learned about how the young child uses their skills in everyday situations (ECTA, n.d.):
1. Having positive social relationships, which includes getting along with other young children and relating well with adults;
2. Acquiring and using knowledge and skills, which refers to thinking, reasoning, problem-solving, and early literacy and early math skills; and
3. Taking appropriate action to meet needs, which includes feeding, dressing, self-care, and following rules related to health and safety.

Reevaluate as Needed

IDEA requires that the IFSP must be evaluated once a year, with a review of the plan at least every 6 months (§ 1436[b]). Although some EI agencies only require reevaluation before the annual IFSP meeting, others may require reevaluation every 6 months to determine ongoing eligibility. Occupational therapy practitioners must be aware of and comply with state and local procedures.

Ongoing data collection during service delivery is necessary to determine progress toward outcomes and provide data for decision making on the effectiveness of intervention. See Chapter 16 for more information about intervention.

SUMMARY

Early childhood evaluations require occupational therapists not only to be familiar with the regulations and provisions of IDEA Part C guidelines that determine best practice in EI but also to focus on the family unit and the context of the natural environments where families and caregivers are. Key concepts and principles that occupational therapists need to incorporate into the evaluation process are family-centered practices, authentic assessment strategies in natural environments, and culturally and linguistically appropriate evaluations. These practices assist occupational

therapists to provide the most comprehensive picture of the young child to evaluate their true abilities and challenges to determine their eligibility for EI services and develop outcomes to direct the intervention process.

Observing the young child in their natural environment with their caregivers and engaging in their typical routines assists the occupational therapist to identify areas of concern for intervention planning. The *OTPF* (AOTA, 2020) advocates for the development of an occupational profile and an occupational performance analysis of the young child and family based on information gathered across a variety of contexts. Focusing on collaboration and partnerships with families during the evaluation process encourages occupational therapists to support families and other caregivers and increase positive outcomes for the child and family.

REFERENCES

American Occupational Therapy Association. (2015). Standards of practice for occupational therapy. *American Journal of Occupational Therapy, 64*(Suppl. 3), S106–S111. https://doi .org/10.5014/ajot.2010.64S106

American Occupational Therapy Association. (2017). Guidelines for occupational therapy services in early intervention and schools. *American Journal of Occupational Therapy, 71*(Suppl. 2), 7112410010. https://doi.org/10.5014/ajot.2017.716S01

American Occupational Therapy Association. (2020). Occupational therapy practice framework: Domain and process (4th ed.). *American Journal of Occupational Therapy, 74*(Suppl. 2), 7412410010. https://doi.org/10.5014/ajot.2020.74S2001

Bagnato, S., & Macy, M. (2010). Authentic assessment in action: A "R-E-A-L" solution. *NHSA Dialog, 13*(1), 42–45. https://doi .org/10.1080/15240750903458121

Bagnato, S., McKeating-Esterle, E., Fevola, A., Bortolamasi, P., & Neisworth, J. (2008). Valid use of clinical judgment (informed opinion) for early intervention eligibility: Evidence base and practice characteristics. *Infants & Young Children, 21,* 334–349. https://doi.org/10.1097/01.IYC.0000336545.90744.b0

Bagnato, S., Neiswoth, J., & Prett-Frontczak, K. (2010). *LINKing authentic assessment and early intervention* (2nd ed). Brookes.

Bayley, N., & Aylward, G. (2019). *Bayley Scales of Infant and Toddler Development*® (4th ed.). Pearson.

Bricker, D., Capt, B., Johnson, J., Pretti-Frontczak, K., Slentz, K., Straka, E., & Wadell, M. (2020). *Assessment, Evaluation, and Programming System for Infants and Children*® (2nd ed.). Brookes.

Brigance, A., & French, B. (2013). *Brigance Inventory of Early Development–III.* North Curriculum Associates.

Child Abuse Prevention and Treatment Act of 1974, Pub. L. 93-247, 42 U.S.C. §§ 5101–5116i.

Cox, J., Holden, J., & Sagovsky, R. (1987). Detection of postnatal depression: Development of the 10-item Edinburgh Postnatal Depression Scale. *British Journal of Psychiatry, 150,* 782–786. https://doi.org/10.1192/bjp.150.6.782

de Sam Lazaro, S. (2017). The importance of authentic assessments in eligibility determination for infants and toddlers. *Journal of Early Intervention, 39,* 88–105. https://doi.org/ 10.1177/1053815116689061

Division for Early Childhood. (2014). *DEC recommended practices in early intervention/early childhood special education 2014.* https://www.dec-sped.org/dec-recommended-practices

Dunn, W. (2014). *The Sensory Profile*™ *2.* Pearson.

Dunst, C. (2002). Family-centered practices: Birth through high school. *Journal of Special Education, 36,* 139–147. https://doi.org/10.1177/00224669020360030401

Dunst, C., Bruder, M., Trivette, C., & Hamby, D. (2006). Everyday activity settings, natural learning environments, and early intervention practices. *Journal of Policy and Practice in Intellectual Disabilities, 3*(1), 3–10. https://doi.org/10.1111/j.1741-1130.2006.00047.x

Early Childhood Technical Assistance Center. (2018). *State approaches to child outcomes measurement Part C APR Indicator 3: FFY 2016 (2016–2017).* https://ectacenter.org/~pdfs/eco/map_partC32018.pdf

Early Childhood Technical Assistance Center. (n.d.). *Family outcomes.* https://ectacenter.org/eco/pages/familyoutcomes.asp

Folio, R., & Fewell, R. (2000). *Peabody Developmental Motor Scales* (2nd ed.). Pro-Ed.

Frolek Clark, G. (2010). Evaluation, assessment, and outcomes in early childhood. In B. Chandler (Ed.), *Early childhood: Occupational therapy services for children birth to five* (pp. 131–177). AOTA Press.

Glover, M., Preminger, J., & Sanford, A. (2002). *Early Learning Accomplishment Profile.* Kaplan Early Learning.

Haley, S., Coster, W., Ludlow, L., Haltiwanger, T., & Andrellos, P. (1992). *Pediatric Evaluation of Disability Inventory.* Pearson.

Hansen, M., & Lynch, E. (2004). *Understanding families: Approaches to diversity, disability and risk.* Brookes.

Improving Head Start for School Readiness Act of 2007, Pub. L. 110-134, 42 U.S.C. §§ 9831.

Individuals With Disabilities Education Improvement Act of 2004, Pub. L. 108-446, 20 U.S.C. §§ 1400–1482.

Jennings, D., Hanline, M., & Woods, J. (2012). Using routines-based interventions in early childhood special education. *Dimensions in Early Childhood, 40*(2), 13–22. https://www.wvsha.org/wp-content/uploads/events-manager-uploads/session-handouts/Handout%20Preschool%20Language%202.pdf

Knox, S. (2008). The Revised Knox Preschool Play Scale. In L. D. Parham. & L. Fazio (Eds.), *Play in occupational therapy for children* (2nd ed., pp. 55–70). Mosby.

Lynch, E., & Hansen, M. (2004). *A guide for working with children and their families: Developing cross-cultural competence* (2nd ed.). Brookes.

Macy, M., Bagnato, S., & Gallon, S. (2016). *Authentic assessment: A vulnerable idea whose time is now.* Washington, DC: ZERO TO THREE.

Macy, M., Bagnato, S., Macy, R., & Salaway, J. (2015). Conventional tests and testing for early intervention eligibility: Is there an evidence base? *Infants & Young Children, 28,* 182–204. https://doi.org/10.1097/IYC.0000000000000032

McWilliam, R. (2010). *Routines-based early intervention: Supporting young children and their families.* Brookes.

McWilliam, R., Casey, A., & Sims, J. (2009). The Routines-Based Interview: A method for gathering information and assessing needs. *Infants & Young Children, 22,* 224–233. https://doi.org/10.1097/IYC.0b013e3181abe1dd

McWilliam, R., & Younggren, N. (2019). *Measurement of Engagement, Independence, and Social Relationships (MEISR™) manual: Research edition.* Brookes.

Miller, L. (2006). *Miller Function and Participation Scales.* Pearson.

Mulligan, S. (2014). *Occupational therapy evaluation for children* (2nd ed.). Lippincott, Williams & Wilkins.

Newborg, J. (2020). *Battelle Developmental Inventory* (3rd ed.). Riverside.

Office of Special Education Programs. (2011). *Part C of the Individuals With Disabilities Education Act: Final regulations: Nonregulatory guidance.* https://sites.ed.gov/idea/files/original_Final_Regulations-_Part_C-DOC-ALL.pdf

Piper, M., & Darrah, J. (1994). *Motor assessment of the developing infant.* Saunders.

Shackelford, J. (2002). *Informed clinical opinion* (NECTAC Notes No. 10). Chapel Hill: University of North Carolina, FPG Child Development Institutes, National Early Childhood Technical Assistance Center. https://ectacenter.org/~pdfs/pubs/nnotes10.pdf

Squires, J., Bricker, D., & Twombly, E. (2015). *Ages & Stages Questionnaires®: Social–Emotional* (2nd ed.). Brookes.

Squires, J., Twombly, E., Bricker, D., & Potter, L. (2009). *Ages & Stages Questionnaires®* (3rd ed.). Brookes.

Voress, J., & Maddox, T. (2013). *Developmental Assessment of Young Children* (2nd ed.). Pro-Ed.

Warsaw, S. (2000). *Hawaii Early Learning Profile.* Vort.

Wilson, L., & Mott, D. (2006). Asset-Based Context Matrix: An assessment tool for developing contextually-based child outcomes. *CASETools, 2*(4), 1–12.

Workgroup on Principles and Practices in Natural Environments, OSEP TA Community of Practice: Part C Settings. (2008). *Seven key principles: Looks like/doesn't look like.* https://ectacenter.org/~pdfs/topics/families/Principles_LooksLike_DoesntLookLike3_11_08.pdf

Best Practices in Intervention Under Part C

16

Pam Stephenson, OTD, OTR/L

KEY TERMS AND CONCEPTS

- Activity analysis
- Authentic assessment
- Capacity
- Coaching
- Collaboration
- Community
- Community integration
- Cultural responsivity
- Displaced families
- Individualized family service plan
- Integrate everyday items and activities
- Interprofessional collaboration
- Natural environments
- Person–Environment–Occupation–Performance model
- Relationship-based practices
- Routines-based interventions
- Self-efficacy
- Strengths-based approach

OVERVIEW

Early intervention (EI) services are provided as a collaborative partnership among families, EI service providers, and other community partners who are important in the life of the child. An essential feature is that services focus on building family capacity through enabling families to participate in everyday activities in everyday places, using everyday routines and objects. These services and activities therefore occur in the context of the child's and family's natural environments.

Natural environments are both defined and mandated ("to the maximum extent appropriate") by Part C of the Individuals With Disabilities Education Improvement Act 2004 (IDEA; P. L. 108-446). They include not only the physical space where everyday activities occur but also the activities themselves and the routines and people that are part of the child's world. Physical, social, and temporal environments are all important considerations for service delivery (American Occupational Therapy Association [AOTA], 2020; Division for Early Childhood [DEC], 2014). A crucial aspect is that natural environments are considered to be settings that are "typical" for same-age young children without disabilities, which allows services to occur in a plethora of home and community contexts (IDEA, 2004, § 303.26).

Furthermore, learning and skills development are more likely to occur when children and families participate in meaningful activities and in natural environments (Workgroup on Principles and Practices in Natural Environments, 2008). Working in the natural environment is consistent with occupational therapy practice. The profession's guiding documents emphasize the importance of both environment and context for participation in meaningful activities (AOTA, 2017, 2020).

The *individualized family service plan* (IFSP) is a legal document that lists not only family priorities, targeted outcomes (goals), and services but also when and where those services will take place. This collaborative document describes the natural environment for service delivery, and should other locations be used, the team must explain why. When creating the occupational therapy intervention plan (AOTA, 2018), practitioners must ensure that it aligns with the IFSP outcomes and that services are occurring with the same frequency and in the same natural environment as stated in the IFSP. The occupational therapy intervention plan includes the occupation-focused goals that are being addressed, intervention approaches, and the types of interventions that are being implemented (AOTA, 2017, n.d.-a).

In addition to acknowledging the various components of the natural environment, EI practice also adopts a *strengths-based approach* to support young children and their families. A strengths-based approach acknowledges what the child and family are doing well, identifies strategies that are already successful, and recognizes diverse potential for further growth (National Council of Teachers of English, n.d.). Helping families to recognize their strengths, including the strengths of their child, is an important foundation for EI practice and one that supports family self-efficacy. A strengths-based approach can help to build family engagement and ultimately foster the collaborative relationship between service providers and families (Gerlach & Gignac, 2019). Identifying strengths in the family's current routines and activities also provides opportunities to expand on these as part of service provision in the natural environment.

Occupational therapy practitioners value client-centered practice and the significance of their clients' occupations, routines, habits, and roles. (*Note. Occupational therapy practitioner* refers to both occupational therapists and occupational therapy assistants.) In the context of EI services, practitioners are able to use their full scope of practice with consideration of the family as the client, not just the individual child who has been referred for services. This is essential when practitioners are working toward outcomes that focus on participation in meaningful activities in meaningful places and contexts.

ESSENTIAL CONSIDERATIONS

EI occupational therapy practitioners need to understand the general principles of providing interventions in natural settings, while recognizing that each family may participate in a variety of different natural environments. Cultural responsivity, collaboration, and reflective practice are essential skills for providing interventions in natural environments. Although practitioners may use a variety of theoretical approaches in EI services, the ***Person-Environment–Occupation–Performance model*** can provide a helpful framework for considering how best to maximize the family's participation in meaningful occupations in the natural environment (Baum et al., 2015). This top-down model helps practitioners consider individual and environmental influences on occupational performance within a client-centered systems perspective. For example, practitioners can consider the intrinsic personal elements of the child and family, such as cognitive and psychological factors and belief systems, in addition to extrinsic environmental elements, such as routines, supports, barriers, and places. Practitioners can also consider the unique characteristics of the child's and family's occupations and their ability to perform them.

Natural Environment

The *natural environment* can be described as "a process, not a place" (Woods, 2008, p. 15), because children learn where they live, play, and interact. As such, the natural environment includes not only the places where young children might naturally spend their time but also the people, activities, and items in those places (Moore et al., 2012). Young children and families engage in a variety of natural environments, including homes, parks, supermarkets, libraries, and child care centers (Campbell et al., 2009; DEC, 2016). Daily activities (i.e., occupations)—including playing, self-care, social participation, and learning—occur in association with caregivers, peers, and siblings. Settings that are not natural environments for young children include clinics, hospitals, and noninclusive contexts.

Occupational therapy practitioners facilitate participation in occupations in the natural environment though partnering with families to build ***capacity*** and ***self-efficacy*** (AOTA, 2015). Building family capacity entails helping caregivers to enhance their skills and knowledge and to acquire adiditonal skills that support their role functioning as parents (DEC, 2016) and the developmental needs of their child (IDEA, 2004). In turn, this leads to increased parental self-efficacy (i.e., an individual's belief in their capacity to succeed in specific situations) and role competence. It is important for practitioners to understand each family's unique routines, activities, and preferences to facilitate participation in the natural environment.

Cultural Considerations

As a result of expanding definitions of the concept of *family* as well as demographic shifts in the population, occupational therapy practitioners need to demonstrate competence in working with families with diverse life experiences, cultural influences, linguistic differences, and world views. To provide inclusive family-centered practice in a changing world, practitioners must take active steps to increase their understanding of and appreciation for the cultural influences on families (Blanche et al., 2015). The process of providing family-centered care that is intentionally inclusive, culturally responsive, and cognizant of diversity requires both ongoing self-reflection by practitioners and also a commitment to skill development.

A dynamic process of ***cultural responsivity*** allows occupational therapy practitioners to embrace the uniqueness of each family they serve. This necessitates learning about the family's culture and heritage and understanding how family traditions and beliefs affect the life, activities, roles, and routines of the family. Collaborating with families to explore how culture affects the family's activities as well as other elements, such as parenting styles, can have a significant impact on facilitating participation in the natural environment. This includes using an assessment process that is culturally sensitive and applying that information to craft culturally responsive practices that best fit the needs of each individual family (Wray & Mortenson, 2011).

In addition to understanding the cultural influences on families, occupational therapy practitioners should also take time to reflect on their own culture and life experiences and to identify any unconscious biases (Wells et al., 2016; Wray & Mortenson, 2011). An ongoing process of reflective practice can assist practitioners to develop their cultural responsivity and to use this to support children and families in natural environments.

Displaced Families

Population shifts, global and environmental upheavals, and economic uncertainty have led to an increase in the number of ***displaced families,*** who are removed from familiar, secure home environments and placed in insecure housing that may not be a good fit physically, psychologically, socially, or geographically. For example, as a result of poverty, families may experience transient or temporary housing as well as disruptions in their preferred routines, activities, and roles (Corr et al., 2016). Refugees and asylum seekers frequently experience disruptions in occupational participation as they adjust to new and unfamiliar environments and possible estrangement from preferred activities or items (Trimboli & Taylor, 2016). Whether displacement is temporary or permanent, it has a significant impact on definitions and experiences of natural environments. Occupational therapy practitioners working in EI settings need to understand the impact of displacement and consider how best to support families to adjust to unfamiliar routines, activities, faces, and spaces.

Collaboration

Collaboration is a key feature of EI services. It requires practitioners to establish a family-centered focus that facilitates joint decision making related to implementing interventions and strategies in natural environments (Adams & Tapia, 2013). Partnering with families to establish a reciprocal and collaborative relationship that fosters discussions around the family's priorities, routines, and environments is a key skill for EI practitioners (AOTA, 2017; DEC, 2016; Holloway & Chandler, 2010). Practitioners need to be able to collaborate with families and support them as active participants in the process of identifying their unique and meaningful natural environments. This includes exploring the family's preferred routines, activities, and venues as well as negotiating how to expand and build on them.

Interprofessional collaboration, in which a variety of providers work together in partnership with the family to provide high-quality care (Interprofessional Education Collaborative, 2016; World Health Organization, 2010), within the EI team and across environments and community agencies, is also important to support the child's development (Frolek Clark & Schlabach, 2013; Salisbury et al., 2010). Occupational therapy practitioners must be able to articulate their scope of practice and define the distinct value of occupational therapy services in the context of EI. As part of the interprofessional team, practitioners must also be able to negotiate how and where services are delivered (e.g., across which specific natural environments) and to resolve any challenges or issues of overlap (Johnson, 2017; Slater & Cusick, 2019).

Payment Sources

Although IDEA ensures that basic screening, IFSP development and review, service coordination, and transition planning are provided at no cost to families (IDEA, 2004), families may be required to explore private pay, private insurance, or Medicaid (if eligible) as options for funding service provision. Some states may also charge families on a sliding fee scale dependent on income. Although children cannot be denied EI services (e.g., occupational therapy) because of the family's inability to pay, Part C funds should only be used as the payer of last resort (IDEA, 2004, § 303.510).

BEST PRACTICES

Occupational therapy practitioners possess a distinct professional skill set that values and maximizes engagement in meaningful occupations in meaningful contexts (AOTA, 2014). This is consistent with the ethos of EI services, which emphasizes supporting families in their natural environments (DEC, 2016). Interventions in the natural environment focus on building participation in family routines and on embedding skills across contexts, people, and activities. Table 16.1 summarizes the best practices for providing services in EI to meet the child's and family's IFSP outcomes.

Provide Ongoing Authentic Assessment in the Natural Environment

Authentic assessment involves observing and evaluating young children when they are engaged in their typical activities, routines, and places, as opposed to solely using standardized, decontextualized evaluation procedures (Macy et al., 2016). Furthermore, it expands opportunities to support families with diverse cultural backgrounds (de Sam Lazaro, 2017). Authentic assessment is a good fit for occupational therapy practice because it emphasizes assessing children and families as they engage in their everyday activities and routines in the context of daily life (Macy et al., 2016). Regarded as an early childhood best practice (Bagnato et al., 2014), it allows ongoing assessment that is both contextualized and dynamic and that responds to the changes that occur in families over time and thereby helps to monitor progress.

Occupational therapy practitioners can use ongoing authentic assessment practice to support functional participation in activities and routines in the family's natural environments (Early Childhood Technical Assistance Center [ECTA], n.d.). For example, practitioners may accompany families during a routine grocery shopping trip to coach them in a real-life context. This offers contextualized opportunities to observe and assess the child's and family's performances and to incorporate both professional judgment and feedback from the family (Macy et al., 2016).

TABLE 16.1. Summary of Best Practices in the Natural Environment

BEST PRACTICE	DESCRIPTION
Activity analysis	Collaborate with families to build their capacity to examine the component parts of everyday activities, to scaffold their child's development and participation
Authentic assessment	Use contextualized and ongoing evaluation of children and families as they participate in the natural environment
Coaching	Explicitly model strategies, coach families to implement them, and provide formative feedback
Community integration	Assist families to establish and strengthen networks in their local communities
Integrate everyday items and activities	Teach families how to use and modify their everyday items and activities to support the child in achieving functional IFSP outcomes
Relationship-based practices	Foster child–family and child–family–practitioner relationships as a foundation for building family capacity and achieving IFSP outcomes
Routines-based interventions	Embed interventions into the family's existing routines; assist families to create routines

Note. IFSP = individualized family service plan.

An authentic assessment approach underpins scheduling therapy services so they occur in the context of the family's natural environment. Using their knowledge of the family's routines, activities, and venues, practitioners should intentionally plan and schedule services to support participation in the natural environment and facilitate families in embedding strategies and supports across activities, routines, and people (e.g., caregivers). For example, working with children and families on mealtime participation is likely to be more authentic and meaningful when it occurs during a routine family meal, rather than in contrived isolation.

Implement Coaching in the Natural Environment

Occupational therapy practitioners must demonstrate skill in coaching families and relevant community partners to build capacity and support participation in the natural environment (Kingsley & Mailloux, 2013; Sawyer & Campbell, 2017; Woods et al., 2011). Coaching is viewed as a best practice in EI (Adams & Tapia, 2013), and coaching strategies should be explicitly communicated and documented (Salisbury et al., 2012). Coaching not only underscores occupational therapy's distinct role in facilitating participation in the natural environment but also assists families in recognizing the strategies they can integrate in their daily routines and activities.

Occupational therapy practitioners use scaffolding strategies in their coaching to help families build on their existing skills and develop new ones (Woods et al., 2011). Scaffolding might include explicitly labeling the strategies that caregivers are using, commenting on events, and providing real-time performance feedback to caregivers. When practitioners emphasize specific strategies, families are able to generalize these strategies across contexts and other caregivers (e.g., extended family).

Coaching through telehealth offers opportunities for practitioners to reach underserved populations, and there is evidence to highlight the efficacy of occupation-based telehealth coaching in supporting children and families to engage in the natural environment (Little et al., 2018).

Integrate Everyday Items and Activities

When working with families in EI, occupational therapy practitioners need to use the everyday items that are naturally a part of the life of the child and the family. Practitioners recognize that bringing specialized items and toys into the home for therapy and then removing them when they leave does not support the family in building their capacity and may give the impression that there is "magic" associated with the practitioner's toys (Workgroup on Principles and Practices in Natural Environments, 2008, p. 2). Going "bagless" is now required in many states and is regarded as a best practice because it not only uses familiar contexts and materials but also is clearly family centered (Williams & Ostrosky, 2019). When using the family's everyday materials and contexts, practitioners enter the home (or community setting) with their professional skill set and knowledge and a coaching, collaborative approach but without a traditional therapy bag. A bagless approach extends beyond physical items and also includes integrating routines and activities that the family engages in or wishes to engage in.

Building family capacity through using everyday items in everyday places is an essential best practice for EI (McWilliam, 2011). Collaborating with families to determine the focus of each session and helping them to identify items and activities that are in their immediate environment offers practitioners opportunities to integrate creativity, flexibility, and professional reasoning. Coaching families in how to use everyday items to support their child allows them to practice strategies on a regular basis and to incorporate them into their everyday life. It also helps families identify incidental learning opportunities to expand on strategies and to generalize them to other activities and routines in the natural environment (Crawford & Weber, 2014; Terrell & Watson, 2018).

For example, occupational therapy practitioners may coach families to incorporate play into a bathtime routine, to use everyday cups and spoons to develop mealtime skills, or to use pillows for positioning. They can assist families to transfer skills and strategies between everyday items or activities that have similar features (e.g., scooping food with a spoon and scooping water in the tub). Practitioners may also work with young children in other environments—for example, during story time at a local library or at child care. In this case, practitioners may coach staff on how best to identify and use the available toys and materials to support the child's development and participation.

Emphasize Routines-Based Interventions

A routines-based approach explores the family's typical activities and routines and uses them as a bedrock for intervention. This approach is a good fit with occupational therapy practice because it emphasizes the importance of using familiar routines and contexts to support learning and participation (Whipple, 2014). Furthermore, recognizing that young children learn best in their natural environments, routines-based interventions offer children and families opportunities to develop skills within individualized contexts that are both functional and relevant. Important features of routines-based interventions are that they are embedded into naturally occurring contexts and that they focus on achieving functional outcomes that are important to the family, including caregiver satisfaction with routines (McWilliam, 2010). Routines-based interventions combined with family coaching have been shown to be more effective in achieving functional outcomes than a traditional child-focused developmental approach (Hwang et al., 2013). Families also report higher satisfaction with routines-based interventions (Kingsley & Mailloux, 2013).

A number of tools can assist occupational therapy practitioners and families in identifying which routines are working well and which ones are not. These include the Scale for Assessment of Family Enjoyment Within Routines (SAFER; Scott & McWilliam, 2000), a semistructured interview tool that asks caregivers to rate their satisfaction with a variety of daily routines, including waking up, mealtimes, dressing, bathtime, and going to the grocery store. This approach allows families to recognize strengths in their current routines while identifying potential areas for intervention. Asking families to describe their typical morning or bedtime routines or eliciting information on what mealtimes look like in a variety of contexts can help families to identify specific concerns and priorities.

Because of their skill set and scope of practice, occupational therapy practitioners are well positioned to support families in expanding their participation in routines and activities and increasing their satisfaction. AOTA (n.d.-b) has developed the Childhood Daily Occupations Toolkit to support this practice. This toolkit includes a number of family-centered information sheets that describe how practitioners support families' occupational performance and participation in routines across the day, including morning, bathtime, bedtime, mealtimes, and toileting. Practitioners can review this information with families and use it as a building block for developing individualized family routines.

Understanding the importance of the family's routines allows practitioners to work with families in a wide variety of contexts. Family-guided routines-based interventions are culturally responsive, individualized, and evidence based, and they lead to functional outcomes in the natural environment (Family Guided Routines Based Intervention, n.d.). For example, occupational therapy practitioners may schedule visits with a family at a grocery store during their regular shopping routine or at pick-up time from child care if those routines are the focus of intervention. Using a routines-based approach, practitioners can assist families to generalize strategies across their routines and activities and to identify naturally occurring opportunities for practice on multiple occasions across the week.

Use Activity Analysis and Environmental Modifications

Occupational therapy practitioners are skilled in analyzing how activities and routines affect a child's participation in natural environments (AOTA, 2020). Through ongoing authentic assessment and both routines-based and strengths-based approaches, practitioners can use activity analysis to tease out the specific supports and barriers to the family's and child's occupational performance. Talking with families about routines (i.e., what families do, how they do it, and who is involved) while using skilled observation during the activity, practitioners elicit a detailed picture of what the activity looks like for a specific family. To the maximum extent possible, practitioners should observe families participating in their routines and activities directly, because this affords opportunities to ask questions in context and to notice small details that may be overlooked or taken for granted in discussion.

Using a collaborative problem-solving approach, occupational therapy practitioners partner with families to identify potential adaptations to facilitate participation (ECTA, n.d.), including adaptations to activities, routines, and everyday items. Although practitioners easily generate adaptive solutions, it is important to actively involve families in this problem-solving process by seeking their input on what options they think might work best for them. Allowing time for this processing is an essential part of building the family's capacity. Practitioners therefore support the development of families' skills and confidence in making environmental and activity adaptations a part of capacity building in the natural environment.

Occupational therapy practitioners help families understand how they can use and adapt everyday items to facilitate participation in activities and routines (Moore et al., 2012). Examples might include adapting activities in terms of complexity, pacing, and location as well as using everyday items, such as pots and pans for play or towels for positioning. Practitioners share information related to activity demands and help families consider how environmental factors affect their child's participation. For instance, discussing how sensory qualities of the mall can affect a child's willingness to go there may assist families to adapt the activity by modifying the time of the visit or by trialing additional supports, such as headphones, baseball caps, or comfort toys.

Enhance Community Integration

Although a key feature of EI services is supporting families' engagement at home, families of young children with disabilities also commonly report challenges in participating in their communities (Khetani et al., 2013). Using a lens of social participation, occupational therapy practitioners play a significant role in assisting families in developing strategies for integrating into their local community (AOTA, 2014). *Community* involves a "group of people with diverse characteristics who are linked by social ties, share common perspectives, and engage in joint action in geographical locations or settings" (MacQueen et al., 2001, p. 1929). Definitions of community vary across families; therefore, practitioners need to take time to find out which communities are important to each individual family.

After identifying the specific barriers to community participation, occupational therapy practitioners and families can explore a variety of options to address these barriers. This may include providing the family with information about resources such as play groups at a local library, exploring transportation options, or developing strategies for supporting the child's behavioral needs in community settings (Khetani et al., 2012). Practitioners can ask probing questions to elicit the family's desired outcome (e.g., "What might it look like if you were able to take part in the play group?") and use the information to develop interventions to support this outcome.

Coaching families in community settings and assisting them to develop and use their skills and strategies in real-life contexts can make a meaningful difference in community participation and integration. In addition, occupational therapy practitioners can use the joint plan with families to facilitate community integration initiatives between sessions. This allows families and practitioners an opportunity to debrief afterward and to reflect on which strategies were helpful and which were not.

Focus on Relationship-Based Practices

People are an integral and essential part of a child's natural environment. Although there are a variety of people in a child's life, including peers, extended family, formal and informal caregivers, neighbors, and community members, the child's immediate family is usually paramount. Relationship-based practices aim to strengthen the relationship between the child and the family to promote engagement and positive interactions. Developing strong attachments and positive parent–child bonding in early childhood has long-term positive effects. Key relationship-based practices include focusing on the child–family relationship, supporting the family's growing competence, clearly describing the child's behaviors, and reflecting on both the family's and the practitioner's perspectives (Early Childhood Learning & Knowledge Center, n.d.).

Strengthen child–family relationships

Relationship-based practices can be embedded into a wide variety of natural environments and activities. As a result, occupational therapy practitioners have multiple opportunities to strengthen the child–family relationship. Explicitly describing positive interactions that have taken place between the child and the family can boost the family's confidence and self-efficacy. Practitioners comment on strategies that they observe caregivers using with their child during everyday activities and routines. For example, during an art activity at home, a practitioner might comment to a caregiver, "I noticed that you did a great job of giving them a choice between the red and blue crayons and that you said, 'You picked blue,' when they picked one." This type of comment highlights a reciprocal interaction between the child and the caregiver and emphasizes how the caregiver is using specific strategies to support the child's development and participation.

Maintaining a strengths-based approach that not only recognizes strengths of both the child and the caregivers but also expresses them clearly and directly is important. Occupational therapy practitioners can help families increase their understanding of their child's behavior by providing alternative viewpoints or hypotheses (Early Childhood Learning & Knowledge Center, n.d.). This may include helping parents read their child's cues and learn how to respond positively to them, to build the child–parent relationship. Practitioners can also help parents build positive parent–child interactions through the use of coaching, modeling, and prompting during naturally occurring play activities (Case-Smith, 2013). In addition, practitioners can partner with families to identify activities that foster child–parent interactions and relationships, such as shared book reading (Terrell & Watson, 2018), arts and crafts, action songs, and play.

Nurture family and practitioner relationships

The relationship between the occupational therapy practitioner and the family is an important aspect of EI practice and can have a significant effect on the efficacy of a coaching approach. Similar to other practice settings, practitioners must invest time, energy, and therapeutic use of self to build and maintain a collaborative relationship with the family. Practitioners use reflective practice to ensure that the practitioner–family relationship continues to be nurtured and strengthened throughout the course of therapy. Using active listening skills, exercising empathy, and being mindful of the practitioner's own emotional responses are key elements in relationship-based practices (Edelman, 2004).

Collect and Analyze Data to Determine Effectiveness of Interventions

As in any other setting, occupational therapy practitioners are required to develop systems to review the child's progress and to evaluate the effectiveness of intervention (AOTA, 2014, 2018). In EI contexts, practitioners should establish a proactive plan for routine data collection and analysis at the start of therapy services to determine whether the IFSP outcomes are being met within the expected time frame. Although parents typically determine whether their child has met the outcome, authentic assessment can be instrumental in assisting practitioners to monitor progress in the natural environment while children and families are engaged in their typical activities, routines, and places. It allows practitioners to track progress over time and to adjust interventions as necessary, confident in the knowledge that their evaluation of the child's performance is dynamic and contextual (Macy et al., 2016). For more on data collection, see Chapter 6, "Best Practices in Data-Based Decision Making."

Discontinuation

The IFSP team reviews progress at least every 6 months and may decide to discontinue services after analysis of the data, including objective measures, authentic assessment practices, and parent and practitioner report. If the child and family have achieved their IFSP outcomes and there is no longer an explicit need for occupational therapy services, then services should be discontinued. Occupational therapy practitioners can contribute to this decision-making process by collecting and analyzing data as well as clearly articulating their full scope of practice.

SUMMARY

The natural environment encompasses places, people, activities, and routines. Occupational therapy practitioners have a crucial role in facilitating child and family participation in the natural environment and in assisting families to build their self-efficacy and capacity. The child–family and family–practitioner relationships are cornerstones of EI practice, and practitioners must invest in both of these simultaneously to maximize outcomes in the natural environment. Using a routines-based approach coupled with their skills in activity analysis and professional reasoning allows practitioners to foster family participation in meaningful, functional activities.

Knowledge of contemporary practices enables practitioners to make informed decisions about building family capacity and success through embedding interventions across the natural environment. Practitioners can collaborate with families to use everyday items, activities, and routines to maximize opportunities to practice and generalize strategies across contexts. Working in the natural environment is a good fit for occupational therapy practice, and practitioners can make a significant impact on family participation in home and community life.

REFERENCES

Adams, R. C., & Tapia, C. (2013). Early intervention, IDEA Part C services, and the medical home: Collaboration for best practice and best outcomes. *Pediatrics, 132,* e1073–e1088. https://doi .org/10.1542/peds.2013-2305

American Occupational Therapy Association. (2015). Occupational therapy's perspective on the use of environments and contexts to facilitate health, well-being, and participation in occupations. *American Journal of Occupational Therapy, 69*(Suppl. 3), 6913410050. https://doi.org/10.5014/ajot .2015.696S05

American Occupational Therapy Association. (2017). Guidelines for occupational therapy services in early intervention and schools. *American Journal of Occupational Therapy, 71*(Suppl. 2), 7112410010. https://doi.org/10.5014/ajot.2017.716S01

American Occupational Therapy Association. (2018). Guidelines for documentation of occupational therapy. *American Journal of Occupational Therapy, 72*(Suppl. 2), 7212410010. https://doi .org/10.5014/ajot.2018.72S203

American Occupational Therapy Association. (2020). Occupational therapy practice framework: Domain and process (4th ed.). *American Journal of Occupational Therapy, 74*(Suppl. 2), 7412410010. https://doi.org/10.5014/ajot.2020.74S2001

American Occupational Therapy Association. (n.d.-a). Learn about occupational therapy for children & youth. *Childhood daily occupations toolkit.* https://www.aota.org/About-Occupational-Therapy/Patients-Clients/ChildrenAndYouth.aspx

American Occupational Therapy Association. (n.d.-b). *FAQs about early intervention.* https://www.aota.org/~/media/Corporate/ Files/Secure/Practice/Children/Member-Questions-about-EI-20170413.pdf

Bagnato, S. J., Goins, D. D., Pretti-Frontczak, K., & Neisworth, J. T. (2014). Authentic assessment as "best practice" for early childhood intervention: National consumer social validity research. *Topics in Early Childhood Special Education, 34,* 116–127. https://doi.org/10.1177/0271121414523652

Baum, C. M., Christiansen, C. H., & Bass, J. D. (2015). The Person–Environment–Occupation–Performance (PEOP) model. In C. H. Christiansen, C. M. Baum, & J. D. Bass (Eds.), *Occupational therapy: Performance, participation, and well-being* (4th ed., pp. 47–55). Slack.

Blanche, E. I., Diaz, J., Barretto, T., & Cermak, S. A. (2015). Caregiving experiences of Latino families with children with autism spectrum disorder. *American Journal of Occupational Therapy, 69,* 6905185010. https://doi.org/10.5014/ajot.2015.017848

Campbell, P. H., Sawyer, B. L., & Muhlenhaupt, M. (2009). The meaning of natural environments for parents and professionals. *Infants & Young Children, 22,* 264–278. https://doi.org/10.1097/ IYC.0b013e3181bc4dd4

Case-Smith, J. (2013). Systematic review of interventions to promote social–emotional development in young children with or at risk for disability. *American Journal of Occupational Therapy, 67,* 395–404. https://doi.org/10.5014/ajot.2013.004713

Corr, C., Santos, R. M., & Fowler, S. A. (2016). The components of early intervention services for families living in poverty. *Topics in Early Childhood Special Education, 36*(1), 55–64. https://doi .org/10.1177/0271121415595551

Crawford, M. J., & Weber, B. (2014). *Early intervention every day! Embedding activities in daily routines for young children and their families.* Brookes.

de Sam Lazaro, S. L. (2017). The importance of authentic assessments in eligibility determination for infants and toddlers. *Journal of Early Intervention, 39,* 88–105. https://doi.org/ 10.1177/1053815116689061

Division for Early Childhood. (2014). *DEC recommended practices with examples.* https://www.dec-sped.org/dec-recommended-practices

Early Childhood Technical Assistance Center. (n.d.). *Practice improvement tools: Performance checklists.* https://ectacenter. org/decrp/type-checklists.asp

Early Childhood Learning & Knowledge Center. (n.d.). *Relationship-based practices.* https://eclkc.ohs.acf.hhs.gov/family-engagement/developing-relationships-families/relationship-based-practices

Edelman, L. (2004). A relationship-based approach to early intervention. *Resources and Connections, 3*(2), 1–9.

Family Guided Routines Based Intervention. (n.d.). *Home page.* http://fgrbi.com

Frolek Clark, G., & Schlabach, T. L. (2013). Systematic review of occupational therapy interventions to improve cognitive development in children ages birth–5 years. *American Journal of Occupational Therapy, 67,* 425–430. https://doi.org/10.5014/ajot.2013.006163

Gerlach, A. J., & Gignac, J. (2019). Exploring continuities between family engagement and well-being in aboriginal Head Start programs in Canada: A qualitative inquiry. *Infants & Young Children, 32,* 60–74. https://doi.org/10.1097/IYC .0000000000000133

Holloway, E., & Chandler, B. E. (2010). Family-centered practice: It's all about relationships. In B. E. Chandler (Ed.), *Early childhood: Occupational therapy services for children birth to five* (pp. 77–107). AOTA Press.

Hwang, A.-W., Chao, M.-Y., & Liu, S.-W. (2013). A randomized controlled trial of routines-based early intervention for children with or at risk for developmental delay. *Research in Developmental Disabilities, 34,* 3112–3123. https://doi.org/10.1016/j .ridd.2013.06.037

Individuals With Disabilities Education Improvement Act of 2004, Pub. L. 108-446, 20 U.S.C. §§ 1400–1482.

Interprofessional Education Collaborative. (2016). *Core competencies for interprofessional collaborative practice: 2016 update.* Author.

Johnson, C. E. (2017). Understanding interprofessional collaboration: An essential skill for all practitioners. *OT Practice, 22*(11), CE1–CE8.

Khetani, M., Graham, J. E., & Alvord, C. (2013). Community participation patterns among preschool-aged children who have received Part C early intervention services. *Child: Care, Health & Development, 39,* 490–499. https://doi.org/10.1111/ cch.12045

Khetani, M. A., Orsmond, G., Cohn, E., Law, M. C., & Coster, W. (2012). Correlates of community participation among families transitioning from Part C early intervention services. *OTJR: Occupation, Participation and Health, 32,* 61–69. https://doi .org/10.3928/15394492-20111028-02

Kingsley, K., & Mailloux, Z. (2013). Evidence for the effectiveness of different service delivery models in early intervention services. *American Journal of Occupational Therapy, 67,* 431–436. https://doi.org/10.5014/ajot.2013.006171

Little, L. M., Pope, E., Wallisch, A., & Dunn, W. (2018). Occupation-based coaching by means of telehealth for families of young children with autism spectrum disorder. *American Journal of Occupational Therapy, 72,* 7202205020. https://doi .org/10.5014/ajot.2018.024786

MacQueen, K. M., McLellan, E., Metzger, D. S., Kegeles, S., Strauss, R. P., Scotti, R., . . . Trotter, R. T., II (2001). What is community?

An evidence-based definition for participatory public health. *American Journal of Public Health, 91*(12), 1929–1938. https://doi.org/10.2105/ajph.91.12.1929

Macy, M., Bagnato, S. J., & Gallen, R. (2016). Authentic assessment: A venerable idea whose time is now. *ZERO TO THREE, 37*(1), 37–43.

McWilliam, R. A. (2010). *Routines-based early intervention: Supporting young children and their families.* Brookes.

McWilliam, R. A. (2011). The top 10 mistakes in early intervention in natural environments—and the solutions. *ZERO TO THREE, 31*(4), 11–16.

Moore, L., Kroger, D., Blomberg, S., McConahy, R., Wit, S., & Gatmaitan, M. (2012). Making best practice our practice: Reflections on our journey into natural environments. *Infants & Young Children, 25,* 95–105. https://doi.org/10.1097/IYC.0b013e31823d0592

National Council of Teachers of English (n.d.) *Strengths-based approach to equity in early childhood* [Policy brief]. https://secure.ncte.org/library/NCTEFiles/StrengthsBased.pdf

Salisbury, C., Cambray-Engstrom, E., & Woods, J. (2012). Providers' reported and actual use of coaching strategies in natural environments. *Topics in Early Childhood Special Education, 32*(2), 88–98. https://doi.org/10.1177/0271121410392802

Salisbury, C. L., Woods, J., & Copeland, C. (2010). Provider perspectives on using collaborative consultation in natural environments. *Topics in Early Childhood Special Education, 30*(3), 132–147. https://doi.org/10.1177/0271121409349769

Sawyer, B. E., & Campbell, P. H. (2017). Teaching caregivers in early intervention. *Infants & Young Children, 30,* 175–189. https://doi.org/10.1097/IYC.0000000000000094

Scott, S., & McWilliam, R. A. (2000). *Scale for Assessment of Family Enjoyment Within Routines (SAFER).* http://www.kansasasd.com/downloads/old_files/SAFER.pdf
Available from https://robinmcwilliam3.wixsite.com/ram-group/about2-c1hux

Slater, C. E., & Cusick, A. (2019). Advocating occupational therapy's distinct value within interprofessional teams. In K. Jacobs & G. L. McCormack (Eds.), *The occupational therapy manager* (6th ed., pp. 321–328). AOTA Press.

Terrell, P., & Watson, M. (2018). Laying a firm foundation: Embedding evidence-based emergent literacy practices into early intervention and preschool environments. *Language, Speech, and Hearing Services in Schools, 49,* 148–164. https://doi.org/10.1044/2017_LSHSS-17-0053

Trimboli, C., & Taylor, J. (2016). Addressing the occupational needs of refugees and asylum seekers. *Australian Occupational Therapy Journal, 63,* 434–437. https://doi.org/10.1111/1440-1630.12349

Wells, S. A., Black, R. M., & Gupta, J. (Eds.). (2016). *Culture and occupation: Effectiveness for occupational therapy practice, education, and research* (3rd ed.). AOTA Press.

Whipple, W. (2014). *Key principles of early intervention and effective practices in natural environments: A crosswalk with occupational therapy literature.* https://www.aota.org/~/media/Corporate/Files/Practice/Children/Crosswalk-12-5-2014.pdf

Williams, C., & Ostrosky, M. (2019). What about my toys? Common questions about using a bagless approach in early intervention. *Young Exceptional Children, 2,* 76–86. https://doi.org/10.1177/1096250619829739

Woods, J. (2008). Providing early intervention in natural environments. *ASHA Leader, 13*(4), 14–23. https://doi.org/10.1044/leader.FTR2.13042008.14

Woods, J. J., Wilcox, M. J., Friedman, M., & Murch, T. (2011). Collaborative consultation in natural environments: Strategies to enhance family-centered supports and services. *Language, Speech, and Hearing Services in Schools, 42,* 379–392. https://doi.org/10.1044/0161-1461(2011/10-0016)

Workgroup on Principles and Practices in Natural Environments. (2008, March). *Seven key principles: Looks like/doesn't look like.* https://ectacenter.org/~pdfs/topics/families/Principles_LooksLike_DoesntLookLike3_11_08.pdf

World Health Organization. (2010). *Framework for action on interprofessional education and collaborative practice.* https://www.who.int/hrh/resources/framework_action/en/

Wray, E. L., & Mortenson, P. A. (2011). Cultural competence in occupational therapists working in early intervention therapy programs. *Canadian Journal of Occupational Therapy, 78,* 180–186. https://doi.org/10.2182/cjot.2011.78.3.6

Best Practices in Documenting Early Intervention Services and Outcomes

17

Ashley Stoffel, OTD, OTR/L, FAOTA, and Lesly Wilson James, PhD, MPA, OTR/L, FAOTA

KEY TERMS AND CONCEPTS

- Child outcomes
- Child Outcomes Summary
- Daily or contact notes
- Developmental progress
- Discharge report
- Documentation
- Evaluation
- Family Educational Rights and Privacy Act of 1974 (FERPA)
- Family engagement
- Health Insurance Portability and Accountability Act of 1996 (HIPAA)
- Health literacy
- IFSP review
- Individualized family service plan
- Individuals With Disabilities Education Improvement Act of 2004 (IDEA)
- Intervention plans (plans of care)
- Lead agency
- Occupational therapy outcomes
- Point-of-service documentation
- Privacy Rule
- Progress report
- Protected health information
- SOAP notes
- Transition report

OVERVIEW

Documentation is electronic and written forms demonstrating the skilled nature of the services provided, the professional reasoning of the occupational therapy practitioner, and the justification for the services related to reimbursement and client outcomes (American Occupational Therapy Association [AOTA], 2018). The ***Individuals With Disabilities Education Improvement Act of 2004*** (IDEA; P. L. 108-446), Part C, requires that state early intervention (EI) programs and providers document multidisciplinary assessment results, family-directed assessment information, and a written ***individualized family service plan*** (IFSP) for each infant and toddler receiving EI services. The IFSP is a key piece of documentation in EI and is a legal, written, family-centered plan for EI services.

Each state's EI program is structured and organized differently, but each state has a designated ***lead agency,*** which sets policies and procedures and ensures the development of an initial IFSP within 45 days from the date of a referral (IDEA, 2004). During this time frame, occupational therapists could be asked to participate in an EI program eligibility evaluation or asked to conduct a discipline-specific initial assessment, because they are listed as qualified personnel in IDEA (IDEA, 2004).

It is important that occupational therapy practitioners ensure that the contents of EI documentation, including the IFSP, have been fully explained and that written parental consent has been documented before providing EI services. (*Note. Occupational therapy practitioner* refers to both occupational therapists and occupational therapy assistants.) Parental consent must be obtained before the provision of any services (e.g., screenings, evaluation, assessment) in EI (IDEA, 2004).

The written IFSP is protected by the ***Family Educational Rights and Privacy Act of 1974*** (FERPA; P. L. 93-380), a federal law that protects the privacy of student education records. Information gathered during the program eligibility evaluation or occupational therapy evaluation could be considered the infant's or toddler's ***protected health information*** (PHI) during billing. Title II of the ***Health Insurance Portability and Accountability Act of 1996*** (HIPAA; P. L. 104-191) includes the ***Privacy Rule,*** which is designed to protect the privacy of individually identifiable health information—referred to in the law as *PHI* (U.S. Department of Health and Human Services [DHHS], 2013). The PHI is health data and information, including physical or mental conditions and demographic information, that is created, received, or stored by a HIPAA-covered entity. Occupational therapy practitioners should be aware of HIPAA requirements related to sharing information and maintaining documentation of information shared related to the provision of services. In addition, practitioners must understand that before they share personal information with anyone who is not an EI participating provider, including reimbursement sources, signed parental consent is required (IDEA, 2004).

The EI program eligibility evaluation, discipline-specific initial assessment, and development of the IFSP should all occur at no cost to the family; however, the state or local EI program should ensure payment to the service provider (e.g., occupational therapist) for these services. If the IFSP team (e.g., family and other team members such as an occupational therapist) determines that services are needed, then Medicaid, other public sources, and private

---

EXHIBIT 17.1.   Common Types of Professional Documentation in Early Intervention

- *Daily or contact notes:* Document the contacts between the client and the occupational therapy practitioner, the goals and the intervention types and approaches used in the occupational therapy process, and the therapy outcomes.
- *Evaluation:* Documents the referral source and data gathered through the occupational therapy evaluation process.
- **Occupational therapy intervention plan** (may be known as **plan of care**): Documents the professional goals and the intervention types and approaches to be used during the occupational therapy process on the basis of the results of evaluation or reevaluation processes. It is typically an occupational therapy document, not part of the IFSP. Physician certification of *Intervention Plans (Plans of Care)* may be required by state practice acts and third-party payers, including Medicare and Medicaid.
- *Progress report:* Documents a summary of the contacts between the client and the occupational therapy practitioner, the goals and the intervention types and approaches used in the occupational therapy process, and the therapy outcomes in accordance with practice guidelines and payer, facility, and state and federal guidelines and requirements.
- *Transition report:* Documents the formal transition plan to support the client's transition from one service setting to another within a service delivery system.
- *Discharge report:* Documents the discharge plan to support the client's discharge from occupational therapy service.

Note. IFSP = individualized family service plan.
Source. Definitions reprinted from "Guidelines for Documentation of Occupational Therapy," 2018, by the American Occupational Therapy Association, *American Journal of Occupational Therapy, 72*(Suppl. 2), 7212410010. Reprinted with permission.

---

insurance can be authorized for billing at the consent of the family. Some states have a sliding fee scale for EI services, whereas other states, known as "birth mandate states," provide EI services at no cost to the parent but may bill Medicaid. Medicaid service delivery, coverage, and reimbursement vary by state, and documentation requirements for billing are also unique to each state Medicaid program (Heider, 2016).

It is important that occupational therapy practitioners be aware of the documentation requirements for Medicaid and other reimbursement sources in their state to ensure reimbursement for services. For example, in most states, Medicaid has specific documentation requirements, such as including time in and out on daily notes, and may also require specific billing codes.

ESSENTIAL CONSIDERATIONS

Occupational therapy practitioners must provide documentation whenever professional, skilled service is provided (AOTA, 2018). This section discusses key considerations for occupational therapy documentation in EI, including documenting skilled occupational therapy, family participation, and the child's developmental progress. Tips and strategies for considering diversity in families, documenting during sessions, and documenting outcomes are also included.

Considerations for Early Intervention Documentation

Documentation in EI may vary on the basis of state and local EI rules, policies, and procedures, and it is the responsibility of each occupational therapy practitioner to identify and abide by those requirements to produce professional and legal documentation (AOTA, 2018). For example, some states require that all EI providers use specific documentation templates. Common types of professional documentation in EI are defined in Exhibit 17.1.

Regardless of the type of documentation, occupational therapy practitioners working in EI should use best practice

strategies, such as documenting skilled occupational therapy service (including family participation and concerns) and capturing the child's developmental progress. Additionally, as a member of the EI team, the occupational therapist participates in completing the child outcomes.

Documenting Skilled Occupational Therapy

To demonstrate skilled occupational therapy, occupational therapy practitioners must document the child's progress and their own role in facilitating that progress, as well as use occupation in the documentation. For example, evaluation, reevaluation, and progress reports should include observation, assessment, and interpretation of occupations and activities such as play, self-care, learning, rest and sleep, and social participation, in addition to reporting on skills related to the EI developmental domains (i.e., physical, adaptive, communication, social or emotional, and cognitive). Use the activity in Exhibit 17.2 to enhance your documentation practices.

EI documentation should demonstrate the importance of the role of the occupational therapy practitioner with the infant or toddler and family as well as the progress of the infant or toddler (Stoffel, n.d.-a). Consider why skilled

---

EXHIBIT 17.2.   Tips for Documentation

Use the verbs found in Table 7 of the *Occupational Therapy Practice Framework: Domain and Process* (AOTA, 2020), titled "Performance Skills for Persons," to document performance of motor, process, and social interaction skills (underlined in the example below) and link to the infant or toddler's participation in areas of occupation (in italics in the example below).

Example: Brian <u>initiates</u> play by grasping a marker and <u>attends</u> to the task of coloring on the paper without looking away, which demonstrates his interest in and motivation for *play exploration* and sustained *play participation*.

occupational therapy is needed for the child and family and how family coaching and education were used in the session. Below is example documentation of family coaching and education in a daily note:

> Michael's mother stated, "He has not been eating except for crackers, 1–2 fries, applesauce, sometimes yogurt, and drinking milk and water." The occupational therapist and Michael's mother discussed strategies to add tastes and textures to his diet, including trying smoothies with milk and yogurt and adding banana and/or avocado and also offering dips such as yogurt or applesauce. Michael was given 6 fries with yogurt dip and ate 4 quickly. His mother fed him yogurt and he ate 2 ounces.

Documenting developmental progress

Documentation of the child's *developmental progress* (i.e., changes the child has made in the EI areas of development such as cognitive, adaptive, physical, social, or emotional development) should align with the infant's or toddler's IFSP outcomes and child outcomes and include measurement to show the infant's or toddler's progress (Stoffel, n.d.-b). Documentation should include the developmental aspects of the task (i.e., skills required by the child), modifications made to the environment or task, and the child's or caregiver's response (e.g., whether the child benefited from a certain type of cue).

SOAP notes are a type of documentation that includes the following sections: Subjective (S), Objective (O), Assessment (A), and Plan (P). Following is an example of SOAP-note-style daily documentation with objective and assessment information:

> Santiago showed awareness of his mealtime (breakfast) routine by raising his arms for his mother to place the highchair tray and by watching his mother fill the bowl. He immediately grasped the spoon when it was placed in front of him, indicating his understanding of the activity. He required the spoon to be filled for him as he lacks the motor planning to do so independently, but once filled, he brought the spoon to his mouth for 10 bites independently throughout the meal and also used his hands to feed himself.

Documenting Family Engagement

Family engagement refers to the "systematic inclusion of families in activities and programs that promote children's development, learning, and wellness, including in the planning, development, and evaluation of such activities, programs, and systems" (DHHS & U.S. Department of Education, 2016, pp. 1–2). Because families are considered critical and essential IFSP team members, it is crucial that occupational therapy practitioners gather information from families to inform documentation and implementation of the occupational therapy process. Families are best suited to provide information about their child's interests, routines, and challenges.

Consider the diversity of the family

Occupational therapy practitioners should be mindful of the family's cultural and linguistic diversity, native language, and any other special considerations (e.g., low English proficiency, hearing or vision impairment) when communicating to gather information during the initial assessment, sharing results, and discussing IFSP outcomes (IDEA, 2004). The EI lead agency should work with all EI providers, including occupational therapy practitioners, to ensure that documents given to the family use their preferred language of the family (IDEA, 2004).

Occupational therapy practitioners should consider *health literacy* when sharing information with families as well as in written documentation. Health literacy includes the ability to obtain, understand, and act on health information and services to make appropriate health decisions as well as the context or environment in which the information is being disseminated (AOTA, 2017; Pleasant et al., 2016). Families may feel less empowered and more overwhelmed by difficulty reading, interpreting, and using unfamiliar EI program forms and documents, which could lead to decreased participation and poorer child outcomes (Pizur-Barnekow et al., 2011).

Suggestions for improving health literacy in EI documentation include the following:

- Assess current EI documents for readability and usability,
- Revise content and wording to be at a fifth–sixth-grade reading level when possible, and
- Involve families in reviewing and revising EI documents (Pizur-Barnekow et al., 2011).

Occupational therapy practitioners can also play a role in promoting health literacy in EI by supporting families in understanding and using the IFSP outcomes that are written for their child and family. Some strategies to enhance the parent's use of the IFSP are included in Exhibit 17.3.

All documentation should show the distinct value of occupational therapy to other IFSP team members and stakeholders. Documentation with outcomes that support enhancing functional participation in everyday routines (e.g., mealtime, bathing, play) and other occupations of interest to the infant or toddler and their family is unique to occupational therapy. Sharing this information in the IFSP team meeting settings can help other disciplines and families to better understand the role of occupational therapy in EI.

Occupational therapy practitioners should document ongoing communication, training, and coaching with families. Documentation should include who is present during the session and any subjective information that the family shares. The following is an example of a statement

---

EXHIBIT 17.3. Strategies to Improve the Family's Use of IFSP Outcome Pages

- Make sure the family has a copy of the IFSP in their home language.
- Encourage the family to post the IFSP Outcome page in a visible location in their home.
- Have the child and siblings decorate the page to make it more meaningful.
- Create a separate occupational therapy intervention plan document to reflect discipline-specific, measurable short-term goals (can be shared with the family if desired).

that could be used in an EI evaluation report: "Timothy was evaluated in his home with his mother and older brother present. Timothy's mother was able to report on his daily routines and participation in activities that were not observed during the evaluation."

Family engagement and participation can be documented with inclusion of the caregiver's response as well as the child's response. At the start of and during the session, discuss with the parent or caregiver what strategies they tried, the child's response, and the progress they have seen since the previous session. On the basis of the conversation, the *Subjective* section of a daily note written in the SOAP-note style might include, "Sebastian's mother reported that he has been eating well and she feels that he is growing. She stated that she has given him a spoon to practice with eggs but he tended to hold the spoon and then use his other hand to feed himself."

Tips for Point-of-Service Documentation

Point-of-service documentation means completing documentation during or at the end of a session in the presence of and while interacting with the client (Waite, 2012). Because EI takes place in natural environments, point-of-service documentation means documenting in the family's home or community setting. Providers might identify challenges to point-of-service documentation in EI, such as feeling disconnected from the family while documenting, disrupting the family's routine, and being concerned about taking time away from working directly with the child and family to document.

Point-of-service documentation also has benefits, such as providing the opportunity for more detailed, accurate, and client-centered documentation (Waite, 2012). It is important that occupational therapy practitioners identify and follow any policies or procedures in their state or local EI programs that would affect point-of-service documentation. Some agencies may require the parent or caregiver to initial or sign daily notes at the end of a session, so in those cases point-of-service documentation is required.

For those who can and want to try point-of-service documentation, the following tips and strategies might be helpful:

- Point-of-service documentation can be an important way to partner with the family. Explain the importance of documentation to the family. Use documentation time to further engage the family by discussing what is being documented. Share observations of the child's responses and progress, and ask the family for their input.
  - What did a parent or caregiver see that was different from a previous session?
- While writing the daily note, engage in conversation with siblings or the child receiving EI, as appropriate, to promote family engagement.
  - "What did we do today? What did you like best? What did your brother or sister do?"
- Use documentation time to discuss the plan for moving forward. Collaborate with the family to plan activities for the next session, and discuss strategies they can continue to use throughout the time in between sessions.
  - What are the next steps to support the child's participation in daily activities and progress toward the IFSP outcomes?

Document Child Outcomes for Federal and State Accountability

IDEA established child outcomes and mandated that all participating states receiving funding for EI and preschool programs develop data-capturing processes. These processes are based on guidelines established by the Office of Special Education Programs (OSEP) to ensure greater accountability. As part of the state performance plan or annual performance report, states are required to report on the percentage of infants and toddlers with IFSPs who demonstrate improved child outcomes (Early Childhood Technical Assistance [ECTA] Center, n.d.-a). Occupational therapy practitioners, as IFSP team members, contribute information gathered during the initial assessment and at transition or discharge by providing a rating during the team rating process regarding the three *child outcomes:*

1. Social–emotional: Positive social relationships;
2. Knowledge and skills: Acquiring and using knowledge and skills; and

TABLE 17.1. Tips for Participating in the Child Outcomes Summary Process

POINT IN TIME DURING THE PROCESS	TIPS FOR PARTICIPATION
Before COS rating	- Discuss the purpose and process for the COS rating process with families. - Identify the sources of information that will be used for the rating and specific examples of the child's progress that could be shared (by you or the family member).
During COS rating	- Ensure everyone has a copy of the outcomes, and read them out loud. - Allow enough time for everyone to read the overall outcomes and the components. - Provide input on each child outcome, with specific examples. - Communicate the sources of information that you are using to justify your input. Work with family members and team members from other disciplines to build consensus. Because the child outcomes are focused on function, multiple perspectives should be considered for each outcome.
After COS rating	- Share success stories and lessons learned from participating in the rating process with other team members. - Discuss how COS ratings can guide the IFSP outcome development.

Note. COS = Child Outcomes Summary; IFSP = individualized family service plan.
Source. Based on James et al. (2016).

3. Meeting needs: Taking appropriate action to meet needs: thinking, problem solving.

The child outcomes are often embedded in the development of the IFSP and should be used to guide development of IFSP outcomes. The **Child Outcomes Summary** (COS) process is a team process using a 7-point scale that is focused on summarizing the functional outcomes achieved by infants and toddlers from participation in EI programming (ECTA Center, n.d.-b). Participation in the COS process helps to highlight the distinct value of occupational therapy services in EI while securing the profession's position as an important service provider (James et al., 2016). Table 17.1 provides some tips for participation in the COS process.

BEST PRACTICES

The *Guidelines for Documentation of Occupational Therapy* (AOTA, 2018) instructs occupational therapy practitioners regarding various actions and documents that are needed during service delivery processes. Guidance is also provided by other official documents, such as the *Occupational Therapy Practice Framework: Domain and Process* (4th ed.; *OTPF*; AOTA, 2020). This section provides discussion of the occupational therapy process and professional forms within the EI process.

Document Evaluation, Assessment, and Reevaluation

Per IDEA, Part C, "the only *evaluation* is the one for program eligibility" (p. 303.321[a][2][i]). In EI, the evaluation includes both eligibility determination and assessment to help identify specific needs and priorities of the infant or toddler and family.

When gathering data to determine eligibility (e.g., on the basis of each state's eligibility criteria), the occupational therapist may not be conducting a "discipline-specific" evaluation. The professionals conducting this eligibility determination must document the assessment tools and methods used as well as their findings regarding eligibility. For occupational therapists conducting an occupational therapy (discipline-specific) evaluation, the *OTPF* identifies the first step in the occupational therapy process (AOTA, 2020) as gathering the occupational profile and then gathering data for analysis of occupational performance.

Evaluation and assessment documentation include referral information and client information (e.g., name, date, date of birth, diagnosis; AOTA, 2018). Documentation of the occupational profile includes client-specific information concerning the infant's or toddler's occupations, personal interests, occupational history, and performance patterns (i.e., roles, routines, habits). The occupational profile documents how the physical and social environments and cultural, personal, temporal, and virtual contexts support or hinder the occupational engagement of infants and toddlers and their families.

Observation and further specific assessment of the infant or toddler and their family provide the opportunity for documenting the analysis of occupational performance, including assessment tools used and factors that support or hinder performance and participation. Because the information in the discipline-specific report is used by the team

to determine service needs, the occupational therapy evaluation should link the infant's or toddler's performance in the EI domains (i.e., physical, adaptive, communication, social or emotional, cognitive) to their participation in occupations and daily routines.

EI evaluation and assessment reports do not typically include recommendations related to frequency, duration, or intensity of occupational therapy services because those are decided at the IFSP meeting by all team members, including the family. Rather, the report should indicate the findings based on strengths and needs of the child and family. See Appendix G, "Sample Early Intervention Team Report," for a sample evaluation report.

Reevaluation

Occupational therapists might also complete a reevaluation, as described in AOTA's (2018) *Guidelines for Documentation of Occupational Therapy,* to contribute to the determination for ongoing occupational therapy services. The IDEA requires that the IFSP be reviewed at least every 6 months (known as the periodic review, or **IFSP review**) and annually. For more information about eligibility, see Chapter 14, "Understanding Part C: Early Intervention Law and the Individualized Family Service Plan (IFSP) Process."

Write Functional, Participation-Based, Measurable IFSP Outcomes

The IFSP includes the child's current development, their strengths, the family's concerns, goals and outcomes for the child and family, and the services needed to help reach those outcomes and therefore support parents or caregivers to make informed decisions and actively participate in their child's program. Occupational therapy practitioners play a key role in writing and implementing the IFSP as part of the EI team. The IFSP outcomes may be written in a variety of ways in different EI programs. A key consideration for practitioners when writing IFSP outcomes is to include outcomes that are

- Functional,
- Participation based, and
- Measurable.

IFSP outcomes are often team based or shared (i.e., multiple providers addressing the same outcome). Occupational therapy practitioners are cognizant of ensuring that the IFSP outcome reflects the need for skilled occupational therapy service. For more information on writing high-quality IFSP outcomes, occupational therapy practitioners can access additional resources through the ECTA Center (n.d.-c) and the AOTA continuing education product, *Best Practice Methods in Early Intervention Documentation* (Stoffel & Pizur-Barnekow, 2018).

Writing functional IFSP outcomes includes centering the outcome on family priorities and making sure the outcomes promote success in everyday activities and environments (Gatmaitan & Brown, 2016; McWilliam, 2010; Pletcher & Younggren, 2013; Workgroup on Principles and Practices in Natural Environments, 2008). Participation-based outcomes are individualized to the infant or toddler and family, incorporate the child's strengths and interests, and use the family's routines and contexts (Foley Hill & Childress, 2015).

TABLE 17.2. Reflective Questions for Writing an IFSP Outcome

ASPECT OF OUTCOME	REFLECTIVE PRACTICE QUESTIONS
Functional and family centered	<ul><li>Does the outcome address the family's concern?</li><li>Does the outcome describe as closely as possible how the parent or caregiver stated the concern?</li><li>Is the outcome based on activities and routines that the family is already doing?</li><li>Can the outcome be addressed during a functional daily activity or routine that already exists for the family?</li><li>Is the outcome impactful across family, child care, and natural environments?</li></ul>
Strengths based and participation based	<ul><li>What are the child's current developmental skills? What is the next developmental step?</li><li>Can you include a child's favorite toy, song, or activity in the outcome?</li><li>How will this IFSP outcome be incorporated into the family's daily activities and routines?</li><li>Can real-life events be used as a timeline (e.g., when school starts, by first birthday)?</li><li>Does the outcome use child and family strengths, resources, and preferences?</li></ul>
Measurable and observable	<ul><li>How will we know when this outcome is met?</li><li>Can the child show achievement across settings and routines?</li><li>Is the outcome meaningful to the child and family?</li></ul>

Note. IFSP = individualized family service plan.
Source. Based on Stoffel & Pizur-Barnekow (2018).

Measurable IFSP outcomes provide the opportunity to show progress over time, use words that are observable and describe action, and avoid passive words (e.g., *improve, tolerate, increase, maintain;* Gatmaitan & Brown, 2016; Shelden & Rush, 2009). For example, instead of, "Alex will improve her fine motor skills," consider, "Alex will play with toys using both hands so that she can hold (stabilize) and move (manipulate) toy parts," or, "We would like Alex to use utensils with minimal spilling while eating so that she can participate in mealtime."

Families are the ultimate decision makers in determining whether an IFSP outcome has been met (Shelden & Rush, 2009); however, including measurable and observable criteria in the IFSP outcomes, such as frequency, duration, and level of assistance, can assist in making sure the outcome is achievable and that progress can be documented over time. Consider adding the following aspects to an IFSP outcome to make it more measurable: when, how often, for how long, where, and under what conditions (e.g., during mealtime; once per week; for the duration of library music time; at Grandma's house; independently, without gagging). Table 17.2 provides additional reflective questions that occupational therapy practitioners can use to write functional, participation-based, and measurable IFSP outcomes, and Table 17.3 provides examples of IFSP outcomes.

Document Intervention

This section includes three parts of intervention: intervention plan, implementation, and review. Each of these parts is documented.

Professional intervention plan (plan of care)

Occupational therapy practitioners are aware of the distinctions between the IFSP and the occupational therapy intervention plan. In EI, the IFSP is developed collaboratively with the family; however, the occupational therapy intervention plan focuses the practitioners' actions and includes specific occupational therapy goals in addition to

describing "the occupational therapy approaches and types of interventions selected for use in reaching clients' targeted outcomes" (AOTA, 2020, p. 25).

Across both the IFSP and the occupational therapy intervention plan, family concerns, priorities, and resources are documented, in addition to transition considerations (i.e., preschool) and referrals to other professionals, to further support the infant or toddler and their family. Given the emphasis on team-oriented outcomes and service delivery in EI, the occupational therapy intervention plan is especially important to demonstrate skilled occupational therapy and may also be required for some reimbursement sources.

Implementation

Occupational therapy interventions are intentionally designed to support infants and toddlers and their families in participating in the daily occupations that occur in their natural learning environments (e.g., home, day care, community). Therefore, the focus of occupational therapy intervention documentation in EI should be on infants' and toddlers' participation in everyday routines, including eating, drinking, bathing, dressing, playing, and sleeping (AOTA, 2014). Occupational therapy intervention documentation includes training, consulting, and collaborating with day care personnel, families (including siblings), caregivers, and other service or medical providers (AOTA, 2014).

Document progress toward outcomes

Ongoing timely documentation of intervention activities is important to highlight the distinct value of occupational therapy to the IFSP team and to demonstrate progress toward established targeted IFSP outcomes. Collecting data does not have to be a cumbersome experience. The first step is to find a system that works best for each individual provider (e.g., clipboard; notebook; counters such as rubber bands moved from wrist to wrist or paperclips moved from pocket to pocket). Consider having older siblings participate as appropriate (e.g., count the number of bites their sibling takes using a spoon, use a watch or smartphone to

TABLE 17.3. Examples of IFSP Outcomes

FAMILY CONCERN AND PRIORITY	EXAMPLE OF IFSP OUTCOMES	CONSIDERATIONS
• We want Omar to use both hands and have fun at the library music class because he likes playing the toy drums at home.	• Omar will play with toys using both hands together during music time at the library or at home one time per week.	• Uses the occupation of play as the primary focus. • Addresses the child's participation across environments, which is a priority for the family. • Incorporates the child's interest in music.
• Kejuan is not sleeping in his own bed.	• Kejuan will fall asleep and remain in his own bed throughout the night for 7 nights in a row.	• Provide family with a data-collection sheet so they can record progress.
• We want Desi to feed herself, eat a variety of foods, and increase her acceptance of vegetables. • We want Desi to be able to eat at restaurants and family gatherings.	• Desi will feed herself with a spoon with minimal spilling for the duration of a mealtime so that she can participate more independently in mealtimes at home and in the community. • Desi will try two new foods at dinner at least 1 time per week for 3 months in order to increase the number of vegetables in her diet.	• Includes family concern and is measurable, so the team will be able to say whether the child has met the outcome.
• We want Elijah to participate with other children at child care. • We want Elijah to know how to color with a crayon so he is ready for preschool.	• Elijah will participate in an art activity with his child care classmates at the table 2 times per week so that he learns to grasp and use a crayon for coloring and be ready for preschool.	• Includes parent priorities (e.g., incorporates day care classmates, "be ready for preschool") and measurement (i.e., 2 times per week).
• We want Ananya to enjoy her birthday party.	• Ananya will participate at her birthday party by blowing out candles, opening gifts with help, and not crying.	• Includes a real-life timeline that is meaningful to the family. • Incorporates several performance skills (e.g., oral–motor and motor planning for blowing; sensory integration and processing for regulation and attention; cognitive understanding of the task) in a family activity.
• We want Daiki to play ball with his brother and understand how to play with toys.	• Daiki will push a ball or toy car back and forth with his brother at least three times during playtime so that he can understand how to play with toys. • Daiki will participate in playtimes with his brother two times per week over 2 months so they can learn to play together.	• Worded as closely as possible to the parents' concerns. • Includes measurement (i.e., at least three times during playtime). • Incorporates sibling per parent priority.
• Parents want resources for community activities.	• The Suarez family will locate one parent–child program in their neighborhood, such as a play group or library story time, so that they feel more connected to their community.	• Family-focused outcome.

Note. IFSP = individualized family service plan.

record how long their sibling stays at the table). The family can also help record data during the time between sessions, such as using a food diary or recording the child's responses to certain activities throughout the week.

Displaying data visually to family and other team members is a beneficial way to show progress. Make simple data collection sheets based on the IFSP outcome to help families collect data with ease (e.g., have families circle a plus or minus sign, use tally marks) or use published data sheets. Collaborate by sharing data collection sheets with team members (see Exhibit 17.4). For more information, see Chapter 6, "Best Practices in Data-Based Decision Making."

Implementation review

Occupational therapy practitioners document ongoing progress and identify opportunities to modify the intervention plan to better support the success of the infant, toddler, or family in their daily routines and natural environment. During intervention, ongoing documentation is important to support whether services should continue or discontinue. During the periodic or annual IFSP review, the IFSP team is responsible for making a collaborative decision regarding progress toward achieving the outcomes, as well as determining modification or revision of the outcomes

EXHIBIT 17.4.   Collecting Data on Child IFSP Outcomes

IFSP Outcome: Erika will use utensils with one or no spills while eating, so that she can participate more independently in mealtime.

Data are collected by the parent during lunch and shared with the occupational therapist during the twice-a-month visit.

Date of session	No. spills	Food and consistency	Utensil used
XX-XX-XX	0 1 2 3 4 5 **6**	Yogurt, sticky	Child-size spoon with shallow bowl
XX-XX-XX	0 1 2 3 4 5 **6**	Yogurt, sticky	Child-size spoon with shallow bowl
XX-XX-XX	0 1 2 3 4 **5** 6	Oatmeal	Child-size spoon with shallow bowl
XX-XX-XX	0 1 2 3 **4** 5 6	Pudding (chocolate)	Child-size spoon with shallow bowl

The occupational therapist showed the family how to connect the highlighted data to visually track changes.

Date of session	No. spills	Food and consistency	Utensil used
XX-XX-XX	0 1 2 3 4 5 6	Yogurt, sticky	Child-size spoon with shallow bowl
XX-XX-XX	0 1 2 3 4 5 6	Yogurt, sticky	Child-size spoon with shallow bowl
XX-XX-XX	0 1 2 3 4 5 6	Oatmeal	Child-size spoon with shallow bowl
XX-XX-XX	0 1 2 3 4 5 6	Pudding (chocolate)	Child-size spoon with shallow bowl

Note. IFSP = individualized family service plan.

or supports and services. The discontinuation of services should be based on the documentation of IFSP outcomes being met or if ongoing services do not produce measurable and meaningful changes (AOTA, 2014).

Documentation of Occupational Therapy Outcomes

The *OTPF* (AOTA, 2020, p. 30) describes *occupational therapy outcomes* as "the results clients can achieve through occupational therapy intervention". As a result of occupational therapy services, the mother may state she feels confident in caring for her child (role competence), or the father may be excited his son is able to eat a variety of foods and they can eat at a restaurant again (participation). Improving the child's and family's quality of life and well-being may also be outcomes that are achieved.

SUMMARY

Occupational therapy documentation in EI is affected by federal, state, and local EI laws, policies, and procedures as well as best practices determined by AOTA. AOTA offers resources to support best practice documentation in EI. Written documentation and communication related to documentation include family considerations, such as

sociocultural factors and health literacy; show the distinct value of occupational therapy to other team members; and comply with the requirements of reimbursement sources and state EI programs. Occupational therapy practitioners advocate for the profession and the role of occupational therapy in EI as well as promote best practices in documentation by linking IFSP outcomes to the OSEP-required child outcomes; writing functional, participation-based, and measurable IFSP outcomes; collecting data to measure progress; and promoting family engagement and participation.

REFERENCES

American Occupational Therapy Association. (2014). *Children & Youth (formerly Early Intervention and School) Special Interest Section FAQs.* https://www.aota.org/Practice/Manage/SIS/Children-Youth/faq.aspx

American Occupational Therapy Association. (2017). AOTA's societal statement on health literacy. *American Journal of Occupational Therapy, 71,* 7112410065. https://doi.org/10.5014/ajot.2017.716S14

American Occupational Therapy Association. (2018). Guidelines for documentation of occupational therapy. *American Journal of Occupational Therapy, 72*(Suppl. 2), 7212410010. https://doi.org/10.5014/ajot.2018.72S203

American Occupational Therapy Association. (2020). Occupational therapy practice framework: Domain and process (4th ed.). *American Journal of Occupational Therapy, 74*(Suppl. 2), 7412410010. https://doi.org/10.5014/ajot.2020.74S2001

Early Childhood Technical Assistance Center. (n.d.-a). *Child outcomes.* https://ectacenter.org/eco/pages/childoutcomes.asp

Early Childhood Technical Assistance Center. (n.d.-b). *Child Outcomes Summary process (COS).* https://ectacenter.org/eco/pages/cos.asp

Early Childhood Technical Assistance Center. (n.d.-c). *Developing high-quality, functional IFSP outcomes and IEP goals training package.* https://ectacenter.org/knowledgepath/ifspoutcomes-iepgoals/ifspoutcomes-iepgoals.asp

Family Educational Rights and Privacy Act of 1974, Pub. L. 93-380, 20 U.S.C. § 1232g; 34 CFR Part 99.

Foley Hill, C., & Childress, D. C. (2015). The individualized family service plan process. In S. A. Raver & D. C. Childress (Eds.), *Family-centered early intervention: Supporting infants and toddlers in natural environments* (pp. 54–74). Brookes.

Gatmaitan, M., & Brown, T. (2016). Quality in individualized family service plans: Guidelines for practitioners, programs, and families. *Young Exceptional Children, 19*(2), 14–32, https://doi.org/10.1177/1096250614566540

Health Insurance Portability and Accountability Act of 1996 (HIPAA), Pub. L. 104-191, 42 U.S.C. § 300gg, 29 U.S.C §§ 1181–1183, and 42 U.S.C. §§ 1320d–1320d9.

Heider, F. (2016). *State Medicaid and early intervention agency partnerships to promote healthy child development.* https://nashp.org/state-medicaid-and-early-intervention-agency-partnerships-to-promote-healthy-child-development/

Individuals With Disabilities Education Improvement Act of 2004, Pub. L. 108-446, 20 U.S.C. §§ 1400–1482.

James, L. W., Stoffel, A., Schefkind, S., & Khetani, M. (2016). Occupational therapy in the Child Outcome Summary process in early intervention and preschool. *OT Practice, 21*(5), 13–16.

McWilliam, R. A. (2010). *Routines-based early intervention: Supporting young children and their families.* Brookes.

Pizur-Barnekow, K., Patrick, T., Rhyner, P. M., Cashin, S., & Rentmeester, A. (2011). Readability of early intervention program literature. *Topics in Early Childhood Special Education, 31,* 58–64. https://doi.org/10.1177/0271121410387676

Pleasant, A., Rudd, R. E., O'Leary, C., Paasch-Orlow, M. K., Allen, M. P., Alvarado-Little, W., . . . Rosen, S. (2016). *Considerations for a new definition of health literacy.* https://nam.edu/considerations-for-a-new-definition-of-health-literacy/

Pletcher, L. C., & Younggren, N. O. (2013). *The early intervention workbook: Essential practices for quality services.* Brookes.

Shelden, M. L., & Rush, D. D. (2009). Tips and techniques for developing participation-based IFSP outcome statements. *BriefCASE, 2*(1), 1–6. https://fipp.org/static/media/uploads/briefcase/briefcase_vol2_no1.pdf

Stoffel, A. (n.d.-a). *How to fix common early intervention documentation mistakes, AOTA Q & A.* http://www.aota.org/practice/manage/reimb/fix-early-intervention-ei-documentation-mistakes.aspx#sthash.YfnlDeac.dpuf

Stoffel, A. (n.d.-b). *Writing pediatric goals: How to document family involvement & developmental progress, AOTA Q and A.* http://www.aota.org/Practice/Manage/Reimb/writing-pediatric-goals-family-involvment-developmental.aspx#sthash.TscQpKxb.dpuf

Stoffel, A., & Pizur-Barnekow, K. (2018). *Best practice methods in early intervention documentation* [AOTA continuing education webinar]. American Occupational Therapy Association.

U.S. Department of Health and Human Services. (2013). *Summary of the HIPAA Privacy Rule.* https://www.hhs.gov/hipaa/for-professionals/privacy/laws-regulations/index.html

U.S. Department of Health & Human Services & U.S. Department of Education. (2016). *Policy statement on family engagement from the early years to the early grades.* https://www2.ed.gov/about/inits/ed/earlylearning/files/policy-statement-on-family-engagement.pdf

Waite, A. (2012). Record time: Point-of-service documentation strategies help practitioners beat the time crunch. *OT Practice, 17*(1), 9–12.

Workgroup on Principles and Practices in Natural Environments. (2008). *Seven key principles: Looks like/doesn't look like.* https://ectacenter.org/~pdfs/topics/families/Principles_LooksLike_DoesntLookLike3_11_08.pdf

Section IV.

Considerations for Preschool:
IDEA Part B

Understanding Preschool Laws and the Individualized Education Program Process

18

Rebecca E. Argabrite Grove, MS, OTR/L, FAOTA

KEY TERMS AND CONCEPTS

- Child Find
- Developmental delay
- Every Moment Counts
- Every Student Succeeds Act of 2015
- Extended school year
- Free appropriate public education
- Individualized education program

- Individuals With Disabilities Education Improvement Act of 2004
- Least restrictive environment
- Local education agency
- Multitiered systems of support
- Positive behavioral supports and interventions

- Preschool grants program
- Prior written notice
- Procedural safeguards
- Related services
- Section 504 of the Rehabilitation Act of 1973
- State performance plan
- Transition planning

OVERVIEW

Young children in the United States receive early education and care across a variety of environments, including at home, in private day care, in public or private preschool settings, or a combination thereof. According to the National Center for Education Statistics (2018), the percentage of children ages 3–5 years attending full-day preschool increased from 47% to 56% between 2000 and 2017 and varied based on parents' education level, race, income, and geographic location (U.S. Department of Education [USDE], 2015).

Federal and state governments have established educational policies to expand public preschool programs, but funding for such programs has decreased. Across the United States, only 33% of 4-year-olds and 5.7% of 3-year-olds attend state-funded preschool programs (Friedman-Krauss et al., 2019). Additionally, there has not been a proportionate expansion of opportunities for children with disabilities to participate in these programs (USDE Office of Special Education Programs [OSEP], 2017). Research has shown that children with and without disabilities who participate in high-quality, inclusive early childhood programs have better outcomes on measures of health, social–emotional status, cognition, and school readiness. These outcomes also extend over time, resulting in improved educational attainment, career success, and future earning potential (U.S. Department of Health and Human Services [DHHS] & USDE, 2015; Yoshikawa et al., 2013).

For children with disabilities, the ***Individuals With Disabilities Education Improvement Act of 2004*** (IDEA; P. L. 108-446) safeguards the opportunity for participation in the public preschool (general education) setting, allowing them access to learn and develop pre-academic and social–emotional skills alongside typical peers. The IDEA, Part B, was established

(a) To ensure that all children with disabilities have available to them a free appropriate public education that emphasizes special education and related services designed to meet their unique needs and prepare them for further education, employment, and independent living;

(b) To ensure that the rights of children with disabilities and their parents are protected;

(c) To assist States, localities, educational service agencies, and Federal agencies to provide for the education of all children with disabilities; and

(d) To assess and ensure the effectiveness of efforts to educate children with disabilities. (34 CFR §300.1)

Under the ***preschool grants program*** of IDEA Part B (hereinafter referred to as Part B), Section 619, all states are required to offer free preschool special education services to children with disabilities who are ages 3–5 years and, at the discretion of the state, to children with disabilities who are age 2 years and will turn age 3 years during the school year. States are not required to provide public preschool programs to all children in the general population; however, many currently do (OSEP, 2017). Many children with disabilities receive special education services in public or private preschool programs, kindergarten, child care facilities, or Head Start to ensure they are educated with typical peers.

Each state is required to submit an annual ***state performance plan*** (SPP) to the USDE OSEP to evaluate its implementation of Part B. States are also required to complete an annual performance report (APR), which tracks the performance of each local education agency (LEA) within its jurisdiction. OSEP (2018) uses a results-driven accountability framework to determine whether states meet the compliance requirements of Part B and demonstrate educational results and functional outcomes that create equal access and opportunity to full participation, independent living, and economic success. These measures are intended to protect children and families by holding states accountable for providing quality preschool education. Table 18.1 outlines OSEP annual performance indicators that specifically target preschool children. Occupational therapy practitioners support their local and state educational agencies by adhering to these outcomes. (*Note. Occupational therapy practitioner* refers to both occupational therapists and occupational therapy assistants.)

Despite legal and regulatory requirements, preschool children with disabilities continue to be at a disadvantage regarding current and future outcomes. Part B SPP/APR 2018 indicator analyses (USDE, 2018) provide evidence over 6 years, from 2011 to 2016, of the following preschool outcomes:

- On average, 51% of children spent time in the general education setting and 21% were in a separate setting, representing only a 1%–2% improvement over 6 years.
- On average, 81% of children substantially increased the rate of growth in positive social–emotional skills, with 59% functioning within age expectations, representing a mere 0%–2% improvement over 6 years.
- On average, 81% of children substantially increased the rate of growth in acquisition and use of knowledge and skills, with 52% exiting preschool at age expectations, representing a 1% improvement in growth rate but a 1% loss in meeting age expectations over 6 years.
- On average, 80% of children substantially increased the rate of growth in use of appropriate behaviors to meet their needs, with 67% exiting preschool at age expectations, representing a 2%–3% improvement over 6 years.

There is much room for improving preschool outcomes given such low rates of longitudinal growth. It is imperative that high-quality, inclusive preschool programs are available, as well as accessible, to all children. Evidence shows that early learning supports, resources, and services can contribute to future academic, social, and career success while also offering a cost benefit through the reduction of need for special education and intersection with the justice system in the future (USDE, 2015). This chapter provides an overview of special education law, regulation, and best practices for demonstrating the distinct value of occupational therapy to ensure quality services and outcomes for preschool age children.

ESSENTIAL CONSIDERATIONS

IDEA, originally enacted in 1975 as the Education for All Handicapped Children Act of 1975 (P. L. 94-142), continues to serve as hallmark legislation for protecting the rights of children to access and participate equally with their peers in public education settings. The law requires that parents and school personnel work together to provide children with a *free appropriate public education* (FAPE). In IDEA, FAPE means that special education and related services

- Are provided at public expense, under public supervision and direction, and without charge;
- Meet the standards of the state education agency, including the requirements of this part;
- Include an appropriate preschool, elementary school, or secondary school education in the State involved; and
- Are provided in conformity with an individualized education program (IEP) that meets the requirements of §§300.320–300.324. (34 CFR §300.17)

For children who have been receiving early intervention (EI) services under IDEA, Part C (for children ages birth–2 years), FAPE must be available no later than the child's third birthday.

Local Education Agency

An *LEA* refers to a public board of education, an institution, or an agency, including charter schools, recognized

---

TABLE 18.1.   Office of Special Education Programs Annual Preschool Performance Indicators

INDICATOR	DESCRIPTION
Indicator 6: Preschool least restrictive environment	Percentage of preschool children with IEPs who received special education and related services in settings with typically developing peers (i.e., early childhood settings, home, and part-time early childhood/part-time early childhood special education settings; 20 U.S.C. 1416[a][3][A])
Indicator 7: Preschool outcome (aka early childhood outcome)	Percentage of preschool children with IEPs who demonstrate improved positive social–emotional skills (including social relationships), acquisition and use of knowledge and skills (including early language/communication and early literacy), and use of appropriate behaviors to meet their needs (20 U.S.C. 1416 [a][3][A])
Indicator 11: Timeframe between evaluation and identification (Child Find)	Percentage of children who were evaluated within 60 days of receiving parental consent for initial evaluation or, if the state establishes a timeframe within which the evaluation must be conducted, within that timeframe (20 U.S.C. 1416[a][3][B])
Indicator 12: Early childhood transition	Percentage of children referred by Part C before age 3 years who are found eligible for Part B and who have an IEP developed and implemented by their 3rd birthdays (20 U.S.C. 1416[a][3][B])

Note. IEP = individualized education program.

by the state, that provides administrative control and oversight of public education (34 CFR §300.28). It is the LEA's responsibility to oversee implementation and compliance with federal and state laws and regulations regarding special education for children and families within its jurisdiction. The LEA must ensure that children with disabilities receive FAPE.

Special Education Process

The special education process, described in this section, is systematic, with multiple safeguards for parents.

Evaluation and eligibility

The first step of the special education process begins with *Child Find* (34 CFR §300.111). Any child who is suspected of having a disability, including homeless or migrant children and children who attend private school, must be identified to determine whether a referral to special education and related services is necessary. Parents, caregivers, school staff, health care providers, or others may initiate a referral, and the educational team must secure written parental permission for an individual evaluation to determine eligibility and must complete this process within 60 calendar days (34 CFR §§300.300 and 300.301).

Evaluation procedures and assessment tools should be carefully selected to gather relevant functional, developmental, and pre-academic information about the child, including input from the parent, to allow determination of whether the child has a disability and the extent to which the child is able to participate in appropriate activities (34 CFR §300.304). A child must not be determined to be a child with a disability based on exclusionary factors such as lack of appropriate instruction or limited English proficiency (34 CFR §300.306), and careful consideration must also be given to the child's physical condition, social or cultural background, and adaptive behavior (34 CFR §300.306[c][1][i]).

Child with a disability

After reviewing the evaluation results, the team determines whether the child is eligible to receive special education and related services as a child with a disability under one of the following categories[1] (34 CFR §300.8[a][1]):

- Intellectual disability
- Hearing impairment (including deafness)
- Speech or language impairment
- Visual impairment (including blindness)
- Emotional disturbance
- Orthopedic impairment
- Autism

- Traumatic brain injury
- Other health impairment
- Specific learning disability
- Deaf blindness
- Multiple disabilities

Additionally, IDEA allows each state to develop evaluation criteria for identifying children between ages 3 and 9 years with a *developmental delay* in one or more areas of development, including physical, cognitive, communication, social–emotional, or adaptive areas of performance (34 CFR § 300.8[b]). There is wide variability in age and significance of delay across states.

Finally, some children do not require special education and, instead, may only need access to related services, such as occupational therapy, to enable them to benefit from their educational program. A few states recognize "related services" such as occupational therapy as a support or instructional service under their state's administrative rules for special education, allowing the service to be the only service on an IEP.

Another way to access occupational therapy services for children in preschool who need educational accommodations or modifications may be through *Section 504 of the Rehabilitation Act of 1973* (29 U.S.C. §794; P. L. 93-112). A child who is identified as having a documented physical or mental impairment that substantially limits one or more major life activities is protected from discrimination under this civil rights legislation. A 504 plan provides accommodations and modifications to ensure a child's access to participation in the educational environment.

Individualized education program

Once a child is deemed eligible for special education, an *IEP* (i.e., a written statement of performance, goals, and services) must be developed. The student's IEP is developed by the IEP educational team and outlines supports and services necessary to provide the child with FAPE. Team members include, but are not limited to, parents; a general education teacher; a special education teacher; an LEA representative; an individual who can interpret the evaluation results (often a school psychologist or educational diagnostician); and others with special expertise, including related services (34 CFR §300.321[a]). For a child transitioning from IDEA Part C to Part B, an invitation should be sent to the Part C service coordinator to ensure a smooth transition (34 CFR §300.321[f]).

It is critically important for parents of preschool children to be provided with the opportunity to participate in and provide input to the IEP (IDEA, 34 CFR §300.322). This involvement includes sharing reports from physicians or health-based occupational therapy practitioners. The team is not required to adhere to the recommendations but must review them for information regarding the child's IEP development. Active participation by the practitioner is essential for information sharing, program planning, and decision making.

The IEP should be developed based on the strengths of the child; concerns of the parents for enhancing the child's education; results of initial or most recent evaluations; and academic, developmental, and functional needs (IDEA, 34 CFR §300.324). Special factors must also be considered by

---

[1]IDEA does not require children to be classified by their disability. OSEP has granted a waiver to one state department of education where children with disabilities are referred to as "eligible individuals" rather than labels since labels do not provide information about instructional needs and are sometimes used for restrictive placement decisions. Teams still must determine if child meets one of these categories (34 CFR § 300.111).

the team when developing an annual IEP, including behavior that impedes the child's learning or that of others, limited English proficiency, blindness or visual impairment, language and communication needs (e.g., of a child who is deaf or hard of hearing), and the need for assistive technology devices and services. IDEA requires that the IEP contain the following seven components for preschool children:

1. A statement of the child's present levels of academic achievement and functional performance, including how the disability affects involvement and progress in the general education curriculum; or for preschool children, how the disability affects participation in appropriate activities
2. A statement of measurable annual goals, including academic and functional goals to include a description of benchmarks or short-term objectives as appropriate
3. A description of how progress toward annual goals will be measured and when periodic reports of progress will be provided
4. A statement of special education, related services, and supplementary aids and services, based on peer-reviewed research to the extent practicable, to be provided to, or on behalf of the child; a statement of program modifications/supports for school personnel to enable participation of the child in the general education curriculum, extracurricular, and other activities with children who have and do not have disabilities
5. An explanation of the extent, if any, to which the child will not participate with children who do not have disabilities in the general education classroom and activities
6. A statement of individual accommodations necessary to measure academic achievement and functional performance on State and districtwide assessments, including a description of why the child may need to take an alternate assessment as appropriate
7. The projected date to begin provision of services and modifications, including anticipated frequency, location, and duration. (34 CFR §300.320)

In addition, the LEA must offer an IEP that is reasonably calculated to enable a child to make progress appropriate in light of the child's circumstances (USDE Office of Special Education and Rehabilitative Services [OSERS], 2017).

Related services

Related services are included in a child's IEP when special education services alone are not enough to provide meaningful benefit and receipt of FAPE. **Related services** are defined as "transportation and such developmental, corrective, and other supportive services as are required to assist a child with a disability to benefit from special education" (34 CFR §300.34). Occupational therapy is considered a related service in some states, whereas in others, it may be defined as specially designed instruction, meaning that it can be provided as a stand-alone IEP service (Schneider & Chandler, 2019). IDEA defines *occupational therapy* as

- Improving, developing, or restoring functions impaired or lost through illness, injury, or deprivation;

- Improving ability to perform tasks for independent functioning if functions are impaired or lost; and
- Preventing, through early intervention, initial or further impairment or loss of function. (34 CFR §300.34(c)(6)(ii)

Other examples of related services include special transportation, speech and physical therapy, counseling, orientation and mobility services, school health and school nurse services, and parent counseling and training as required for a child to benefit from special education (34 CFR §300.34).

Although IDEA does not expressly require the IEP to specify the exact amount of services in terms of hours and minutes, according to the U.S. Department of Education, precision is preferable to the extent that the nature of a child's disability and needed services can be quantified daily by hours and minutes (OSEP, 1994). Related services must be documented based on the child's unique needs and in a manner that clearly outlines the number (frequency) and duration (length) of sessions. This documentation provides clarity for school staff and parents and can help avoid future misunderstandings over service delivery.

Least restrictive environment

IDEA Part B requires the LEA to educate children in the *least restrictive environment* (LRE), that is,

- To the maximum extent appropriate, children with disabilities, including those in public or private institutions or other care facilities, are educated with children who are nondisabled; and
- Special classes, separate schooling, or other removal of children with disabilities from the regular educational environment occurs only if the nature or severity of the disability is such that education in regular classes with the use of supplementary aids and services cannot be achieved satisfactorily. (34 CFR §300.114[a][2])

Furthermore, the LEA must ensure that a continuum of placement options be available to meet the individual needs of the child for special education and related services, such as instruction in regular classes, special classes, special schools, the home, and hospitals and institutions as well as supplementary services (e.g., resource room, itinerant instruction) that are provided in conjunction with regular class placement (34 CFR §300.115). The IEP team may not determine initial placement or make a change in educational placement without written parental consent (34 CFR §300.327). Consideration of services provided in the LRE under Part B is like the requirements in IDEA Part C in which services must be provided in the natural environment where the child participates (e.g., home, child care settings, preschool).

Any potential harmful effect on the child or impact on the quality of the IEP service provided must be considered when determining a child's placement in the LRE. The DHHS and USDE (2015) joint policy *Statement on Inclusion of Children With Disabilities in Early Childhood Programs* supports the presumption that the first placement option discussed and considered by the IEP team is a regular public preschool program that a child would attend if they did not have a disability.

Related services should also be delivered within the context of daily activities and routines of the classroom with typical peers to the maximum extent possible, based on the child's individual needs. Any removal from the classroom to other locations away from typical peers for one-on-one services or small group settings that only include children with disabilities constitutes a removal from the regular preschool setting and should be minimized (OSEP, 2017). Removal of a child from the general education program must be documented on the student's IEP and reported by the state to OSEP. Occupational therapy within the child's natural context and routine builds supports for the child within their environment, instruction, and curriculum.

Extended school year

Most public preschool programs operated by the LEA follow a traditional school schedule, offering services for 36 weeks per year. However, IEP teams must ensure that *extended school year* (ESY) services, including special education and related services, are available during school breaks if necessary, to provide FAPE. ESY services must be determined based on the individual needs of the child as outlined in the IEP and may not be limited to

- Specific disability categories;
- Type, amount, or duration of services; or
- Time of the year in which services are provided. (34 CFR §300.106)

ESY must be provided at no cost to the parents and may occur during any break in school instruction, including holidays and summer months, based on consideration of the following criteria:
- Regression and recoupment
- Degree of progress toward IEP goals and objectives
- Emerging skills and breakthrough opportunities
- Interfering behavior
- Nature or severity of disability
- Special circumstances.
The IEP team should conduct an analysis of whether learning that occurred during the regular school year will be significantly jeopardized if ESY services are not provided (OSEP, 2003).

Procedural safeguards

The rights of parents and their children are protected through the LEA's provision of procedural safeguards (34 CFR §300.504) and prior written notice (34 CFR §300.503). *Procedural safeguards* outline the rights parents have as participants and decision makers for their children's education and must be provided at least once per school year. Many LEAs maintain a copy of procedural safeguards on their website. Procedural safeguards must be provided in understandable language and may be translated to ensure parents' native language needs are met.

Prior written notice must be given to parents each time the LEA proposes or refuses to initiate or change the identification, evaluation, educational placement of the child, or the provision of FAPE and must include

- A description of the action proposed or refused by the agency;
- An explanation of why the agency proposes or refuses to take the action;
- A description of each evaluation procedure, assessment, record, or report the agency used as a basis for the proposed or refused action;
- A statement that the parents of a child with a disability have protection under the procedural safeguards of this part and, if this notice is not an initial referral for evaluation, the means by which a copy of a description of the procedural safeguards can be obtained;
- Sources for parents to contact to obtain assistance in understanding the provisions of this part;
- A description of other options that the IEP Team considered and reasons why those options were rejected; and
- A description of other factors relevant to the agency's proposal or refusal. (34 CFR §300.503[b])

Prior written notice must be provided in the parents' native language or translated, so that it is understandable prior to parents providing consent for the LEA to implement the proposed IEP (34 CFR §300.503[c]).

Early childhood outcomes

The process of determining early childhood outcomes remains family centered with parents serving as an important source of information. Occupational therapy practitioners work with the education team to define outcomes, describe how data will be collected, and provide multiple methods for engaging families using a strengths-based, individualized approach to obtain data in natural environments (e.g., home, community, preschool) from adults involved with the child (Early Childhood Technical Assistance [ECTA] Center, 2012). Three common areas of performance are measured, including social–emotional skills (social interaction, play, emotional expression, and following rules and routines), acquisition and use of knowledge and skills (language and communication, early literacy and numeracy, and problem solving), and use of appropriate behavior to meet individual needs (self-care, transitions from place to place, and shift toward independent functioning; ECTA Center, 2012).

BEST PRACTICES

Occupational therapy practitioners working in preschools should understand educational laws, complete their responsibilities during transition planning using inclusive practices in evaluation and intervention, and implement multitiered systems of supports within their agency.

Assist in Transition Planning

Transition planning is a set of coordinated activities, based on the strengths and needs of the child, designed to facilitate movement from one service setting to another (34 CFR §303.209). Occupational therapy practitioners are often members of the receiving educational team when children transition from IDEA Part C, EI, to Part B, preschool services. The involvement of the practitioner to communicate and collaborate with EI professionals and parents builds a relationship of trust and support to ensure the child's smooth and successful transition (Teeters Myers et al., 2011). It also allows the occupational therapist to contribute to evaluation and planning for an appropriate IEP based on the strengths and anticipated needs of the child within the context of an inclusive preschool classroom.

The occupational therapy practitioner can modify and accommodate the classroom and greater school environment to enhance the child's performance, allowing learning, socialization, and participation in school routines and activities to occur with ease (Teeters Myers & Podvey, 2019). Frequent communication with parents is helpful to assist the family in adjusting to changes inherent in the transition from the family-focused approach in EI to the educational team approach in preschool, during which parents may feel that their input is minimized and legal requirements are difficult to understand (Frolek Clark & Hanft, 2016).

Use Inclusive Practices

Khetani and colleagues (2015) found that children with disabilities participated less and were perceived to have less environmental support for participation in child care and preschool activities than children without disabilities. The delivery of related services such as occupational therapy within the natural context supports a child's integration of performance skills and strategies into the daily routines of the classroom, thus enhancing participation in learning and social activities (Bazyk & Cahill, 2015; Cahill, 2019). The joint policy statement on inclusion of children with disabilities (DHHS & USDE, 2015) establishes an expectation that high-quality, inclusive preschool programs should enable the full participation and success of all children. Evidence exists to support cognitive and communication development, social–emotional skills, higher test scores over the educational career, and lower rates of absenteeism for children with disabilities who participate in inclusive settings.

Children without disabilities may also benefit developmentally, socially, and attitudinally because occupational therapy supports the diverse needs of all children who participate as equals in the preschool classroom and other school settings such as hallways, cafeterias, school buses, restrooms, playgrounds, and art or music rooms. Although case law and administrative decisions afford school districts with flexibility in interpreting implementation of the LRE requirement, the removal of children to separate settings should be minimized and should occur only when individualized instruction for acquisition of new skills is documented as necessary and beneficial for the provision of FAPE (Bazyk & Cahill, 2015; Frolek Clark, 2016).

Provide Multitiered Systems of Support

The most essential aspects of quality preschool learning include a language- and literacy-rich, interactive social environment that effectively incorporates a developmentally appropriate and engaging multisensory curriculum.

Occupational therapy practitioners can provide curricular support, accommodations, and modifications by incorporating occupational therapy–related concepts. For example, practitioners can use developmentally appropriate, play-based preschool activities that strengthen fine and visual motor skills to facilitate new learning and increase participation and social interactions across routines for all students (Dessoye et al., 2017). At arrival, children can sign their name or first letter of their names on a vertical surface such as a chalkboard, which strengthens shoulder muscles, enhances wrist stability for writing, works on early literacy skills, and provides a sense of belonging, which promotes social–emotional development). Preschool teachers can benefit from occupational therapy support to implement and accommodate this type of inclusive learning environment.

The *Every Student Succeeds Act of 2015* (P. L. 114-95) identifies occupational therapy practitioners as *specialized instructional support personnel* (SISP), allowing them to provide *multitiered systems of support* (MTSS) to all children with and without disabilities. MTSS is a framework that uses evidence-based, systemic practices designed to support a rapid response to a child's needs with regular observation and data collection to facilitate instructional decision making (OSEP, 2016). MTSS involve a tiered system of interventions, most commonly at three levels, that are designed to provide increasingly intense instruction and intervention (Cahill, 2019). MTSS can target early literacy and numeracy skill development, but they may also apply to children with social and behavioral challenges in need of *positive behavioral supports and interventions* (PBIS). PBIS offer a multitiered approach for social, emotional, and behavioral support to all students, including students with disabilities, whose behavior may interfere with their learning or the learning of others (OSEP Technical Assistance Center on PBIS, 2019). The use of MTSS and PBIS may not take the place of the LEA's obligation to conduct an evaluation, including a functional behavior assessment, of a child who is suspected of having a disability once a referral has been received (OSEP, 2016).

Occupational therapists who work in inclusive preschool settings can easily serve on intervention or problem-solving teams to screen, identify pre-academic or behavioral areas of concern to target, develop and implement tiered interventions, and design and analyze data systems that allow progress monitoring and decision making to achieve desired educational outcomes. The partnership that coexists between teaching staff and occupational therapy practitioners working in an inclusive classroom can lead to beneficial and meaningful change in professional behaviors and the long-term educational and social outcomes of children (Cahill, 2019; DHHS & USDE, 2015). The contributions that practitioners can make as SISP complement the natural routines, activities, and participation of preschool children in the general school community. These contributions can include

- Consulting with teachers and families to support effective teaching and assessment strategies for learning;
- Developing a safe and positive school climate;
- Providing supportive systems for classroom management, transitions from one school location to another,

healthy social relationships, and positive mental health; and

- Working collaboratively to promote professional development and instructional integration with general and special education teaching staff (Cahill, 2019).

Every Moment Counts is a mental health promotion initiative that provides exemplar models and toolkits developed by occupational therapists working within an MTSS framework (USDE, 2014).

SUMMARY

Occupational therapy practitioners bring added value in support of educational policy decisions, administrative oversight, and preschool educational teams. The role of practitioners may include advocacy, consultation, professional development, collaboration, innovation, and direct service that involve

- Contributing to state early learning and development standards,
- Developing and modifying early learning curriculum,
- Establishing and expanding inclusive practices in general education classrooms,
- Creating partnerships with organizations and agencies that support innovation through preschool development grants,
- Promoting professional development for general and special education staff,
- Building relationships with parents and providing them with resources,
- Problem solving with interdisciplinary teams using MTSS and progress monitoring, and
- Supporting IEP teams to ensure that children have appropriately ambitious standards with more than "de minimis" educational benefit (OSERS, 2017; USDE, 2015).

Although IDEA cannot and does not promise any particular outcome, occupational therapy practitioners must demonstrate knowledge and skills for enhancing learning in all children, provide quality services in preschool programs, and demonstrate outcomes that ensure equity for all children's current and future needs.

REFERENCES

Bazyk, S., & Cahill, S. (2015). School-based occupational therapy. In J. Case-Smith & J. O'Brien (Eds.), *Occupational therapy for children* (7th ed., pp. 664–703). Elsevier.

Cahill, S. (2019). Best practices in multi-tiered systems of support. In G. Frolek Clark, J. Rioux, & B. Chandler (Eds.), *Best practices for occupational therapy in schools* (pp. 211–217). AOTA Press.

Dessoye, J., Davis, L., Mahon, E., Rehrig, S., & Robinson, T. (2017). The effectiveness of a multisensory center-based learning curriculum in prekindergarten students. *American Journal of Occupational Therapy, 71,* 71115203161. https://doi.org/10.5014/ajot.2017.71S1-PO6155

Early Childhood Technical Assistance Center. (2012). *Talking with families.* Chapel Hill, NC: Frank Porter Graham Child Development Institute. Retrieved from https://ectacenter.org/eco/pages/talking.asp

Education for All Handicapped Children Act of 1975, Pub. L. 94-142, reauthorized as the Individuals With Disabilities Education Improvement Act of 2004, codified at 20 U.S.C. §§ 1400–1482.

Every Student Succeeds Act of 2015, Pub. L. 114-95, 129 Stat. 1802 (2015).

Friedman-Krauss, A. H., Barnett, W. S., Garver, K. A., Hodges, K. S., Weisenfeld, G. G., & DiCrecchio, N. (2019). *The state of preschool 2018: State preschool yearbook.* National Institute for Early Education Research. http://nieer.org/wp-content/uploads/2019/04/YB2018_Full-ReportR2.pdf

Frolek Clark, G. (2016). Collaboration within the paces: Structures and routines. In B. Hanft & J. Shepherd (Eds.), *Collaborating for student success: A guide for school-based occupational therapy* (pp. 177–207). AOTA Press.

Frolek Clark, G. & Hanft, B. (2016). Collaboration in preschool: Family, school, and community partners. In B. Hanft & J. Shepherd (Eds.), *Collaborating for student success: A guide for school-based occupational therapy* (pp. 283–303). AOTA Press.

Individuals With Disabilities Education Improvement Act of 2004, Pub. L. 108-446, 20 U.S.C. §§ 1400-1482. 1232g, 34 CFR Part 99.

Khetani, M., Little, L., Lucas-Thompson, R., Davies, P., & Benjamin, T. (2015). Participation disparities between children with and without disabilities in early childhood educational environments. *American Journal of Occupational Therapy, 69,* 6911505028. https://doi.org/10.5014/ajot.2015.69S1-PO2098

National Center for Education Statistics. (2018). *Preschool and kindergarten enrollment 2000–2017.* https://nces.ed.gov/programs/coe/indicator_cfa.asp

Office of Special Education and Rehabilitative Services. (2017, December 7). *Questions and answers (Q&A) on U.S. Supreme Court case decision* Endrew F. v. Douglas County School District Re-1. https://sites.ed.gov/idea/files/qa-endrewcase-12-07-2017.pdf

Office of Special Education Programs. (1994). *Letter to Copenhaver,* 21 IDELR 1183. https://www.education.nh.gov/instruction/special_ed/memos/documents/fy16_memo_12_copenhaver_letter.pdf

Office of Special Education Programs. (2003, February 4). *Letter to Given.* https://www2.ed.gov/policy/speced/guid/idea/letters/2003-1/given020403iep1q2003.pdf

Office of Special Education Programs. (2016, April 29). *Memo 16-07—Response to intervention (RTI) and preschool services.* https://www2.ed.gov/policy/speced/guid/idea/memosdcltrs/oseprtipreschoolmemo4-29-16.pdf

Office of Special Education Programs. (2017, January 9). *Dear colleague letter: Preschool least restrictive environment.* https://www2.ed.gov/policy/speced/guid/idea/memosdcltrs/preschool-lre-dcl-1-10-17.pdf

Office of Special Education Programs Technical Assistance Center on Positive Behavioral Interventions and Supports. (2019). *Positive Behavioral Interventions & Supports* [Website]. https://www.pbis.org/

Rehabilitation Act of 1973, Pub. L. 93-112, 29 U.S.C. §§ 701–796l.

Schneider, E., & Chandler, B. E. (2019). Laws that affect occupational therapy in schools. In G. Frolek Clark, J. Rioux, & B. Chandler (Eds.), *Best practices for occupational therapy in schools* (pp. 19–26). AOTA Press.

Teeters Myers, C., & Podvey, M. (2019). Best practices in transition planning for preschoolers. In G. Frolek Clark, J. Rioux, & B. Chandler (Eds.), *Best practices for occupational therapy in schools* (pp. 187–192). AOTA Press.

Teeters Myers, C., Schneck, C., Effgen, S., McCormick, K., & Brandenburger Shasby, S. (2011). Factors associated with therapists' involvement in children's transition to preschool. *American Journal of Occupational Therapy, 65,* 86–94. https://doi.org/10.5014/ajot.2011.09060

U.S. Department of Education, Office of Special Education Programs. (2014). *Every Moment Counts:* https://everymoment-counts.org/

U.S. Department of Education. (2015, April). *A matter of equity: Preschool in America.* https://www2.ed.gov/documents/early-learning/matter-equity-preschool-america.pdf

U.S. Department of Education. (2018). *Part B state performance plan/annual performance report 2018 indicator analyses.* https://osep.grads360.org/services/PDCService.svc/GetPDC DocumentFile?fileId=33061

U.S. Department of Education's Office of Special Education and Rehabilitative Services Office of Special Education Programs. (2018, July 24). *2018 Determination letters on state implementation of IDEA.* https://sites.ed.gov/idea/files/ideafactsheet-determinations-2018.pdf

U.S. Department of Health and Human Services and U.S. Department of Education. (September 14, 2015). *Policy statement on inclusion of children with disabilities in early childhood programs.* https://www2.ed.gov/policy/speced/guid/earlylearning/joint-statement-full-text.pdf

Yoshikawa, H., Weiland, C., Brooks-Gunn, J., Burchinal, M., Espinosa, L., Gormley, W. T., . . . Zaslow, M. (2013, October). *Investing in our future: The evidence base on preschool.* Society for Research in Child Development. https://www.fcd-us.org/the-evidence-base-on-preschool/

19

Best Practices in Preschool Screening and Evaluation

Debi Hinerfeld, PhD, OTR/L, FAOTA

KEY TERMS AND CONCEPTS

- Authentic assessment
- Child-centered evaluation
- Child Find
- Child Outcomes Summary
- Education evaluations
- Effective, collaborative partnerships
- Hypotheses
- IEP goals
- Individuals With Disabilities Education Improvement Act of 2004
- Multitiered systems of support
- Occupational profile
- Occupational therapy evaluation
- Ongoing assessment
- Reevaluation

OVERVIEW

Occupational therapy practitioners who work with young children in preschool settings provide distinctly valuable screening, evaluation, and intervention supports to enhance the participation of all children, with and without disabilities, so they can achieve educational success. (*Note. Occupational therapy practitioner* refers to both occupational therapists and occupational therapy assistants.) As key members of educational evaluation teams, occupational therapists conduct contextual assessments that lead to valid identification of children's strengths and needs, which is foundational to determining shared educational goals and appropriate interventions.

The ***Individuals With Disabilities Education Improvement Act of 2004*** (IDEA; P. L. 108-446) is federal legislation that specifically includes occupational therapy as a related service for children with disabilities who are eligible for special education. Occupational therapy practitioners who work in preschool settings are instrumental in supporting all children in their performance of important educational and developmental tasks and activities (American Occupational Therapy Association [AOTA], 2017b).

Occupational therapists are members of the multidisciplinary educational teams who conduct screenings to identify and respond to young children who require ***multitiered systems of support*** (MTSS). MTSS is an educational framework that provides a proactive approach to early identification, assessment, and intervention of children with educational or behavioral needs. It includes universal screening to identify children who may be struggling in academic or behavioral areas and to prevent delayed development by targeting critical foundation skills. The MTSS framework is built on three additive tiers of graded supports and evidence-based interventions that respond to each child's unique needs. Additional key components include a strengths-based problem-solving process, ongoing data collection and continuous progress monitoring, a programwide approach, and systematic planning for parent engagement.

Tier 1, universal outcomes and supports, encompasses all children who learn together through core curriculum and basic interventions. Tier 2, targeted outcomes and interventions, is for small groups of children who need extra supports or intensity in order to meet educational goals (and includes supports from Tier 1). Tier 3, highly individualized outcomes and interventions, is for children who do not respond to supports provided in Tiers 1 and 2 and who require more individualized supports to meet their educational goals. Within an MTSS service delivery system, children with disabilities might receive instruction and support at any tier in a blended inclusive classroom. However, children do not need to go through the MTSS process in order to be referred for special education and related services.

Occupational therapists consult with educators and families on strategies to enhance children's occupational performance when there are motor, sensory, social–emotional, cognitive, or adaptive skill challenges and serve on multidisciplinary teams that evaluate children to determine eligibility for special education and related services. In classrooms and on evaluation teams, occupational therapy practitioners collaboratively contribute to the understanding of a child's strengths and needs relative to participation in educational activities and routines in the context of the preschool setting (AOTA, 2017b).

Engagement and participation take place in familiar social and physical environments situated in contexts that influence children's access to occupations and satisfaction with performance (AOTA, 2020). When screening and evaluation occur within typical routines and in natural environments, children demonstrate their personal strengths, and evaluators have an opportunity to identify how the context of the tasks and the environment supports or creates barriers to occupational performance. Using a top-down, multimodal, and ecological approach to screening and evaluation explicitly identifies what the child can do and how these skills can be used as building blocks to enhance participation in meaningful occupations (Case-Smith, 2015).

This chapter discusses the process and methods used in preschool screening and evaluation from referral to determine eligibility for special education and related services and the development of shared goals in the individualized education program (IEP). It emphasizes the use of ecological, authentic, and team-based approaches that include members of the child's family to determine appropriate goals, services, and supports.

ESSENTIAL CONSIDERATIONS

To be purposeful, when selecting the appropriate methods and tools, occupational therapists must understand the intent of the request (Frolek Clark & Kingsley, 2013). The preschool *occupational therapy evaluation* is a comprehensive assessment of the child, focused on performance in typical occupations of young children, such as ADLs, play, social participation, education, and rest and sleep, and how participation in these occupations occurs in the context of the preschool environment (Frolek Clark & Kingsley, 2013). Working on teams, occupational therapists gather information, perform appropriate assessments, and synthesize data to develop logical hypotheses based on the strengths and needs of the child. The occupational therapy evaluation strengthens team-based decision making that optimizes a child's engagement and participation in preschool and community activities and routines in natural settings.

Preschool Supports

There are several options for children who may need additional supports in preschool. These include MTSS, Child Find, and referral for a full and individual initial evaluation.

Multitiered Systems of Support

IDEA's early intervention (EI) services and the Every Student Succeeds Act of 2015 (P. L. 114-195) made it possible for all children struggling with learning and behaviors to receive MTSS. Although IDEA allows states to use up to 15% of their special education funds for educational and behavioral evaluations, services, and supports for children in kindergarten through Grade 12 (IDEA § 1413[f]), some states have extended this process to preschools.

The request for occupational therapy is typically focused on specific areas of concern in the general education environment. Professional development for educators and school administrators, and child evaluations, services, and supports are provided to promote learning and performance in the general education environment (Bazyk & Cahill, 2015) and are not to be seen as screening or evaluation for special education. After formally observing the child during preschool activities and routines and interviewing teachers and other adults, the occupational therapist may provide appropriate recommendations to enhance the child's success in general education. The therapist provides ongoing assessment to systematically monitor the child to determine progress in an effort to prevent further gaps in learning and development; however, if progress-monitoring data indicate that strategies and supports are not sufficient or if the child is suspected of having an educational disability, the child may be referred for a full and individualized eligibility evaluation for special education.

Child Find

IDEA's **Child Find** mandate requires school districts to have a process for identifying and evaluating children (from ages birth–21 years) who may need EI or special education and related services, such as occupational therapy. Each state must have policies and procedures in place that ensure all children with disabilities and those who are suspected of having disabilities, and who reside in the state, are identified, located, and evaluated (IDEA, 2004). This includes children with disabilities who attend private schools or programs, those that are homeless or wards of the state, and children of migrant workers; and establishes a method to determine eligibility for special educational services.

Referral for full and individual initial evaluation

Children may be referred for an evaluation by a parent, state agency, or local educational agency to determine whether they meet the state's eligibility criteria (Bazyk & Cahill, 2015; Frolek Clark & Kingsley, 2013). Children transitioning from EI (Part C of IDEA) may be referred for a full and individualized evaluation completed by a multidisciplinary team to determine eligibility for special education and related service needs in preschool (Part B of IDEA). Once a referral is made, IDEA stipulates that "each public agency must conduct a full and individual initial evaluation," which is completed before the child is provided with special education and related services (IDEA § 300.301[a]).

As written in the law, before any evaluation procedures are conducted, prior written consent must be obtained from the parents of the child with a disability (IDEA § 300.304). The team has 60 days from the signed parent referral to complete the evaluation; determine eligibility; and, if the child is eligible, complete the child's IEP. In accordance with IDEA, a single assessment measure or method cannot be used as the sole criterion for determining whether a child has a disability or for determining appropriate programs for the child (IDEA § 300.304[b][2]). Using a range of assessment methods focused on measuring a child's performance skills and abilities in different contexts supports decision-making processes, such as determining eligibility for special education and related services (e.g., occupational therapy).

Partner With Families

The role of families is significant during the evaluation and identification of their child's strengths and needs. As equal partners throughout the evaluation process, families provide valuable information (e.g., sleep patterns, social interactions in the community, toileting routines, activity preferences) and increase the richness of assessment data (Coster, 1998; Neisworth & Bagnato, 2004). Beginning when the initial referral is made, it is important to keep the family involved in activities and meetings throughout the process. Families need to understand the purpose and process of the evaluation and to have opportunities to ask questions and offer suggestions based on their knowledge of their child. Acknowledging and having respect for family cultures and backgrounds leads to a strong rapport and more robust collaborations. IDEA mandates that assessments are provided and administered in the child's and family's native language or by other modes of communication (IDEA § 300.304[c][1][ii]), and therefore a translator may be necessary if the family speaks a different language.

Child-centered evaluation means evaluation that is focused on the child but also on the family's priorities and concerns. Parents may share copies of medical reports or information from health care or community providers. It is best practice to ask open-ended questions during the evaluation process to encourage family members to "tell their child's story," point out the child's strengths and interests, and elaborate on the types of supports they provide to the child during daily activities and routines. As parents discuss their child, the occupational therapy practitioner listens intently to identify any red flags that point to factors that may affect the child's ability to effectively engage with others and the environment. Parents can also confirm that evaluation and assessment results throughout the process are actual reflections of their child's abilities.

Form Effective, Collaborative Partnerships With Educational Staff

Effective, collaborative partnerships with interdisciplinary team members (e.g., parents, teachers, psychologists, speech pathologists, physical therapists, social workers) are essential (AOTA, 2017b). The occupational therapy practitioner works collaboratively with the child's family and other members of the educational team to gather and share information that contributes to the best understanding of the "nature and extent of the child's strengths and needs" (AOTA, 2017b, p. 7). Throughout the screening and evaluation process, the practitioner demonstrates effective communication and interpersonal skills that lead to collaboration, takes responsibility for leading assessments in areas related to occupation, shares assessment results, and is an active participant in team decision making (AOTA, 2017b; Handley-More et al., 2013). Each team member should be flexible in their roles and responsibilities as their involvement in the assessment process changes (Linder, 2008).

BEST PRACTICES

Evaluation of young children in preschool settings should be a partnership with the family and the evaluation team, so that information is shared for the express benefit of the child's development and well-being (Division for Early Childhood [DEC], 2007). Evaluation is an individualized process designed to discover a child's strengths and needs

through authentic, developmentally appropriate, culturally responsive, and multimodal assessment methods. Best practices in the evaluation of young children must be ecologically based, match the purpose of the assessment, and support valid and reliable methods necessary to inform the decision-making process.

Comprehensively Evaluate the Child

As members of the multidisciplinary team, occupational therapists may participate in full and individual *education evaluations.* The purpose of these evaluations is to determine whether the child is eligible for special education and related services on the basis of educational needs (IDEA, 2014); whether the child needs occupational therapy services to benefit from their education program (IDEA, 2014); and whether the child may be eligible under Section 504 Plan for accommodations, modifications, and services (Rehabilitation Act of 1973, P. L. 93-112). The occupational therapy evaluation process includes the completion of the *occupational profile* and analysis of occupational performance (AOTA, 2020). The occupational profile is a unique and important part of the occupational therapy evaluation (Whitney, 2019). It is the process of gathering information about why the client is seeking services and the client's occupational history and experiences that also takes into consideration the client's "patterns of daily living, interests, values, needs, and relevant contexts" (AOTA, 2017a, as cited in AOTA, 2020, p. 21). This process collaboratively identifies priorities and desired outcomes that will lead to the client's engagement and participation in life's activities.

After gathering the occupational profile through parent and teacher interview, the occupational therapist formulates and tests their hypotheses.

Formulate and test hypotheses during the evaluation process

Hypotheses are proposed statements about why the child has occupational challenges and are based on consideration of different frames of reference. Occupational challenges may be described differently on the basis of the different perspectives offered by each frame of reference (Candler et al., 2007). The hypotheses are refuted or supported on the basis of the data that were collected. The more data are collected, the greater the chance that conclusions will be valid and reliable.

Analyze occupational performance: observation and assessment tools

On the basis of an understanding of the preschool routine, the type of curriculum being taught, and the method of instruction, as well as aspects of the environment such as the classroom, playground, bathrooms, dining areas, and indoor play areas that may support or limit the child's participation and engagement in typical preschool activities and routines (Frolek Clark & Kingsley, 2013), the occupational therapy practitioner has an understanding of the expectations during the preschool program and where to focus assessment methods. Children with disabilities are often not included in standardization processes of assessment tools, and, depending on the tool, their scores may not be a true reflection of their actual abilities in the preschool routines. Young children may be difficult to test depending on their developmental and cognitive level and may not perform well on standardized assessments, especially when they are done in unfamiliar environments and by unfamiliar adults (DEC, 2007; Frolek Clark & Kingsley, 2013).

Practitioners also should conduct assessments in the child's dominant language (DEC, 2014). With young dual-language learners, discerning between typical developmental language differences and potential developmental delays can be difficult. For example, if a child is asked to "put the block on top of the table" and they pick up the block and just hold it, it may be difficult to determine whether the child does not understand the concept or does not have the English vocabulary to correctly respond.

Make observations in child's environment and routines. The DEC (2014) recommends family-centered, team-based, and ecologically valid evaluation methods that are designed to identify the child's unique strengths and needs in the context of typical activities, environments, and routines. Ecological evaluation methods are naturalistic assessments of a child's behavior across multiple domains, which result in a richer understanding of how the child performs in multiple domains and across contexts (DEC, 2007; Frolek Clark & Kingsley, 2013). An ecological approach embeds observation and, when appropriate, standardized assessment into methods that are conducted while the child is participating in typical activities and routines and in the natural environment. Repeated observations and assessments while the child participates in different contexts and environments allow a child more opportunities to demonstrate their individual strengths and needs (Frolek Clark et al., 2019).

Use authentic assessment methods. The *Occupational Therapy Practice Framework: Domain and Process* (4th ed.; *OTPF;* AOTA, 2020) and the DEC (2007) both recommend that assessment data should be gathered from naturalistic settings where children spend their time and while children are engaged in typical activities and routines (Jiban, 2013). Although conventional standardized assessments are useful to identify skill deficits, a holistic picture of the child's strengths and needs is best obtained through the process of authentic assessment.

Authentic assessment is the process of "collecting information about the naturally occurring behaviors of young children and families in their daily routines" (Neisworth & Bagnato, 2004, p. 204). Also known as *play based, naturalistic,* and *performance based,* authentic assessment is an ecological and functional approach that leads not only to valid and reliable data about the child but also to evaluation results that can serve as building blocks for the development of functional goals and interventions (Dennis et al., 2013). The use of authentic assessment is purposeful and rich beyond standardized testing because of the way it allows the team to make inferences about the child's functioning beyond the particular assessment items and scenarios (Neisworth & Bagnato, 2004). It is the "collection

of information from familiar caregivers about the child's behavior and functional abilities as they are naturally occurring" (Dennis et al., 2013, p. 190).

If standardized assessments are used, best practice is to use occupation-based, curriculum- or criterion-based tools that provide information that can be analyzed and useful across disciplines and used to measure ongoing progress. Providing the child with multiple naturalistic opportunities to demonstrate individual strengths, authentic assessment practices also include the collection of the child's work samples, videos, and photographs of the child that can be used to develop a portfolio of artifacts ready to be examined by the team. These products can then be used later to document changes over time and can be shared with family and other stakeholders (Dennis et al., 2013).

Throughout this process, observations may also lead the occupational therapy practitioner to identify potential opportunities to adapt tasks or environments to promote a child's increased participation. For example, the occupational therapy practitioner might suggest the use of sensory-based supports that promote attention or might recommend adapted tools that allow a child to participate in preschool activities such as painting. Environmental considerations may include placing an adapted swing on the playground or adding playground structures that are wheelchair accessible. In the classroom, the practitioner may suggest that a corner of the room be reserved as a calming area where children may go to take a self-regulation break or to spend time with a peer looking at books or listening to soft music.

Authentic assessment is developmentally appropriate and relies on strong parent–professional partnerships. It is dynamic and purposeful and accounts for children's developmental variability. Authentic assessment also promotes the development of functional shared goals with the intent of embedding goals in routines with a focus on participation and engagement rather than goals focused on the development of isolated skills. Most important, it is a developmentally appropriate practice that is sensitive to children's opportunities to learn.

Assessment tools. Although standardized assessment measures are often used to identify skill development and needs, professional judgment is important to ensure valid results. Therapists use assessment tools and strategies that accommodate young children's cultural, linguistic, social, and emotional characteristics (DEC, 2014). Table 19.1 provides examples of commonly used tools for screening and evaluation.

Participate in Determining Eligibility and Need for Special Education

Occupational therapy practitioners often serve on IEP teams to determine the child's eligibility for special education and related services and to assist in the transition from EI to preschool educational settings. The IEP team reviews the existing evaluation data; evaluations and information from the parents; current classroom-based, local, or state assessments; and observations by the teachers and related service providers to determine whether the child has an

TABLE 19.1. Common Assessment Tools

PURPOSE	MEASURE	POPULATION	AREAS INCLUDED
Screening	Early Screening Inventory (3rd ed.) for preschool and kindergarten ages (Meisels et al., 2019)	Preschool: 3 years–4 years, 5 months Kindergarten: 4 years, 6 months–5 years, 11 months	Visual–motor, adaptive, language, cognition, and gross motor skills
	First Step Screening Test for Evaluating Preschoolers (Miller, 1993)	Ages: 2 years, 9 months–6 years, 2 months	Cognition, communication, and motor skills (optional testing includes social–emotional and adaptive functioning)
	Developmental Indicators for the Assessment of Learning (4th ed.; Mardell & Goldenberg, 2011)	Ages: 2 years, 6 months–5 years, 11 months	Motor, cognition, language, and self-help skills, and social–emotional development
Evaluate occupations	Pediatric Evaluation of Disability Inventory (Haley et al., 1992)	Ages: 6 months–7 years, 6 months	Self-care, mobility, and social functioning; also assesses level of need for caregiver assistance
Evaluate performance skills	Bruininks–Oseretsky Test of Motor Proficiency (2nd ed.; Bruininks & Bruininks, 2005)	Ages: 4–21 years	Fine motor precision, fine motor integration, manual dexterity, bilateral coordination, balance, running speed, upper-limb coordination
	Hawaii Early Learning Inventory for Preschoolers (2nd ed.; Teaford, 2010)	Ages: 3–6 years	Cognitive, language, gross motor, fine motor, social, and self-help skills
	Miller Function and Participation Scales (Miller, 2006)	Ages: 2 years–7 years, 11 months	Hand function, motor free visual perceptual skills, postural control, and executive functioning
	Movement Assessment Battery for Children (2nd ed.; Henderson et al., 2007)	Ages: 3 years–6 years, 11 months	Manual dexterity, ball skills, and balance
	Peabody Developmental Motor Scales (2nd ed.; Folio & Fewell, 2000)	Ages: Birth–5 years	Reflexes, stationary–equilibrium, locomotion, object manipulation, grasping, and visual–motor integration skills
	Vineland Adaptive Behavior Scales (3rd ed.; Sparrow et al., 2016)	Ages: Birth–90 years	Communication, ADLs, socialization, and motor skills as well as maladaptive behaviors

Note. ADLs = activities of daily living.

educational disability and educational needs (IDEA, 2004, § 1414).

If the team determines that the child is eligible for preschool special education services, the occupational therapy practitioner works collaboratively with the team to develop the child's IEP. Focusing on educational and family priorities, the team determines functional and measurable *IEP goals* that are aligned with the curriculum and based on the child's participation in activities such as learning (including early math and literacy), performing classroom expectations and routines, promoting social engagement, developing play skills, managing self-help skills, and following directions. Related service recommendations, such as the need for occupational therapy, are based on the needs of the child in the context of preschool activities and routines, not solely on the need to improve discrete skills. The educational team determines the priority educational needs of the child, which may or may not require occupational therapy services.

Participate in Reporting Early Childhood Outcomes

Teams working in state preschool special education agencies are also required to report children's progress through outcomes to the U.S. Office of Special Education Programs. The *Child Outcomes Summary* is the team process for reporting the status of a child's functioning and any additional progress achieved in the following three outcome areas:

1. The development of positive social–emotional skills the child needs to have good social relationships with peers and adults and to follow rules when interacting with others in groups;
2. The acquisition and use of knowledge and skills, including language and communication and early literacy, so the child is able to think, learn, reason, memorize, solve problems, understand symbols, and understand the world around them; and

3. The use of appropriate behaviors to meet the child's needs (e.g., caring for oneself, using words to communicate needs and wants) and to master everyday activities (e.g., eating, dressing, brushing teeth, toileting).

Preschool teams report progress toward these outcomes on entrance to and exit from the special education program through the Child Outcomes Summary Form, which is based on a 7-point scale that ranges from "overall skills are not age-appropriate" (1–5) to "overall skills are age-appropriate" (6–7). Child outcome ratings are determined by the team members, who synthesize information from multiple sources and across different settings and who must include perspectives and input from the family (Early Childhood Technical Assistance Center, n.d.).

The occupational therapy practitioner plays a valuable role on the team in the analysis and interpretation of a child's ability to integrate skill sets and their performance and is a vital member of the team in helping to inform the early childhood outcomes. As guided by the *OTPF* (AOTA, 2020), social participation (being able to relate to individuals and in groups), participation in education (thinking, learning, reasoning, problem solving), and participation in ADLs (caring for self, eating, dressing, toileting) are all identified as occupations within the domain of the occupational therapy practitioner, who identifies client factors, performance patterns, and performance skills that prevent or promote the child's engagement.

Conduct Ongoing Assessment

Occupational therapy practitioners participate in program planning and program evaluation. As members of the educational team, practitioners collaboratively participate in identifying the child's individualized educational goals and determining whether the child would benefit from occupational therapy services. Throughout the period of the child's intervention, **ongoing assessment** is conducted to determine whether interventions are effective in meeting the desired goals, as well as to determine ongoing eligibility for special education (Frolek Clark & Kingsley, 2013).

Occupational therapists in educational settings use formative and summative ongoing assessment. Formative assessment is the collection and analysis of data conducted throughout a continuum of time during an intervention period to determine whether the current interventions are effective at improving the child's performance. Summative assessment is an evaluation of cumulative data at a specific point in time (such as the end of the school year in preparation for an annual IEP meeting) and answers the question of whether the intervention plan worked overall (Frolek Clark & Kingsley, 2013).

Reevaluate and Transition

Reevaluation is a continuous and integral part of ongoing assessment while evaluating the effectiveness of intervention. Reevaluation may include re-administering assessments used at the time of the initial evaluation, conducting parent or teacher interviews, or the completion of questionnaires. Results of reevaluation support decision making about the need for future occupational therapy services and referrals to other agencies and professionals (Frolek Clark & Kingsley, 2013).

Occupational therapy practitioners play an integral role in the process of transitions because they have specialized knowledge and can serve as a valuable resource to the team and families as decisions are made regarding the least restrictive environment where the child will have opportunities to thrive. Practitioners are also instrumental in helping families navigate the new roles, routines, and performance skills they need in the next environment and context (Frolek-Clark & Kingsley, 2013). For more detailed information, refer to Chapter 10, "Best Practices in Early Childhood Transitions."

SUMMARY

Occupational therapy practitioners have critical roles as members of educational evaluation teams that serve preschool children and their families to optimize inclusion at school, at home, and in the community. When occupational therapists evaluate children using ecological and authentic methods that include family members as equal members of the team, young children are afforded with opportunities to demonstrate individual strengths and needs, particularly when they are observed and evaluated in typical preschool contexts. The occupational therapist supports the evaluation process by being client and family centered and purposeful when selecting evaluation methods and assessment tools. The team works collaboratively to analyze assessment results, make decisions regarding the child's eligibility, and identify services and supports that best promote the child's opportunities to engage and participate in typical preschool educational activities and routines.

REFERENCES

American Occupational Therapy Association. (2017a). AOTA's occupational profile template. *American Journal of Occupational Therapy, 71*(Suppl. 2), 7112420030. https://doi.org/10.5014/ajot.2017.716S12

American Occupational Therapy Association. (2017b). Guidelines for occupational therapy services in early intervention and schools. *American Journal of Occupational Therapy, 71*(Suppl. 2), 7112410010. https://doi.org/10.5014/ajot.2017.716S01

American Occupational Therapy Association. (2020). Occupational therapy practice framework: Domain and process (4th ed.). *American Journal of Occupational Therapy, 74*(Suppl. 2), 7412410010. https://doi.org/10.5014/ajot.2020.74S2001

Bazyk, S., & Cahill, S. (2015). School based occupational therapy. In J. Case-Smith & J. O'Brien (Eds.), *Occupational therapy for children and adolescents* (7th ed., pp. 664–703). Elsevier.

Bruininks, R. H., & Bruininks, B. D. (2005). *Bruininks–Oseretsky Test of Motor Proficiency* (2nd ed.). Pearson.

Candler, C., Clark, G., & Swinth, Y. (2007). School-based services: What does OT bring to the IFSP and IEP table? *Journal of Occupational Therapy, Schools, and Early Intervention, 1*, 17–23. https://doi.org/10.1080/19411240802060959

Case-Smith, J. (2015). Foundations and practice models for occupational therapy with children. In J. Case-Smith & J. O'Brien (Eds.), *Occupational therapy for children and adolescents* (7th ed., pp. 27–64). Elsevier.

Coster, W. (1998). Occupation-centered assessment of children. *American Journal of Occupational Therapy, 52,* 337–334. https://doi.org/10.5014/ajot.52.5.337

Dennis, L., Rueter, J., & Simpson, C. (2013). Authentic assessment: Establishing a clear foundation for instructional practices. *Preventing School Failure, 57,* 189–195. https://doi.org/10.1080/1045988X.2012.681715

Division for Early Childhood. (2007). *Promoting positive outcomes for children with disabilities: Recommendations for curriculum, assessment and program evaluation [Position paper].* https://www.decdocs.org/position-statement-promoting-positi

Division for Early Childhood. (2014). *DEC recommended practices in early intervention/early childhood special education 2014.* https://www.dec-sped.org/dec-recommended-practices

Early Childhood Technical Assistance Center. (n.d.). *Child Outcomes Summary (COS) process.* https://ectacenter.org/eco/pages/cos.asp

Every Student Succeeds Act of 2015, Pub. L. 114-195, 20 U.S.C. §6301 *et seq.*

Folio, M. R., & Fewell, R. R. (2000). *Peabody Developmental Motor Scales* (2nd ed.). Pro Ed.

Frolek Clark, G., & Kingsley, K. (2013). *Occupational therapy practice guidelines for early childhood: Birth through 5 years.* AOTA Press.

Frolek Clark, G., Watling, R., Parham, D., & Schaaf, R. (2019). Occupational therapy interventions for children and youth with challenges in sensory integration and sensory processing: A school-based practice case example. *American Journal of Occupational Therapy, 73,* 7303390010. https://doi.org/10.5014/ajot.2019.733001

Haley, S. M., Coster, W. J., Ludlow, L. H., Haltiwagner, J. T., & Andrellos, P. J. (1992). *Pediatric Evaluation of Disability Inventory.* San Antonio: Pearson.

Handley-More, D., Wall, E., Orentlicher, M., & Hollenbeck, J. (2013). Working in early intervention and school settings: Current views of best practice. *Early Intervention and Schools Special Interest Section Quarterly, 20,* 1–4.

Henderson, S. E., Sugden, D. A., & Barnett, A. (2007). *Movement Assessment Battery for Children* (2nd ed.). Pearson.

Individuals With Disabilities Education Improvement Act of 2004, Pub. L. 108-446, 20 U.S.C. §§ 1400–1482.

Jiban, C. (2013). *Early childhood assessment: Implementing effective practice.* http://info.nwea.org/rs/nwea/images/EarlyChildhoodAssessment-ImplementingEffectivePractice.pdf

Linder, T. (2008). *Transdisciplinary Play-Based Assessment 2.* Brookes.

Mardell, C., & Goldenberg, D. S. (2011). *Developmental Indicators for the Assessment of Learning* (4th ed.). Pearson.

Meisels, S. J., Marsden, D. B., Wiske, M. S., & Henderson, L. W. (2019). *Early Screening Inventory* (3rd ed.). Pearson.

Miller, L. J. (1993). *First Step Screening Test for Evaluating Preschoolers.* Pearson.

Miller, L. J. (2006). *Miller Function and Participation Scales.* Pearson.

Neisworth, J., & Bagnato, S. (2004). The mismeasure of young children: The authentic assessment alternative. *Infants and Young Children, 17,* 198–212. https://doi.org/10.1097/00001163-200407000-00002

Rehabilitation Act of 1973, Pub. L. 93-112, 29 U.S.C. §§ 701–796l, as amended 29 U.S.C. § 794 (2008).

Sparrow, S. S., Cicchette, D. V., & Saulnier, C. A. (2016). *Vineland Adaptive Behavior Scales* (3rd ed.). Pearson.

Teaford, P. (2010). *Hawaii Early Learning Inventory for Preschoolers (HELP) 3-6 Assessment Strands* (2nd ed.). VORT.

Whitney, R. (2019). *The occupational profile as a guide to clinical reasoning in early intervention: A detective's tale* [American Occupational Therapy Association Continuing Education Product No. CEA0419]. https://www.aota.org/~/media/Corporate/Files/Publications/CE-Articles/CE-article-April-2019-Occupational-Profile.pdf

Best Practices in Intervention in Preschool 20

Terry Giese, MBA, OT/L, FAOTA

KEY TERMS AND CONCEPTS

- Activities
- Advocacy
- Coaching
- Consultation
- Context
- Co-occupations
- Create
- Data collection
- Discharge planning
- Education

- Embedded learning opportunities
- Environmental factors
- Establish or restore
- Group interventions
- Individualized education program
- Intervention plan
- Interventions to support occupations
- Least restrictive environment
- Maintain

- Modify
- Multitiered systems of support
- Occupations
- Personal factors
- Preschool programs
- Prevent
- Training
- Universal design for learning

OVERVIEW

According to Barnett and colleagues of the National Institute for Early Education Research (Barnett et al., 2016), nearly 1.5 million children attend preschool in the United States (Covert, 2018). *Preschool programs* are defined by the National Center for Education Statistics (2019) as "groups or classes that are organized to provide educational experiences for children" (p. 1). With the growing body of evidence that supports better life outcomes for children who are prepared for primary education through preschool attendance, more states are pushing for required preschool education. Publicly funded preschools are available in almost every state.

This chapter discusses the fundamental requirements of best practices in the ever-evolving area of occupational therapy service delivery in preschool programs. Public health models that use multitiered systems of support (MTSS) and principles of universal design for learning (UDL) are examined. Intervention plans and individualized education programs (IEP) are differentiated as complementary tools that are used in tandem to identify chosen therapeutic methods and meaningful functional performance outcomes. The collaborative service delivery approach to coaching, consulting, and establishing parent partnerships is deliberated as it relates to defining desired outcomes and monitoring progress toward identified goals. Additional resources to support culturally competent and collaborative practice are provided.

ESSENTIAL CONSIDERATIONS

Occupational therapy practitioners provide skilled intervention to children who have disabilities or who are at risk of developing disabilities to promote developmental skills and enhance performance of daily life skills in home, child care, and preschool environments (Frolek Clark & Schlabach, 2013). (*Note. Occupational therapy practitioner* refers to both occupational therapists and occupational therapy assistants.) This section covers preschool interventions, including MTSS, UDL, the importance of providing intervention in the least restrictive environment, and considerations in educating others to provide practice opportunities throughout the day.

Multitiered Systems of Support in Early Childhood

Current best practices in early childhood education follow the principles of a public health model of service delivery. *MTSS* uses various levels (tiers) of support, which typically include three tiers:

1. All children;
2. Children requiring supplemental assistance; and
3. Children who need intensive assistance, which may include evaluation to determine eligibility for special education services.

Through the practices of collaboration, coaching, and engagement in meaningful occupations, this model of service delivery strives to improve outcomes by embedding intervention into naturally occurring and created routines, sequences, and activities in the least restrictive environment. Preschools and child care centers have also been shown to be effective environments for collaborative service delivery to effect change in foundational large motor development (Bellows et al., 2013; Larson et al., 2011; Ward et al., 2010).

Environmental Factors

Daily life activities occur within a ***context***, defined as a person's environmental and personal factors that affect engagement and participation (AOTA, 2020b). ***Environmental factors*** are aspects of the physical, social, and attitudinal surroundings of a person (AOTA, 2020b). Physical aspects include physical geography, light, and sound and can be promoted through universal design or may limit access to participation (e.g., steps in place of ramps, narrow doorways that prevent entry to children in wheelchairs). The social aspect reflects the support, assistance, and relationships (e.g., people, animals). The attitudinal aspect is focuses on how children are received and supported in communities and family units.

    Personal factors comprise the features and background of the person's life (AOTA, 2020b). These include age, education, race, cultural identification, and social status. The cultural attitudes in which a child is raised may shape and influence the child's identity and choice of occupations that are meaningful to the child. Activity choices and patterns, as well as performance expectations, may be influenced by personal factors. Fine motor development may be different for children who eat with chopsticks than for children who first learn to use a spoon or fork. Socioeconomic status may affect opportunities for the development of play skills with differing access to toys and playful environments. Resources for building culturally competent services for children are provided at the end of this chapter.

    Studies have found that child-rearing and play practices are the most divergent elements of cultural context affecting the occupations of young children (Lindsay et al., 2014; Williams & McLeod, 2012). One of the greatest cultural barriers that may affect practice is the cultural pressure in some communities to "fix" a child with a disability rather than learn to live with and manage the disability (Grandpierre et al., 2018). Occupational therapy practitioners should not assume that ethnicity or religion imparts one common set of beliefs and expectations on children and families. Implicit bias can become an unintended consequence of limited exposure to or understanding of cultural context (Darawsheh et al., 2015; Suarez-Balcazar et al., 2013).

Universal Design for Learning

UDL promotes practices that make a curriculum accessible to **all** learners, regardless of ability, disability, age, gender, and cultural and linguistic differences, by intentionally planning a variety of ways to gain access, engage, and process new information. Three guiding principles are the foundation of UDL (see Exhibit 20.1).

Collaborating Across Diverse Early Childhood Approaches

The importance of consulting and collaborating with preschool personnel has been recognized since the early days of inclusive service delivery models of practice (Dunn, 1988; Hanft & Place, 1998). Although many early childhood programs have fundamental learning approaches and contexts

---

EXHIBIT 20.1.	Guiding Principles of Universal Design for Learning

- *Multiple means of representation:* The "what" of learning; guiding children in recognizing, processing, and building patterns about concepts (e.g., verbally giving directions paired with a picture of the steps in the task and modeling how to use the tools)
- *Multiple means of engagement:* The "why" of learning; deliberately planning strategies to recruit children's interest and maintain attention often by utilizing children's interests and offering choices when designing learning activities (e.g., offering choices of the superhero they want to be during role play activity addressing social–emotional development)
- *Multiple means of expression:* The "how" of learning; allowing various formats for showing what they have learned (e.g., let children express their ideas by speaking the story into a recording device, telling it to a peer, or voicing it to a favorite stuffed animal)

---

in common, occupational therapy practitioners need to understand the varying components, roles of adults, and contextual features of the curriculum approach and philosophy utilized in each setting. Many early childhood curricular approaches have distinct features that reflect varying developmental theories and educational philosophies. For example, in the Montessori Approach, often 2–3 hours of independent work time are required, so the supports and temporal adaptations needed for a child in a Montessori setting may be very different than in a setting that uses 45–60 minutes of center time. For a comparison of selected early childhood approaches across components, roles, and contextual features see Table 2.1 in Chapter 2, "Influences From Early Childhood Professional Organizations and Technical Assistance Centers."

BEST PRACTICES

Early childhood inclusion embodies the values, policies, and practices that support the right of all young children to participate in a broad range of activities and contexts as full members of their communities. The joint policy statement on inclusion of children with disabilities (U.S. Department of Health and Human Services & U.S. Department of Education, 2015) establishes an expectation that high-quality, inclusive preschool programs should enable the full participation and success of all children. Providing services, including occupational therapy, to young children with identified delays and disabilities in inclusive early childhood settings within the natural context supports a child's integration of skills and strategies into the daily routines of the classroom, thus enhancing participation in learning and social activities (Bazyk & Cahill, 2015; Cahill, 2019).

    Interventions are chosen for each child on the basis of the child's strengths and needs, individualized education program (IEP) goals, the least restrictive environment, and contextual factors that affect the changes and modifications needed to close the functional performance gap with peers. Although research has shown that embedding therapeutic approaches into naturally occurring activities that have meaning to the child is the most effective approach for promoting occupational performance, individual interventions must match the needs of the child, because no single intervention method is appropriate for all children (Case-Smith & Holland, 2009).

Implement the Child's Individualized Education Program With Fidelity

The child's *IEP* constitutes a legal agreement for the provision of services in the preschool setting. The IEP must be implemented with fidelity to ensure that children progress toward meeting their educational goals. Collaborative strategies facilitate the attainment of IEP goals by avoiding discipline-specific goals and instead partnering with teachers and other team members to purposely identify and pursue a unified set of shared goals aimed at increasing participation within the routines and sequences of the school day. Data are collected to monitor the child's progress and systematically examine the effectiveness of the intervention. It is the responsibility of the occupational therapy practitioner to participate in the development of the IEP and to provide services to enhance the child's ability to benefit from their educational program.

Develop and Implement an Occupational Therapy Intervention Plan

The *intervention plan* is a professional document that guides the occupational therapy practitioner in the selection of interventions that will best meet the child's needs. It is used to determine guiding frames of reference for chosen intervention approaches and is combined with research evidence to support proposed interventions (AOTA, 2014, 2020b; Lopez et al., 2008). The therapy intervention plan outlines the related challenge and targeted outcomes, identifies the hypothesized cause underlying the occupational dissonance, and specifies possible interventions and precautions associated with the proposed therapeutic techniques. The plan also anticipates client-readiness indicators for discharge.

The occupational therapy intervention plan not only ties theory to practice but also may be an important communication tool among practitioners as children move from one classroom to another or as they transition out of preschool to kindergarten. The intervention plan not only includes what will be done to achieve desired outcomes but also anticipates what will determine the child's need for continuation or discontinuation of occupational therapy services. The intervention plan should include the occupational therapy intervention approaches and methods for delivering services, including the person, types of interventions, and service delivery models to be used. These are discussed in further detail below.

Occupational Therapy Practice Framework *intervention approaches*

The following intervention approaches are identified in the *Occupational Therapy Practice Framework: Domain and Process* (4th ed.; *OTPF*; AOTA, 2020b; Dunn et al., 1998): create (i.e., promote, health promotion), restore and

---

| EXHIBIT 20.2. | Examples of Occupational Therapy Intervention Approaches |

Establish: Studies have demonstrated that a focus on fine motor skill development for in-hand manipulation, eye–hand coordination, and grasp strength is correlated with improvements in the functional performance of preschoolers with moderate fine motor delays for self-care performance, mobility, and social function (Case-Smith, 2000). The effectiveness of occupational therapy intervention to improve visual–motor skills among preschoolers has also been demonstrated (Dankert et al., 2003).

Maintain: Participation in formal and informal activities is important for the development and maintenance of social skills, self-esteem, resilience, and fine motor skills (Law, 2002).

Prevent: The Pack It Light, Wear It Right backpack public health initiative launched by AOTA in 2000 has been successfully implemented for many years in the United States and abroad (Jayaratne et al., 2012). School-based prevention approaches have been shown to have long-lasting positive effects well into adulthood (Ball, 2018; Ialongo et al., 2019).

---

establish, maintain, modify, and prevent. Examples can be found in Exhibit 20.2 and include the following:

- *Create* (also known as *promote* and *health promotion*) does not assume the client has a disability; rather, the occupational therapy practitioner provides an enriched contextual experience and activities to enhance performance (e.g., provide an all-school education in-service on self-regulation to enhance attention for learning).
- *Establish or restore* (also known as *remediation*) focuses on client variables to establish or restore a skill or ability (e.g., use specially designed games or cooking activities to develop grasp and coordination abilities for a child with cerebral palsy).
- *Maintain* assumes performance will be lost without ongoing intervention; it supports the child's ability to continue to perform at the same level (e.g., providing ongoing intervention for a child with muscular dystrophy to continue self-feeding and dressing performance).
- *Modify* revises the current context or activity demands to support the child's performance (e.g., attaching visual task strips of the morning routine to the child's cubby to organize their performance).
- *Prevent* addresses the needs of any child who is at risk for problems with occupational performance (e.g., decrease sensory stimuli in the classroom—visual, auditory—to minimize distractibility, which may interfere with learning).

Occupational Therapy Practice Framework *intervention types*

According to the *OTPF*, "occupational therapy intervention types include occupations and activities, interventions to support occupations, education and training, advocacy, group interventions … [that] facilitate engagement in occupations to enable persons, groups, and populations to achieve health, well-being, and participation in life" (AOTA, 2020b, p. 59). These are further described as the following:

- *Occupations* are client-directed daily life activities that address participation goals (e.g., puts on coat for recess; eats lunch, then plays on playground).
- *Activities* support the development of performance skills and patterns to facilitate engagement in occupations (e.g., focus on coat and backpack fasteners so child will be independent).
- *Interventions to support occupations* include methods and tasks used to prepare the person for or during activities and occupations or home therapy programs. Examples include PAMs and mechanical modalities; orthotics and prosthetics (e.g., hand splint to enable grasp); assistive technology and environmental modifications (e.g., modified cup for drinking); wheeled mobility; and self-regulation (e.g., breathing strategies).
- *Education* imparts specialized knowledge to enhance understanding (e.g., providing information about developmental progression of fine motor skills).
- *Training* supports specific skill development in techniques to enhance performance (e.g., train in proper body mechanics for lifting, transfers, positioning).
- *Advocacy* promotes occupational justice and empowers clients to support health, well-being, and participation (e.g., include accommodations in the IEP, support the child in requesting support for bullying prevention).
- *Group interventions* may include activity groups or social groups that encourage children to explore and develop participation skills (e.g., self-regulation group, play groups).

Planning for discharge at the beginning

Discharge planning is an essential element of developing an intervention plan. *Discharge planning* supports the rationale for determining when and under what conditions a child is ready to discontinue occupational therapy services in the preschool setting. It guides the child's trajectory toward greater participation in meaningful occupations. The discharge plan provides the vision of what successful participation will look like for each individual child.

Discharge planning is not only a professional practice responsibility, it is an ethical consideration stated in the *2020 Occupational Therapy Code of Ethics* as a moral obligation to "terminate occupational therapy services in collaboration with the service recipient or responsible party when the services are no longer beneficial" (AOTA, 2020a, p. 7). Under the Individuals With Disabilities Education Improvement Act of 2004 (IDEA; P. L. 108-446), the occupational therapist does not make the decision to terminate therapy services in isolation. The decision is made in collaboration with the child's IEP members (e.g., parent, teacher). Current performance data gathering during the preschool day can determine the child's ongoing need for services. Occupational therapy practitioners can facilitate this task by initiating discharge planning at the initial evaluation of eligibility for services.

Complete Service Delivery in Natural Context and Routines

IDEA Part B requires services to be provided in the *least restrictive environment (LRE; 34 CFR §300.114[a][2]).

This means that children with disabilities should spend as much time as possible with peers without disabilities in natural environments (e.g., child care centers, community early childhood classrooms). Best practices support the provision of occupational therapy services in natural learning contexts with active collaboration with teachers and team members, inclusive of parents as equal partners in the collaborative process (Giese, 1993; Giovacco-Johnson, 2009; Laverdure et al., 2017). Related services, such as occupational therapy, should be delivered within the context of daily activities and routines of the setting with typical peers to the maximum extent possible based on the child's individual needs. Because service delivery in natural contexts demonstrates how occupational therapy interventions support curriculum expectations and preschool practices, this further increases the visibility and distinct value of occupational therapy.

Effective collaboration

Professional relationships built through collaborative efforts and the presence of therapy practitioners in the preschool environment enhance the effectiveness of therapeutic interventions and outcomes. The focus on collaboration has been shown to increase the child's participation and learning and to increase the satisfaction of team members working as a unified group, with better decision making and increased opportunities for practicing skills in the naturally occurring activities, routines, and sequences of the preschool program (Case-Smith & Cable, 1996; Fairbarn & Davidson, 1993).

Although best practices support the use of collaborative and contextual service delivery in preschool programs, there are many perceived barriers to successful implementation. Ineffective communication, scheduling difficulties, and employment of a caseload rather than a workload staffing model contribute to the challenges of implementing best practices (Frolek Clark et al., 2019; Gaylord, 2016). Successful collaboration and consultation require time to plan, communicate, and develop relationships; however, the inclusive model of practice faces only barriers to implementation, not inclusive practice (Giese, 1991; Villeneuve, 2009; Villeneuve & Shulha, 2012).

Embed learning opportunities

Intervention is most effective when opportunities to acquire and practice skills occur across the day during functional, meaningful routines and activities (Dinnebeil & McInerney, 2011). In addition to direct service delivery, effective occupational therapy service delivery should incorporate a consultative approach to plan for practice opportunities embedded throughout routines.

Embedded learning opportunities (ELOs) are a recommended practice for addressing individualized education interventions to meet goals for young children in preschool settings. (Division for Early Childhood, 2014). When collaborating and planning activities with early childhood teachers, the team members, including occupational therapy practitioners, use an ELO approach to support the implementation of the IEP goals in typical classroom routines and activities. ELOs are brief intervention episodes

EXHIBIT 20.3. Example of an Embedded Learning Opportunity Activity Matrix

Child's Name _____SHANA_____

SCHEDULE ↓	IEP GOALS/LEARNING OBJECTIVES		
	REQUEST (WORDS AND GESTURES)	TRANSITION—STAY WITH GROUP	PLAY WITH PEERS 5 MIN
Arrival		Stay with adult and classmates	
Circle	Provide opportunities to request song		
Small groups	Provide opportunities to request materials		
Outside play		Stay with adult and classmates	Encourage play with peers (sandbox, tire swing)
Snack	Provide two opportunities to request snack		
Centers	Present toys in containers with lids so that child needs to request		Join peers in dramatic play, sensory table, or game center
Book	Provide two opportunities to comment		
Dismissal		Stay with adult and classmates	

Note. IEP = individualized education program.
Source. Adapted from Horn et al. (2016).

designed to address children's IEP goals and learning objectives using the natural temporal and physical context of the preschool classroom routines (Horn et al., 2016; Sandall & Schwartz, 2008).

Together, teams develop an ELO matrix to organize and plan when and how interventions and opportunites to address shared goals will be embedded throughout the child's preschool day (see Exhibit 20.3). A matrix allows all team members to understand when and where the IEP goals will be addressed. For example, the occupational therapy practitioner may choose to work on social intervention during outside play or center time.

Coaching and consultation

Service delivery in natural contexts and routines requires the effective use of coaching and *consultation* skills in addition to effective collaboration. Traditional consultative approaches involve provision of expert opinions and recommendations from the perspective of the occupational therapy practitioner, whereas coaching extracts solutions from the client. A diversity of methods and approaches to this aspect of practice have been used, with no singular method showing greater effectiveness over others (Giese, 2002; Kessler & Graham, 2015). Flexibility in providing direct and consultative services has shown benefit by allowing practitioners to meet the demands of ever-changing program dynamics (Case-Smith & Holland, 2009). This fluid model of service delivery optimizes benefits to children as priorities shift, and teachers' needs are considered in addition to the goals of the child. Teachers have expressed a preference

for the coaching and consultative model because it enables them to learn new strategies and ways to embed these strategies into their daily routines (Wilson & Harris, 2018).

Occupational performance *coaching* focuses on strengths of the child and team members (Graham et al., 2013). This coaching method uses a goal-focused, conversational format to elicit perceptions about occupational performance and contextual factors that would benefit from embedded strategies to improve participation and performance. Occupational therapy practitioners provide emotional support during the process of information exchange and offer systematic procedures for problem solving. The collaborative performance analysis clarifies barriers to desired outcomes and elicits solutions from participating team members. Four questions guide this process:

1. What priority issues are creating gaps in learning, occupational engagement, and participation?
2. What strategies are available to close the gap, and how will they be implemented?
3. What data will be collected to measure progress, and how will they be collected?
4. What outcomes have been achieved, and do they match expectations (Fairbairn & Davidson, 1993)?

Distinguishing characteristics of coaching and consultation have been identified in business communities and can be extrapolated for consideration in occupational therapy service delivery. Exhibit 20.4 highlights the benefits and features of each method. Occupational therapy practitioners must determine when to use each approach to elicit successful outcomes. Additional resources for successful coaching strategies are provided at the end of the chapter.

EXHIBIT 20.4.	Comparing Coaching and Consulting Models

COACHING	CONSULTING
▪ Maximizes commitment to implementing solutions	▪ Limited commitment to implementing solutions
▪ Elicits answers from the client	▪ Provides expert advice to the client
▪ Assists the client in discovering solutions	▪ Offers technical assistance as an expert
▪ Builds capacity for future problem solving	▪ Helps resolve specific challenges through provision of answers
▪ Explores possibilities	▪ Provides options
▪ Equal input toward creating solutions	▪ Expert analysis of situations and performance
▪ Provides guidance	▪ Provides authoritative solutions
▪ Requires good listening skills	▪ Requires good analytic skills
▪ Focuses on the client	▪ Focuses on the problem
▪ Recognizes teaching expertise	▪ Relies on therapeutic knowledge and expertise

Note. Adapted from Forbes Coaching Council (2018).

Develop a Partnership With the Parents

The family is typically an active member of the team. Because many childhood occupations are actually *co-occupations* (i.e., occupations that children share with caregivers to implement successful occupational performance; e.g., feeding, bathing, dressing), the inclusion of family members in decision making and implementation is critical for generalization of skills across environments. For example, although a teacher may be struggling with convincing a preschooler with autism spectrum disorder to eat various snacks, the parent may provide multiple strategies that are successful at home. Building an effective relationship and partnership with parents is easier during positive times and will be beneficial if conflicts arise.

Conduct Ongoing Data Collection During Intervention

Data collection is an ongoing and critical element for measuring progress toward desired outcomes for children receiving occupational therapy services in the preschool setting.

State data

The Office of Special Education Programs requires each state to develop a state performance plan and submit an annual performance report that evaluates the state's ability to implement IDEA requirements (U.S. Department of Education [USDE], n.d.). The USDE uses these data to submit an annual report to Congress on the progress made toward providing a free, appropriate public education to all children with disabilities.

Collect data on child's response to intervention

Monitoring progress aligns with the requirement for reporting progress on the child's IEP goals to parents on a periodic basis (e.g., quarterly, trimester). Ongoing data collection regarding children's performance during occupational therapy interventions is critical. Specific, measurable data are necessary for accurately assessing the effectiveness of occupational therapy interventions and the need to modify or adjust approaches. Data expressed in the form of graphs or work samples provide visual illustrations of a child's response to therapeutic intervention and can be provided by teachers and practitioners in a collaborative effort to demonstrate progress and to implement strategies with fidelity (Bayona et al., 2006). Evidence of the effectiveness of interventions guides professional reasoning and enhances outcomes by encouraging reflection on practice to support opportunities for a child's growth, occupational equanimity, and performance (AOTA, 2020b; see Chapter 6, "Best Practices in Data-Based Decision Making").

Occupational therapy practitioners use data collection to help determine when a child has met all targeted outcomes; plateaued in skill development; or failed to meet objectives in spite of multiple program, task, or contextual modifications and adaptations. When these discharge situations are considered and expressed at the time of the initial evaluation, the advanced planning assists in reducing barriers to discharge when the time arrives.

Occupational therapy practitioners face a variety of challenges when recommending discharge. The overarching goal of occupational therapy in preschool is to promote the child's occupational performance in the preschool environment. When the practitioner considers potential discharge needs from the beginning of service delivery and communicates those needs effectively, team members create shared expectations and are more prepared to hold authentic discussions about discharge along the way. Practitioners must consider whether additional supports or modification of therapeutic approaches are warranted or whether the child's needs may be met by other educators or related service professionals.

SUMMARY

Preschool programs provide important foundations for learning, with the goals of preventing disability and promoting healthy lifestyles for young children and their families. As program design and regulations evolve, occupational therapy service delivery in preschools is a growing area of occupational therapy practice.

Collaborative coaching and decision-making models of service delivery promote authentic practice in the naturally occurring routines and sequences of preschool programs. Teams collaborate to determine the strengths of the child, identify gaps in performance expectations, and prioritize desired outcomes for effective participation. The occupational therapy practitioner works with team members to use valid and reliable data collection methods to measure progress toward identified goals. Discharge planning begins with the initial evaluation so that team members can discuss and share a common vision for the child.

RESOURCES

▪ *Building Culturally and Linguistically Competent Services to Support Young Children, Their Families and*

School Readiness, by Kathy Seitzinger Hepburn: https://www.aecf.org/resources/building-culturally-linguistically-competent-services/
This toolkit provides resources and strategies on how to build culturally and linguistically competent services, in particular for young children and their families, and is available through the Annie E. Casey Foundation.

- National Center for Pyramid Model Innovations (NCPMI) ***Classroom Coaching Log*** and ***Definitions of Classroom Coaching Strategies:*** https://challengingbehavior.cbcs.usf.edu/docs/coaching_log.pdf
This resource provides an algorithm for coaching teachers and implementing a coaching model of practice.

- NCPMI ***Inventory of Practices for Promoting Social Emotional Competence:*** https://challengingbehavior.cbcs.usf.edu/docs/inventory_of_practices.pdf
This tool is designed to help teams identify student needs and develop action plans in the areas of building positive relationships, designing supportive environments, developing social emotional teaching strategies, and creating individualized intensive interventions.

REFERENCES

American Occupational Therapy Association. (2014). Guidelines for supervision, roles, and responsibilities during the delivery of occupational therapy services. *American Journal of Occupational Therapy, 68*(Suppl. 3), S16–S22. https://doi.org/10.5014/ajot.2014.686S03

American Occupational Therapy Association. (2020a). 2020 occupational therapy code of ethics. *American Journal of Occupational Therapy, 74*(Suppl. 3), 7413410005. https://doi.org/10.5014/ajot.2020.74S3006

American Occupational Therapy Association. (2020b). Occupational therapy practice framework: Domain and process (4th ed.). *American Journal of Occupational Therapy, 74*(Suppl. 2), 7412410010. https://doi.org/10.5014/ajot.2020.74S2001

Ball, M. A. (2018). Revitalizing the OT role in school-based practice: Promoting success for all students. *Journal of Occupational Therapy, Schools, & Early Intervention, 11*, 263–272. https://doi.org/10.1080/19411243.2018.1445059

Barnett, W. S., Friedman-Krauss, A. H., Weisenfeld, G. G., Horowitz, M., Kasmin, R., & Squires, J. H. (2016). *The state of preschool: State preschool yearbook.* National Institute for Early Education Research.

Bayona, C. L., McDougall, J., Tucker, M. A., Nichols, M., & Mandich, A. (2006). School-based occupational therapy for children with fine motor difficulties: Evaluating functional outcomes and fidelity of services. *Physical and Occupational Therapy in Pediatrics, 26*, 89–119. https://doi.org/10.1080/J006v26n03_07

Bazyk, S., & Cahill, S. (2015). School-based occupational therapy. In J. Case-Smith & J. O'Brien (Eds.), *Occupational therapy for children* (7th ed., pp. 664–703). Elsevier.

Bellows, L. L., Davies, P. L., Anderson, J., & Kennedy, C. (2013). Effectiveness of a physical activity intervention for Head Start preschoolers: A randomized intervention study. *American Journal of Occupational Therapy, 67*, 28–36. https://doi.org/10.5014/ajot.2013.005777

Cahill, S. (2019). Best practices in multi-tiered systems of support. In G. Frolek Clark, J. Rioux, & B. Chandler (Eds.), *Best practices for occupational therapy in schools* (pp. 211–217). AOTA Press.

Case-Smith, J. (2000). Effects of occupational therapy services on fine motor and functional performance in preschool children. *American Journal of Occupational Therapy, 54*, 372–380. https://doi.org/10.5014/ajot.54.4.372

Case-Smith, J., & Cable, J. (1996). Perceptions of occupational therapists regarding service delivery models in school-based practice. *Occupational Therapy Journal of Research, 16*, 23–44. https://doi.org/10.1177/153944929601600102

Case-Smith, J., & Holland, T. (2009). Making decisions about service delivery in early childhood programs. *Language, Speech, and Hearing Services in Schools, 40*, 416–423. https://doi.org/10.1044/0161-1461(2009/08-0023)

Covert, B. (2018, May 1). A new deal for day care: Can America change the way it takes care of kids? *The New Republic.* https://newrepublic.com/article/147802/new-deal-day-care-america-change-care-kids

Dankert, H. L., Davies, P. L., & Gavin, W. J. (2003). Occupational therapy effects on visual–motor skills in preschool children. *American Journal of Occupational Therapy, 57*, 542–545. https://doi.org/10.5014/ajot.57.5.542

Darawsheh, W., Chard, G., & Eklund, M. (2015). The challenge of cultural competency in the multicultural 21st century: A conceptual model to guide occupational therapy practice. *Open Journal of Occupational Therapy, 3*(2). https://doi.org/10.15453/2168-6408.1147

Dinnebeil, L. A., & McInerney, W. F. (2011). *A guide to itinerant early childhood special education services.* Brookes.

Division for Early Childhood. (2014). *DEC recommended practices in early intervention/early childhood special education 2014.* https://www.dec-sped.org/dec-recommended-practices

Dunn, W. (1988). Models of occupational therapy service provision in the school system. *American Journal of Occupational Therapy, 42*, 718–723. https://doi.org/10.5014/ajot.42.11.718

Dunn, W., McClain, L. H., Brown, C., & Youngstrom, M. J. (1998). The ecology of human performance. In M. E. Neistadt & E. B. Crepeau (Eds.), *Willard and Spackman's occupational therapy* (9th ed., pp. 525–535). Lippincott Williams & Wilkins.

Fairbairn, M., & Davidson, I. (1993). Teachers' perceptions of the role and effectiveness of occupational therapists in schools. *Canadian Journal of Occupational Therapy, 60*, 185–191. https://doi.org/10.1177/000841749306000404

Forbes Coaching Council. (2018, June 14). Key differences between coaching and consulting (and how to decide what your business needs). *Forbes Magazine.* https://www.forbes.com/sites/forbescoachescouncil/2018/06/14/key-differences-between-coaching-and-consulting-and-how-to-decide-what-your-business-needs/#2d1c6c013d71

Frolek Clark, G., Rioux, J., & Chandler, B. (2019). *Best practices for occupational therapy in schools* (2nd ed.). AOTA Press.

Frolek Clark, G., & Schlabach, T. L. (2013). Systematic review of occupational therapy interventions to improve cognitive development in children ages birth–5 years. *American Journal of Occupational Therapy, 67*, 425–430. https://doi.org/10.5014/ajot.2013.006163

Gaylord, H. C. (2016). *Factors associated with school based occupational therapy service delivery* (Unpublished doctoral project). University of Oklahoma Health Sciences Center, Oklahoma City, OK.

Giese, T. (1991). *School-based practice: Current issues, future directions.* Illinois Occupational Therapy Association.

Giese, T. (1993). *The S.U.C.C.E.S.S. program for school-based therapy.* Paper presented at the 17th congress of the Australian

Association of Occupational Therapy, Darwin, New Territories, Australia.

Giese, T. (2002). *Kinetic educational approaches for developing therapeutic rapport: Giese's holistic theory of human development*. World Federation of Occupational Therapy.

Giovacco-Johnson, T. (2009). Portraits of partnership: The Hopes and Dreams Project. *Early Childhood Education Journal, 37,* 127–135. https://doi.org/10.1007/s10643-009-0332-1

Graham, L., Rodger, S., & Ziviani, J. (2013). Effectiveness of occupational performance coaching in improving children's and mothers' performance and mothers' self-competence. *American Journal of Occupational Therapy, 67,* 10–18. https://doi.org/10.5014/ajot.2013.004648

Grandpierre, V., Sikora, L., Fitzpatrick, E., Thomas, R., & Potter, B. (2018). Barriers and facilitators to cultural competence in rehabilitation services: A scoping review. *BMC Health Services Research 18,* 23. https://doi.org/10.1186/s12913-017-2811-1

Hanft, B., & Place, P. (1998). *The consulting therapist: A guide for OTs and PTs in schools*. Therapy Skill Builders.

Horn, E. M., Palmer, S. B., Butera, G. D., & Lieber, J. (2016). *Six steps to inclusive preschool curriculum: A UDL-based framework for children's school success*. Brookes.

Ialongo, N. S., Domitrovich, C., Embry, D., Greenberg, M., Lawson, A., Becker, K. D., & Bradshaw, C. (2019). A randomized controlled trial of the combination of two school-based universal preventive interventions. *Developmental Psychology, 55,* 1313–1325. https://doi.org/10.1037/dev0000715

Individuals With Disabilities Education Improvement Act of 2004, Pub. L. 108-446, 20 U.S.C. §§ 1400–1482.

Jayaratne, K., Jacobs, K., & Fernando, D. (2012). Global healthy backpack initiatives. *Work, 41*(Suppl. 1), 5553–5557. https://doi.org/10.3233/WOR-2012-0880-5553

Kessler, D., & Graham, F. (2015). The use of coaching in occupational therapy: An integrative review. *Australian Occupational Therapy Journal, 62,* 160–176. https://doi.org/10.1111/1440-1630.12175

Larson, N., Ward, D. S., Neelon, S. B., & Story, M. (2011). What role can child-care settings play in obesity prevention? A review of the evidence and call for research efforts. *Journal of the American Dietetic Association, 111,* 1343–1362. https://doi.org/10.1016/j.jada.2011.06.007

Laverdure, P., Cosbey, J., Gaylord, H., & LeCompte, B. (2017). Providing collaborative and contextual service in school contexts and environments. *OT Practice, 22*(15), CE1–CE8. https://www.aota.org/~/media/Corporate/Files/Publications/CE-Articles/CE-Article-August-2017.pdf

Law, M. (2002). Participation in the occupations of everyday life. *American Journal of Occupational Therapy, 56,* 640–649. https://doi.org/10.5014/ajot.56.6.640

Lindsay, S., Tétrault, S., Desmaris, C., King, G. A., & Piérart, G. (2014). The cultural brokerage work of occupational therapists in providing culturally sensitive care. *Canadian Journal of Occupational Therapy, 81,* 114–123. https://doi.org/10.1177/0008417413520441

Lopez, A., Vanner, E. A., Cowan, A. M., Samuel, A. P., & Shepherd, D. L. (2008). Intervention planning facets—four facets of occupational therapy intervention planning: Economics, ethics, professional judgment, and evidence-based practice. *American Journal of Occupational Therapy, 62,* 87–96. https://doi.org/10.5014/ajot.62.1.87

National Center for Education Statistics. (2019). *Preschool and kindergarten enrollment*. https://nces.ed.gov/programs/coe/pdf/coe_cfa.pdf

Sandall, S. R., & Schwartz, I. S. (2008). *Building blocks for teaching preschoolers with special needs* (2nd ed.). Brookes.

Suarez-Balcazar, Y., Friesema, J., & Lukyanova, V. (2013). Culturally competent interventions to address obesity among African American and Latino children and youth. *Occupational Therapy in Health Care, 27,* 113–128. https://doi.org/10.3109/07380577.2013.785644

U.S. Department of Education. (n.d.). *Data*. https://sites.ed.gov/idea/data/

U.S. Department of Health and Human Services & U.S. Department of Education. (2015). *Policy statement on inclusion of children with disabilities in early childhood programs*. https://www2.ed.gov/about/inits/ed/earlylearning/inclusion/index.html

Villeneuve, M. (2009). A critical examination of school-based occupational therapy collaborative consultation. *Canadian Journal of Occupational Therapy, 76,* 206–218. https://doi.org/10.1177/000841740907600s05

Villeneuve, M. A., & Shulha, L. M. (2012). Learning together for effective collaboration in school-based occupational therapy practice. *Canadian Journal of Occupational Therapy, 79,* 293–302. https://doi.org/10.2182/CJOT.2012.79.5.5

Ward, D. S., Vaughn, A., McWilliams, C., & Hales, D. (2010). Interventions for increasing physical activity at child care. *Medicine and Science in Sports and Exercise, 42,* 526–534. https://doi.org/10.1249/MSS.0b013e3181cea406

Williams, C. J., & McLeod, S. (2012). Speech–language pathologists' assessment and intervention practices with multilingual children. *International Journal of Speech Language Pathology, 14,* 292–305. https://doi.org/10.3109/17549507.2011.636071

Wilson, A. L., & Harris, S. R. (2018). Collaborative occupational therapy: Teachers' impressions of the Partnering for Change (P4C) model. *Physical & Occupational Therapy in Pediatrics, 38,* 130–142. https://doi.org/10.1080/01942638.2017.1297988

Best Practices in Documentation of Preschool Services and Outcomes

21

Francine Seruya, PhD, OTR/L, FAOTA

KEY TERMS AND CONCEPTS

- Analysis of occupational performance
- Annual progress report
- Approaches to intervention
- Confidentiality
- Contact report
- *Current Procedural Terminology*
- Documentation
- Early Child Outcomes
- Evaluation report
- Family Educational Rights and Privacy Act of 1974
- IEP goals
- IEP progress note
- Individualized education program
- *International Classification of Diseases*
- Intervention goals
- Occupational profile
- Occupational therapy intervention plan
- Outcomes
- Plan for discharge
- Reevaluation report
- Screening report
- Service delivery mechanisms
- Therapy log
- Types of interventions

OVERVIEW

Documentation is an essential component in the provision and ongoing review of occupational therapy service delivery. The American Occupational Therapy Association (AOTA; 2018) has developed guidelines related to minimum and typical requirements for documentation of services (see Exhibit 21.1). As noted in the guidelines, *documentation* provides a means for communicating the need for occupational therapy services, the professional reasoning process used in determining intervention and service delivery models, a perspective on the client through an occupational lens, and a chronological account of service provision. Effective documentation allows occupational therapy practitioners in preschool settings to determine initial and ongoing eligibility for services, evaluate the appropriateness of goals and effectiveness of intervention, and provide evidence for determining whether and when to discontinue services. (*Note. Occupational therapy practitioner* refers to both occupational therapists and occupational therapy assistants.)

Occupational therapy practitioners must take the time to educate themselves and remain knowledgeable about the specific documentation requirements used by their state educational agency (SEA) and local educational agency (LEA), as well as the guiding professional (AOTA, 2018, 2020a) and legal documents (Individuals With Disabilities Education Improvement Act of 2004 [IDEA], P. L. 108-446), to ensure they complete all expected and required documentation. Within early childhood settings, required documentation may include screening, referral, and evaluation reports; collaboratively developed individualized education programs (IEPs); documentation of occupational therapy intervention, including annual progress reports; reevaluation reports; documentation of outcomes, including Early Child Outcomes; and documentation of discharge and transitions. This chapter reviews both AOTA guiding documents and IDEA requirements for documentation of services within preschools.

ESSENTIAL CONSIDERATIONS

Prior to service delivery, occupational therapy practitioners need to be aware of and follow federal, state, and local regulations and professional guidelines for generating, maintaining, and destroying documents. Documentation in preschool settings may include not only district and agency paperwork but also Medicaid billing forms, other types of payment documentation, and professional required documentation. Practitioners must recognize that documentation is not only a means of noting progress and providing information regarding service delivery but also consists of legal records that can be used in a court of law. Therefore, practitioners need to follow standards for basic formatting and presentation (AOTA, 2018; Sames, 2015). Additionally, documentation is a means of communicating with all members of the child's educational team, including parents or caregivers, teachers, and support personnel. The use of medical terms or jargon is discouraged, and the language used must be appropriate to the health literacy levels and cultural diversity of all team members, including families.

Confidentiality of Records

All documentation must be considered confidential, and guidelines regarding *confidentiality* must be followed when keeping records. The *Family Educational Rights and*

EXHIBIT 21.1.   Fundamentals of Documentation

- Documentation practices and storage and disposal of documentation must meet all state and federal regulations and guidelines, payer and facility requirements, practice guidelines, and confidentiality requirements.
- Client's full name, date of birth, gender, and case number, if applicable, are included on each page of the documentation.
- Identification of type of documentation and the date service is provided and documentation is completed are included in the documentation.
- Acceptable terminology, acronyms, and abbreviations are defined and used within the boundaries of the setting.
- Clear rationale for the purpose, value, and necessity of skilled occupational therapy services is provided. The client's diagnosis or prognosis is not the sole rationale for occupational therapy services.
- Professional signature (first name or initial, last name) and credential; cosignature and credential when required for documentation of supervision; and, when necessary, signature of the recorder are included with each documentation entry.
- All errors are noted and initialed or signed.

Source. From "Guidelines for Documentation of Occupational Therapy," by American Occupational Therapy Association, 2018, *American Journal of Occupational Therapy, 72*(Suppl. 2), 7212410010, p. 2. Used with permission.

Privacy Act of 1974 (FERPA) provides specific protocols related to maintaining the confidentiality of school records. FERPA affords families the right to inspect and review their child's records and provides guidelines for amending and allowing outside access to records and documentation pertaining to a child (34 CFR § 300.613[b]). Guidelines for confidentiality outlined in FERPA must be followed for all documentation, including evaluation protocols and work samples kept as part of ongoing progress reporting. State practice acts (i.e., licensure laws) may also include directives regarding documentation and confidentiality.

As LEAs continue to expand their use of electronic platforms for documentation, practitioners need to be mindful that FERPA guidelines for confidentiality and record maintenance also apply to electronic records. If Medicaid is billed, elements of the Health Insurance Portability and Accountability Act of 1996 (HIPAA; P. L. 104-191) must also be followed (e.g., inclusion of a national provider identifier [NPI]). Practitioners must be aware of the need to maintain confidential records and follow guidelines for maintenance and destruction of all documents and artifacts used as part of documentation regardless of the media used in the creation of those documents.

Electronic Documentation Platforms

Many LEAs use electronic platforms for the development and ongoing updates of the IEP as well as for documentation of services provided. Some electronic IEP and contact report platforms offer practitioners predetermined goal or checkbox templates. Practitioners need to gauge the appropriateness of these templates to ensure they adequately reflect service delivery that is tailored to the specific needs of the child and individualized goals as developed by IEP teams. Understanding the LEA's policy regarding the use of predetermined goals and the flexibility to create and add individually written goals is essential when developing appropriate goals that are individualized and personally relevant to the child and family.

Billing for Services

Documentation has an essential role in billing for services. Although schools receive funding through IDEA, Part B, Sec. 619 for children with educational disabilities, they may also receive Medicaid reimbursement to assist in supporting preschool programs. To maintain confidentiality, LEAs must comply with state Medicaid guidelines regarding documentation for all children. Some agencies require practitioners to complete the documentation requirements for all children to whom they provide services without knowing which children receive Medicaid, whereas other agencies provide practitioners with forms to complete each month based on children who were receiving Medicaid that month. Compliance with state Medicaid rules is essential, and practitioners are advised to seek state resources for assistance.

Billing requires use of codes from the ***International Classification of Diseases,*** *Tenth Revision, Clinical Modification (ICD-10-CM)* and ***Current Procedural Terminology (CPT®)***. The *ICD* system, developed by the World Health Organization (2019), is used to classify and track diagnostic categories of diseases and health conditions around the world. The *ICD-10-CM* coding system helps agencies in the United States track trends in health care and assists in billing and reimbursement (Centers for Disease Control and Prevention, 2010). Because the *ICD-10-CM* codes are considered treatment diagnoses, occupational therapists may be required to include the appropriate code in documentation (AOTA, n.d.). When assigning *ICD-10-CM* codes, therapists must follow the appropriate procedures set forth in their state practice act and LEA guidelines. Although documentation may require diagnostic codes, practitioners need to be mindful that these codes are not considered educational diagnoses and that medical diagnosis differs from classification for the purposes of eligibility for services as part of IDEA Part B.

CPT codes are the standard medical codes used to report all medical, surgical, and diagnostic procedures and services in the United States (American Medical Association, 2020). This information is shared with health insurance companies and accreditation organizations to track types of services and procedures and facilitate billing. On the basis of the type of intervention provided, practitioners select and document the relevant codes. AOTA has provided general guidelines on the use of *CPT* codes (AOTA, 2016) and more specific guidelines for practitioners working with pediatric populations (Brennan & Glennon, 2017). Practitioners must ensure that they are being precise in determining diagnostic and procedural codes and that the codes accurately reflect the services provided.

Documentation Requirements for Initiating Services

Some state practice acts require occupational therapists to have a physician's referral before initiating screening, evaluation, and intervention, and IDEA requires written consent from a parent before an evaluation is conducted. In addition, the LEA may have formal or informal documentation procedures that must be followed. If the IEP team has determined that a child is eligible for occupational therapy services and these services are included on the IEP, therapists need to ensure they have completed the necessary evaluation and documentation before initiating intervention. The LEA may have written policies regarding missed and makeup sessions for child illness, school vacations, or holidays, including the amount of time allowed to provide makeup sessions.

Differences Between a State Practice Act and Education-Based Documentation

Occupational therapy practitioners need to understand and adhere to their state practice act to ensure that the documentation of services aligns with legal mandates. In some cases, practitioners may need to advocate for the inclusion of appropriate documentation. For example, some LEAs, community programs, or agencies may not consider contact reports (e.g., daily treatment notes) to be necessary. Practitioners must follow professional guidelines for all documentation, including contact reports and progress reports (AOTA, 2018). Advocating for best practices related to documentation is an essential skill for practitioners working in preschool settings.

Within team reports, practitioners also need to ensure that the distinct value of occupational therapy services is reflected in documentation and in agencies using electronic platforms for IEPs, including those that use a goal template. The ability to articulate occupational therapy's scope of practice in school settings outside of traditional fine motor, handwriting, and sensory processing skills is essential in providing individualized and meaningful services to children. Being well versed in their state practice act and AOTA (2014b, 2017, 2018) documents enables practitioners to successfully advocate for appropriate service delivery and documentation.

BEST PRACTICES

In addition to federal, state, and local requirements for documentation, occupational therapy practitioners need to follow basic documentation requirements that are typical within the context of preschool services. As part of the documentation process, practitioners should be aware of health literacy levels and cultural diversity. Documentation should be provided in a manner that allows parents, caregivers, and other members of the educational team to have a clear understanding of occupational therapy's distinct value under IDEA Part B. Using AOTA and IDEA guidelines as a framework, this section outlines best practices in typical documentation required at various stages along the service delivery continuum from screening and referral to discharge.

Document Screening, Referral, and Evaluation

Frequently, occupational therapists' first contact with a child is made via screening or referral. To identify and assist children at risk for problems in their preschool, an occupational therapist may be asked to complete a screening by a teacher or child because of concerns in the preschool setting or curriculum and for the purpose of identifying strategies to enhance the child's performance in the preschool education classroom. If a child is suspected of an educational disability as part of IDEA's Child Find mandate or if the family completes a referral for a full and individualized educational evaluation of their child, an education team must determine if a child is eligible and needs special education and related services. Based on the concerns, an occupational therapy evaluation may be necessary to provide data as part of that determination. Sometimes a child with an educational disability who has been receiving special education services is referred for an occupational therapy evaluation to determine whether occupational therapy services are necessary.

Occupational therapists need to be mindful of timelines from requests for screening or referral for evaluation to ensure timely documentation. For example, a preschool program may have a policy regarding the amount of time allotted between a therapist's receipt of referral for screening and when the documentation and reporting to the caregiver is due. Likewise, IDEA requires that an IEP meeting must be conducted within 60 days of receiving the parental consent for the initial evaluation. When conducting an educational evaluation, practitioners therapists also need to select the appropriate *CPT* intervention codes if their state allows Medicaid billing (AOTA, 2016).

Screening report

An occupational therapy screening may be requested for a whole general education class or an individual child as part of screening for instructional purposes (34 CFR § 300.302). Under IDEA, screening is not considered an evaluation for eligibility for special education and related services. Education teams may request a screening to provide specific strategies and resources for children who appear to need additional academic or behavioral support or at-risk learners. Obtaining parent consent prior to initiation of screening is essential, and this process may vary among LEAs.

If screening a child is allowable under state professional regulations (e.g., licensure), occupational therapists may conduct direct observations in the context in which the child is having difficulty. They may also use standardized screening tools consistent with their agency's policy and protocols. The ***screening report*** typically summarizes the concerns noted by caregiver or teacher and provides resources and strategies to address these concerns. Typically, the teacher implements the strategies and meets with the occupational therapist in 2–4 weeks to discuss the child's performance. Sometimes the child's performance has improved, while sometimes additional strategies are provided. If a child's performance does not improve with these general education interventions and the child is suspected of having an educational disability, an evaluation should be pursued (IDEA, 1412[a][3]).

Referral for special education evaluation

Under IDEA, a *referral* for a full and individual education evaluation begins the formal process of determining eligibility for special education services. The LEA must obtain informed written consent from the parent or legal guardians to initiate this process. If parents request an evaluation, but there is no evidence to suspect that the child has an educational disability, the LEA may decline to conduct an evaluation (34 CFR § 300.300[c][iii]). The school is required to provide parents with a written explanation of their actions in response to the referral and their reasons to deny the request for evaluation.

Evaluation report

When occupational therapists evaluate children as part of the determination for special education eligibility or to determine the need for occupational therapy, they must gather and document the *occupational profile,* which includes information from the parent or caregiver and teacher and, when appropriate, the child. Developing the occupational profile is an essential component of evaluation and provides an opportunity for the therapist to identify the occupations, assessment methods, and environments in which the child has strengths as well as challenges. Next, the therapist conducts an *analysis of occupational performance* by identifying the child's strengths and needs through formal observations in the natural context and routines, and the use of standardized and nonstandardized assessment. Appendix H, "Sample Initial Preschool Team Evaluation Report," provides a sample.

The occupational therapy *evaluation report* should contain the following components (AOTA, 2018, p. 3):

- *Referral information:* Date, source, and reason for referral.
- *Client information:* Description of child's occupational history, experiences, and performance; health status and previous services required and accessed; and applicable medical, educational, and developmental diagnoses.
- *Occupational profile:* Information gathered through discussion with the educational team and child, if appropriate, including areas of occupation in which the child is successful and areas in which the child is challenged; the contexts in which the child is expected to perform and level of performance in those contexts; contexts and environments that support and hinder occupational performance; relevant medical, psychosocial, and educational history; occupational priorities; and suggested goal areas.
- *Assessments used and results:* Detail on all assessments, both formal and informal, used to perform the evaluation, including, when appropriate, a brief description of the assessment, its intended use as part of the evaluation, and results obtained.
- *Analysis of occupational performance:* Based on standardized and informal assessment results and information from the occupational profile, an analysis of the child's strengths and challenges and their impact on occupational performance within the school context.
- *Summary and analysis:* Concise summary and interpretation of the occupational profile and analysis of occupational performance.
- *Recommendations:* Areas to be addressed to improve the child's ability to access or participate in the educational context and specific suggestions for the educational team. Therapists need to be aware of specific SEA and

LEA guidelines regarding recommendations for specific services as part of the evaluation report; determination of eligibility for services should not occur until the IEP team meeting.

Most licensure laws require an occupational therapist evaluation report to be written. If the educational team uses a team report, the occupational therapists' evaluation should be explicit (i.e., identifies the information from the occupational therapist). Another method is for the occupational therapist to write their report and then incorporate pertinent information into the team report, thus satisfying both the licensure and LEA requirements.

Collaboratively Develop Individualized Education Programs

Occupational therapy practitioners, as part of the educational team, help create the *IEP,* including appropriate *IEP goals,* to facilitate the child's ability to access the curriculum and participate in the educational program. According to IDEA Part B § 1414(d), the following information must be included in a child's IEP:

- Present level of performance, including strengths and challenges (from parent concerns, evaluation results)
- Special education and related services to be provided to the child, including type of classroom setting and need for and frequency of related and other support services (e.g., occupational therapy, technology supports)
- Indication of restriction to the least restrictive environment (LRE)
- Any need for accommodations specific to the classroom and other academically related settings (e.g., visual supports, specialized seating)
- Annual goals related to access and participation in the preschool setting
- Indication of the means by which progress toward goals will be assessed and the frequency with which objective measures will be administered
- Specific start and end dates of services, specific location of service provision, and frequency and duration of services.

The IEP is considered a legal document and all components are very important, including the child's goals. As part of the team, occupational therapists participate in the development of measurable annual goals that should enable the child to access, participate, and make progress in the general education curriculum as well as meet other needs resulting from the educational disability (IDEA Part B § 1414[d][1][A][II]). Occupational therapists do not contribute discipline-specific goals focused on discrete skill development to the IEP; rather, the child's IEP goals should lead to functional outcomes and improved participation for the child. Some LEAs use electronic platforms for IEPs, which may be challenging as they frequently offer predetermined goals rather than those individualized for the child's specific needs. Therapists need to advocate for individualized goals that accurately reflect the occupational needs of the child within the school setting. See Exhibit 21.2 for examples of IEP goals.

Although not all states encourage occupational therapy practitioners to attend IEP meetings, their contribution is valuable. Attendance by members of the IEP team is not

<table>
<tr><td>

EXHIBIT 21.2. Individualized Education Program Goal Samples

1. **Current Performance:** *During peer groups, Joe is not participating in music and movement opportunities, nor shared book reading experiences. When given at least 4 opportunities each day, Joe participated 30 seconds per 10 minutes of group time over 5 days.*
   Goal: During group activities, Joe will attend to an appropriate object, person, or event that is the focus of the activity and participate (e.g., sing, imitate motions, comment on book) for at least 8 minutes during 4 groups each day for 3 days.

2. **Current Performance:** *During classroom activities (e.g., drawing, story time), Joe runs away from the class rather than engaging. Data indicate he remains in the work area for an average of 35 seconds before he runs.*
   Goal: Given choices and preferences based on his interests, Joe will remain in the work area and actively engage in activities for at least 10 minutes (without running away) for 5 consecutive days.

3. **Current Performance:** *Joe consistently forgets steps and impulsively skips parts of the handwashing routine. Baseline data indicate he independently (without adult support or prompts) completes 10% of steps in the classroom's 10-step routine.*
   Goal: With visual support for the 10-step handwashing routine present (posted near sink), Joe will independently complete 80% of the ten steps for five consecutive data collections.

</td></tr>
</table>

required if the parent and the LEA agree that a team member's attendance is not necessary because the related service is not being modified or discussed at the meeting (IDEA Part B § 1414[d][1][C]). However, if a modification or discussion of the related service is to occur at the IEP meeting and the team member cannot attend, the parent and the LEA must consent to the excusal, and the member must submit written input to the parent and team prior to the meeting. Practitioners should educate themselves about their LEA's policies related to meeting attendance. Decisions made at the team meetings are documented on the IEP, which is a legal document.

Document Occupational Therapy Intervention

Documentation related to occupational therapy intervention includes the occupational therapy intervention plan, contact reports, IEP progress notes, and annual progress reports.

Occupational therapy intervention plan

The **occupational therapy intervention plan** is the occupational therapy practitioner's professional document guiding the interventions they will use as part of the occupational therapy process (Frolek Clark & Handley-More, 2017). This document may appropriately include professional jargon to describe specific interventions the practitioner will provide, similar to a teacher's daily plan or a plan of care in health care. It also lists the areas that are delegated to the occupational therapy assistant. According to AOTA (2018) guidelines, the intervention plan includes the following components:

- *Client information:* As indicated in the evaluation report.
- *Intervention goals:* Specific outcomes for occupational therapy services (e.g., "will develop in-hand manipulation skills," "will extend arm") that contribute to the functional IEP goals (e.g., "will complete journal writing," "will hang up coat"). The IEP goals may also be listed in the intervention plan but are not considered the intervention goals.
- *Approaches to intervention* and *types of interventions* to be used: Approaches to intervention to be used for the child, which may include create/promote, establish/restore, maintain, modify, and prevent, as well as types of interventions, which may include therapeutic use of occupations and activities, education and training, advocacy, and consultation (AOTA, 2020b). Intervention approaches and types are not specified in the IEP.
- *Service delivery mechanisms:* Service provider, location, and frequency and duration of services, as specified in the IEP.
- *Plan for discharge:* In the preschool setting, transition planning for either the continuation of services through IDEA Part B as the child transitions to kindergarten or the discontinuation of services.
- *Outcomes:* Changes as a result of occupational therapy (e.g., increased occupational performance, improved health and wellness, improved quality of life, self-advocacy) and tools to be used to measure ongoing progress.

Contact reports

A **contact report** is the documentation of the services provided (e.g., interventions, phone calls, attended meetings). Occupational therapy practitioners need to follow professional guidelines and SEA and LEA procedures when documenting service contacts. The following are basic components of contact reports (AOTA, 2018):

- *Client information:* Specific information unique to the child (e.g., name, *ICD-10-CM* code) and contraindications and precautions, if appropriate.
- *Therapy log:* Detailed information about services provided, including date and specific time (some billing requires time in and time out to be documented); location; delivery model; number of children in the session; goal areas addressed; child's actual performance; level of support provided; modifications provided; specific intervention techniques; progress toward achievement of goals; and *CPT* code if required.
- *Signature of service provider and cosignature for documentation of supervision (if applicable):* Handwritten or electronic signature.

See Exhibit 21.3 for an example of a contact report.

Individualized education program progress report to family

IDEA requires that the child's progress on the IEP goals be reported to the parent using the same time frame the LEA uses for report cards (e.g., quarterly, trimester). An **IEP progress note** is the LEA's documentation related to the child's current status and progress toward goals documented as part of the IEP. SEAs and LEAs may differ in requirements related to ongoing documentation of progress, and occupational therapy practitioners providing services for children in multiple

EXHIBIT 21.3. Sample Occupational Therapy Contact Report

Occupational Therapy Service Record   Page: __1__
Child Name: ___Nikita Johnsen___   Birthdate: ___9-9-2016___   District: Springfield_

Contact Type Key: C = child/contact; E = evaluation/email; M = meeting; O = other (describe); P = parent/phone; T = text message.

DATE	TIME IN TIME OUT	CONTACT TYPE	BILLING CODES	SUMMARY OF CONTACT OR SERVICE
11-10-19	--	M	--	Team meeting. New referral received from parent for girl age 38 months. A time for team evaluation was set for 11-22-19 at 10 a.m. at her Head Start preschool. [OT electronic signature]
11-22-19	9:00–10:05	E	97166	Evaluation at Head Start with Nikita's parent (Junnie) present. OT interviewed Junnie to develop occupational profile and reviewed medical records from local hospital. Additionally, OT involved in evaluation of physical, adaptive, and social–emotional skills, while early childhood teacher evaluated communication and cognitive skills. Analytical complexity moderate and comorbidities are present that affect performance. OT to return on 11-29-19 to continue evaluation of child strengths and needs. [OT electronic signature]

Note. OT = occupational therapist.

LEAs need to be aware of the requirements for each LEA. Some LEAs require service providers to complete these IEP progress notes directly on the paper or electronic version of the IEP. Practitioners must collect ongoing data on the child's performance and record this in their notes or on graphs. Graphs that include student performance data can be used to visually report progress on the IEP goals to parents. (Refer to Chapter 6, "Best Practices in Data-Based Decision Making," for further information on data collection.) Electronic IEP formats may allow progress reporting only via checkboxes related to level of child progress toward goal areas. See Exhibit 21.4 for an example of a quarterly IEP progress note.

Annual progress report

The ***annual progress report*** provides an in-depth summary of occupational therapy services provided, documents the child's progress, and records decisions about ongoing services or discontinuation. The annual progress report differs from IEP progress notes in that it provides a review of the child's progress over an entire year (e.g., period of IEP, school year). The annual report may be written and shared prior to the annual IEP meeting to help the team, including the family, reflect on the child's progress on their annual IEP goals; identify the child's current access, participation, and performance in the preschool setting; and recommend areas of strength and need for the upcoming academic year. Eligibility for IDEA Part B is always determined by the IEP team, based on the child's ongoing educational diagnosis and need for special education and related services (e.g., occupational therapy).

The annual progress report includes the following components (AOTA, 2018):
- *Client information:* As indicated in the evaluation report.
- *Summary of services provided:* Brief statement of the frequency and duration of occupational therapy services, approaches to and types of interventions provided, data

EXHIBIT 21.4. Sample Quarterly Individualized Education Program Progress Report

Happy Valley PreSchool District IEP Progress Report
2019-2020 School Year   Quarter: _2nd___

Child's Name: Joe Smith   **DOB:**   7-8-2014

Parent: Adam & Harlow Nelson (guardians)

Persons Completing Report: Andrew Green (teacher) and Shantell Smith, OT/L

Summary of Services Provided: Joe has attended all scheduled preschool four afternoons per week, with one absence (weather). He has received all scheduled OT sessions (once weekly for 30 minutes within the classroom; 15 minutes per month teacher–OT collaboration) and is making steady progress on these IEP goals. Focus is on attention/participation, social skills, and self-care.

Current Progress: Joe continues to need prompting to engage in and follow adult-directed tasks. He responds well to positive reinforcement at times but this is not consistent. Increasing compliance and ability to cooperatively play with peers is a continued area of need.

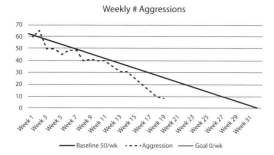

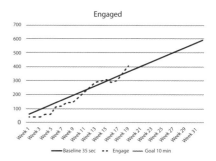

Progress on Goal #1: Joe will participate in group activities for an average of 4.9 minutes over 3 days (goal is 8 minutes). His performance ranges from 4–6 minutes most days. He seems to enjoy singing and imitates 3 of the motions for his favorite songs (e.g., Wheels on the Bus).

Progress on Goal #2: He will remain in work area and engage in classroom activities. Running away has decreased. He will now work for 5–7 minutes (baseline was 35 seconds; goal is 10 minutes). His rate of progress is steady with his goal line (black) so he should complete this goal on time.

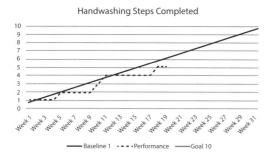

Plan or Recommendations: Joe is making progress on his IEP goals. Programming and interventions appear effective. No changes recommended at this time. Please let us know if you have any questions!

Progress on Goal #3: He has completed 4 steps in the handwashing program (baseline was 1 step); however, in order to meet his goal, he should have mastered 6 steps. The changes you suggested helped— he did complete 5 steps the last 2 weeks. Thank you for working on this at home, as well.

Note. IEP = individualized education program; OT = occupational therapy.

collection procedures, results showing measurable progress or lack thereof, environmental or task modifications provided, adaptive equipment provided, pertinent medical or other contextual updates, the child's response to services, and education or training provided to the child or educational team.

- *Current performance:* Child's goal achievement and current performance in areas of occupations, including progress on IEP goals that were addressed and reasons any IEP goals were not addressed during the year.
- *Plan or recommendations:* Proposed continuation of the occupational therapy intervention plan and services or

changes to the intervention plan reflecting ongoing clinical reasoning and the child's progress toward IEP goals.

Complete a Reevaluation Report

When no new evaluation data are collected

Occupational therapists may be part of a child's reevaluation to determine ongoing eligibility for special education. IDEA considers existing evaluation data to include evaluations and information provided by the parents; current classroom-based, local, or state assessments; classroom-based observations; and observations by teachers and related service providers (IDEA, 300.305[a]). If no additional evaluation data are required to determine whether the child continues to have an educational disability and determine educational needs, the LEA notifies the child's parent of the determination.

When new data are collected

Under IDEA, formal reevaluation is required only if one of three conditions is met: (1) the LEA has determined a need for reevaluation, (2) the educational team has determined a need for reevaluation, or (3) 3 years have passed since the initial determination of eligibility or evaluation. In addition, therapists may deem reevaluation to be warranted to respond to a specific change in the child's performance or to justify the need to change service delivery frequency or intensity. Additionally, reevaluation reporting as part of a child's transition from preschool to kindergarten is a typical practice in some LEAs. Collection of new information (e.g., new goal area, more in-depth information) may require written parent notification.

Occupational therapists completing a *reevaluation report* to summarize new evaluation information can follow the format for the evaluation report outlined earlier in this chapter. Important additions would be to note changes in performance on assessments (e.g., observation, tools) as an indication of progress in targeted skill areas and to update the occupational profile with information from the child, when appropriate, and the educational team related to classroom performance since the last evaluation report. Ongoing evidence of progress plays an essential role in completing reevaluation and should be documented.

Document Occupational Therapy Outcomes

As part of the occupational therapy process, assessing outcomes allows evaluation of the occupational therapy intervention (AOTA, 2020b). Assessing outcomes enables occupational therapy practitioners to determine the child's progress toward intervention and IEP goals and overall participation in their classroom settings. Documenting a child's lack of progress toward goals may indicate the need to reassess and adjust intervention methods and goals accordingly (e.g., further services may not be beneficial, the intensity or frequency may not match the child's needs). Likewise, accurately documenting a child's achievement of goals may suggest the need to assess the appropriateness of continued occupational therapy services. Practitioners need to be aware of the procedures and documentation necessary for both changing goals and discharging from services.

Document Early Childhood Outcomes

The U.S. Office of Special Education Programs requires all states to submit, as part of the state performance plan/ annual performance report, the percentage of preschoolers with IEPs who demonstrate improvement in three *Early Child Outcomes* (ECOs) as a measure of progress in facilitating children's ability to actively participate and learn within their preschool setting as a result of services provided to the children and families (Early Childhood Technical Assistance Center, n.d.). The ECOs are as follows:

1. Positive social–emotional skills (including social relationships)
2. Acquisition and use of knowledge and skills (including early language, communication, and literacy)
3. Use of appropriate behaviors to meet their own needs.

The ECO reporting process allows program evaluation and improvement of preschool programs. This is required for preschool children with an IEP (upon entering and exiting preschool). Many states collect information related to these outcomes using a team process to summarize information about children's functioning across multiple sources. Occupational therapy practitioners working with preschoolers who have IEPs assist in the gathering of this information as part of the educational team and should educate themselves about their agency's procedures regarding the ECO process and documentation.

Document Transitions or Discharge From Services

The need for ongoing service delivery can be a problematic issue to address because preschool children are developing and their potential is difficult to assess. Transitions from preschool to kindergarten or when a child no longer needs special education are common in the early years. Some SEA and LEA guidelines require updated evaluations as children transition from early childhood programs to kindergarten. The use of these evaluations can also assist in determining need for discharge or to develop a new IEP if continued eligibility is determined. It is best practice to provide the receiving teams with current information about each child.

Discharge planning should be considered during the initial evaluation to establish when and under what conditions to discontinue occupational therapy services. When determining the need for occupational therapy services, occupational therapists need to be mindful of the intent of related services: "to assist a child with a disability to benefit from special education" (34 CFR § 300.34). The intent is not to provide occupational therapy until a child reaches "typically developing" skill levels or graduates from school. When children are able to access and participate in their curriculum and meet their other educational needs resulting from the disability, therapists should reassess the appropriateness of the service delivery frequency and model of delivery as well as the need to continue providing services.

Monitoring and documenting progress toward the IEP goals is one way to determine the need for modification or discontinuation of occupational therapy services. Providing contextually based services and documenting the child's ability to access and participate in their school environment assists practitioners in making professional judgments and determinations related to continuation of services. Practitioners need to follow professional and SEA and LEA guidance related to discontinuation of services.

SUMMARY

Documentation is an essential part of occupational therapy service delivery within early childhood settings.

Ensuring that documentation requirements are properly fulfilled provides occupational therapy practitioners and all educational stakeholders with important information related to needs justification and service efficacy and provides the means by which educational agencies verify delivery of and obtain payment for services. Practitioners need to be aware of and educate themselves regarding the various federal, state, and local mandates and professional requirements when completing all documentation across the service continuum from initial referral to discontinuation of services.

REFERENCES

American Medical Association. (2020). *CPT® 2020 professional edition.* American Medical Association Press.

American Occupational Therapy Association. (n.d.). *Can occupational therapists assign ICD-10 codes?* https://www.aota.org/advocacy-policy/federal-reg-affairs/icd-10-diagnosis-coding/can-occupational-therapists-assign-icd-10-codes.aspx

American Occupational Therapy Association. (2020a). Guidelines for supervision, roles, and responsibilities during the delivery of occupational therapy services. *American Journal of Occupational Therapy, 74,* 7413410020. https://doi.org/10.5014/ajot.2020.74S3004

American Occupational Therapy Association. (2020b). Occupational therapy practice framework: Domain and process (4th ed.). *American Journal of Occupational Therapy, 74*(Suppl. 2), 7412410010. https://doi.org/10.5014/ajot.2020.74S2001

American Occupational Therapy Association. (2016). *New occupational therapy evaluation coding overview.* https://www.aota.org/~/media/Corporate/Files/Advocacy/Reimb/Coding/final%20version%2010%20page%20article.pdf

American Occupational Therapy Association. (2017). Guidelines for occupational therapy services in early intervention and schools. *American Journal of Occupational Therapy, 71*(Suppl. 2), 7112410010. https://doi.org/10.5014/ajot.2017.716S01

American Occupational Therapy Association. (2018). Guidelines for documentation of occupational therapy. *American Journal of Occupational Therapy, 72*(Suppl. 2), 7212410010. https://doi.org/10.5014/ajot.2018.72S203

Brennan, C., & Glennon, T. J. (2017). *Frequently asked questions (FAQs) for correctly choosing new evaluation codes for pediatric OTs.* https://www.aota.org/Advocacy-Policy/Federal-Reg-Affairs/News/2017/Frequently-Asked-Questions-FAQs-For-Correctly-Choosing-New-Evaluation-Codes-for-Pediatric-OTs.aspx

Centers for Disease Control and Prevention. (2010). *International Classification of Diseases, Tenth Revision, Clinical Modification (ICD-10-CM).* https://www.cdc.gov/nchs/icd/icd10cm.htm

Early Childhood Technical Assistance Center. (n.d.). *Child outcomes.* https://ectacenter.org/eco/pages/childoutcomes.asp

Family Educational Rights and Privacy Act of 1974, 20 U.S.C. § 1232g; 34 CFR Part 99.

Frolek Clark, G., & Handley-More, D. (2017). *Best practices for documenting occupational therapy services in schools.* AOTA Press.

Health Insurance Portability and Accountability Act of 1996, Pub. L. 104-191, 42 U.S.C. § 300gg, 29 U.S.C §§ 1181–1183, and 42 U.S.C. §§ 1320d–1320d9.

Individuals With Disabilities Education Improvement Act of 2004, Pub. L. 108-446, 20 U.S.C. §§ 1400–1482.

Sames, K. (2015). *Documenting occupational therapy practice* (3rd ed). Pearson Education.

World Health Organization. (2019). *International statistical classification of diseases and related health problems* (10th rev., 2019 version). https://icd.who.int/browse10/2019/en

Section V.

Considerations for Medical and Health Care

Understanding Health Care Requirements, Process, and Billing

22

Janice Flegle, MA, OTR/L, BCP, and Sara O'Rourke, MOT, OTR/L, BCP

KEY TERMS AND CONCEPTS

- *Current Procedural Terminology* codes
- Evaluation
- Habilitation
- *International Classification of Diseases*
- Managed care
- Medical necessity
- National Provider Identifier
- Protected health information

OVERVIEW

Occupational therapy practitioners working in a children's hospital, pediatric rehabilitation setting, home health, or private outpatient facility need to understand how the service delivery model in their practice setting, ethical and legal imperatives, and payer rules govern how young children with (or at risk for) disabilities access occupational therapy services. (*Note. Occupational therapy practitioner* refers to both occupational therapists and occupational therapy assistants.) To successfully advocate for a child's needs, occupational therapy practitioners must be able to interpret and define *medical necessity* in the context of their particular practice setting (Stover, 2016).

The Patient Protection and Affordable Care Act (ACA; P. L. 111-148), signed into law in March 2010, did not offer a concise definition of *medical necessity,* but it did establish an expectation that insurance coverage should be available when the client[1] is expected to benefit from medical treatment. Stover (2016) referred to a glossary that was created by the U.S. Department of Health and Human Services (DHHS) in an effort to provide consumers with a better understanding of medical and insurance terms while choosing their health care plan. This glossary defines *medically necessary* as "health care services or supplies needed to prevent, diagnose, or treat an illness, injury, condition, disease, or its symptoms and that meet accepted standards of medicine" (Healthcare.gov, n.d., p. 6).

Occupational therapy services to young children in health care settings are generally *habilitative,* in that the focus of intervention is on helping children acquire, retain, and improve performance skills that will promote their participation in daily occupations and routines in natural environments and on building the capacity of families to support positive outcomes. The DHHS glossary defines *habilitation* as follows: "health care services that help you keep, learn, or improve skills and functioning for daily living" (Healthcare.gov, n.d., p. 4). This chapter provides essential considerations and best practices for occupational therapy practitioners working with young children in medical settings that bill third-party payers.

ESSENTIAL CONSIDERATIONS

This section provides an overview of the credentialing process and basic information on how to select appropriate diagnosis and procedure codes when billing for services provided in a medical setting.

Credentialing

The Health Insurance Portability and Accountability Act of 1996 (HIPAA; P. L. 104-191) Privacy Rule was published by DHHS to address the use and disclosure of *protected health information* (PHI) by covered entities. Health care providers must use caution when electronically transmitting information either directly or through a third party to inquire about a person's benefit eligibility, facilitate a referral authorization request, or file a claim for payment of services rendered because these are considered HIPAA-covered entities. The Privacy Rule defines *PHI* as individually identifiable health information, including demographic data that relate to

- Past, present, or future physical or mental health conditions of a person;
- Provision of health care to a person; or
- Previous, current, or future payment for the provision of health care to a person (DHHS, 2013).

All health care providers who are HIPAA-covered entities, whether individuals or organizations, must obtain a *National Provider Identifier* (NPI), which is a unique 10-digit numeric identifier that is used in HIPAA standard transactions, including, but not limited to, referrals

---

[1]Because the young child is dependent on an adult, the term *client* refers to both the child and the caregiver or parent.

https://doi.org/10.7139/2021.978-1-56900-610-8.022

and authorizations, claims, and encounter information. Once assigned, an NPI follows occupational therapy practitioners throughout their career (Centers for Medicare & Medicaid Services [CMS], 2016).

Additional licensure and certifications required by employers or third-party payers vary regionally. Most hospital and outpatient clinics employ personnel dedicated to credentialing the occupational therapy practitioners working in that setting with the primary insurance carriers in that region. Private practitioners who provide medical therapy independently can either pursue in-network status with their clients' insurance carrier and submit their invoices and documentation directly to that carrier or invoice the family directly. In the latter context, occupational therapy practitioners are considered out-of-network providers. *Without exception,* the occupational therapy provider whose NPI and professional license is attached to an insurance claim is accountable for the documentation included with that claim.

Payer Requirements Vary

Every insurance company or payer network offers a wide range of policies to a variety of consumer groups and individuals, so predicting the limits of a policy's coverage for occupational therapy evaluation or intervention on the basis of carrier or network alone is not possible. Group insurance plans offered through employers typically offer tiered cost and coverage options, and individual plans vary widely. The wallet-sized card that carriers issue to enrollees will have a member ID and group or policy numbers that providers can refer to when contacting that carrier for information about a client's coverage. When possible, the enrolled member should contact the insurance carrier directly, because enrollees will be able to obtain more detailed information about their plan's coverage of occupational therapy services than occupational therapy providers or their delegate.

Managed Care Organizations

In general terms, *managed care* is a health care delivery system organized to manage the cost, utilization, and quality of services through contractual arrangements between state Medicaid agencies and managed care organizations (MCOs) that accept a set per-member, per-month (capitation) payment for these services (Medicaid.gov, 2019). Currently, 38 states are using MCOs to cover at least 50% of their Medicaid beneficiaries. In 2017, more than two thirds (69.3%) of all Medicaid beneficiaries were enrolled in MCOs (Medicaid.gov, 2019)

In states whose comprehensive MCO offers one to three different coverage networks, occupational therapy practitioners need to be particularly diligent about monitoring their clients' enrollment status. Medicaid beneficiaries who choose to transition from one provider network to another within their MCO during their annual reenrollment period might not be aware of how that decision will affect provider authorizations already in place. (The importance of educating family members about the complexities of their health care coverage is discussed again in the Best Practices section of this chapter.) Table 22.1 offers contact information for the largest health care provider networks.

Coding and Billing

Obtaining payment for services rendered is largely dependent on occupational therapy practitioners' ability to assign diagnostic and evaluation or intervention codes to their documentation in a manner that is consistent with the payment policies established by payer networks (Umphred, 2013). Occupational therapy practitioners must take responsibility for learning how to apply diagnosis codes using the *International Classification of Diseases* (10th revision; *ICD–10-CM;* World Health Organization [WHO], 1990), which defines and classifies diseases, disorders, injuries, and

TABLE 22.1.   Contact Information for Major Health Care Provider Networks

NETWORK	CONTACT INFORMATION (NATIONAL PHONE NUMBERS LISTED, CHECK STATE LISTINGS FOR LOCAL NUMBERS)
Aetna (Coventry)	1-800-US-AETNA (1-800-872-3862) 8:00 a.m.–6:00 p.m. Eastern time
BlueCross BlueShield	1-888-630-2583; https://www.bcbs.com/member-services
Centers for Medicare & Medicaid Services	1-800-318-2596; 24 hours a day, 7 days a week (except holidays)
Cigna Health	1-800-997-1654; 24 hours a day, 365 days a year
Health Net Federal Services— (administers TriCare West)	https://www.tricare-west.com/content/hnfs/home/tw/common/contact_us.html
Humana Group (administers TriCare East)	Insurance through employers 1-800-448-6262; Medicaid Customer Service 1-800-477-6931; Monday–Friday, 8:00 a.m.–8:00 p.m.
Kaiser Permanente	1-800-488-3590
Oscar Health	1-855-672-2788; https://www.hioscar.com/providers/resources
Physicians Mutual	1-800-228-9100 for policy-related questions; https://www.physiciansmutual.com/cs/contactus/contactus.html
United Healthcare	1-866-414-1959 for general information; 1-877-542-9239 for Medicaid, if unable to log into member site

other related health conditions. WHO has supported ongoing revision of the *ICD* so that health information can be shared and compared regionally and around the world. The *ICD–10-CM* also supports evidence-based decision making and provides data on the incidence and prevalence of diseases, reimbursement, and resource allocation trends and helps monitor safety and quality guidelines (WHO, n.d.).

A physician must assign the *ICD–10-CM* code that describes the child's medical diagnosis. Occupational therapists assign therapy diagnosis codes, and they should do so as specifically as possible to reflect the performance deficit being addressed. Occupational therapy practitioners' documentation must reflect the value of the service provided and clearly connect the need for therapy to the diagnosis (American Occupational Therapy Association [AOTA], 2020c).

Although *ICD–10-CM* codes allow occupational therapy practitioners to communicate the conditions and injuries being treated to third-party payers, ***Current Procedural Terminology (CPT®) codes*** identify and communicate the interventions being used during the course of treatment. *CPT* is a code set that is trademarked, maintained, updated, and published by the American Medical Association (AMA; 2020; Umphred, 2013). Selecting the appropriate *CPT* code can be daunting because there are five-digit codes for both evaluation and treatment, some of which are timed (vs. untimed), and there are rules about which *CPT* codes can be combined.

Evaluation Codes

By definition, an ***evaluation*** initiates a plan of care. This is the first step in determining what occupational therapy services are needed. The *Occupational Therapy Practice Framework: Domain and Process* (4th ed.; *OTPF*; AOTA,

TABLE 22.2. *CPT* **Evaluation Codes and Descriptors**

CPT CODE	*CPT* DESCRIPTORS FOR OT EVALUATION CODES
97165—occupational therapy evaluation, low complexity	▪ An occupational profile and medical and therapy history, which contains a brief history, including review of medical and therapy records relating to the presenting problem ▪ An assessment that identifies 1–3 performance deficits (i.e., relating to physical, cognitive, or psychosocial skills) that result in activity limitations, participation restrictions, or both ▪ Clinical decision includes an analysis of the occupational profile, analysis of data from problem-focused assessments, and consideration of a limited number of treatment options. Patient presents with no comorbidities that affect occupational performance. Modification of tasks or assistance (e.g., physical or verbal) with assessment is not necessary to enable completion of evaluation component.
97166—occupational therapy evaluation, moderate complexity	▪ An occupational profile and medical and therapy history, which includes an expanded review of medical and therapy records and additional review of physical, cognitive, or psychosocial history related to current functional performance ▪ An assessment that identifies 3–5 performance deficits (i.e., relating to physical, cognitive, or psychosocial skills) that result in activity limitations, participation restrictions, or both. ▪ Clinical decision making of moderate analytic complexity, which includes an analysis of the occupational profile, analysis of data from detailed assessments, and consideration of several treatment options. Patient may present with comorbidities that affect occupational performance. Minimal to moderate modification of tasks or assistance (e.g., physical or verbal) with assessment is necessary to enable patient to complete evaluation component.
97167—occupational therapy evaluation, high complexity	▪ An occupational profile and medical and therapy history, which includes review of medical and therapy records and extensive additional review of physical, cognitive, or psychosocial history related to current functional performance ▪ An assessment that identifies 5 or more performance deficits (i.e., relating to physical, cognitive, or psychosocial skills) that result in activity limitations, participation restrictions, or both ▪ Clinical decision making of high analytic complexity, which includes an analysis of the patient's occupational profile, analysis of data from comprehensive assessment, and consideration of multiple treatment options. Patient presents with comorbidities that affect occupational performance. Significant modification of tasks or assistance (e.g., physical or verbal) with assessment is necessary to enable the patient to complete the evaluation component.
97168—reevaluation of occupational therapy established plan of care	▪ An assessment of changes in patient functional or medical status with revised plan of care ▪ An update to the initial occupational profile to reflect changes in condition or environment that affect future interventions, goals, or both ▪ A revised plan of care. A formal reevaluation is performed when a documented change in functional status occurs or a significant change to the plan of care is required.

Note. CPT = Current Procedural Terminology; OT = occupational therapy.

Source. Codes shown refer to *CPT 2017* (American Medical Association, 2020, *CPT 2020 standard,* Chicago: American Medical Association Press) and do not represent all of the possible codes that may be used in occupational therapy evaluation and intervention. After 2020, refer to the current year's *CPT* code book for available codes. *CPT* codes are updated annually and become effective January 1. *CPT* is a trademark of the American Medical Association. *CPT* five-digit codes, two-digit codes, modifiers, and descriptions are copyright © 2020 by the American Medical Association. All rights reserved.

2020e) describes the evaluation process as one in which the occupational therapist establishes an occupational profile, gathers relevant history, obtains appropriate assessment data, and develops a plan of care. When coding occupational therapy evaluations, several additional factors should be considered. The level of complexity of the evaluation is determined by the child's condition; the level of clinical decision making; and the depth of the child's performance deficits, or occupations (AOTA, 2016).

Low-complexity evaluations require a brief occupational profile and history, one to three performance deficits resulting in participation restrictions, and a low level of decision making. Moderate-complexity evaluations include a more expanded medical review, three to five performance deficits, and more detailed decision making with several treatment options. Last, high-complexity evaluations include an extensive medical history review and occupational profile, five or more performance deficits, and a high level of analysis directing decision making. The last code in this grouping is reevaluation. A reevaluation occurs when a change in status or function leads to a revised plan of care. See Table 22.2 for further descriptions.

Treatment Codes

Intervention, as described in the *OTPF,* is the "process and skilled actions taken by occupational therapy practitioners in collaboration with the client to facilitate engagement in occupation related to health and participation" (AOTA, 2015, p. 2, as cited in AOTA, 2020e, p. 78).

Most of the codes used by occupational therapy practitioners fall under the Physical Medicine and Rehabilitation section of the *CPT* manual. These codes are often time based, which allows variable billing in 15-minute increments. Each year, practitioners should review the codes available through AMA or professional organizations. Not all codes are accepted by all payers, and limitations on the use of these codes are established by payer policy. Reimbursement rates vary among the codes. Reviewing information from third-party payers concerning codes and state rules is recommended (AOTA, 2020a). See Table 22.3 for common treatment codes and definitions.

Modifiers

The Medicare National Correct Coding Initiative (NCCI) includes Procedure-to-Procedure edits that describe the use of modifiers to indicate that the *CPT* codes reported together truly represent services that are separate and distinct. Modifier 59 is used by occupational therapy practitioners providing services to indicate that two codes from the NCCI list are actually distinct services. Documentation should support the modifier by clearly describing

- A different session,
- A different procedure,
- A different site or organ system, or
- Service not ordinarily performed by the same occupational therapy practitioner on the same day (AOTA, 2020d).

For example, Modifier 59 is needed for a co-treatment. In addition, Modifier 59 is needed for self-care or home management training if billed with another *CPT* code (CMS, 2019) specifically to show that there was no overlap in the timed services and they were performed sequentially.

BEST PRACTICES

The rapidly changing health care environment presents new and complex challenges to pediatric occupational therapy practitioners whose practice depends on third-party payment to survive and thrive. Best practice takes a commitment to ethical practice and an understanding of the service delivery model in which one works.

TABLE 22.3.   Common *CPT* Codes for Occupational Therapy Treatment

CPT CODE	DEFINITION
97110—therapeutic exercise	- Therapeutic exercises to develop strength and endurance, range of motion, and flexibility - Timed code
97112—neuromuscular reeducation	- Reeducation in movement, balance, coordination, kinesthetic sense, posture, or proprioception for sitting or standing activities - Timed code
97530—therapeutic activities	- Use of activities to improve functional performance - Timed code
97533—sensory integrative techniques	- To enhance sensory processing and promote adaptive responses to environmental demands - Timed code; some payers routinely deny this code
97535—self-care or home management	- Activities of daily living and compensatory training, meal preparation, safety procedures, and instructions in the use of assistive technology devices or adaptive equipment - Timed code

Note. CPT = Current Procedural Terminology.

Source. Codes shown refer to *CPT 2020* (American Medical Association, 2020, *CPT 2020 standard,* Chicago: American Medical Association Press) and do not represent all of the possible codes that may be used in occupational therapy evaluation and intervention. After 2020, refer to the current year's *CPT* code book for available codes. *CPT* codes are updated annually and become effective January 1. *CPT* is a trademark of the American Medical Association. *CPT* five-digit codes, two-digit codes, modifiers, and descriptions are copyright © 2020 by the American Medical Association. All rights reserved.

Commit to Ethical Practice

Persch et al. (2013) named federal laws, state regulations, autism insurance mandates, and essential health benefit definitions and limits as factors that complicate implementation of the ACA in pediatric settings. Using an interview format to explore the implications and impact of the ACA on the perceptions and practice of occupational therapy practitioners, Yuen et al. (2017) found that practitioners have to be more conscientious about clients' insurance coverage when developing treatment plans than they might have been in the past. Increasingly stringent workplace expectations were identified as a factor reducing opportunities to collaborate, and changing reimbursement patterns were discussed as a potential threat to the long-term viability of private practices and outpatient clinics.

Altruism, truth, and prudence are among the aspirational core values put forward as a guide toward ethical action in all aspects of professional practice in the *2020 Occupational Therapy Code of Ethics* (AOTA, 2020b). Occupational therapy practitioners whose practice is supported by third-party payers should know that it will sometimes be difficult to balance a concern for the welfare of others (altruism) against an ethical obligation to be truthful and prudent in all client documentation and decision making about the expected benefit of initiating or continuing therapy.

Know Payer Requirements

Occupational therapy practitioners whose documentation and billing practices adhere to the rules and regulations described by CMS are likely to meet the requirements of most other payers because CMS is generally viewed as having the most stringent regulations in the industry. However, every payer network has the right to establish its own standards for authorization and documentation. Occupational therapy practitioners or their delegate must stay abreast of the policies established by every network plan pertinent to their practice and be ready to incorporate changes into their practice policies as soon as changes are forecast in a bulletin from that network. Following are some requirements that might vary from one payer to another:

- Physician (MD or DO) script may be required to complete an initial evaluation.
  - State occupational therapy licensure law and payer requirements may differ. Comply with both.
- Prior authorization might be required for initial evaluation and intervention.
  - Authorization for intervention may depend on the occupational therapist's ability to justify need in the evaluation plan of care.
- Standardized testing may be a required element of all evaluations.
- Allowable *CPT* codes may be provided with authorization from the payer network.

Communicate With the Medical Home Provider

The primary care medical home provider is generally called on to coordinate the services provided for children with disabilities in school, hospital, and community settings (American Academy of Pediatrics, 2014). In a clinical report published by the American Academy of Pediatrics, Houtrow and Murphy (2019) strongly advocated for ongoing communication between care team members about a child's functional status, achievement of therapy goals, identification of new goals, when cessation of therapy might be appropriate, and family functioning and concerns. Care team members include the child's parents or caregivers, medical home providers, therapists, educators, and subspecialists.

Because physicians are often called on to determine the medical necessity for therapy services, Houtrow and Murphy also advocated for pediatric medical home providers to provide a high level of detail when writing prescriptions for therapy and to remain the locus of communication and coordination of services. The pediatric occupational therapy practitioner must commit to ongoing, positive, and professional communication with clients' medical home providers and their delegates if they hope to sustain a successful practice.

Document and Write Goals

Every payer network provides guidelines for documentation. These networks employ professionals charged with reviewing claims for payment and requests for authorization for an episode of care. These reviewers base their decisions about payment and authorization on how well occupational therapy practitioners have described the child's status and need for skilled services in the documentation submitted (AOTA, 2018). It is incumbent on occupational therapy practitioners to support their requests with unambiguous data and to clearly articulate a decision-making process that supports medical necessity and the frequency and duration of services proposed. Houtrow and Murphy (2019) stated that

> information about the trajectory of disability associated with the condition, the evidence of the value of therapies to improve functioning, and how the individual child is expected to benefit from the interventions is also important when providing written medical justification. (p. 8)

A second key component of documentation and justifying the need for services is goal writing. The goals submitted with the occupational therapy practitioner's documentation must be meaningful and occupation based, with time frames associated with completion that reflect the performance deficits identified. Establishing a template for documentation can assist practitioners in ensuring all elements of documentation meet both practice guidelines and payer, state, and federal requirements.

Manage Denials

The decision to pay for services is often made after the care has been given and reviewed by the payers (Umphred, 2013). There are multiple reasons why payers deny claims. When a claim comes back as a denial, it has a denial code. This code helps practitioners determine how to review or correct the claim. For example, therapy could not be a covered service, or a more specific *ICD–10-CM* code may be needed. There is a process for appeals, which may require a peer-to-peer review that is determined by the payer.

When addressing a denial in any capacity, Houtrow and Murphy (2019) suggested that four key pieces of information are needed to justify medical necessity: (1) the diagnosis for which the service is needed, (2) how the service addresses the disabling condition, (3) that an effective less costly option is not available, and (4) any other medical history relevant to the case.

Occupational therapy practitioners are often the first resource contacted by families when they receive notification of an insurance denial. It is important to empower families for success with information to successfully navigate these systems. This can include providing them with the diagnosis and *CPT* codes used during treatment so families can discuss in advance what their payer network is willing to cover.

SUMMARY

Occupational therapy practitioners have a responsibility to know and understand the service delivery models in which they work and how these models affect children's access to care. Navigating payment for services has many facets, including understanding payer requirements, coding and billing, and documentation that supports the medically necessary need for skilled care by an occupational therapy practitioner.

REFERENCES

American Academy of Pediatrics, Council on Children With Disabilities and Medical Home Implementation Project Advisory Committee. (2014). Patient- and family-centered care coordination: A framework for integrating care for children and youth across multiple systems. *Pediatrics, 133,* e1451–e1460. https://doi.org/10.1542/peds.2014-0318

American Occupational Therapy Association. (2015). Standards of practice for occupational therapy. *American Journal of Occupational Therapy, 69*(Suppl. 3), 6913410057. https://doi.org/10.5014/ajot.2015.696S06

American Occupational Therapy Association. (2016). *Occupational therapy evaluations as described in CPT Code Manual®.* https://www.aota.org/~/media/Corporate/Files/Advocacy/Federal/coding/Descriptors-of-New-CPT-Occupational-Therapy-Evaluation-Codes.pdf

American Occupational Therapy Association. (2018). Guidelines for documentation of occupational therapy. *American Journal of Occupational Therapy, 72*(Suppl. 2), 7212410010. https://doi.org/10.5014/ajot.2018.72S203

American Occupational Therapy Association. (2020a). *2020 CPT codes for occupational therapy.* https://www.aota.org/~/media/corporate/files/secure/advocacy/federal/coding/2020-selected-occupational-therapy-cpt-codes.pdf

American Occupational Therapy Association. (2020b). 2020 occupational therapy code of ethics. *American Journal of Occupational Therapy, 74*(Suppl. 3), 7413410005. https://doi.org/10.5014/ajot.2020.74S3006

American Occupational Therapy Association. (2020c). *Can occupational therapists assign ICD-10 codes?* https://www.aota.org/Advocacy-Policy/Federal-Reg-Affairs/ICD-10-Diagnosis-Coding/can-occupational-therapists-assign-icd-10-codes.aspx

American Occupational Therapy Association (2020d). *Occupational therapists should continue modifier 59 use.* https://www.aota.org/Advocacy-Policy/Federal-Reg-Affairs/Coding/Occupational-Therapists-Should-Continue-Modifier-59-Use.aspx

American Occupational Therapy Association. (2020e). Occupational therapy practice framework: Domain and process (4th ed.). *American Journal of Occupational Therapy, 74*(Suppl. 2), 7412410010. https://doi.org/10.5014/ajot.2020.74S2001

Centers for Medicare & Medicaid Services. (2016). *NPI: What you need to know.* https://www.cms.gov/Outreach-and-Education/Medicare-Learning-Network-MLN/MLNProducts/downloads/NPI-What-You-Need-To-KnowText-Only.pdf

Centers for Medicare & Medicaid Services. (2019). *National correct coding initiative edits.* https://www.cms.gov/Medicare/Coding/NationalCorrectCodInitEd/index.html

Healthcare.gov. (n.d.). *Glossary.* https://www.healthcare.gov/glossary/

Health Insurance Portability and Accountability Act of 1996, Pub. L. 104-191, 42 U.S.C. § 300gg, 29 U.S.C. §§ 1181-1183, and 42 U.S.C. §§ 1320d-1320d9.

Houtrow, A., & Murphy, N.; Council on Children With Disabilities. (2019). Prescribing physical, occupational, and speech therapy services for children with disabilities. *Pediatrics, 143,* e20190285. https://doi.org/10.1542/peds.2019-0285

Medicaid.gov. (2019). *Managed care.* https://www.medicaid.gov/medicaid/managed-care/index.html

Patient Protection and Affordable Care Act, Pub. L. 111-148, 42 U.S.C. §§ 18001–18121 (2010). https://www.congress.gov/111/plaws/publ148/PLAW-111publ148.pdf

Persch, A. C., Braveman, B. H., & Metzler, C. A. (2013). P4 medicine and pediatric occupational therapy. *American Journal of Occupational Therapy, 67,* 383–388. https://doi.org/10.5014/ajot.2013.674002

Stover, A. D. (2016). Client-centered advocacy: Every occupational therapy practitioner's responsibility to understand medical necessity. *American Journal of Occupational Therapy, 70,* 7005090010. https://doi.org/10.5014/ajot.2016.705003

Umphred, D. A. (2013). *Umphred's neurological rehabilitation.* Elsevier/Mosby.

U.S. Department of Health and Human Services. (2013). *Summary of the HIPAA Privacy Rule.* https://www.hhs.gov/hipaa/for-professionals/privacy/laws-regulations/index.html

World Health Organization. (1990). *International classification of diseases, 10th revision.*: Author.

World Health Organization. (n.d.). *International classification of diseases (ICD) information sheet.* https://www.who.int/classifications/icd/factsheet/en/

Yuen, H. K., Spicher, H. S., Semon, M. R., Winwood, L. M., & Dudgeon, B. J. (2017). Perceptions of occupational therapists on the Patient Protection and Affordable Care Act: Five years after its enactment. *Occupational Therapy in Health Care, 31,* 84–97. https://doi.org/10.1080/07380577.2016.1270480

Best Practices in Evaluation in Health Care Settings

Kaitlin Hagen, MOT, OTR/L; Alaena McCool, MS, OTR/L, CPAM; and Rebecca Martin, OTR/L, OTD

KEY TERMS AND CONCEPTS

- Acquired diagnoses
- Analyzing occupational performance
- Client-centered goals
- Client factors
- Developmental disabilities
- Hypothesis
- Interdisciplinary team
- Occupational profile
- Occupational therapy evaluation
- Performance patterns
- Performance skills
- Planning for discharge

OVERVIEW

Occupational therapy practitioners have an important role in supporting the health and well-being of children from birth to age 5 years served in health care settings: acute hospital, inpatient rehabilitation, outpatient rehabilitation, and home health settings. (*Note. Occupational therapy practitioner* refers to both occupational therapists and occupational therapy assistants.) According to the American Occupational Therapy Association (AOTA; 2020) workforce survey, 11.3% of occupational therapy assistants and 28.6% of occupational therapists work in hospital settings, 8.3% of occupational therapy assistants and 13.3% of occupational therapists work in outpatient settings, 7.8% of occupational therapy assistants and 7.3% of occupational therapists work in home health settings, and about 1.6% of both occupational therapy assistants and occupational therapists work in other settings.

In health care settings, occupational therapists conduct a thorough evaluation to capture the context, capacity, and impairments with which a child presents so that a comprehensive treatment plan can be developed and the child can safely function in their living situation. During evaluation, occupational therapists glean information on functional skills (e.g., mobility, self-care), impairments (e.g., strength, range of motion, balance, tone, vision, cognition), and child and family treatment priorities. Depending on the child's age, arousal, and cooperation level, this information may be captured through chart review, clinical observation, caregiver report, or standardized assessment. From this information and with input from the interdisciplinary team, occupational therapists use their professional judgment to define priority interventions, goals, and discharge disposition.

Occupational therapy practitioners are uniquely positioned in an interdisciplinary medical team to make determinations about safe return to home, equipment needs, and caregiver support. Occupational therapy practitioners' input on self-care, school, play activity capacity, and necessary modifications is critical in successful return to home for young children.

Acquired and Developmental Conditions

Acquired diagnoses are conditions that affect a child during development and most commonly are the result of illness or injury. Some common diagnoses occupational therapy practitioners see while working in pediatric health care practice include

- Acquired neurological conditions, such as injuries of the brain and spinal cord;
- Neurological birth injuries, including brachial plexus injury;
- Cancer;
- Burns; and
- Postsurgical care.

Developmental disabilities are defined by the Centers for Disease Control and Prevention (2019) as "a group of conditions due to an impairment in physical, learning, language, or behavior areas" (para. 1). These conditions include developmental delays, autism spectrum disorder, cerebral palsy, and other learning and language disorders. These conditions may develop during developmental periods and persist throughout the child's lifetime.

Although both acquired and developmental conditions may differ in etiology and treatment planning, each occupational therapy practitioner uses a client-centered approach to evaluate and treat this population. Although a diagnosis may give guidelines on how one may treat the symptoms to initiate a plan of care, an occupational therapy evaluation provides the therapist with the whole picture of the child so they can formulate goals and intervention ideas to provide the best care to the child. The process includes conducting a chart review as appropriate in the clinician's setting (e.g., medical chart for hospital settings, past occupational therapy evaluations and treatment notes for outpatient clinics, preschool individualized education programs and available past occupational therapy notes for preschool settings, referral information for home health settings), interviewing the child and caregiver, obtaining home set-up and current equipment, and performing formal and informal assessments of the child to obtain a baseline of ADLs and functional mobility. This information will help the practitioner formulate a treatment plan with goals and recommendations for frequency of therapy.

ESSENTIAL CONSIDERATIONS

Before processing the occupational therapy evaluation, the therapist communicates with other members of the team to ensure the child and family's needs are being met. This collaboration is crucial to ensure everyone's goals are being achieved, as is effectively communicating with the family and child during this process. On the basis of this communication, the occupational therapist determines what frames of reference will be most appropriate to use during the child's evaluation and ongoing care.

Interdisciplinary Teaming and Collaboration

Occupational therapy practitioners in health care settings are members of an *interdisciplinary team.* Although this team may look different depending on where the occupational therapy practitioner works, the team is an essential part of the child's plan of care. The interdisciplinary team may include doctors, nurses, occupational therapy practitioners, physical therapists, speech-language pathologists, behavioral psychologists, neuropsychologists, social workers, case managers, respiratory therapists, educational specialists, child life specialists, and certified recreation therapists as well as the child and family.

Occupational therapy practitioners need to understand the whole picture of their client,[1] including past and current medical history, medical plans, other rehabilitation practitioners' goals, possible behaviors that may interfere with their own treatment plan, family dynamics, and the client's interests. In the health care field, practitioners may further understand their client by communicating in person during team rounds, by email, or through other hospital applications, depending on the setting. Clients may also obtain therapy outside the hospital and clinic environment—for example, in more natural environments, such as the school system and at home.

The team may look somewhat different in each environment but often contains multiple professionals, including rehabilitation disciplines, teachers, family, and paraprofessionals. In natural settings, different behaviors, interests, and interactions may be observed that are not typical in the rehab environment. It is important to collaborate with other professionals and family members to ensure carryover is consistent for the child and family to obtain their goals.

Communication among the treatment team, including the family, is key to ensuring proper follow-up, care, and to be aware of a potential change in treatment plan for the child's session. Given the variety of individuals on the team, communication and collaboration within the team is critical to guide the occupational therapy practitioner's service provision. For example, if a child has been having pain in a localized limb, they may have an acute fracture, be overworked, or need a change in medication.

Communication is important for any changes in medical care that may affect the evaluation or treatment plan. Above all, the child and their family are an essential part of the team, and their goals need to be considered during formulation of a treatment plan. This ensures there is buy-in from the family and motivation from the child to achieve their goals and progress toward functional independence and developmental milestones.

Hospital teams

Before or after an occupational therapy evaluation, a team meeting is recommended to outline findings, determine the family and child's needs, formulate a tentative plan of care with the team, and start planning for discharge from the beginning of the admission. Depending on the acuity and severity of the child's diagnosis, daily meetings or rounds may be more typical in this setting, because the child's medical status may guide therapy and other team members during the hospital stay. Meetings held at the beginning of the admission, weekly, and closer to discharge are typical.

At the initial meeting, the team sets goals that can lead the occupational therapy practitioner's plan of care. Concerns raised by the team, including barriers to discharge, are discussed, and goals are updated to assist in getting the child home. Family members are also present in this meeting to include any other cultural, family dynamics, and environmental factors that may affect the child's admission, current plan of care, or discharge disposition. During the meeting, the family can agree with the practitioner's plan of care, make suggestions, identify motivators and barriers, and express their own goals for care, which might not have come up in the initial occupational therapy evaluation. Throughout the admission, weekly rounds are held to update the team on the child's progress, and daily communication occurs with family during therapy. Closer to discharge, the practitioner informs the case manager of equipment needs and initiates training for a home rehabilitation program with the family.

Communication is also done through a daily medical chart review, including a review of recent scans, new concerns, and any acute changes. Follow-up clarification from a team member can be communicated by telephone, a clinical communication online platform application, or pager system, depending on the hospital system. Communication with the medical team is essential to provide the optimum care and to best prepare the child and family for discharge from the hospital to rehab or home.

---

[1]Because young children are dependent on an adult, the term *client* refers to the child and caregiver or parent.

Community, home, and outpatient health care teams

When working in home health, outpatient, and community settings, the team members may include a small group of providers. The occupational therapist is typically in the position of making decisions, seeking consultation, and coordinating care in compliance with the payer source. The child and family remain at the center of the team, and clear communication remains critical. Frequent contact among all team members is important, to adjust goals and help the child progress toward their functional independence and developmental milestones. Open communication is helpful (e.g., what works for one team member to challenge the child may be helpful to another). Occupational therapy practitioners should provide strategies and training to assist the family in home program activities and exercises.

Occupational Therapy Practice Framework: Domain and Process

The *International Classification of Functioning, Disability and Health* (World Health Organization, 2001) and AOTA's (2002) *Occupational Therapy Practice Framework: Domain and Process (OTPF)*, which were being developed at the same time, are interwoven and guide occupational therapy practitioners during the evaluation and intervention process.

The *OTPF*, now in its fourth edition, includes both the occupational therapy domain and the process. The *domains* are the "profession's purview and areas in which its members have an established body of knowledge and expertise"; they include occupations, client factors, performance skills, performance patterns, and contexts and environments (AOTA, 2020b, p. 85). The *service delivery process* is how practitioners use their expertise to provide services to children and families. The process includes evaluation, intervention, and outcomes. More on the service delivery process is covered in the next section.

During the evaluation, the occupational therapist develops and refines a **hypothesis** on the basis of the child's performance limitations and strengths (AOTA, 2020b). Hypotheses are based on typical occupational therapy frames of reference and theory used with this population. These may include occupation-based models, such as the Model of Human Occupation (Kielhofner, 2002), the Person–Environment–Occupation model (Law et al., 1996), developmental and behavioral models, or performance deficit models (e.g., biomechanical, rehabilitation).

BEST PRACTICES

A comprehensive, holistic evaluation is important to set the stage for a client-centered plan of care in health care settings. The purpose of the **occupational therapy evaluation** is to identify what a client (i.e., child and family) want and need to do, and then identify supports and barriers to health and participation (AOTA, 2020b).

Initiate the Evaluation

When completing an evaluation, occupational therapists focus on developing an occupational profile and analyzing occupational performance. For further information on writing evaluation reports in health care settings, refer to Chapter 26, "Best Practices in Documentation of Health Care Services and Outcomes." Developing an occupational profile and analyzing occupational performance consist of gathering useful data through informal methods of interview, clinical observations, and formal methods of standard and appropriate occupational therapy assessments.

Develop an occupational profile

The **occupational profile** is a summary of a child and family's "occupational history and experiences, patterns of daily living, interests, values, and relevant contexts" (AOTA, 2020b, p. 24). Using a client- and family-centered approach, the occupational therapist gathers information through interview and record review to understand the family's priorities and desired outcomes connected to the child's engagement in occupations. See Exhibit 23.1 for some questions therapists may ask when developing the occupational profile. The questions vary on the basis of the child's diagnosis, the health care setting, and the age of the child.

The occupational profile also includes asking about the family's experiences, interests, values, and social and cultural items of importance to the family. This allows the occupational therapist to provide the best care to the child and family while respecting any cultural, religious, or social contexts that the family discloses. For example, is an interpreter needed? Does the family's religion require them to adhere to certain standards that might affect the time they can do therapy or even the order in which they can get dressed? It is important to keep in mind that gathering this comprehensive history, current home set-up, and current level of function and participation provides the therapist with a starting point to understanding the child and family's occupational profile, which can greatly affect their occupational performance.

In addition, the interview and data collection associated with creating the occupational profile process allows the occupational therapist to observe and develop rapport with the family and child. During this time, it is important to identify the health literacy of the caregiver and child to ensure that they fully understand the nature of occupational therapy, the child's diagnosis, and other medical terms that may come up during the evaluation process. By targeting and understanding the family's health literacy skills, practitioners can provide education and teaching in different ways, such as offering visual handouts or using more clear, concise, and basic language to ensure full understanding and participation in the occupational therapy process.

Last, gathering further information about the services and technology that the child currently has is important. This includes low-tech items, such as splints and orthotics, as well as high-tech items, such as communication boards and power mobility. Having this information again provides the occupational therapy practitioner with a baseline for what the child has and what they may need to increase independence, decrease caregiver burden, and improve safety for the child and family members.

Analyze occupational performance

Analyzing occupational performance is the second part of the occupational therapy evaluation process. During the evaluation process, the occupational therapist should be

EXHIBIT 23.1.   Sample Questions for Gathering the Occupational Profile

Questions and prompts regarding the need for evaluation and intervention
- "Tell me about your current concerns."
- "What are the goals for this bout of care?"
- "What services has your child previously received?"
- "Did you self-refer for an evalution? If referred by a doctor or other licensed practitioner, why?"

Questions about the child's occupations —strengths and barriers
- "What are your child's interests?"
- "Does your child attend preschool or child care?"
- "How does your child interact during the day with peers and other adults?"
- "Do you have any concerns about participation in daily activities or age-appropriate play?"

Questions about aspects of the environment or context that support or inhibit engagement
- "Do you live in an apartment, townhome, or house?" (If adaptations to the home need to be made, ask whether the family rents or owns the property.)
- "Can your child currently access all the rooms in the home (e.g., bathroom, bedroom)? If not, what are the barriers?" An option is to ask the family to bring in pictures if physical barriers are present.
- "Are there any safety concerns in the home (e.g., kitchen, steps)?"

Questions about prenatal, birth, and developmental history
- "Tell me about your (or the birth mother's) pregnancy. Were there complications during pregnancy or with the birth?"
- "Tell me about your child's development (motor, speech, self-care, learning, social skills)." If the child's development was delayed, ask when the family noticed.
- "What have you done to help your child learn new skills?"
- "Does your child have a history of cardiac, respiratory, or other health concerns?"

Questions about current services, equipment, and assistive technology
- "Does your child currently have any assistive equipment (e.g., wheelchair, bathroom equipment, specialized stroller)?"
- "Does your child wear splints, casts, or orthotics (i.e., upper extremity, lower extremity, trunk, or cervical)?"
- "Does your child have any specialized rehabilitation equipment in the home?"
- "Do you have any equipment that your child has outgrown or that you no longer use?"

Questions about the child and family's priorities and desired targeted outcomes for the child and their family
- "What would you like your child to accomplish during this bout of care?"
- "What would you like your child to accomplish within the next year or even 5 years?"

strengths based, client centered, and participation based as they observe the child for who they are, not what their medical reports or diagnosis indicate. Therapists often use multiple methods during this process to assess the child, environments or context, and occupational performance.

Assess the child's activity and participation in occupations. Activity and participation may be assessed with a combination of interview, clinical observation, and standardized instruments. Components of assessment at this level should include functional mobility, self-care, play, and preschool. To further assess participation, occupational therapists should evaluate all age-appropriate occupations that a child is involved in. This includes basic ADLs and IADLs, if appropriate.

For an infant, this may just mean looking at their ability to swallow and eventually self-feed. For an older child, it includes their ability to dress, bathe, complete personal hygiene, and so forth. An area often overlooked is the child's activities related to sleep and rest. From infants to adults, this is important information because it supports the client's (i.e., child and family's) participation in the more active ADLs. Last, it is important to assess the child's participation in educational settings, both formal and informal, and how they are performing in this environment.

Assess client factors, performance skills, and performance patterns. Depending on the child's diagnosis and concerns, areas that may need to be assessed include client factors, performance skills, and performance patterns (AOTA, 2020b). ***Client factors*** include body functions and structures, such as pain, sensory functions, neuromusculoskeletal functions, bowel and bladder functions, and oral–motor functions. In addition, the beliefs, values, and spirituality of the child and family are identified, because these may be used in a strengths-based approach.

Pain, sensory function, and cognitive status are common areas that should be documented to provide a baseline for a child's care. Occupational therapists typically ask about pain with all children, unless they have a pain diagnosis, such as conversion disorder, for which asking about pain may not be warranted with the treatment plan. Conversion disorder is a psychological condition in which a patient's physical appearance or function is altered without identifiable organic cause (Murgai et al., 2019). Pain should not be the focus of a session for a child with a pain diagnosis; however, it should still be documented as appropriate with a standardized scale, such as the numeric or faces scales that are commonly used (Cohen et al., 2008).

The child's sensory function may include proprioception, kinesthesia, and stereognosis testing. If a child's sensation is limited, such as with some spinal cord injuries, understanding whether they have impairments to light touch, pin prick, or temperature will assist the occupational therapist in providing appropriate recommendations and planning interventions appropriately.

Occupational therapists may be able to evaluate cognitive status by observing the child. Typically, however, they address the following areas during an evaluation, if appropriate: orientation, attention to tasks, short-term memory, long-term memory, ability to follow directions (e.g., one step, two steps, with or without prompts), problem solving, overall behavior and cooperation, and communication (including how the child communicates if they use adaptive strategies). Therapists may be able to assess some of these areas through observation, whereas others may need more formal assessment during evaluation.

Neuromusculoskeletal and movement-related function may include range of motion, manual muscle testing to assess strength, and postural tone assessments. For the hand, additional measures, such as grip and pinch strength, should be assessed. Developmental tests (e.g., Peabody Developmental Motor Scales—2; Folio & Fewell, 2000) may be used for younger children to identify their strength and coordination abilities. Standardized tools can be used to provide a baseline, which assists in establishing goals and tracking progress.

Oral–motor function should be assessed, including oral–motor skills, feeding, and drinking. Although some agencies divide this up between occupational therapy and speech–language pathologists, occupational therapists should educate the team that eating and feeding are within their professional domain.

Performance skills include motor skills, process skills, and social interaction skills and are based on the child's abilities. Children learn and progress in these skills as they age; among typically developing children, the skills follow a developmental trajectory. Motor skills, such as imitating, sequencing, and constructing, are affected by many other body functions, including cognitive abilities (AOTA, 2020b). Emotional regulation and perception are also factors that affect a child's ability to develop and perform motor skills. Last, the environment can greatly affect a child's performance skills and the subcategories that are outlined above.

The third domain is *performance patterns,* which include habits, routines, roles, and rituals. These patterns need to be assessed and taken into account during the occupational therapy evaluation, because they may affect the child and family's goals and the child's current function in various settings. *Habits* are specific and automatic behaviors. *Routines* help to establish structure in a client's daily life and are sequences of occupations or activities. *Roles* are typically defined by society, correlating with the child's current age and set behaviors that are expected by society. Occupational therapists need to take into account the child's current environment (e.g., whether they live in a rural neighborhood or a city) to understand how the child's role may change over time as they develop and age.

TABLE 23.1. Commonly Used Assessments in Pediatric Health Care Practice

ASSESSMENT	DESCRIPTION	OTHER
Bayley Scales of Infant and Toddler Development (Bayley & Aylward, 2019)	An assessment of global development for infants ages 1–42 months. The instrument is intended to assist in diagnosis and treatment planning for infants with developmental delays.	Includes cognitive, language, and motor scales administered by a clinician, and social–emotional and adaptive behavior scales administered by a caregiver. Scores are used to monitor developmental growth over time and are compared with provided norms for the purposes of developmental screening.
Canadian Occupation Performance Measure (COPM; Law et al., 1990, 2005, 2019; Verkerk et al., 2006)	An interview assessment intended to quantify performance and satisfaction in self-care, leisure, and productivity tasks.	Caregivers rank the importance of functional activities, which are repeatedly scored for performance and satisfaction over time. The COPM has been shown to be reliable, valid, and sensitive to change in many diagnoses across the life course.
Functional Independence Measure for Children (Wee-FIM; Chen et al., 2005; Msall et al., 1994)	Measures the degree of independence in self-care, sphincter control, transfers, locomotion, communication, and cognition for children ages 6 months–7 years.	Aggregate data are maintained by the Uniform Data System for Medical Rehabilitation, which sets rehab standards across the country. The Wee-FIM scores patients on a 7-point Likert scale on 18 items across the six domains. Typically administered through interview; assessor training is preferred.
Peabody Developmental Motor Scales–2 (PDMS-2; Folio & Fewell, 2000; Gill et al., 2018)	Measures a child's development of gross and fine motor skills for ages birth–5 years (Folio & Fewell, 2000). There are six subtests: four for gross motor, and two for fine motor.	The PDMS–2 allows the practitioner to compare the child's motor competence with that of other children the same age and determine disparity in gross and fine motor skills.
Pediatric Evaluation of Disability Inventory (PEDI; Haley et al., 1992, 2012)	Measures current functional capabilities and changes in performance over time. Limited to the functional age range of ages 6 months–7.5 years, the PEDI may be used for older children whose functional capacity is less than that of a typically developing 7-year-old.	The original PEDI was revised into a computer adaptive test (CAT) and associated short form (SF). The PEDI-CAT is appropriate for use with children ages birth–20 years across diagnoses and settings. The instrument measures capability (what the child can do) and performance (what the child typically does) across daily activities, mobility, and social–cognitive domains.

This helps the therapist to understand the child's expected occupation during each stage of life and activities that may be accepted as appropriate during this time. *Rituals* have a spiritual, cultural, or symbolic meaning for the child and family and need to be identified within the context of the child's culture.

As stated before, these patterns develop over a child's life course and are influenced by client factors and performance skills. The child needs to use those factors and skills to engage in productive patterns in society to have a positive effect on their health, well-being, and participation. For example, if a child has the skills to socialize with peers but does not engage with other peers appropriately in their society, the child may become isolated from their peers and not participate in socially acceptable extracurricular activities that facilitate their development from childhood into early adolescence.

Use assessment tools. Selecting appropriate objective measures is an important part of the assessment process. Objective measures, including standardized tests, should be reliable and valid in the population being tested. For example, a standardized test that has validity with a specific adult population would not be applicable to children. Objective measures corroborate professional judgment, ensuring accurate and meaningful measurement of change, which is central to responsible service delivery. Many resources exist to assist practitioners in selecting appropriate outcome measures; see the list at the end of this chapter and Table 23.1 for commonly used assessments in pediatric health care practice. Also see Appendix F, "Examples of Assessments for Early Childhood (Birth–5 Years)."

Develop goals and plan for discharge

The final steps in the evaluation process include creating **client-centered goals,** goals that are relevant and meaningful to a patient and family's unique circumstance, needs, and capabilities, and **planning for discharge,** deciding on the ultimate disposition and supports necessary for the child to leave the hospital. This is extremely important to discuss with the family at evaluation to determine their goals for the child during occupational therapy intervention. Collaborative goal development leads to setting expectations with the family as to what is achievable in the short term versus the long term. Last, it is important to plan for discharge. This planning should start the first day of therapy to best serve the child and family in preparation for discharge.

SUMMARY

Comprehensive evaluation is central to occupational therapy intervention and care for young children and their families in health care settings. Using a combination of record review, interview, clinical observation, and standardized assessment allows the occupational therapist to set meaningful, reasonable goals and quantify important progress. Occupational therapists bring important assessment information to the medical team, across settings. As always, the family and child are the center of the team and have

an important role in the establishment of goals and plan of care. Occupational therapists are uniquely positioned to synthesize evaluation information across providers to create cohesive, relevant plans of care.

RESOURCES

- The **National Institutes of Health** (NIH) maintains an online toolbox (NIH, 2019) that includes comprehensive neurobehavioral measurements in the domains of cognition, emotion, sensory, and motor function. Practitioners can use the tool box for a nominal fee to administer electronic assessments and store and analyze data.
- **NIH and the National Institute of Neurological Disease and Stroke** (NINDS) have published common data elements (CDEs; NIH & NINDS, n.d.) for select pediatric diagnoses, including, but not limited to, brain injury, cerebral palsy, muscular dystrophy, and spinal cord injury. The CDEs are intended to standardize data collection and allow data sharing and aggregate analysis. CDEs are developed by working groups of international experts convened by the NINDS. They provide information on the psychometric properties of given instruments, data standards, and accompanying tools, at no cost when possible, for assessments across the *International Classification of Functioning, Disability and Health* (WHO, 2001) continuum.
- The **Shirley Ryan Ability Lab** maintains www.rehab-measures.org, a database of instruments, associated psychometrics, and professional recommendations for clinician reference.

REFERENCES

American Occupational Therapy Association. (2002). Occupational therapy practice framework: Domain and process. *American Journal of Occupational Therapy, 56,* 609–639. https://doi.org/10.5014/ajot.56.6.609

American Occupational Therapy Association. (2020a). *2019 workforce & salary survey.* https://www.aota.org/Education-Careers/Advance-Career/Salary-Workforce-Survey.aspx

American Occupational Therapy Association. (2020b). Occupational therapy practice framework: Domain and process (4th ed.). *American Journal of Occupational Therapy, 74*(Suppl. 2), 7412410010. https://doi.org/10.5014/ajot.2020.74S2001

Bayley, N., & Aylward, G. P. (2019). *Bayley Scales of Infant and Toddler Development* (4th ed.). Pearson.

Centers for Disease Control and Prevention. (2019). *Facts about developmental disabilities.* https://www.cdc.gov/ncbddd/developmentaldisabilities/facts.html

Chen, C. C., Bode, R. K., Granger, C. V., & Heinemann, A. W. (2005). Psychometric properties and developmental differences in children's ADL item hierarchy: A study of the WeeFIM® instrument. *American Journal of Physical Medicine & Rehabilitation, 84,* 671–679. https://doi.org/10.1097/01.phm.0000176439.32318.36

Cohen, L. L., Lamanek, K., Blount, R. L., Dahlquist, L. M., Lim, C. S., Palermo, T. M., . . . Weiss, K. E. (2008). Evidence-based assessment of pediatric pain. *Journal for Pediatric Psychology, 33,* 939–955. https://doi.org/10.1093/jpepsy/jsm103

Folio, M. R., & Fewell, R. R. (2000). *Peabody Developmental Motor Scales.* Pro-Ed.

Gill, K., Osiovich, A., Synnes, A., Agnew, J. A., Grunau, R. E., Miller, S. P., & Zwicker, J. I. G. (2018). Concurrent validity of the Bayley–III and the Peabody Developmental Motor Scales–2 at 18 months. *Physical & Occupational Therapy in Pediatrics, 39,* 514–524. https://doi.org/10.1080/01942638.2018.1546255

Haley, S. M., Coster, W. J., Dumas, H. M., & Fragala-Pinkham, M. A. (2012). *Pediatric Evaluation of Disability Inventory Computer Adaptive Test (PEDI-CAT), Version 1.3.6: Development, standardization and administration manual.* CRECare.

Haley, S. M., Coster, W. J., Ludlow, L. H., & Haltiwanger, J. T. (1992). *Pediatric Evaluation of Disability Inventory: Development, standardization, and administration manual* (Version 1.0). Pearson Assessments.

Kielhofner, G. (2002). *A model of human occupation: Theory and application.* Lippincott Williams & Wilkins.

Law, M., Baptiste, S., McColl, M., Opzoomer, A., Platajko, H., & Pollock, N. (1990). The Canadian Occupational Performance Measure: An outcome measure for occupational therapy. *Canadian Journal of Occupational Therapy, 57,* 82–87. https://doi.org/10.1177/000841749005700207

Law, M., Baptiste, S., Carswell, A., McColl, M. A., Polatajko, H. J., & Pollock, N. (2005). *Canadian Occupational Performance Measure* (4th ed.). CAOT Publications ACE.

Law, M., Baptiste, S., Carswell, A., McColl, M., Polatajko, H. & Pollock, N. (2019). *Canadian Occupational Performance Measure* (5th ed., rev.). COPM Inc.

Law, M., Cooper, B., Strong, S., Stewart, D., Rigby, P., & Letts, L. (1996). The Person–Environment–Occupation model: A transactive approach to occupational performance. *Canadian Journal of Occupational Therapy, 63,* 9–23. https://doi.org/10.1177/000841749606300103

Msall, M. E., DiGaudio, K., Rogers, B. T., LaForest, S., Catanzaro, N. L., Campbell, J., . . . Duffy, L. C. (1994). The Functional Independence Measure for Children (Wee-FIM): Conceptual basis and pilot use in children with developmental disabilities. *Clinical Pediatrics, 33,* 421–430. https://doi.org/10.1177/000992289403300708

Murgai, R. R., Vandenberg, C., Stevanovic, M., & Lightdale-Miric, N. (2019). Upper extremity conversion disorder in children. *Journal of Shoulder and Elbow Surgery, 28,* 175–181. https://doi.org/10.1016/j.jse.2018.10.027

National Institutes of Health. (2019). *NIH toolbox®.* https://www.healthmeasures.net/explore-measurement-systems/nih-toolbox

National Institutes of Health and National Institute of Neurological Disease and Stroke. (n.d.). *NINDS common data elements.* https://www.commondataelements.ninds.nih.gov

Verkerk, G. J., Wolk, M. J., Louwers, A. M., Meester-Delver, A., & Nollet, F. (2006). The reproducibility and validity of the Canadian Occupational Performance Measure in parents of children with disabilities. *Clinical Rehabilitation, 20,* 980–988. https://doi.org/10.1177/0269215506070703

World Health Organization. (2001). *International classification of functioning, disability and health.* Author.

Best Practices in Health Care Interventions for Developmental Conditions

24

Bonnie Riley, OTD, OTR/L, and Molly Connor-Hall, MS, OTR/L

KEY TERMS AND CONCEPTS

- Developmental conditions
- Discharge
- Health care
- Home health
- Inpatient setting
- Neonatal intensive care unit setting
- Outpatient clinic settings
- Parent coaching
- Plan of care
- Progress monitoring
- Secondary settings
- Sensory Stories®
- Social Stories™
- Video modeling

OVERVIEW

Health care services strive to provide family-centered and interdisciplinary care to children and their families. According to the Federal Interagency Forum on Child and Family Statistics (2018), **health care** "comprises the prevention, treatment, and management of illness and the preservation of mental and physical well-being through services offered by health professionals" (p. 4). Children and their families pursue developmental health care services to promote overall health and well-being, address acute illnesses, and manage chronic conditions. **Developmental conditions** include a broad range of diagnoses, including "[attention deficit hyperactivity disorder]; cerebral palsy; autism; seizures; stammering or stuttering; intellectual disabilities; blindness; learning disorders; and other developmental delays" (Boyle et al., 2011, p. 1035).

Many developmental disabilities are not diagnosed until after age 3 years, and some diagnoses may not be noted until children are school age. Researchers have found children with developmental disabilities are more likely to require health and special education services, compared with children without developmental disabilities (Boyle et al., 2011).

Occupational therapy practitioners offer screening, evaluation, and intervention services in primary and secondary health care settings. (*Note. Occupational therapy practitioner* refers to both occupational therapists and occupational therapy assistants.) In primary care settings, such as a pediatrician's office, therapists offer developmental screening and contextual interventions for promoting healthy daily routines. The occupational profile reveals important information for the practitioner to support performance patterns through coaching in the primary care setting.

A child with a developmental condition may encounter and receive health care services in a variety of **secondary settings** throughout their childhood, including the neonatal intensive care unit (NICU), hospital, outpatient, and home health setting. Secondary settings are necessary when the child has a condition that requires specialized care that cannot be offered in their primary care setting. In a secondary setting, occupational therapy practitioners address individual and group developmental needs of children and their families through tailored activities. Emphasis is placed on the individual client's[1] needs to minimize activity limitations and restore functional participation and developmental acquisition. Services provided in both primary and secondary settings support the child and family in developmental and functional skill acquisition for increased participation in daily occupations.

ESSENTIAL CONSIDERATIONS

Developmental needs and considerations vary by condition and individual child and family contexts. Occupational therapy practitioners are guided by the *Occupational Therapy Practice Framework: Domain and Process* (4th ed.; American Occupational Therapy Association [AOTA], 2020). In health care settings, practitioners work on interprofessional teams, relying on the *International Classification of Functioning, Disability and Health: Children and Youth Version* (World Health Organization, 2007) during collaboration. Practitioners should be aware of the role of other professionals who may contribute to the health care team (see Table 24.1). Understanding the etiology and characteristics of the range of developmental conditions as well as the prognosis and presence of coexisting conditions is important for practitioners who are considering the child's occupational profile and anticipating the needs the child may experience during intervention.

---

[1]Because young children are dependent on an adult, the term *client* refers to the child and caregiver or parent.

TABLE 24.1.   Contributions of Interprofessional Team Members in Health Care

TEAM MEMBER	CONTRIBUTIONS
Applied behavioral analysis provider	Collaborates on specific behaviors to increase positive behaviors and decrease negative behaviors.
Counselor	Works with children and family to promote emotional regulation and mental health
Developmental pediatrician or other specialist	Manages medications and interventions specific to developmental condition
Occupational therapy practitioner	Works with children and families to improve participation in activities of everyday life (e.g., address cognitive, physical, psychosocial, sensory skills); addresses needs for adaptive equipment and assistive technology
Orthotist	Provides braces and orthotics to promote stability and support body structures
Optometrist or ophthalmologist	Provides visual aids and services to support visual skills
Parent	Advocates integration of community resources (advocacy and support groups)
Physical therapist	Works with children and families to improve coordination, strength, and balance; addresses needs for adaptive mobility equipment
Physician or nurse	Assesses medical stability, treats illness, and manages chronic conditions
Preschool teacher or service provider	Provides early educational experiences, including learning and socializing; may include early intervention providers
Speech therapist	Works with children and families to improve language, articulation, and oral motor skills; addresses needs for adaptive communication devices
Social worker or case manager	Supports families to obtain waivers for services and durable medical equipment; assists with finding appropriate child care or preschool; helps manage insurance benefits

Occupational Therapy Role in Health Care Settings

Medical services are traditionally problem focused. However, modern health care emphasizes the need for predictive, personalized, preventive, and participatory services; systematically integrating information from the occupational profile and occupational performance analysis is an important part of this process (Persch et al., 2013). See Table 24.2 for key concepts in health care. In each setting, children are expected to participate in a home program with caregivers between appointments to carry over skills and make progress toward goals.

TABLE 24.2.   Key Concepts in Delivering Health Care Services

CONCEPT	EXAMPLES
Predictive	Provide expertise related to prognosis and effective interventions on interdisciplinary teams
Personalized	Provide interventions sensitive to child's individual contexts and abilities (i.e., just-right challenge, activity analysis to support performance)
Preventive	Develop healthy habits for eating and sleeping, exercise, self-regulation, and play promotion
Participatory	Encourage active engagement in therapy process (e.g., parent coaching) and promote participation in occupations during interventions

Source. Concepts from Persch et al., 2013.

Neonatal intensive care unit setting

The *NICU setting* is designed for infants in need of intensive medical care resulting from premature birth or other health problems requiring specialized care. In the NICU, developmental care initiatives begin with family-centered care achieved through provision of consistent medical providers whenever possible and flexible care supportive of the parent–child relationship in developmentally supportive individualized environments (Pressler et al., 2010). Developmentally coordinated care in the NICU promotes neurodevelopment for infants born preterm or with significant medical complications. NICU interventions prioritize brain homeostasis for optimal short- and long-term outcomes. Interventions focus on sleep protection, assessment and management of pain, positioning, infant-driven feeding, control of environmental light and noise, and touch massage and skin-to-skin contact with parents (Lavallée et al., 2019).

Inpatient hospital setting

The hospital setting is an *inpatient setting* for individuals to recover from illness or procedures who may need around-the-clock care and services that cannot be provided from home. Hospital settings vary by the type of care provided: A general hospital provides medical services for the community, a trauma center provides treatment for injuries for those in critical care, and a children's hospital provides specialized developmental care. In the hospital setting there are different levels of care, depending on the severity of the care needed; occupational therapy practitioners may provide services at all levels.

In both the NICU and hospital settings, children receive occupational therapy services as needed to support goals related to becoming medically stable. A child with a developmental diagnosis may require hospital services because of a new injury or illness; however, they may also need services for ongoing chronic conditions and comorbid diagnoses. Occupational therapy practitioners may provide consultation to caregivers and nursing staff on improving the child's performance for basic ADLs, such as positioning and feeding.

When health care services are provided outside of the NICU and hospital setting, the child is likely to be medically stable. This offers the opportunity to focus on a wide range of functional outcomes using a variety of intervention models and strategies. Health care in outpatient, home, and community settings may address social skills, feeding skills, play skills, ADLs, sleep training and routines, and IADLs (including transitions, community safety, and health management).

Home health setting

Home health services are delivered by health care and medical professionals in the child's home environment because the child is homebound. This differs from early intervention services, which are services are provided to children from birth to age 3 years in their natural environment, including the home and community locations, to optimize development. Children who are homebound and require home health services may be limited in their ability to leave the home because of ongoing illnesses, conditions, or injuries. Occupational therapy practitioners providing treatment in the home emphasize developmentally appropriate ADLs, play, and social participation using items and people in the home environment to improve children's functional participation in daily occupations.

Therapy clinic settings

Outpatient clinic settings may be affiliated with a hospital or a privately owned clinic children travel to for appointments. In this setting, children are able to use specialized equipment during treatment and may be exposed to a variety of resources to optimize progress toward goals. The length of the plan of care and frequency of treatment can vary greatly in this setting. Many children with developmental diagnoses participate in episodes of care in the clinic setting, during which the children, their families, and the occupational therapy practitioner focus on specific goals during a determined time period (Gee et al., 2016). Children often take breaks from services in clinic settings and return later to work on new goals.

Collaborating With Others

Parents and caregivers are encouraged to monitor developmental milestones (Centers for Disease Control and Prevention, 2019) and advocate for their children's developmental needs. A child may be referred to occupational therapy services by primary care providers or by physical therapists, speech therapists, preschool teachers, child care providers, social workers, or occupational therapists in other settings. Occupational therapy practitioners collaborate with the referral source, other professionals on the interdisciplinary health care team, and others as invited by the family throughout the intervention.

Payment Sources

Occupational therapy services in the health care setting may be funded by private insurance, government funding (i.e., Medicaid), or private pay when other options have been exhausted. Funding sources may place certain stipulations on the provision of services, such as requiring preapproval of intervention goals and only including coverage for certain interventions. Limits imposed by funding sources also may affect how occupational therapy services are delivered, such as requiring documentation of progress toward established goals and preestablished limits on the number of visits.

Scheduling

Scheduling in health care settings is challenged by hospital productivity requirements and busy family schedules. When scheduling occupational therapy services, one must consider the parents' work and family members' schedules, the child's school schedule and medical appointments, and the best time of day to address the targeted occupations. After a schedule is set for services, schedule adherence is easily challenged by weather, holidays, illness, and transportation issues. Decreased ability to participate in regular appointments can limit a child's progress and ability to reach their maximum potential during therapy services. Engaging parents in the intervention process so the benefit of each visit is apparent, keeping appointments on the same day and at the same time, and sending appointment reminders are helpful strategies to help parents keep appointments.

BEST PRACTICES

It is important to support families by empowering parents and caregivers through interventions and home programs with exercises and functional activities.

Establish the Occupational Therapy Intervention Plan

A *plan of care,* or treatment plan, with functional goals and a time frame for providing services, the frequency of services, and length of intervention sessions is established during the occupational therapy evaluation. Intervention approaches frequently used in health care settings propose to restore, modify, or prevent the impact of developmental challenges (AOTA, 2020). Intervention provided in primary or secondary, NICU, hospital, outpatient, or home health settings should focus on restoring body functioning, finding alternative use of environmental resources, or promoting a different degree of participation (Simeonsson & Lee, 2018). The plan of care guides intervention and is frequently modified during intervention as circumstances such as illness, transportation barriers, busy parent schedules, or accelerated progress toward goals unfold. The length of the intervention session is determined with consideration for the child's medical stability and activity tolerance. Throughout the intervention process, occupational therapy practitioners collaborate and possibly cotreat with others on the health care team.

In health care settings, occupational therapy practitioners attempt to maximize contexts in preparation for intervention. It is imperative that the practitioner be mindful of imitating the child's natural physical and social contexts as well as possible, which includes involving families and siblings whenever they can. Additionally, intervention should consider natural temporal contexts, such as avoiding the young child's nap time or prioritizing a feeding intervention during mealtime. During intervention, the practitioner makes ongoing recommendations for supporting the child's daily routine in their natural contexts, which may include a home activity program, strategies and modifications, or referral to other services.

Intervention planning may include preparatory activities to support the child's ability to further participate in intervention activities. Intervention activities may be selected to increase occupational engagement; alternatively, performance in occupation areas may be the emphasis during intervention (see Table 24.3). When planning for occupational therapy intervention in health care settings, occupational therapy practitioners need to be aware of the funding source, which may dictate which developmental occupation areas can be addressed and which approaches can be used.

Implement Intervention

Intervening early when a developmental challenge is identified is essential to promote the best outcome for the child as well as to support the parent–child relationship and parent well-being. Engaging parents while providing intervention for client factors, such as sensory functions, is effective for increasing function and adaptive behaviors (Schoen et al., 2018). When providing developmental care, occupational therapy practitioners commonly use therapeutic activities and the Occupation Adaptation model (Palisano, 2012; Valvano & Rapport, 2006).

A challenge in health care settings is that clients are not likely to be in their natural setting. Therefore, occupational therapy practitioners may use the Person–Environment–Occupation model (Law & Dunbar, 2007) to deliver individual, contextual interventions to children and their families. Practitioners select the best approach to address the needs of the person (child and family) and are mindful

TABLE 24.3.   Occupations to Consider During Program Planning With Families

OCCUPATIONS	INTERVENTION CONSIDERATIONS
ADLs	*Dressing:* Management of clothing (donning–doffing and manipulating clothing fasteners); tolerance for wearing different fabrics and changes in seasonal clothing
	Bathing: Performing range of motion, integrating sensory input, and maintaining postural stability for bathing tasks; bathing environment (shower vs. bath); bathing equipment (infant bathtub or shower chair)
	Grooming and hygiene: Awareness of appearance (overall presentation of cleanliness); participation in trimming fingernails, washing hands, brushing hair, cleaning face
	Toileting: Attention and postural stability for seated tasks (sitting on toilet); frequency and consistency of bowel movements; ability to position for diaper changes
	Self-feeding: Using feeding tube, bottle, cup, straw, and utensils; recording diet; performing range of motion and coordination; integrating sensory input for manipulating food and drink
	Functional mobility: Mobility throughout evaluation, including rolling, sitting, crawling, and walking, as well as ability to transition across different surfaces; use of adaptive mobility equipment, such as wheelchair or walker
	Personal device care: Coordination and tolerance in donning and doffing personal devices, such as orthotics and hearing aids
Community safety and participation	Safety awareness during transitions in parking lots and in the community; ability to respond to name in the community and follow other emergency procedures
Leisure	Ability to pursue preferred toys and favorite activities; ability to engage in variety of activities in addition to electronics
Play	Play initiation and self-regulation; ability to explore new play material and develop imaginary play schemes; interaction with others while playing
Preschool and child care participation	Ability to functionally attend to learning and play activities; ability to maintain self-regulation during transitions
Religious and spiritual activities, participation, and expression	Ability to attend to seated tasks and integrate sensory input during spiritual routines
Sleep	Activities for sleep preparation and bedtime routine; sleep schedule (amount of time spent sleeping at night and during naps); sleep cycles (ability to fall asleep and sustain sleep state)
Social	Ability to engage in reciprocal play and activities with family members and peers; ability to respond to verbal and nonverbal communication from others and express oneself

Note. ADLs = activities of daily living.

to implement interventions similar to the way they will occur in the person's natural setting.

Intervention theories and approaches in health care

Depending on the performance skills and occupations identified by the child and family as problematic, different frames of reference may be used during intervention to address occupation performance and participation. Sensory processing affects participation in education, leisure, social participation, mealtime, and sleep (Ismael et al., 2018), and sensory modifications to the child's natural environments can support participation (Bodison & Parham, 2018).

Several theories are available to occupational therapy providers addressing a range of performance skills and client factors during intervention. Neurodevelopment and motor acquisition theories guide upper-limb training for achieving goals determined to be meaningful to the child and family (Sakzewski et al., 2009). Applying cognitive process theories when working with children and partnering with families promotes self-awareness, organization, and joint attention while developing independence in daily activities (Frolek Clark & Schlabach, 2013; Tanner et al., 2015). Relationship theories further assist occupational therapy practitioners who are working with children and their families on social interaction skills. Likewise, practitioners should also consider Synactive Development Theory and the interaction of dynamic systems, because children present with varying motor abilities and behavioral responses (Maltese et al., 2017). Theories for addressing performance skills during intervention are outlined in Table 24.4.

In health care settings, occupational therapy practitioners may simultaneously use a "modify" compensatory approach and an "establish" approach when providing intervention services (AOTA, 2020). While attempting to develop (habilitation) or restore (rehabilitation) skills to achieve developmental progress, practitioners may use a compensatory approach to support more immediate gains in occupational participation. The practitioner selects the intervention approach that best fits the person's (child's and family's) needs. The practitioner may emphasize motor skills, process skills, or social interaction skills during the intervention.

When addressing developmental conditions in the health care setting, occupational therapy practitioners often need to balance compensatory and remediation approaches to support children in increased occupation participation while promoting development. Additional approaches may be warranted, depending on the results of the evaluation (AOTA, 2020). As intervention is implemented, practitioners may use specific strategies to support the intervention approach. Strategies introduced through education and training during the intervention are expected to be carried over in the home setting through parent or caregiver coaching.

Coach the caregiver

Family-centered practice is an ethical obligation supported by legal mandates when occupational therapy practitioners provide developmental services to children across health care settings (Kuo et al., 2012). As discussed in previous chapters, families play a critical role in the daily development of the young child and should be engaged throughout the occupational process in health care settings. ***Parent coaching***, when the practitioner collaboratively guides the caregiver to support the child's occupational performance in goal areas, is one intervention tool the practitioner may use to engage parents and caregivers (King et al., 2017).

Health care services are offered in settings where numerous members of the family may be present; it is important to engage other family members, including siblings, grandparents, and relatives, as they are available. Family members play a critical role in the child's daily life and natural social context. Cognitive and occupation-based interventions in collaboration with families and other professionals can improve self-regulation across contexts (Pfeiffer et al., 2018).

Because parents are collaboratively engaged from evaluation to discharge, occupational therapy practitioners have numerous and ongoing opportunities to understand the evolving family milieu and provide education to parents. They can choose from a continuum of approaches to address family needs in health care settings, from education and information resources to service coordination and support groups (King et al., 2017). However, active participation is best achieved through parent coaching (Kessler & Graham, 2015). Through parent coaching, parents have the opportunity to learn more about their child's difficulties while emphasizing their strengths to support their performance in daily activities important to the family. Parent coaching is important for decreasing parent stress and increasing child performance (Miller-Kuhaneck & Watling, 2018).

TABLE 24.4.   Theories for Addressing Performance Skills

PERFORMANCE SKILL AREA WITH EXAMPLES	THEORIES
Motor skills - Coordination, posture, balance - Movement functions (reflexes) - Muscle functions (strength, range of motion) - Neuromuscular functions	- Motor Skill Acquisition (Case-Smith et al., 2013; Zwicker & Harris, 2009) - Biomechanical (Gates et al., 2016)
Process skills - Safety awareness - Self-regulation and arousal - Attention	- Cognitive Orientation to daily Occupational Performance (Dawson et al., 2017) - Social–Emotional Learning (Arbesman et al., 2013)
Social interaction skills - Approaches, starts - Takes turns - Accommodates	- DIRFloortime® (Pajareya & Nopmaneejumruslers, 2011) - Relationship-based interventions (Case-Smith, 2013)

Video modeling

Video modeling can be a helpful strategy used during intervention in health care settings that can be easily integrated in other settings and a home program. ***Video*** *modeling* involves children watching a model of themselves or another individual performing a behavior or activity to learn and imitate the model in self-help, social, and play activities. These types of interventions have been found to be more beneficial for individuals who are able to both attend to the model and imitate modeled behavior immediately as well as after a time delay (Drysdale et al., 2015).

Sensory Stories® and Social Stories™

Sensory Stories® and Social Stories™ are individualized stories written to instruct a child. *Sensory Stories* teach the reader sensory strategies to increase participation in daily activities. *Social Stories* describe required behaviors in specific social situations. Research has shown Sensory Stories can be effective in reducing target behaviors in a preschool class by cueing use of sensory strategies (Marr et al., 2007). Social Stories can be a useful tool for teaching appropriate ways to overcome social behaviors and participate in social situations (Thompson & Johnston, 2013).

Review Intervention

Occupational therapists should begin to consider the parameters for discharge with the child and family during the evaluation.

Consistently monitor progress

Progress monitoring is the ongoing assessment of a child's performance and response to intervention activities to determine progress toward established goals. As individual contextual interventions are implemented, it is critical that the occupational therapy practitioner monitor progress. During the intervention process, evidence is generated as the child responds to intervention. Subjective reports of improved functional performance, objective measurements during intervention, and artifacts produced during intervention are important to document progress (Tomlin & Dougherty, 2014). It is important to observe and monitor this evidence to evaluate the outcomes of the intervention (Bennett et al., 2016).

Additionally, progress monitoring should occur throughout intervention to ensure intervention remains within payer guidelines (i.e., insurance certification period). Data collection may rely on narrative review of documentation or use of a summary table. It is important to collect data in a manner that documents progress toward established goals and allows the effectiveness of specific interventions to be determined. Progress may be monitored with daily notes, weekly or monthly progress notes, or both. See Chapter 6, "Best Practices in Data-Based Decision Making," for more information.

Discharge

Discharge may occur when goals are met or when the child is no longer receiving skilled therapy. For example, if a caregiver can be educated on and carry out activities from sessions, the child is no longer receiving skilled therapy. When treating children with a developmental diagnosis, occupational therapy practitioners also may need to consider when the child has reached their maximum potential as an individual and given their diagnosis, which may be different than the potential appropriate for the child's age. In health care settings, discharge may also occur because of limited insurance authorization for services; however, this should be anticipated when the intervention plan is established. Other reasons for discharge may include limited or no progress resulting from poor attendance, poor adherence to the home program, or a child's decreased ability to participate in sessions resulting from underlying medical conditions or changes in medical condition or behaviors.

SUMMARY

Occupational therapy services in health care settings support healthy occupation development and participation for children with developmental diagnoses. Children with developmental disabilities are more likely to receive health care services because they may have comorbid diagnoses, client factors, and performance skill deficits that require them to be seen in different health care settings. Therefore, occupational therapy practitioners working in health care should be prepared to plan, implement, and review intervention for a wide range of unique needs for this population. The intervention emphasis depends on the health care setting and payment source.

Engaging families is critical for the success and carryover of occupational therapy in all health care settings. Occupational therapy practitioners work on interprofessional teams to provide services promoting participation in areas prioritized by the child and family using a variety of intervention models and approaches. Systematic progress monitoring is important for providing effective services and making decisions.

REFERENCES

American Occupational Therapy Association. (2020). Occupational therapy practice framework: Domain and process (4th ed.). *American Journal of Occupational Therapy, 74*(Suppl. 2), 7412410010. https://doi.org/10.5014/ajot.2020.74S2001

Arbesman, M., Bazyk, S., & Nochajski, S. M. (2013). Systematic review of occupational therapy and mental health promotion, prevention, and intervention for children and youth. *American Journal of Occupational Therapy, 67*, e120–e130. https://doi.org/10.5014/ajot.2013.008359

Bennett, S., Whitehead, M., Eames, S., Fleming, J., Low, S., & Caldwell, E. (2016). Building capacity for knowledge translation in occupational therapy: Learning through participatory action research. *BMC Medical Education, 16*(1), 257. https://doi.org/10.1186/s12909-016-0771-5

Bodison, S., & Parham, D. (2018). Specific sensory techniques and sensory environmental modifications for children and youth with sensory integration difficulties: A systematic review. *American Journal of Occupational Therapy, 72*, 7201190040. https://doi.org/10.5014/ajot.2018.029413

Boyle, C., Boulet, S., Schieve, L., Cohen, R., Blumberg, S., Yeargin-Allsopp, M., . . . Kogan, M. (2011). Trends in the prevalence of developmental disabilities in US children, 1997–2008. *Pediatrics, 127*, 1034–1042. https://doi.org/10.1542/peds.2010-2989

Case-Smith, J. (2013). Systematic review of interventions to promote social–emotional development in young children with or at risk for disability. *American Journal of Occupational Therapy, 67,* 395–404. https://doi.org/10.5014/ajot.2013.004713

Case-Smith, J., Frolek Clark, G., & Schlabach, T. (2013). Systematic review of interventions used in occupational therapy to promote motor performance for children ages birth–5 years. *American Journal of Occupational Therapy, 67,* 413–424. https://doi.org/10.5014/ajot.2013.005959

Centers for Disease Control and Prevention. (2019, May 28). *Learn the signs. Act early.* https://www.cdc.gov/ncbddd/actearly/index.html

Dawson, D. R., McEwen, S. E., & Polatajko, H. J. (Eds.). (2017). *Cognitive Orientation to daily Occupational Performance: Using the CO–OP Approach™ to enable participation across the lifespan.* AOTA Press.

Drysdale, B., Lee, C., Anderson, A., & Moore, D. (2015). Using video modeling incorporating animation to teach toileting to two children with autism spectrum disorder. *Journal of Developmental & Physical Disabilities, 27,* 149–165. https://doi.org/10.1007/s10882-014-9405-1

Federal Interagency Forum on Child and Family Statistics. (2018, September). *America's children: Key national indicators of well-being.* Government Printing Office.

Frolek Clark, G., & Schlabach, T. (2013). Systematic review of occupational therapy interventions to improve cognitive development in children ages birth–5 years. *American Journal of Occupational Therapy, 67,* 425–430. https://doi.org/10.5014/ajot.2013.006163

Gates, D., Walters, L., Cowley, J., Wilken, J., & Resnik, L. (2016). Range of motion requirements for upper-limb activities of daily living. *American Journal of Occupational Therapy, 70,* 7001350010. https://doi.org/10.5014/ajot.2016.015487

Gee, B. M., Lloyd, K., Devine, N., Tyrrell, E., Evans, T., Hill, R., . . . Magalogo, K. (2016). Dosage parameters in pediatric outcome studies reported in 9 peer-reviewed occupational therapy journals from 2008 to 2014: A content analysis. *Rehabilitation Research and Practice, 2016,* 3580789. https://doi.org/10.1155/2016/3580789

Ismael, N., Lawson, L., & Hartwell, J. (2018). Relationship between sensory processing and participation in daily occupations for children with autism spectrum disorder: A systematic review of studies that used Dunn's sensory processing framework. *American Journal of Occupational Therapy, 72,* 7203205030. https://doi.org/10.5014/ajot.2018.024075

Kessler, D., & Graham, F. (2015). The use of coaching in occupational therapy: An integrative review. *Australian Occupational Therapy Journal, 62,* 160–176. https://doi.org/10.1111/1440-1630.12175

King, G., Williams, L., & Hahn Goldberg, S. (2017). Family-oriented services in pediatric rehabilitation: A scoping review and framework to promote parent and family wellness. *Child: Care, Health and Development, 43,* 334–347. https://doi.org/10.1111/cch.12435

Kuo, D., Houtrow, A., Arango, P., Kuhlthau, K., Simmons, J., & Neff, J. (2012). Family-centered care: Current applications and future directions in pediatric health care. *Maternal and Child Health Journal, 16,* 297–305. https://doi.org/10.1007/s10995-011-0751-7

Lavallée, A., De Clifford-Faugère, G., Garcia, C., Oviedo, A., Héon, M., & Aita, M. (2019). Part 2: Practice and research recommendations for quality developmental care in the NICU. *Journal of Neonatal Nursing, 25,* 160–165. https://doi.org/10.1016/j.jnn.2019.03.008

Law, M., & Dunbar, S. (2007). Person-Environment-Occupation Model in Occupational Therapy. In S. Dunbar (Ed.), *Models for Intervention with Children and Families* (pp. 27–49). Slack.

Maltese, A., Gallai, B., Marotta, R., Lavano, F., Lavano, S. M., Tripi, G., . . . Salerno, M. (2017). The synactive theory of development: The keyword for neurodevelopmental disorders. *Acta Medica Mediterranea, 33,* 1257–1263. https://www.actamedicamediterranea.com/archive/2017/special-issue-2/the-synactive-theory-of-development-the-keyword-for-neurodevelopmental-disorders

Marr, D., Mika, H., Miraglia, J., Roerig, M., & Sinnott, R. (2007). The effect of sensory stories on targeted behaviors in preschool children with autism. *Physical and Occupational Therapy in Pediatrics, 27,* 63–79. https://doi.org/10.1080/J006v27n01_05

Miller-Kuhaneck, H., & Watling, R. (2018). Parental or teacher education and coaching to support function and participation of children and youth with sensory processing and sensory integration challenges: A systematic review. *American Journal of Occupational Therapy, 72,* 7201190030. https://doi.org/10.5014/ajot.2018.029017

Pajareya, K., & Nopmaneejumruslers, K. (2011). A pilot randomized controlled trial of DIR/Floortime™ parent training intervention for pre-school children with autistic spectrum disorders. *Autism, 15,* 563–577. https://doi.org/10.1177/1362361310386502

Palisano, R. J. (2012). Activity-focused motor interventions for children with neurological conditions. In R. J. Palisano (Ed.), *Movement sciences: Transfer of knowledge into pediatric therapy practice* (pp. 91–120). Routledge.

Persch, A., Braveman, B., & Metzler, C. (2013). P4 medicine and pediatric occupational therapy. *American Journal of Occupational Therapy, 67,* 383–388. https://doi.org/10.5014/ajot.2013.674002

Pfeiffer, B., Frolek Clark, G., & Arbesman, M. (2018). Effectiveness of cognitive and occupation-based interventions for children with challenges in sensory processing and integration: A systematic review. *American Journal of Occupational Therapy, 72,* 7201190020. https://doi.org/10.5014/ajot.2018.028233

Pressler, J., Turnage-Carrier, C., & Kenner, C. (2010). Developmental care: State of the science. In C. Kenner & J. McGrath (Eds.), *Developmental care of newborns and infants* (2nd ed., pp. 1–17). National Association of Neonatal Nurses.

Sakzewski, L., Ziviani, J., & Boyd, R. (2009). Systematic review and meta-analysis of therapeutic management of upper-limb dysfunction in children with congenital hemiplegia. *Pediatrics, 123,* e1111–e1122. https://doi.org/10.1542/peds.2008-3335

Schoen, S., Miller, L., & Flanagan, J. (2018). A retrospective pre–post treatment study of occupational therapy intervention for children with sensory processing challenges. *Open Journal of Occupational Therapy, 6*(1), 4. https://doi.org/10.15453/2168-6408.1367

Simeonsson, R., & Lee, A. (2018). *International Classification of Functioning, Disability and Health*—children and youth: A universal resource for education and care of children. In S. Castro & O. Palikara (Eds.), *An emerging approach for education and care: Implementing a worldwide classification of functioning and disability* (pp. 5–22). Routledge.

Tanner, K., Hand, B. N., O'Toole, G., & Lane, A. E. (2015). Effectiveness of interventions to improve social participation, play, leisure, and restricted and repetitive behaviors in people with autism spectrum disorder: A systematic review. *American Journal of Occupational Therapy, 69,* 6905180010. https://doi.org/10.5014/ajot.2015.017806

Thompson, R. M., & Johnston, S. (2013). Use of social stories to improve self-regulation in children with autism spectrum disorders. *Physical & Occupational Therapy in Pediatrics, 33,* 271–284. https://doi.org/10.3109/01942638.2013.768322

Tomlin, G., & Dougherty, D. (2014). Decision-making and sources of evidence in occupational therapy and other health professions: Evidence-informed practice. *International Journal of Health Professions, 1,* 13–19. https://doi.org/10.2478/ijhp-2014-0001

Valvano, J., & Rapport, M. J. (2006). Activity-focused motor interventions for infants and young children with neurological

conditions. *Infants & Young Children, 19,* 292–307. https://doi.org/10.1097/00001163-200610000-00003

World Health Organization. (2007). *International classification of functioning, disability and health: Children and youth version (ICF-CY).* Author.

Zwicker, J. G., & Harris, S. R. (2009). A reflection on motor learning theory in pediatric occupational therapy practice. *Canadian Journal of Occupational Therapy, 76,* 29–37. https://doi.org/10.1177/000841740907600108

Best Practices in Health Care Intervention for Acquired Conditions

Kaitlin Hagen, MOT, OTR/L; Rebecca Martin, OTR/L, OTD; and Alaena McCool, MS, OTR/L, CPAM

25

KEY TERMS AND CONCEPTS

- Acquired brain injuries
- Acquired conditions
- Autonomic dysreflexia
- Brain tumors
- Burns
- Chemical burns
- Child and family education
- Childhood stroke
- Compensatory training
- Decreased bone density
- Diffuse axonal injury
- Dysautonomia
- Electrical burns
- Encephalitis
- First-degree burn
- Glasgow Coma Scale
- Habilitation
- Hemorrhagic stroke
- Infectious diseases
- Interprofessional collaborative practices
- Ischemic stroke
- Joint preservation
- Mental health conditions
- Mental status
- Neuroplasticity
- Nontraumatic brain injuries
- Orthopedic precautions
- Orthostatic hypotension
- Perinatal stroke
- Physical trauma injuries
- Radiation burns
- Rehabilitation
- Restore function
- Scoliosis
- Second-degree burn
- Spinal cord injuries
- Stroke
- Thermal burns
- Third-degree burn
- Traumatic brain injuries
- Viral meningitis

OVERVIEW

Occupational therapy practitioners have a large role in serving children with acquired conditions across a variety of settings. (*Note. Occupational therapy practitioner* refers to both occupational therapists and occupational therapy assistants.) This chapter discusses interventions aimed at children with *acquired conditions* (i.e., conditions that are not congenital or developmental and arise during childhood as the result of injury or illness). The conditions most commonly seen in pediatric practice include nontraumatic or traumatic brain injuries (TBIs), including stroke and diffuse axonal injuries; spinal cord injuries (SCIs) and related disorders; burns; cancer; physical trauma; and mental health issues.

Occupational therapy practitioners must understand the diagnosis, mechanism of injury, and progression since injury to get a holistic picture of the child's strengths and needs. Acquired condition diagnoses offer a wide range of symptoms, severity, and prognosis. The wide range in premorbid status and presentation creates significant heterogeneity in this population. Beyond the physical and cognitive aspects of the child, acquired conditions affect a child's quality of life, social and community reintegration, family and peer dynamics, and environment. The progress made in therapy can be quick or slow, which the practitioner can adjust by grading activities up or down to offer the just-right challenge to achieve the child's and family's goals.

Common types of acquired conditions, population statistics, and the role of occupational therapy are addressed in this section.

Brain Injuries

In a review of literature, worldwide incidences of pediatric TBI ranged from 47 to 280 per 100,000 children. Rates of hospital admission vary widely and are higher in the United States than in other countries (Dewan et al., 2016). Boys have a higher rate of TBIs compared with girls. Zaloshnja et al. (2008) estimated that 145,000 children from birth to 19 years of age are living with lasting impairments from a TBI. These issues affect the child as well as the child's family and community (Zaloshnja et al., 2008). Brain injury can result in a wide range of deficits and symptoms. Children with a brain injury require a comprehensive, neurologically focused assessment (see Chapter 23, "Best Practices in Evaluation in Health Care Settings"), which includes the child's past and current cognition, behaviors, movement, sensation, vision, hearing, and emotional functioning.

Causes of brain injuries

Acquired brain injuries (ABIs) can be categorized by their etiology: traumatic or nontraumatic. According to the Brain Injury Association of America (n.d.), *nontraumatic brain injuries* cause damage to the brain by internal factors, such as lack of oxygen, pressure from tumors, and exposure to toxins, whereas *TBIs* result from an alteration in the brain caused by an external force. ABIs include stroke, aneurysm, tumors, and infectious diseases such as meningitis. TBIs may be caused by falls, motor vehicle accidents, sports injuries, and assaults. TBIs are the leading cause of disability and death among children from birth to age 4 years, with injuries primarily from falls, abuse, and motor vehicle accidents (Araki et al., 2017).

Classification of brain injuries

Understanding the differences in the types of brain injuries, as well as a typical brain injury progression, may help occupational therapy practitioners develop measurable and reliable goals as the child is healing. The *Glasgow Coma Scale* (GCS; Reith et al., 2016) is the most common measure to describe level of consciousness after brain injury (Mesfin & Taylor, 2019). The GCS assesses eye opening, verbal response, and motor response to determine the severity of an acute injury. An initial GCS score helps indicate the severity of injury to practitioners, who then assess, set goals, and plan for the patient.

An ABI may also be described by the location and mechanism of damage. *Diffuse axonal injury* (DAI), common in car accidents, results from a shearing effect in the white matter of the brain. Most often, these tracts are affected in the brainstem and corpus collosum. Nearly 10% of brain injuries include some amount of even mild DAI (Mesfin & Taylor, 2019). A mild DAI may be similar to a concussion, with symptoms including headaches, dizziness, fatigue, and vomiting. A child with a more severe DAI may present in a coma and remain in a vegetative state.

During the acute management of DAI, treatment is focused on stabilizing the child by providing medical and neurological care to constantly monitor and reassess the child as needed. Children in this setting may have additional neurological management to consider, including intracranial pressure monitoring to measure the pressure in the brain during the acute phase of hospitalization. Once the child is stable, medically and neurologically, occupational therapy can begin at the bedside and move to an inpatient, outpatient, or home setting to progress the child toward their functional goals.

Pediatric stroke

Stroke is a focal brain infarction or hemorrhage with acute-onset neurological signs and symptoms (Ferriero et al., 2019). The stroke incidence among children is about 3–25 per 100,000 children per year (Ferriero et al., 2019). Children with stroke present differently than adults, and often there is a delay in the diagnosis, especially in the neonatal phase (Tsze & Valente, 2011). Pediatric stroke is one of the top 10 causes of death among children, including infants, toddlers, adolescents, and teens (American Stroke Association, 2020).

Strokes can be classified as ischemic, hemorrhagic, or both. *Ischemic stroke* occurs from an infarction or occlusion of blood vessels, resulting in oxygen loss, whereas a *hemorrhagic stroke* is a result of bleeding from an arterial rupture. Certain medical conditions, including sickle cell disease, moyamoya disease, arterial dissection, autoimmune disorders, congenital heart disease, and blood clotting disorders, are all associated with stroke in children. *Perinatal stroke* occurs from 28 weeks gestation to 28 days of life. Any stroke from age 1 month to 18 years is referred to as *childhood stroke* (Ferriero et al., 2019).

Early indicators of common clinical presentations of stroke include hemiplegia and seizures. Infants present with lethargy, apnea spells, or hypotonia. Toddlers often have increased crying, sleepiness, irritability, feeding difficulties, vomiting, and sepsislike symptoms with cold extremities. Older children's symptoms are comparable to adults' symptoms of hemiparesis, language and speech difficulties, visual deficits, and headache (Tsze & Valente, 2011). Acute management of this diagnosis is similar to other brain injuries, with medical and neurological management of symptoms as well as possible surgical intervention.

Tumors and infections

An ABI may also be caused by tumor or infection. *Brain tumors* are an abnormal growth of cells in the brain that may be cancerous (i.e., malignant) or noncancerous (i.e., benign) and are the second most common type of cancer among children (National Cancer Institute, 2019). Although these tumors rarely spread to other tissues, malignant tumors grow quickly and press on areas of the brain. Both types of tumors may cause headaches; nausea; vomiting; loss of balance; trouble walking; problems with vision, hearing, or speech; increased sleepiness; personality changes; seizures; and changes in infant head sizes. Treatment for pediatric brain tumors depends on the location, size, and development of the tumor as well as the child's age.

Possible interventions include a biopsy of the tumor, surgery to remove all or part of the brain tumor, radiation, and chemotherapy. Postradiation or chemotherapy side effects may include cognitive deficits and continued symptoms of the tumor secondary to the brain still being swollen or the tumor not being fully removed. Intervention during the acute phase involves ensuring the child is medically stable. Rehabilitation begins when the child is out of the acute, medically unstable phase. Close communication with the child's family, the medical team, and the child is critical before occupational therapy intervention. The occupational therapy practitioner may focus on cognitive and physical development, depending on the severity of the child's symptoms.

Infectious diseases include viruses and bacterial infections, such as meningitis and encephalitis, that may alter the child's cognitive function. Meningitis is inflammation of brain tissues or meninges; it can be bacterial or viral. Risk factors include recent infections, travel to areas where bacterial meningitis is common, serious head injury, immune system problems, cochlear implants, and certain anatomic abnormalities (Kaplan & Pentima, 2019). *Viral meningitis* is commonly caused by an enterovirus. In the United States it is typically seen from June to October and can be spread through airborne droplets, direct contact, and animal or bug bites (Kaplan & Pentima, 2019). Symptoms among newborns include decreased feeding needs, vomiting, diarrhea, rash, stiff neck, irritability, restlessness, and lethargy.

Older children may experience a fever, headache, nausea, vomiting, confusion, stiff neck, and light sensitivity.

Bacterial meningitis is a medical emergency that is treated in the hospital with a blood culture, lumbar puncture to analyze the cerebral spinal fluid, and imaging. Bacterial infections need to be treated quickly, typically with intravenous antibiotics; however, there can still be long-term complications, even with treatment. Most children recover from both types of meningitis, but there is a chance of brain damage that can cause long-term complications, such as deafness, developmental and learning disabilities, spastic or paralyzed muscles, and seizures (Kaplan & Pentima, 2019).

Similar in its presentation, *encephalitis* is inflammation of the brain by a virus, fungus, or parasite, with symptoms of altered mental status, confusion, disorientation, fever, and seizures (National Institute of Neurological Disorders and Stroke, 2018). Mild flulike symptoms are common, with severe complications, including muscle weakness, partial paralysis in upper or lower extremities; impaired executive functioning skills; and seizures. Treatment can include antiviral drugs; however, no specific treatment is currently available. Once the child becomes medically stable, rehabilitation can begin with a team approach. The occupational therapy practitioner's role is to treat the symptoms and progress the child toward their developmental milestones if delays are noted, through cognitive and physical rehabilitation.

Spinal Cord Injuries

SCIs can be traumatic or nontraumatic in the pediatric population. Injuries can result in tetraplegia or paraplegia and may be complete or incomplete. Nontraumatic SCIs can be acquired by spinal stroke, transverse myelitis, acute flaccid myelitis, or other causes (e.g., surgical, tumor). According to the American Spinal Injury Association (ASIA; n.d.), 20% of SCIs occur in children and adolescents. In early childhood, the rate of SCI is higher among girls compared with boys, which changes with age. Younger children are more likely to sustain complete injuries when compared with older adults.

When working with children with SCIs, occupational therapy practitioners' focus is on recovery but also on the secondary effects of an injury. Research indicates that 90% of children with an SCI before puberty will develop scoliosis (ASIA, n.d.). Skin integrity, urinary tract infections, autonomic function, and atrophy of the muscles should all be addressed during occupational therapy.

The plasticity of children's neurological system can help them to have a faster and improved recovery (ASIA, n.d.) and can be a critical part of their recovery when receiving a neurological diagnosis. Additional information on plasticity is addressed later in this chapter. Acute management is focused on medical stability, including stabilizing blood pressure and mean arterial pressure before initiation of therapy. Therapy is critical in the early phase of the acute hospitalization to educate the child and family about the benefits of getting out of bed, preventing pressure wounds, maintaining range of motion (ROM), and providing information about the next step in the rehabilitation phase.

Burns

Burns are a common diagnosis seen in the pediatric population. Among children, 75% of burns could have been prevented (e.g., car accident, house fire; Children's National Hospital, n.d.). *Burns* are a type of injury caused by heat, which can be thermal, chemical, electrical, or caused by electromagnetic energy (i.e., radiation). *Thermal burns* are due to external heat sources, such as hot metals, scalding liquids, steam, or flames. *Chemical burns* are caused by strong acids, alkaline detergents, or solvents that come into contact with the skin or eyes, whereas *electrical burns* are from electrical currents (Children's National Hospital, n.d.). *Radiation burns* are caused by prolonged exposure to ultraviolet rays of the sun or other sources, such as X rays. Burns and fires are the fifth most common cause of accidental death among children and adults. However, the rate of burns among children has decreased over the years with the help of increased safety provisions, such as smoke detectors and consumer product flammability guidelines (Johns Hopkins Medicine, 2019).

Burns are classified by cause and severity. This classification is useful for occupational therapy practitioners to define their assessment, interventions, and modifications. A *first-degree burn* affects only the outer layer of the skin and presents with blisters. These blisters should not be popped, and the burn usually heals itself within 3–7 days. A *second-degree burn* affects the outer layer of skin (epidermis) and inner layer of skin (dermis). Most heal within 2–3 weeks; however, deeper second-degree burns take more than 3 weeks to heal and may require a skin graft. With a *third-degree burn,* immediate medical attention is needed, and the burn affects the outer and inner layers of skin. The burn may look shiny and white, and the child may not report much pain because of damaged nerves. These burns require skin grafts and 3–6 weeks to heal (Children's National Hospital, n.d.).

Working alongside the medical team, occupational therapy practitioners are consulted when the child is ready to tolerate and is appropriate for a splint or cast as well as a ROM protocol. Once the practitioner initiates this treatment in the acute phase, the parent or caregiver is highly involved to ensure good carryover of the ROM protocol. The practitioner also monitors for skin breakdown from the splint and ensures proper healing. If changes arise, the practitioner notifies the medical team to ensure proper healing. As the child is ready to discharge, the practitioner educates the family on making environmental modifications to ensure access and independence at home and promote healing to decrease the long-term effects of the burn. Outpatient therapy is typically recommended to continue monitoring the splint or cast as well as increase the ROM of the affected extremity to progress independence in ADLs.

Cancer

Cancer is the second leading cause of death among children ages 1–14 years (American Cancer Society [ACS], 2019). Leukemia, brain, and other nervous system cancers rank as the leading types of childhood cancer. It is estimated that 11,050 children between birth and age 14 years will be diagnosed with new cases of cancer in 2020, with

1,190 deaths occurring in 2020 (ACS, 2019). Survival rates have improved over the last 30 years as a result of new and improved treatments available, with survival rates higher than 80% among children (ACS, 2019). However, these rates vary depending on type and stage of cancer, patient age, and other characteristics.

Acute management of cancer is focused mostly on medical treatments for survival. Many of these treatments, including radiation therapy, chemotherapy, and immunotherapy, can affect children well past their treatment for the cancer itself (Sparrow, 2020). A child's chance of having these secondary effects depends on the type of cancer, its location, and what treatment they received. The child may have higher risk for second cancers or a different cancer that occurs at least 2 months after primary cancer treatment. Occupational therapy practitioners provide holistic interventions and assess organs, tissues, body function, development, emotions, cognition, and social adjustment (National Cancer Institute, 2020).

Communication with the medical team through chart reviews or daily rounds is critical for occupational therapy practitioners to stay informed of lab results and provide appropriate interventions for the child. For example, if the child has an extremely low platelet count, strengthening activities or intervention out of bed may be contraindicated. Practitioners must understand the medical and therapeutic guidelines when treating this population in the acute hospitalization phase. Most of these guidelines are specific to the practitioner's hospital or attending physician. After the initial hospitalization phase, rehabilitation in the home, outpatient, or inpatient setting may be recommended for the child to build strength and endurance to get back to daily activities, roles, and community involvement. Continued collaboration with the caregivers, the child, and the medical team is needed to appropriately progress the child back to functional independence.

Physical Trauma

Physical trauma injuries are a leading cause of death and disability among children ages 1–18 years in the United States (American Academy of Pediatrics, 2016). One in six children present to the emergency room each year for trauma-related injuries (McFadyen et al., 2012). *Physical trauma injuries* include orthopedic injuries from falls, sports injuries, and motor vehicle injuries. Acute management of these injuries often happens in a trauma hospital, with the medical team working on stabilizing the child medically. Once the child is medically stable and appropriate for therapy, the occupational therapy practitioner communicates with the child's medical team, which may include orthopedics, cardiology, neurology, and other medical team members, depending on the severity of the injury. Communication is key with these team members to ensure medical and neurological stability, proper ROM, weight bearing, and level of activity appropriateness.

Occupational therapy practitioners then follow the medical team's protocols for out-of-bed mobility, ROM if there is an affected extremity, and strengthening, and they contact providers if a discrepancy is noted in the medical chart. The practitioner provides constant education to the child and family on the medical doctor's protocols and discharge recommendations. If psychosocial factors are present, the practitioner may request a referral to social work or another type of psychology provider to ensure proper follow-up from the trauma the child has experienced.

At discharge, the child may be recommended to continue rehabilitation at an inpatient level before going home or may be discharged home with home or outpatient services, with the goal of reintegrating the child back into their own community and leisure activities. The occupational therapy practitioner assists the case manager in ensuring a safe discharge home while the child is in the hospital setting. Overall, occupational therapy is critical to continue to promote healing, decrease the psychological impact of the injury, and help with return to preferred activities through inpatient, outpatient, or home therapies, depending on the severity of the injury (McFadyen et al., 2012).

Mental Health Conditions

Mental health diagnoses are becoming more common at younger ages as further research and awareness about mental health increases (Whitney & Peterson, 2019). Unlike other acquired conditions, *mental health conditions* change the way a child learns, behaves, or handles emotions and causes stress and role disruption. They can be diagnosed in early childhood but may not be caused by a significant event. Though not all mental health conditions are acquired, common pediatric mental health diagnoses may include emotional and behavioral diagnoses, disruptive behaviors, and attention-related diagnoses. Among very young children, extreme disruptive behavior, increased tantrums, and difficulty meeting social–emotional developmental milestones may be indicators that mental health interventions could be needed. Poverty and low socioeconomic status increase a child's risk for developing these disorders secondary to limited access to the health care system or limited education about the diagnosis (Center on the Developing Child, 2007). Often children are not diagnosed until they are school age.

For mental health diagnoses, the focus of occupational therapy not only is with the child and managing behaviors but also involves educating the parents or caregivers of the child on how to respond to these behaviors as well as provide carryover in other settings. This approach helps to manage the behaviors and prevent them from increasing (Ogundele, 2018). Occupational therapy practitioners can work with children in school, outpatient, home health, and possibly inpatient settings if needed. Communication is important for carryover of behavioral protocols and goals to help the child achieve developmental and age-appropriate milestones.

The majority of children who are diagnosed with mental health conditions will require lifelong care, and occupational therapy practitioners need to consider the transitions children will go through during their lifetime. Young children with mental health conditions may develop mentally, physically, and emotionally differently than a typical child because of the way they explore and access their environment. Working with an interdisciplinary team to identify, address these changes, and meet the child and family's needs at the child's current developmental stage, as well as prepare the family and child for the next transitional stage, is critical.

ESSENTIAL CONSIDERATIONS

After understanding the child's diagnosis, occupational therapy practitioners must also consider the child's current age and developmental milestones achieved before the onset of diagnosis, as well consider adjustments to the child's natural environment, including home, school, and community.

Habilitation Versus Rehabilitation

Occupational therapy practitioners can use many different frames of reference for treatment for pediatric patients. Since the mid-1900s, practitioners have focused on the idea of rehabilitation versus habilitation. *Rehabilitation* is restoring skills that were lost. *Habilitation* is intervention for a child who is learning skills for the first time. Habilitation may be necessary for children born with an injury or diagnosis as well as children who acquire a condition before they have completed critical developmental stages. This is an important factor for practitioners to keep in mind during interventions, because a child's nervous system may not have knowledge of what "normal" or "near normal" patterns are. It may be beneficial to guide the child's biomechanical structures to help them learn normal patterns.

Occupational therapy practitioners may need to balance teaching a normal pattern with compensatory training. Whereas traditional therapy often teaches compensations to make a child independent, newer models teach the idea of retraining for long-term recovery. Often both concepts can be worked into interventions with children who have acquired conditions. For example, when working with a child with a cervical-level SCI, practitioners may provide the child with adaptive utensils to promote independence with self-feeding and simultaneously work on grasp and release during therapy, with the long-term goal being that the child can use typical utensils.

Plasticity

For children who have neurological conditions, such as brain injuries or SCIs, the plasticity of the brain and spinal cord among young children can actually enhance recovery. Recovery after an injury for a child at any age stems from changes in *neuroplasticity.* Young neuronal circuits have the capacity to make structural and functional changes on the basis of experience (Su et al., 2016). The brain adjusts after acquiring an injury through remyelination and reorganization of circuits (Dennis et al., 2013).

However, without appropriate rehabilitation or habilitation to learn the right patterns, children may learn maladaptive behaviors. There are critical times as the brain is developing that may influence its plasticity after the child acquires an injury. Intervention after an acquired neurological injury is critical to enhance the plastic reorganization of the child.

Age-Specific Considerations

Although the focus of interventions for children may be driven by their diagnosis, occupational therapy practitioners should consider a client-centered, holistic approach. This involves considering the child's age and interests.

Children acquire conditions at different ages and in different stages of development and therefore require different goals. For example, a child who is age 2 years is focused on parallel play, exploration of their environment, and meeting developmental milestones for a 2-year-old. A child who is age 5 years, however, is starting kindergarten, so their goals may be more focused on learning to draw shapes, starting to write, playing with peers, and being independent with ADLs such as dressing, toileting, and self-feeding. As children continue to grow, these goals will change, as will their interests and participation in activities.

The family, child, and occupational therapy practitioners collaboratively develop the goals and treatment plan (American Occupational Therapy Association [AOTA], 2020). It is important to gather from the child and family the child's interests and activities. The practitioner can then incorporate these interests into treatment sessions to keep the child's interest in therapy while the practitioner focuses on their goals.

For example, to increase a child's ability to transition from supine to tall kneeling to play with their peers on the floor, the occupational therapy practitioner can use the child's interest in coloring. The practitioner places the crayons or markers on the floor, with the paper on a bench. This facilitates the child reaching for the writing utensil on the floor and moving into tall kneeling to reach the paper on the bench to color. Client-centered activities during interventions can achieve developmental goals, improve independence with functional mobility, and increase upper extremity and core strength.

Interprofessional Coordination of Care

Children with acquired conditions often work with multiple professionals, and maintaining good communication with each other is critical to provide the best care to the child and their family. *Interprofessional collaborative practices* allow professionals to update each other on progress or problems and may identify problem areas for the occupational therapy practitioner to address. For example, a speech therapist may be addressing feeding and note that the child is having trouble coordinating movements without spilling when bringing their hand to their mouth. The occupational therapy practitioner can incorporate that into the therapy plan. Collaboration ultimately allows the child and family to receive optimal care and achieve the best outcome for the child.

Family Adjustment and Setting Expectations

Family and child adjustment to an acquired condition can greatly affect the plan of care and recommendations. The family may be grieving their child's condition and learning to accept the new diagnosis. Practitioners must respect the family's emotional state and may need to adjust education, interventions, and recommendations. These conversations will take place with the family over the full plan of care and may continue to the next bout of care, depending on the emotional state of the child and family at that time.

Depending on the therapy setting, a social worker or another mental health professional may be available to guide the family as they learn to cope with their "new normal," which may include making home modifications, adapting new activities for the child, and learning to navigate the world outside of the home and therapy as a family. Occupational therapy practitioners have a mental health background and can educate and guide the family as well during the child's bout of care; however, having those conversations outside of therapy may help with the family's coping and grieving.

Throughout the planning process for interventions, the goals should align with the child's developmental progress to continue to meet milestones while also facilitating recovery. For example, as noted by Jones et al. (2012), it is important for children to have access to powered mobility to explore their environment independently, which is how young children develop. Although a power wheelchair may seem to contradict the idea of walking and recovery, it helps the child continue to develop cognitively, keep up with peers, decrease caregiver burden, and engage in daily occupations. While the child has their power wheelchair at home and in the community, the occupational therapy practitioner can work on other interventions that may focus more on recovery.

Payment Sources

Once a child has been given a diagnosis and treated medically, a doctor may refer them to occupational therapy if there are occupational performance concerns or performance skill deficits related to strength or ROM that impede the child's developmental achievements, ADLs, or age-appropriate leisure participation. In the United States, once the referral is in place, the family provides information regarding private (e.g., insurance, private pay) or government (e.g., Medicaid) payment sources to cover the costs of therapy. (See Chapter 26, "Best Practices in Documentation of Health Care Services and Outcomes," for more information.)

If the family chooses to use insurance, the clinic's financial team lets the family and occupational therapy practitioner know whether there is a set number of visits in a year, as well as whether there are any other stipulations. For example, for inpatient care, the child may be approved for unlimited days depending on medical necessity, whereas for outpatient care, the child may get 50 occupational therapy and physical therapy visits combined for a year. This affects the occupational therapy treatment plan. Occupational therapy practitioners need to be in open communication with other disciplines (e.g., if the child is also receiving physical therapy).

BEST PRACTICES

This section addresses intervention planning and implementation and reviews the acute versus chronic phases of acquired conditions in general. This includes medical precautions, orthopedic considerations, appropriate interventions during these phases, and patient and family education.

Attend to Medical Complications and Precautions

Medical complications and precautions are prevalent in the pediatric population and must be considered before, during, and after intervention has occurred. Next are common complications and precautions associated with the diagnoses in this chapter.

Blood pressure

Blood pressure issues, such as *autonomic dysreflexia* (AD), a sudden elevation of blood pressure, related to an irritation below the level of injury, and orthostatic hypotension, can be common, especially among children who have a T6-level SCI or above. It is important to first establish the patient's baseline blood pressure and resting heart rate. Children with SCI, for example, often present with different baselines compared with healthy children because of changes in their autonomic system (Hwang et al., 2013).

It is important to be aware of the signs and symptoms of AD, which include facial flushing, sweating, blotchiness above the level of injury, goosebumps below the level of injury, headaches, blurred vision, and increase in systolic blood pressure (Hickey et al., 2004). Typically, among pediatric patients with SCIs, an increase of 15–20 mm Hg warrants consideration for AD (Eldahan & Rabchevsky, 2018). When a child presents with AD, the body is indicating something is wrong. Most often it is related to bowel or bladder issues, but it can also be caused by problems such as tight clothing, a wrinkle, or an ingrown toenail, which children with SCI often cannot feel.

Orthostatic hypotension occurs when there is a decrease in blood pressure, often when a child cannot tolerate an upright position. This is especially important for children who have been in bed for many days, weeks, or months. When they are first supported to sit up or to stand, their blood pressure may drop, which can lead to fainting or loss of consciousness (Tanaka et al., 1999). Lifting the child's legs in supine or using elastic compression wraps around the child's legs, an abdominal binder, or functional electrical stimulation on larger muscle groups can help improve circulation and help the child improve their tolerance for upright positioning. In general, if a child's blood pressure is increased (up), support the child in sitting up; however, if the child's blood pressure is decreased (down), lay the child down.

Dysautonomia

Dysautonomia is dysregulation of the autonomic nervous system associated with neurological injury. It is also referred to as *storming* or *paroxysmal sympathetic hyperactivity* and presents with a combination of fever, tachypnea, hypertension, tachycardia, diaphoresis, and dystonia (Kirk et al., 2012). Dysautonomia is more prevalent among patients with ABIs. Children who present with these symptoms typically have a more severe brain injury and may be minimally conscious. Children who present with dysautonomia are shown to have worse outcomes, as demonstrated by longer inpatient stays and worse results on outcome measures such as the Wee-FIM (Kirk et al., 2012).

Changes in mental status

Any acute change in *mental status,* including increased confusion, decreased alertness, or change in personality, among children with a neurological condition is concern for a possible rebleed, infection, or even a sign of AD among children with SCI. Changes in mental or cognitive status can include that the child (if old enough) is unable to report their current location, name, or date of birth. Changes can also be visually observed, as with eye changes or inability for the child to attend to task on one side of body, as well as any other physical changes, such as facial droop, weakness in upper or lower extremities, decreased ability to maintain balance while sitting, and frequent falls. These are all signs of an acute change in mental status and need to be addressed immediately.

Orthopedic concerns

Among children who have an acquired condition from a trauma, such as a car accident, or have been through surgery, it is important to consider their **orthopedic precautions.** These should be clarified by the surgeon or medical team. These precautions may include limited weight bearing as well as limited passive or active ROM to an extremity that was affected in the trauma. This may be especially important for children who have traumatic SCIs or TBIs or who have sustained a multitrauma. Patients who have sustained two or more separate injuries throughout their body, with one injury endangering their life, are considered to have multitrauma (Frink et al., 2017).

The medical team provides a protocol about weight-bearing or ROM limitations, which is important to start in therapy as early as possible. The child may have limited tolerance to these positions or certain ranges at first, but it is critical to continue to work with them to regain positions and range to prevent further complications. Building rapport early on with the child and family is crucial to ensure good carryover at home or continued carryover while in the hospital.

Decreased bone density

Children with acquired conditions are often at risk for fractures as a result of **decreased bone density,** or loss of bone mineralization. This is most common in conditions in which the child has decreased weight bearing (e.g., SCI, TBI, ABI), has previous fractures, or has a history of cancer, dependent on their treatment. Using caution when moving children in and out of positions safely is critical, especially with a history of fractures (National Institute of Arthritis and Musculoskeletal and Skin Diseases, 2018). However, activity through weight bearing is beneficial to increase bone mineral density, and it is critical that the practitioner educate the family about the risks and benefits of this intervention (Dolbow et al., 2015).

Weight bearing

Joint preservation is a precaution that should be taken with children who have an acquired condition affecting their ability to move. Joints can quickly become partially or completely dislocated, especially at the shoulder or hip. Weight bearing through these joints is important, especially for children from birth to age 5 years. Weight-bearing conditions include unilateral weight bearing through one upper extremity, posterior propping, prone, tall kneeling, quadruped, standing, and walking. Young children's joints develop as they start crawling and weight bearing during typical development. If a child is limited in development, the development of their joints may be affected. Practitioners should teach the child and their family how to achieve these weight-bearing positions to facilitate development.

Scoliosis

Children who acquire an injury before they are fully grown are also at a high risk to develop **scoliosis,** or curvature of the spine. Proper positioning in a wheelchair, weight bearing, bracing, and functional electrical stimulation to the core muscles can help to decrease the development of scoliosis. Bracing may be used to prevent the progression of the scoliosis once it is present; however, because of the nature of the pediatric population, tolerance and compliance may be low (Melicosta et al., 2019).

Provide Effective Care During the Acute Phase

When working with a child in the acute phase, practitioners must prioritize medical needs. Often children are more fragile, and medical needs may take priority to stabilize a patient.

Provide intervention

Intervention, including movement and activity, is critical, as tolerated, during this phase because it can help to decrease a child's complications long term. Working closely with the child's medical team is very important in this phase to ensure that limitations and precautions are understood. However, current research shows that early mobility is achievable in the acute phase, including bed mobility and walking, and may lead to better outcomes (Walker & Kudchadkar, 2018).

Prevent secondary complications

Preventing secondary complications is an acutely important part of therapy. ROM at all joints is essential so that as the child continues to medically stabilize, their joints and body are functionally ready for intervention. Often children may need orthotics, splints, and prosthetics acutely to maintain joint, muscle, and tendon lengths. Positioning protocols are important and may be completed by the occupational therapy practitioner to prevent wounds and to keep the child tolerating different positions. This may mean turning every 2 hours in bed from right side-lying, left side-lying, and supine, unless a position is not permitted medically.

Education of the team and family regarding the importance of out-of-bed activity is essential. This can also help with preventing pressure sores and can help optimize the child's earlier recovery, which leads to better outcomes overall. If the child tolerates being out of bed but is not able to stand and walk, they may require a seating system for support while out of bed. Practitioners should optimize the child's seating and positioning for joint preservation, weight bearing through the feet and forearms when possible, and keeping a child's pelvis and spine as neutral as possible. These basic interventions can lead to better outcomes and help the child tolerate therapy in the long term with decreased complications.

Maximize independence with compensatory training

Compensatory training to maximize independence (as developmentally appropriate) is an important part of acute rehabilitation. Compensatory training involves teaching modified skills or modifying environments to help increase independence in daily skills. The needs of each child are different depending on their age and presentation but may include compensatory techniques to regain independence with self-care, communication, or developmental play. A child with a cancer diagnosis or burn may need compensatory techniques to continue age-appropriate play while in a sterile hospital room. This can include playing dress-up in protective isolation gowns to work on self-care. A child with a brain injury or high SCI may need compensatory ways to communicate, push a call bell, use age-appropriate technology, or do self-care tasks. For children with cognitive deficits, visual schedules can be made, whereas various types of adaptive call bells can be obtained for children with physical deficits.

Occupational therapy practitioners can design creative ways to encourage safe participation in preferred tasks and help children stay developmentally engaged while decreasing secondary complications that happen with immobility. Although this can be challenging acutely if a child is connected to multiple lines and wires, occupational therapy practitioners' skill set allows them to think creatively.

Restore function

Interventions to *restore function,* or return to preinjury function, such as activity-based restorative therapy, include high-intensity training, functional electrical stimulation for neuromuscular recovery, and weight bearing (Bosques et al., 2016). As noted above, a child who has acquired a neurological injury may need interventions to direct their nervous system how to move again and work toward restoring function. For example, with self-feeding, the child may initially use adapted utensils and a plate with sides, while resting their elbow on a table if they have difficulty reaching against gravity. However, with intervention, passive and active ROM of the shoulder, elbow, wrist, and fingers may be addressed to increase the child's independence with these tasks using the least restrictive equipment.

Educate the child and family

Child and family education are critical parts of the acute phase. Child and family education involves providing developmentally appropriate information to children and their caregivers about their injury or disease and prognosis. In this phase, the family is still coming to terms with a new injury that their child has sustained, which may limit their ability to learn new information. Education should start as early as possible, using hands-on training with the family for better retention. With the families, practitioners prioritize what is important for the family to learn so that the most important skills are taught and carried over the long term.

Some examples of family and child education include how to perform pressure reliefs to prevent pressure wounds, how to recognize signs of blood pressure dysfunctions, and how to complete ROM. Further education and carryover typically continue into the chronic phase. Providing written resources allows the family to review the information and may increase their understanding. A simple, realistic home rehabilitation program should be provided to the family. Studies have shown that families are more inclined to carry out the home program when practitioners incorporate the exercises into a daily routine (Medina-Mirapeix et al., 2017). Communication with the occupational therapy practitioners who will be taking over the child's care is important so they are aware of the child and family's needs.

Provide Effective Care During the Chronic Phase

Children in the chronic phase (typically more than 6 months out from injury) continue to evolve developmentally and with recovery.

Provide intervention

Occupational therapy goals change and interventions evolve with recovery. As children move into the chronic phase, they may be able to tolerate more aggressive interventions. The more interventions are set up with play and preferred activities, the better the child will tolerate intervention.

Prevent secondary complications

Occupational therapy practitioners should continue to consider prevention of secondary complications, including what was discussed in the acute phase: splinting, orthotics or prosthetics, and seating and positioning. As children naturally age and stabilize medically, precautions become lifted, and needs evolve. Interventions should reflect these changes.

Although children may achieve milestones in different ways, practitioners should emphasize continued growth and development. Part of this growth may also be the acceptance of the child's condition by the family. For example, a family might not have agreed with a power or manual wheelchair initially, but as they accept the diagnosis, they may come to terms with this idea.

Maximize independence with compensatory training

Continued compensatory training to maximize independence is important, as developmentally appropriate for the child. These needs will change again with age and natural recovery from an acquired condition. This may mean finding different adaptive equipment, using environmental controls, and ensuring the child has the least restrictive devices for their current status.

Restore function

Continued interventions to restore function can be completed in this phase to keep the child's body as healthy as possible and prevent secondary complications, such as atrophy. These interventions may look similar to what was done in the acute phase, but the intensity may increase, and the goals of the training may change as the child becomes more medically stable and returns to the community in the chronic phase. Continued high-intensity training, functional electrical stimulation, and weight bearing can be completed in therapy and possibly carried over at home, depending on the family situation and the child.

As a child approaches preschool and then school age, it is important for the occupational therapy practitioners to help the child and family start to plan for school. Attending school can be scary for a family, because it means germs, separating from their child, and starting a new phase. However, school is important for emotional, social, and cognitive development if the child is medically stable.

Homebound school services may be considered. These may be provided at the hospital or home (e.g., if the child has a depressed immune system, is unable to physically tolerate school). Support from the team can be critical to arrange accommodations and make sure the child is set up for success in this environment. Communication with the current team and school team is critical at this phase.

Educate the child and family

Overall, family and child education are important to help the family continue to carry over the work done in therapy and guide the child to continue to grow, develop, and meet developmental milestones. Education can include family training during the child's therapy session, either hands on, through a handout, or both. Depending on the child's age, they may be able to demonstrate good understanding of their home exercise program; however, the family should be included for accountability and to progress the child toward functional independence.

Document progress

Depending on the setting, occupational therapy practitioners may use SOAP (Subjective, Objective, Assessment, Plan) notes, electronic documentation systems, or written notes. Practitioners need to document the date and time of the session as well as record the child's current progress toward their short- and long-term goals. This information should be documented clearly in case another practitioner needs to cover, so they can fully understand the plan of care. This is also critical for insurance companies to see the child's progress to continue skilled occupational therapy services.

Plan discharge

Discharge planning starts the day of evaluation and continues until the child is discharged from services. The occupational therapy practitioner considers the equipment, home program, and follow-up recommendations, depending on multiple factors of the child and family. These factors include motivation, home set-up, community participation, the child's roles and occupations in their daily routines, and the parent or caregiver's ability to carry out the recommendations. Discharge planning is a continued conversation that occurs throughout the child's bout of care to ensure a successful transition back home and to the community and a successful progression toward the child's goals.

SUMMARY

Overall, occupational therapy practitioners play an important role in the interdisciplinary team, and their role may change depending on the practitioner's setting. Practitioners need to collaborate and communicate with their team members to ensure the child is getting the best care for the best possible outcome. This communication assists in developing goals during the child's episode of care in a health care setting and ensuring the child is safely performing all activities during therapy.

Once a plan is in place, the occupational therapy practitioner needs to think about appropriateness of interventions. Again, collaborating with the team helps the practitioner understand what is or what is not appropriate for that child. This can include avoiding weight bearing because of possible fractures or encouraging full ROM to prevent contractures. Once the intervention begins, the practitioner involves the family in preparation for discharge home and encourages the family to assist in the child's therapy services. The family plays a role in follow-up recommendations and ensuring a safe discharge home and back into the child's daily routines, with the support and input of the rest of the team.

REFERENCES

American Academy of Pediatrics. (2016). Management of pediatric trauma. *Pediatrics, 138*(2), e20161569. https://doi.org/10.1542/peds.2016-1569

American Cancer Society. (2019). *Cancer facts & figures 2019.* https://www.cancer.org/content/dam/cancer-org/research/cancer-facts-and-statistics/annual-cancer-facts-and-figures/2019/cancer-facts-and-figures-2019.pdf

American Occupational Therapy Association. (2020). Occupational therapy practice framework: Domain and process (4th ed.). *American Journal of Occupational Therapy, 74*(Suppl. 2), 7412410010. https://doi.org/10.5014/ajot.2020.74S2001

American Spinal Injury Association. (n.d.). *Facts on pediatric spinal cord injury.* https://asia-spinalinjury.org/committees/pediatric/pediatric-committee-news-and-resources/pediatric-spinal-cord-injury-facts

American Stroke Association. (2020). *Pediatric stroke infographic.* https://www.stroke.org/en/about-stroke/stroke-in-children/pediatric-stroke-infographic

Araki, T., Yokota, H., & Morita, A. (2017). Pediatric traumatic brain injury: Characteristic features, diagnosis, and management. *Neurologia Medico-Chirurgica, 57*(2), 82–93. https://doi.org/10.2176/nmc.ra.2016-0191

Bosques, G., Martin, R., McGee, L., & Sadowsky, C. (2016). Does therapeutic electrical stimulation improve function in children with disabilities? A comprehensive literature review. *Journal of Pediatric Rehabilitation Medicine, 9,* 83–99. https://doi.org/10.3233/PRM-160375

Brain Injury Association of America. (n.d.). *What is the difference between an acquired brain injury and a traumatic brain injury?* https://www.biausa.org/brain-injury/about-brain-injury/nbiic/what-is-the-difference-between-an-acquired-brain-injury-and-a-traumatic-brain-injury

Center on the Developing Child. (2007). *InBrief: The impact of early adversity on child development.* https://developingchild.harvard.edu/resources/inbrief-the-impact-of-early-adversity-on-childrens-development/

Children's National Hospital. (n.d.). *Burns.* https://childrensnational.org/visit/conditions-and-treatments/skin-disorders/burns

Dennis, M., Spiegler, B. J., Juranek, J. J., Bigler, E. D., Snead, O. C., & Fletcher, J. M. (2013). Age, plasticity, and homeostasis in childhood brain disorders. *Neuroscience and Biobehavioral Reviews, 37,* 2760–2773. https://doi.org/10.1016/j.neubiorev.2013.09.010

Dewan, M. C., Mummareddy, N., Wellons, J. C., III, & Bonfield, C. M. (2016). Epidemiology of global pediatric traumatic brain injury: Qualitative review. *World Neurosurgery, 91,* 497–509. https://doi.org/10.1016/j.wneu.2016.03.045

Dolbow, D. R., Gorgey, A. S., Recio, A. C., Stiens, S. A., Curry, A. C., Sadowsky, C. L., . . . McDonald, J. W. (2015). Activity-based restorative therapies after spinal cord injury: Inter-institutional conceptions and perceptions. *Aging and Disease, 6,* 254–261. https://doi.org/10.14336/AD.2014.1105

Eldahan, K. C., & Rabchevsky, A. G. (2018). Autonomic dysreflexia after spinal cord injury: Systemic pathophysiology and methods of management. *Autonomic Neuroscience, 209,* 59–70. https://doi.org/10.1016/j.autneu.2017.05.002

Ferriero, D. M., Fullerton, H. J., Bernard, T. J., Billinghurst, L., Daniels, S. R., Debaun, M. R., . . . Smith, E. R. (2019). Management of stroke in neonates and children: A scientific statement from the American Heart Association/American Stroke Association. *Stroke, 50,* e51–e96. https://doi.org/10.1161/STR.0000000000000183

Frink, M., Lechler, P., Debus, F., & Ruchholtz, S. (2017). Multiple trauma and emergency room management. *Deutsches Arzteblatt International, 114,* 497–503. https://doi.org/10.3238/arztebl.2017.0497

Hickey, K. J., Vogel, L. C., Willis, K. M., & Anderson, C. J. (2004). Prevalence and etiology of autonomic dysreflexia in children with spinal cord injuries. *Journal of Spinal Cord Medicine, 27,* S54–S60. https://doi.org/10.1080/10790268.2004.11753786

Hwang, M., Zebracki, K., Betz, R. R., Mulcahey, M. J., & Vogel, L. C. (2013). Normative blood pressure and heart rate in pediatric spinal cord injury. *Topics in Spinal Cord Injury Rehabilitation, 19,* 87–95. https://doi.org/10.1310/sci1902-87

Johns Hopkins Medicine. (2019). *Burns and wounds.* https://www.hopkinsmedicine.org/health/conditions-and-diseases/burns

Jones, M. A., McEwen, I. R., & Neas, B. R. (2012). Effects of powered wheelchairs on the development and function of young children with severe motor impairments. *Pediatric Physical Therapy, 24,* 131–140. https://doi.org/10.1097/PEP.0b013e31824c5fdc

Kaplan, S. L., & Pentima, C. D. (2019). *Patient education: Meningitis in children (beyond the basics).* https://www.uptodate.com/contents/meningitis-in-children-beyond-the-basics

Kirk, K. A., Shoykhet, M., Jeong, J. H., Tyler-Kabara, E. C., Henderson, M. J., Bell, M. J., & Fink, E. L. (2012). Dysautonomia after pediatric brain injury. *Developmental Medicine and Child Neurology, 54,* 759–764. https://doi.org/10.1111/j.1469-8749.2012.04322.x

McFadyen, J. G., Ramaiah, R., & Bhananker, S. M. (2012). Initial assessment and management of pediatric trauma patients. *International Journal of Critical Illness and Injury Science, 2,* 121–127. https://doi.org/10.4103/2229-5151.100888

Medina-Mirapeix, F., Lillo-Navarro, C., Montilla-Herrador, J., Gacto-Sánchez, M., Franco-Sierra, M. Á., & Escolar-Reina, P. (2017). Predictors of parents' adherence to home exercise programs for children with developmental disabilities, regarding both exercise frequency and duration: A survey design. *European Journal of Physical and Rehabilitation Medicine, 53,* 545–555. https://doi.org/10.23736/S1973-9087.17.04464-1

Melicosta, M. E., Dean, J., Hagen, K., Oppenheimer, K., Porter, C., Rybczynski, S., & Sadowski, C. (2019). Acute flaccid myelitis: Rehabilitation challenges and outcomes in a pediatric cohort. *Journal of Pediatric Rehabilitation Medicine, 12,* 245–253. https://doi.org/10.3233/PRM-180549

Mesfin, F. B., & Taylor, R. S. (2019). *Diffuse axonal injury (DAI).* StatPearls.

National Cancer Institute. (2019). *Cancer facts and figures 2019.* https://www.cancer.org/content/dam/cancer-org/research/cancer-facts-and-statistics/annual-cancer-facts-and-figures/2019/cancer-facts-and-figures-2019.pdf

National Cancer Institute. (2020). *Childhood Brain and Spinal Cord Tumors Treatment Overview (PDQ®)–Patient Version.* https://www.cancer.gov/types/brain/patient/child-brain-treatment-pdq

National Institute of Arthritis and Musculoskeletal and Skin Diseases. (2018). *Juvenile osteoporosis.* https://www.bones.nih.gov/health-info/bone/bone-health/juvenile/juvenile-osteoporosis

National Institute of Neurological Disorders and Stroke. (2018). *Meningitis and encephalitis fact sheet.* https://www.ninds.nih.gov/Disorders/Patient-Caregiver-Education/Fact-Sheets/Meningitis-and-Encephalitis-Fact-Sheet

Ogundele, M. O. (2018). Behavioural and emotional disorders in childhood: A brief overview for paediatricians. *World Journal of Clinical Pediatrics, 7,* 9–26. https://doi.org/10.5409/wjcp.v7.i1.9

Reith, F. C., Van den Brande, R., Synnot, A., Gruen, R., & Maas. A. I. (2016). The reliability of the Glasgow Coma Scale: A systematic review. *Intensive Care Medicine, 42,* 3–15. https://doi.org/10.1007/s00134-015-4124-3.

Sparrow, J. (2020). Special considerations for children with cancer. In B. Braveman & R. Newman (Eds.), *Cancer and occupational therapy: Enabling participation across the lifespan* (pp. 43–66). AOTA Press.

Su, Y. R. S., Veeravagu, A., & Grant, G. (2016). Neuroplasticity after traumatic brain injury. In D. T. Laskowitz & G. Grant (Eds.), *Translational research in traumatic brain injury* (Ch. 8). CRC Press/Taylor and Francis. https://www.ncbi.nlm.nih.gov/books/NBK326735/

Tanaka, H., Yamaguchi H., Matushima, R., & Tamai, H. (1999). Instantaneous orthostatic hypotension in children and adolescents: A new entity of orthostatic intolerance. *Pediatric Research, 46,* 691–696. https://doi.org/10.1203/00006450-199912000-00022

Tsze, D. S., & Valente, J. H. (2011). Pediatric stroke: A review. *Emergency Medicine International, 2011,* 734506. https://doi.org/10.1155/2011/734506

Walker, T., & Kudchadkar, S. R. (2018). Early mobility in the pediatric intensive care unit: Can we move on? *The Journal of Pediatrics, 203,* 10–12. https://doi.org/10.1016/j.jpeds.2018.08.058

Whitney, D. G., & Peterson, M. D. (2019). U.S. national and state-level prevalence of mental health disorders and disparities of mental health care use in children. *JAMA Pediatrics, 173,* 389–391. https://doi.org/10.1001/jamapediatrics.2018.5399

Zaloshnja, E., Miller, T., Langlois, J., & Selassie, A. (2008). Prevalence of long-term disability from traumatic brain injury in the civilian population of the United States, 2005. *The Journal of Head Trauma Rehabilitation, 23,* 394–400. https://doi.org/10.1097/01.HTR.0000341435.52004.ac

Best Practices in Documentation of Health Care Services and Outcomes

26

Stephanie L. de Sam Lazaro, OTD, OTR/L

KEY TERMS AND CONCEPTS

- *Current Procedural Terminology* codes
- Demographic information
- Discharge reports
- Documentation
- Evaluation report
- Goals
- *Guidelines for Documentation of Occupational Therapy*

- Health care settings
- Health literacy
- Home care
- Inpatient hospital settings
- Neonatal intensive care units
- Occupational profile
- *2020 Occupational Therapy Code of Ethics*

- Occupational therapy intervention plan
- *Occupational Therapy Practice Framework: Domain and Process*
- Outpatient settings
- Prior authorization
- Progress reports
- Session treatment notes

OVERVIEW

Documentation of skilled occupational therapy services in *health care settings* (i.e., inpatient and outpatient hospitals, clinics, home care) is required by state regulatory boards and third-party payers (e.g., Medicaid, health maintenance organizations [HMOs], preferred provider organizations [PPOs]). The types of documentation commonly used in these settings include evaluation and reevaluation reports, intervention plans, progress reports, daily or session treatment notes, and discharge notes. All of these forms of documentation are generally provided to referring providers, third-party payers, caregivers, and team members in other practice settings (e.g., preschools, early intervention programs).

When documentation or other personal information is shared across practice settings, it is imperative that parental consent be obtained in adherence with the Health Insurance Portability and Accountability Act of 1996 (HIPAA; P. L. 104-191). In addition, the typical recipients of services in early childhood health care settings fall into the category of children with special health care needs, and optimal outcomes for this population rely on coordinated health care, which is often the caregivers' responsibility (Pizur-Barnekow et al., 2011). Therefore, health literacy in all forms of documentation is a critical consideration in early childhood occupational therapy practice in health care settings.

Several American Occupational Therapy Association (AOTA) documents assist occupational therapy practitioners in understanding the purpose of documentation and the responsibilities of practitioners in documentation of services in early intervention. (*Note. Occupational therapy practitioner* refers to both occupational therapists and occupational therapy assistants.) The *Guidelines for Documentation of Occupational Therapy* (AOTA, 2018a) outlines the following four purposes of documentation:

- To communicate information from an occupational therapy perspective (e.g., the occupational profile)
- To provide justification for the necessity of occupational therapy services
- To establish a chronological record of services provided
- To document the child's response to intervention (AOTA, 2018a).

The *2020 Occupational Therapy Code of Ethics* (AOTA, 2020a) outlines expectations for all occupational therapy practitioners with regard to documentation for reimbursement purposes and its adherence to laws, guidelines, and regulations.

This chapter reviews AOTA documents along with health care resources to support occupational therapy practitioners working in health care settings with infants and children between birth and age 5 years. This includes neonatal intensive care unit (NICU), inpatient hospital, outpatient hospital and clinic, and home care settings. Resources and information are shared to support early childhood practitioners' abilities to adhere to best practices and legal and ethical requirements of the profession.

ESSENTIAL CONSIDERATIONS

As in other areas of occupational therapy practice, the documentation process for children in health care settings begins with a referral. It is the responsibility of the occupational therapist to review the referral information and establish an evaluation plan based on the reason for referral, service competence of the clinician, and access and availability of the services required for the child in the practice setting.

Ethical and Legal Considerations

Occupational therapy practitioners must maintain confidentiality in all communications regarding the referral, services, and interventions provided to the child in alignment with HIPAA. This includes password-protected documentation in electronic health care records (EHR) and secure storage of paper documentation. It is best practice in interdisciplinary settings for the occupational therapy records to be stored in a common client file with all the child's other records. Although many health care settings serving young children have moved to EHR, many continue to use and store paper charts and files.

Billing and Reimbursement

There are generally three categories for reimbursement of occupational therapy services in early childhood health care settings: (1) government funded (Medicaid), (2) private insurance (e.g., HMO, PPO), and (3) private pay from the caregiver. It is the responsibility of the occupational therapy practitioner to verify and understand what types of services are covered by the third-party payer for the child.

Regardless of the payment method, services are billed through *Current Procedural Terminology (CPT) codes* (American Medical Association [AMA], 2020a).[1] Table 26.1 contains the three levels for coding occupational therapy evaluations and one code for occupational therapy reevaluations (AMA, 2020a). In addition, occupational therapy practitioners commonly use nonoccupational therapy–specific evaluation codes as well as intervention codes with children in health care settings.

Health Literacy in Documentation

The majority of occupational therapy documentation in health care settings is provided to the families of young children, which makes health literacy a crucial consideration. *Health literacy* encompasses the client's[2] ability to gather, interpret, and use information received from health care providers to make informed decisions as well as the communication skills of the health care provider and context in which the information is shared (AOTA, 2017b). Thus, health literacy is a partnership between the client and the practitioner to ensure understanding of documentation shared.

The language used in all documentation must be consistent with the expectations of the practice setting itself and easily translatable across multiple disciplines and team members, including the families. Pizur-Barnekow et al. (2011) found that families identified the need to retain information shared by health care providers and then learn and understand it. Only after these aspects are completed can the family apply new knowledge for the care of their child and determine the best course of action on the basis of treatment plans and recommendations (Pizur-Barnekow et al., 2011).

Best practice strategies to improve the health literacy of occupational therapy documentation include
- Tailoring documentation to the audience (including families);
- Providing clear messages while limiting the number of messages given at one time;
- Using active voice and positive messages;
- Avoiding jargon and using culturally familiar words; and
- Formatting the document so it is easy to read and follow, with clear headings and a minimum of 12-point font (Niebaum et al., 2015).

It is the responsibility of occupational therapy practitioners to ensure that caregivers have a clear understanding of the information being presented and the risks and benefits of any services recommended. Practitioners must match their documentation and information sharing to the literacy, verbal, cognitive, and social skill level of the caregivers while also being sensitive to cultural and linguistic differences that affect health literacy to ensure optimal outcomes (AOTA, 2017b).

Types of Settings and Documentation in Health Care Early Childhood Practice

This chapter outlines documentation in four health care early childhood practice settings, (1) the NICU, (2) the inpatient hospital, (3) the outpatient hospital or clinic, and (4) home care for medically fragile children not funded through the Individuals With Disabilities Education Improvement Act of 2004 (P. L. 108-446).

NICUs are also referred to as *special care nurseries.* The levels of care in these units range from
- Well-newborn nurseries that monitor newborn infants at low risk to
- Specialty NICUs that provide care for newborn infants with moderate levels of risk but expectation for rapid improvement to
- Subspecialty NICUs that have around-the-clock specialty personnel of all disciplines to care for infants with extreme prematurity (28 weeks gestation or less; American Academy of Pediatrics, 2004).

Occupational therapists are typically part of the team in specialty and subspecialty NICU settings. The role in these settings focuses on co-occupations of the child and caregiver, early parenting skills, and any factors that may be affecting participation in early occupations (AOTA, 2018b). Documentation in this setting is often cyclical in nature with assessment and reassessment, because rapid changes often occur for children and caregivers in the NICU environment (AOTA, 2018b).

Inpatient hospital settings include a range of levels of care, including intensive care units, medical units, surgical

---

[1]Codes shown refer to *CPT 2020* (American Medical Association, 2020, *CPT 2020* standard, Chicago: American Medical Association Press) and do not represent all of the possible codes that may be used in occupational therapy evaluation and intervention. After 2020, refer to the current year's *CPT* code book for available codes. *CPT* codes are updated annually and become effective January 1. *CPT* is a trademark of the American Medical Association. *CPT* five-digit codes, two-digit codes, modifiers, and descriptions are copyright © 2020 by the American Medical Association. All rights reserved.

[2]Because the young child is dependent on an adult, the term *client* refers to the child and caregiver or parent.

TABLE 26.1.   Common *CPT* Codes Used in Early Childhood Health Care Settings

CPT CODE NUMBER	DESCRIPTION
97165	OT evaluation, low complexity
97166	OT evaluation, moderate complexity
97167	OT evaluation, high complexity
97168	OT reevaluation
97530	Therapeutic activities, such as play, to promote functional performance
97533	Sensory-integrative techniques (note that many third-party payers do not cover this code)
97535	ADLs
97542	Wheelchair management, including assessment and fitting
97755	Assistive-technology assessment
97760, 97763	Orthotic management and training
92526	Treatment for swallowing or oral dysfunction
92605, 92606	Evaluation and services for nonspeech-generating communication devices
92610	Evaluation of oral and pharyngeal swallowing
92611	Fluoroscopic evaluation of swallowing
92612, 92613, 92614, 92615	Flexible endoscopic evaluation, interpretation, and reporting of swallowing or laryngeal sensory testing
95831, 95832, 95833, 95834	Manual muscle testing
95851, 95852, 95992	Range of motion measurements
96110	Developmental screening
96112	Developmental test administration
96127	Emotional and behavioral assessment
99366, 99368	Medical team conferences
97153, 97154, 97155, 97156, 97157, 97158, 0373T	Adaptive behavior interventions

Note. ADLs = activities of daily living; *CPT* = *Current Procedural Terminology*; OT = occupational therapy.
Source. CPT is a trademark of the American Medical Association. *CPT* five-digit codes, two-digit codes, modifiers, and descriptions are copyright © 2020 by the American Medical Association. All rights reserved.

units, cardiac units, transplant units, and oncology units. Hospitals that provide this level of care may also provide outpatient pediatric rehabilitation services as part of the team that includes occupational therapy practitioners, physical therapists, speech therapists, social workers, child and family life specialists, and additional health care team members. In addition to hospital-affiliated *outpatient settings* (freestanding independently or privately owned outpatient clinics) may provide occupational therapy services in addition to other allied health services. Finally, many children who are discharged from inpatient hospital settings have medical diagnoses that put them in a high-risk or fragile state. They may receive services from a *home care* team, including occupational therapy. Home care services are provided by allied health professionals in the client's home to support participation in daily life activities (Medicare.gov, n.d.).

Across the four health care practice settings, there are documentation similarities and differences based on the practice setting (see Table 26.2).

BEST PRACTICES

All documentation in early childhood health care settings must align with the *Guidelines for Documentation in Occupational Therapy* (AOTA, 2018a) and the **Occupational Therapy Practice Framework: Domain and Process** (*OTPF;* AOTA, 2020b). The process itself starts with a referral and then moves through screening or evaluation (and reevaluation if needed), prior authorization (if required), intervention planning, session notes, progress reports, and discharge plans. Regardless of the type of documentation, there are several key aspects required in all types of documentation.

Obtain Prior Authorization, When Required

On some occasions, ***prior authorization*** is required before an evaluation is conducted. Prior authorization, or prior approval, is a process in which health care providers are required to obtain approval for their proposed or planned

TABLE 26.2.   Documentation Descriptions and Practice Settings

TYPE OF DOCUMENTATION	SETTINGS	DESCRIPTION
Prior authorization	▪ Outpatient settings ▪ Home care	Depending on the payer source, prior authorization may be required before an evaluation or before intervention. This form is completed and sent to the third-party payer before services can be initiated.
Initial evaluation	▪ NICU ▪ Inpatient hospital ▪ Outpatient settings ▪ Home care	An initial evaluation includes background information, reason for referral, occupational profile, assessment of functional performance, analysis of occupational performance, summary, and recommendations.
Reevaluation	▪ NICU ▪ Inpatient hospital ▪ Outpatient settings ▪ Home care	A reevaluation includes background information; occupational profile; and results of the reevaluation, analysis of occupational performance, summary, and recommendations. In the NICU and inpatient hospital settings, this is generally completed when there is a change in medical status. In the outpatient and home care settings, reevaluations are completed with a change in status but also as required by the third-party payer, typically every 90 days or 6 months.
Intervention plan (or plan of care)	▪ NICU ▪ Inpatient hospital ▪ Outpatient settings ▪ Home care	This plan for services is based on the initial evaluation or reevaluation. It includes the goals for services; plan for setting; and intensity, frequency, and duration recommended. In the outpatient and home care settings, the occupational therapy intervention plan may also be updated when a progress report occurs.
Contact report (e.g., Daily or session treatment notes)	▪ NICU ▪ Inpatient hospital ▪ Outpatient settings ▪ Home care	Most frequently, this takes the format of a SOAP or a DAP note. These are completed after each intervention session and also may be used as a method for documentation of caregiver education, phone contacts, or a team meeting.
Progress report	▪ Outpatient settings ▪ Home care	Progress reports are not generally completed in the NICU or inpatient hospital setting because of the length of stay in those settings. For the outpatient and home care settings, these are generally completed to provide an update on progress toward achievement of goals and the establishment of new goals. This typically occurs every 60–90 days, depending on third-party payer requirements.
Discharge report	▪ NICU ▪ Inpatient hospital ▪ Outpatient settings ▪ Home care	Documents reason for discharge, beginning level of functioning, interventions provided, child's progress toward goals and ending level of functioning, and referrals and recommendations.

Note. DAP = Data, Assessment, Plan; NICU = neonatal intensive care unit; SOAP = Subjective, Objective, Assessment, Plan.

services from the payor (insurance provider) before they can deliver the service (AMA, 2020b). Most often, prior authorization is required after an initial evaluation or reevaluation before intervention services can occur. Some third-party payers require prior authorization before any services are provided; others do not require prior authorization until after a certain number of visits have been used in a calendar year. The information required for prior authorization varies from payer to payer, but in general the following information is required:

▪ Demographic information about the recipient of services;
▪ Reason for referral for services and referring provider's information;
▪ *International Statistical Classification of Diseases and Related Health Problems* (10th ed.; World Health Organization, 2010) code;
▪ *CPT* code and description of services to be provided as well as location for these services; and
▪ Intensity, frequency, and duration of services requested.

If prior authorization is required, services can only be provided after authorization for services is received or payment is denied.

Include Demographic Information

There are several pieces of ***demographic information*** commonly included in all documentation in early childhood health care settings. The child's name, date of birth, and chronological age or adjusted age and the date of service are included in all documentation notes. In addition, parent or caregiver information is included because caregivers are typically recipients of copies of the records. The child's medical diagnosis, referral source, and reason for referral are key pieces of information in the demographic section and are important for reimbursement purposes. Occupational therapy practitioners should include any precautions or contraindications for working with the child. This is important to communicate to interdisciplinary team members to provide safe and effective care for the child. Finally, the setting in which services are provided and the practitioner's name and credentials should be evident on all documentation notes in health care settings.

Document Initial Evaluation

The *OTPF* (AOTA, 2020b) outlines two sections of the evaluation: the (1) occupational profile and (2) analysis of occupation. To obtain this information, occupational therapy practitioners use a multistep process. The occupational profile includes a summary of the child's history, daily living routines within their environments and contexts, personal interests and values, and client needs (AOTA, 2020b). The analysis of occupational performance includes analyzing interview and occupational profile information, observing, administering assessments, interpreting the results, and creating goals based on the synthesis and analysis of information (AOTA, 2020b). The *evaluation report* documents the process of data collection and results as well as interprets the need for intervention planning (AOTA, 2020b).

Document occupational profile

The first step in this process is to gather background information from the family and referral source to plan the evaluation (AOTA, 2020b; Richardson, 2015). The *occupational profile* is a critical aspect of all evaluation and reevaluation plans because it summarizes the child's and family history, strengths and needs across occupational performance and environments, interests, priorities, and desired outcomes. Once that information has been collected, the initial evaluation commences with building rapport with the child and their caregivers, conducting informal observations, and interviewing the caregivers to develop an occupational profile (Richardson, 2015). AOTA (2017a, n.d.) has developed an occupational profile template tool in fillable PDF and Microsoft Word versions with examples for various client populations.

Document analysis of occupation

Information in the occupational profile assists in determining which standardized and nonstandardized assessments will be used to evaluate occupations, performance skills, performance patterns, activity demands, and environmental and contextual factors (Richardson, 2015). This section of the report should include persons interviewed, records reviewed, and a summary of the occupational profile.

Guided by the data in the occupational profile, the therapist completes observations and, if needed, uses formal assessment tools for occupational performance and sometimes performance skills. This may include a description of informal or systematic observations and standardized and nonstandardized assessment tools, including the psychometric properties of these tools. The Description of Assessments section also includes a description of where the evaluation was conducted.

The results of these assessments provide a description of the supports and hindrances to occupational performance and participation for the child, with objective and measurable information to support those statements. Occupational therapy evaluations in the NICU and inpatient hospital setting may use standardized assessment measures in some instances but not all. In the outpatient and home care settings, standard test scores are often required by third-party payers for reimbursement of services on the intervention plan.

The next section of the report provides an interpretation of the objective data, with a summary of occupational performance deficits and targeted occupational performance areas to be addressed in intervention. A statement providing a rationale for why and how skilled occupational

therapy services will support occupational participation for the child is also included.

The final aspect of the evaluation report includes the plan of care, with recommendations for frequency, intensity, and duration of skilled occupational therapy services. This is followed by a signature and date. Appendix I, "Sample Occupational Therapy Evaluation in Health Care" outlines an abbreviated evaluation report in a health care setting. AOTA (2017c) has also developed a PERFORM template that can be used to integrate the initial evaluation into the EHR.

Complete the Occupational Therapy Intervention Plan (Plan of Care)

The initial evaluation or reevaluation report drives the *occupational therapy intervention plan,* sometimes called the *occupational therapy plan of care.* Depending on the practice setting, the intervention plan or plan of care may be in the same document or report as the evaluation or reevaluation report or may be a separate document. The components of the intervention plan include (1) child information; (2) intervention goals (long-term and short-term goals); (3) provider information, provider location, frequency, intensity, and duration of services; (4) plan for discharge or discharge criteria and setting; (5) outcome measures; and (6) signature and date.

The long-term and short-term *goals* must be developed collaboratively with the family, occupation based, measurable, and linked directly to the summary and analysis in the evaluation or reevaluation plan, the justification for services, and the occupational performance priorities identified on the occupational profile. Health care in early childhood settings may include child goals as well as caregiver goals to support occupation-based outcomes for the child.

Before writing intervention plans, occupational therapy practitioners should consult with the third-party payer to ensure that goal areas are covered in the child's plan. In addition, the third-party payer dictates in many ways the length for establishing long-term goals. Long-term goals are generally 60 days or 90 days in length for outpatient and home care settings, with short-term goals 3–6 weeks in length to build to the long-term goals. In inpatient and NICU settings, long-term goals are generally written for the expected length of stay (1–2 weeks to 3–4 months). These may be rewritten more frequently than in other health care settings, and generally short-term goals are for 1 week or less and rewritten every 7 days.

There are many formats for writing goals in health care settings. RUMBA (relevant, understandable, measurable, behavioral, achievable) and COAST (client, occupation, assist level, specific condition, timeline) are both formats that may be used in early childhood health care settings (Sames, 2015). Regardless of the setting, the number of long-term and short-term goals should be reasonable for the setting and the length of time available (Park, 2012). Examples of goals can be seen in Table 26.3.

Provider information, frequency, intensity, and duration of services as well as discharge criteria, anticipated discharge setting, and discharge needs are included in the intervention plan. The statement indicating why occupational therapy services are needed and the plan for monitoring and evaluating progress are also required before the signature and date of the report.

TABLE 26.3.   Long- and Short-Term Goal Examples by Setting

PRACTICE SETTING	LONG-TERM GOAL	SHORT-TERM GOALS
NICU	In 3 weeks, D. will maintain homeostasis in his respiration, oxygen saturation, and temperature during his bath at least once a week.	In 3 days, D. will maintain homeostasis on 90% of diaper changes. In 2 weeks, D. will maintain homeostasis 90% of the time while clothed or blanketed in a variety of positions (held in supine, side lying, or at caregiver's shoulder; lying supine, side lying, or prone).
Inpatient hospital	In 2 weeks, M. will independently feed herself 75% of a meal at least one time a day.	In 3 days, M. will reach for items on her plate or tray to indicate a preferred food item one time a day. In 5 days, M. will scoop with a spoon and bring a sticky or lumpy food (e.g., oatmeal, mashed potatoes, macaroni and cheese) to her mouth at one meal each day.
Outpatient hospital or clinic	In 3 months, J. will increase his play skills, as evidenced by independently obtaining and playing with toys in his home and child care environments at least twice a day.	In 2 weeks, J. will choose a preferred toy from three options presented by caregivers on 75% of opportunities. In 4 weeks, J. will move across the room independently to obtain an item of interest at least one time each day.
Home care	In 2 months, S. will increase her ability to interact with her environment, as evidenced by independently holding her head up in supported sit for at least three reciprocal turns in a social game with her sibling or caregiver.	In 2 weeks, S. will visually attend to three to five pages of a board book without interruption on 80% of opportunities. In 4 weeks, S. will hold her head up in a prone position for the duration of a short song sung by her sibling (e.g., "Twinkle, Twinkle Little Star") once a week.

Note. NICU = neonatal intensive care unit.

Complete Contact Report (Daily or Session Treatment Notes)

The majority of early childhood health care settings use the SOAP note format for daily or *session treatment notes.* The statements in the *O* and the *A* sections should relate directly to progress toward the child's achievement of goals. Here is a brief description:

- **S (Subjective):** Statement of what the child, caregiver, or both said during the session
- **O (Objective):** Objective information to describe the child's reaction and participation during the session
- **A (Assessment):** The child's progress toward their goals and therapy potential
- **P (Plan):** Frequency, duration, and intensity of continued services and the plan for the next intervention session.

For many early childhood health care practice settings, treatment notes are written in a narrative format. However, with the growth of EHR, table formats that are aligned with goals increasingly are being used for daily treatment or session notes. The same components of SOAP are still used, but they are merged together in some ways. Exhibit 26.1 shows an example of what this might look like in an EHR.

Complete Progress Report

Progress reports are a summary of progress of the client on their goals and include a modification of the goals and plan as needed (AOTA, 2018). Some NICU and inpatient settings may complete progress reports every 7–10 days. In outpatient and home care settings, the third-party payer dictates the frequency of progress reports, generally every 60 or 90 days. The required components of progress reports include client information, goals that were set for the intervention period, a summary of the services provided, the child's current occupational performance, and the plan or recommendation for upcoming and future services. Goals are frequently rewritten in this document. If discontinuation of services is recommended, then a discharge or discontinuation note is written in place of a progress report. Exhibit 26.2 provides an example of the format of a progress report.

Complete Discharge or Discontinuation Report

Discharge reports for early childhood health care settings are written when a child is discharged from the NICU or inpatient hospital setting, when a plateau in progress occurs, when the child's goals are met, if the child is not attending sessions, or when transition to a different practice setting or discipline is recommended. Discharge notes may take many formats, but the required components are the same: child information, summary of the intervention process (including frequency, intensity, and duration of services received), progress on goals or achievement of goals (i.e., beginning and ending occupational performance), and the child's response to interventions provided. Follow-up recommendations, referrals to other services, and home programming recommendations should also be included, as well as the signature and date of the report. In the NICU and inpatient hospital setting, these may be very brief (e.g., child might have received 1–2 days of service). However, in the home care or outpatient setting, these may be extensive notes, because duration of services may be 18 months to 2 years before discharge occurs.

EXHIBIT 26.1. Sample Daily Note Grid

Occupational Therapy Contact Report
Child: Joey Miller   Birthdate: 11-25-17
Date: 12/20/19   Session # 4   Time: 10–10:45 a.m.

Joey was seen in the outpatient clinic with his mother and older brother for 45 minutes. The first 20 minutes were spent in play activities. Mom reports Joey's increased interest in people and objects in his environment. During the session, Joey was presented with options of items to play with, including bubbles, a beach ball, and a shape sorter. Joey chose the bubbles and engaged in reciprocal turns of attempting to blow and popping bubbles from sitting for 5 minutes (previously sat for 3.5 minutes). Joey only popped bubbles in his immediate reach. He moved from sitting to his stomach and scooted on his stomach about 5 feet to reach a preferred singing/musical toy (previously scooted 3 feet).

The remainder of the session (25 minutes) was spent in the therapy kitchen for a snack. Before and after the meal, he used a washcloth to wipe his hands and face with minimal assistance (last session he required physical assistance). Joey attempted to scoop pudding onto his spoon 5 times (3:5 accurate; 60%) and brought a preloaded spoon of pudding to his mouth when prompted by the therapist or his mother in 60% of attempts. This is an improvement from the last session, when he refused to scoop foods and had 40% accuracy on bringing the preloaded spoon to his mouth. He drank 4 sips of water from a nosey cup presented by his mom or therapist with moderate spilling/leakage. He independently fed himself 3 graham cracker strips (new skill).

Summary: Joey is progressing toward his goals. He requires adult prompts and encouragement for participation in play and mealtime.

Plan: Home programming to practice putting preferred items just out of reach in play and continue practice with self-feeding with sticky/thick consistencies. Large motor skills in play and a preferred snack will be used next session.

Signature ____[electronic signature]____   *Date* ___12/20/19___

EXHIBIT 26.2. Progress Report Template Example

Occupational Therapy Progress Report

Client name: **Client DOB:**   **Date of report:**
Diagnosis: **Precautions/medical history:**
Reason for referral to occupational therapy:
Occupational therapist (and occupational therapy assistant, if applicable):
Summary of services provided:
[This section includes frequency, intensity, and duration of services provided since the last intervention plan or progress report and the number of visits attended and missed. It also includes measurement data collected, results, equipment provided, any medical or educational updates for the child, the child's response to intervention, home programming, and caregiver training.]
Child's current performance:

GOAL	INITIAL PERFORMANCE	CURRENT PERFORMANCE	REVISED GOALS
LTG 1			
STG 1			
STG 2			
LTG 2			
STG 3			
STG 4			
LTG 3			
STG 5			
STG 6			

Summary and recommendations:
[Assessment of progress, potential for improvement and benefit from services provided, and recommendations for continued services are listed here. This section may also include a skilled occupational therapy statement, home program recommendations, and any recommended referrals or community services.]
Signature and Date

Note. LTG = long-term goal; STG = short-term goal.

SUMMARY

In health care settings, occupational therapy documentation is separate from the documentation of other interdisciplinary team members. However, it is important to note that occupational therapy documentation will be used by other members of the health care team in supporting the outcomes for the child and family receiving services. It is critical that the occupational therapy practitioner's analysis and recommendations be clear to these other health care providers to best establish interprofessional coordinated care for the child and family in alignment with family-centered and client-centered practices.

Documentation is a vital piece of occupational therapy practice across settings. AOTA's occupational profile template (AOTA, 2017a) and the PERFORM documentation template (AOTA, 2017c) can be a useful place to start in developing documentation templates for early childhood health care settings. These templates can be used to support increased efficiency in documentation while also meeting legal and ethical requirements. These tools are particularly useful when time for documentation is limited and the need for high-quality documentation remains high because of continued use of medical records in legal cases. Using AOTA resources such as these can help support occupational therapy practitioners in working with their employer's EHR and data privacy teams to keep documentation as updated as possible to support the valued role of early childhood occupational therapy in health care settings.

REFERENCES

American Academy of Pediatrics. (2004). Levels of neonatal care. *Pediatrics, 114,* 1341–1347. https://doi.org/10.1542/peds.2004-1697

American Medical Association. (2020a). *Current procedural terminology (CPT®) 2020 standard.* American Medical Association Press.

American Medical Association. (2020b). *Prior authorization practice resources.* https://www.ama-assn.org/practice-management/sustainability/prior-authorization-practice-resources

American Occupational Therapy Association. (2017a). AOTA occupational profile template. *American Journal of Occupational Therapy, 71,* 7112420030. https://doi.org/10.5014/ajot.2017.716S12

American Occupational Therapy Association. (2017b). AOTA's societal statement on health literacy. *American Journal of Occupational Therapy, 71*(Suppl. 2), 7112410065. https://doi.org/10.5014/ajot.2017.716S14

American Occupational Therapy Association. (2017c). *PERFORM documentation templates.* https://www.aota.org/~/media/Corporate/Files/Secure/Advocacy/Federal/Perform-Documentation-Templates.pdf

American Occupational Therapy Association. (2018a). Guidelines for documentation of occupational therapy. *American Journal of Occupational Therapy, 72*(Suppl. 2), 7212410010. https://doi.org/10.5014/ajot.2018.72S203

American Occupational Therapy Association. (2018b). Occupational therapy's role in the neonatal intensive care unit. *American Journal of Occupational Therapy, 72*(Suppl. 2), 7212410060. https://doi.org/10.5014/ajot.2018.72S204

American Occupational Therapy Association. (2020a). 2020 occupational therapy code of ethics. *American Journal of Occupational Therapy, 74*(Suppl. 3), 7413410005. https://doi.org/10.5014/ajot.2020.74S3006

American Occupational Therapy Association. (2020b). Occupational therapy practice framework: Domain and process (4th ed.). *American Journal of Occupational Therapy, 74*(Suppl. 2), 7412410010. https://doi.org/10.5014/ajot.2020.74S2001

American Occupational Therapy Association. (n.d.). *Improve your documentation with AOTA's occupational profile template.* https://www.aota.org/Practice/Manage/Reimb/occupational-profile-document-value-ot.aspx

Health Insurance Portability and Accountability Act of 1996, Pub. L. 104-191, 42 U.S.C. § 300gg, 29 U.S.C. §§ 1181–1183, and 42 U.S.C. §§ 1320d–1320d9.

Individuals With Disabilities Education Improvement Act of 2004, Pub. L. 108-446, 20 U.S.C. §§ 1400–1482.

Medicare.gov. (n.d.). *What's home health care?* https://www.medicare.gov/what-medicare-covers/whats-home-health-care

Niebaum, K., Cunningham-Sabo, L., & Bellows, L. (2015). Developing effective educational materials using best practices in health literacy. *Journal of Extension, 53*(4), 1–4.

Park, S. (2012). Setting goals that express the possibilities: If we don't know where we're going, how will we know when we get there? In S. J. Lane & A. C. Bundy (Eds.), *Kids can be kids: A childhood occupations approach* (pp. 349–367). F. A. Davis.

Pizur-Barnekow, K., Darragh, A., & Johnston, M. (2011). "I cried because I didn't know if I could take care of him": Toward a taxonomy of interactive and critical health literacy as portrayed by caregivers of children with special health care needs. *Journal of Health Communication, 16,* 205–221. https://doi.org/10.1080/10810730.2011.604386

Richardson, P. K. (2015). Occupational therapy evaluation in pediatrics. In J. Case-Smith & J. C. O'Brien (Eds.), *Occupational therapy for children and adolescents* (7th ed., pp. 163–192). Elsevier Mosby.

Sames, K. (2015). *Documenting occupational therapy practice* (3rd ed.). Pearson Education.

World Health Organization. (2010). *International statistical classification of diseases and related health problems* (10th ed.). Author.

Section VI.

Evidence-Guided Practice: Addressing Evaluation and Intervention

Best Practices in Supporting Activities of Daily Living and Sleep (Adaptive Skills)

27

Meredith Gronski, OTD, OTR/L, CLA

KEY TERMS AND CONCEPTS

- Activities of daily living
- Backward chaining
- Caregiver education and coaching
- Chaining
- Context
- Delayed toileting skills
- Dressing and undressing
- Forward chaining
- Interoception
- Kangaroo care
- Nocturnal enuresis
- Occupational performance coaching
- Rapid Toileting Training
- Sleep
- Sleep challenges
- Toilet training
- Toileting readiness skills
- Visual schedule

OVERVIEW

The ability to perform activities of daily living (ADLs) is critical to overall child development and quality of life. *ADLs* are basic self-care skills, including dressing, personal hygiene and grooming, toileting, personal device care, and bathing or showering (American Occupational Therapy Association [AOTA], 2020). Although the *Occupational Therapy Practice Framework* (4th ed.; AOTA, 2020) lists rest and sleep separately from ADLs, this chapter includes sleep because it was part of a systematic review. Feeding and eating are also ADLs and are addressed in depth in Chapter 28, "Best Practices in Supporting Mealtimes and Nutritional Needs (Adaptive Skills)."

In addition to functional independence in self-care skills, young children learn to self-soothe, sleep through the night, take naps, and participate in rest time over their first 5 years of life. Sleep preparation, sleep hygiene, sustained sleep states, and resting or napping are essential occupations across the life course (AOTA, 2020). Development of self-care and adaptive skills is propelled by the child's functional ability in performance skills and opportunity to practice the targeted daily living skills. Occupational therapy practitioners often provide interventions for adaptive and self-care skills in the context of the neonatal intensive care unit (NICU), early intervention, inpatient hospital programs, early childhood education programs (child care, preschool, Head Start and Early Head Start), and pediatric outpatient clinics. (*Note. Occupational therapy practitioner* refers to both occupational therapists and occupational therapy assistants.)

ESSENTIAL CONSIDERATIONS

Children's ability to develop independence in self-care skills is supported by intrinsic capacity and affordance of opportunity. Children with health conditions, developmental delays, and acquired disabilities may experience barriers to full ADL independence related to poor motor coordination, strength, and stamina; atypical sensory registration or sensitivities; or limitations in perception, initiation, concentration, and sequencing. Further barriers to independence may include a child's self-efficacy, their motivation to be independent, a caregiver's expectation of independence, and schedules and routines that limit practice opportunities and independent skill development.

Toileting

For young children, *toilet training* is a major developmental milestone that affects the family's habits and routines for a significant period of time at home, at child care or preschool, and in the community. It is common for toileting independence and continence training to begin between ages 21 and 36 months in the United States, with daytime toileting independence typically achieved by ages 3–4 years (Blum et al., 2003). The age at which toilet training is accomplished is strongly linked to culture and ethnicity.

Child care or preschool attendance may also be an important influential factor in childhood toileting independence. Children who attend traditional child care facilities are often required to be independent in toileting by age 3 years. A child who demonstrates *toileting readiness skills* can typically indicate when wet or soiled, sit comfortably on a commode, manage donning and doffing pants and undergarments, communicate the need to eliminate (through words, sign, or adaptive communication system), stay dry for a period of at least 1 hour, and demonstrate a predictable bowel movement schedule (Anderson et al., 2007; LaVesser & Hilton, 2010). Aspects of *delayed toileting skills,* including difficulty with lying

---

still during diapering, incontinence, stool toileting refusal, and daytime or nocturnal out-of-toilet elimination, can have a significant impact on a child's personal hygiene, self-confidence, independence, and social acceptance; caregiver burden of care; and parenting stress (Cicero & Pfadt, 2002; Keen et al., 2007).

Children with developmental disabilities may have more difficulty achieving interest and independence in toilet training and may never achieve full continence (Lomas Mevers et al., 2018). Children with motor performance deficits may have challenges with manipulating clothing and fasteners, achieving seated and dynamic balance, getting on and off of the commode, maneuvering and approaching the bathroom with enough efficiency to prevent toileting accidents, and achieving toileting hygiene (e.g., wiping oneself). Children with atypical sensory processing patterns may have difficulty with registering when they are wet or soiled. Some children, especially those with autism spectrum disorder (ASD), may have difficulty with *interoception,* or recognizing and responding to the internal urge to go to the bathroom (Garfinkel et al., 2016). Some children may further exhibit stool refusal or other maladaptive responses during the toilet training process.

Children with intellectual disabilities or with deficits in concentration or sequencing may take more time to learn the routine of toileting or to remember to complete all the steps. It is also important to be aware that children who have been exposed to trauma or have experienced poor attachment may express fear, anxiety, or other negative reactions during diapering and toileting (Shepherd, 2019). Children who lack toileting independence and continence are more likely to have more difficulty with adaptive skills later in life, be victims of bullying (Joinson et al., 2007), and have reduced quality of life (Cicero & Pfadt, 2002).

Dressing

Independence in *dressing and undressing* begins to emerge around age 12 months. Full independence, including manipulation of fasteners, is typically achieved around age 6 years (Barnes, 2020). The development of independence in dressing is related to a number of personal factors, including hand strength, balance, and sensitivity to fabric textures. Additionally, when children are afforded more time and opportunity for practice to dress and undress, they become more confident and independent in these self-care skills sooner.

A child's readiness to start learning independent dressing skills begins with the ability to attend to a task for 5–10 minutes, follow simple one-step directions, imitate the actions of others, participate in adult assistance with dressing and undressing, and demonstrate emerging body awareness and concepts of front–back and left–right (Anderson et al., 2007). A family's cultural values may influence the development of independence in dressing. Many cultures place high value on interdependence in dressing, and parents use the activity to share time, care, and affection with the child (LaVesser & Hilton, 2010).

Children with developmental disabilities, such as ASD, often have greater rates of atypical sensory processing patterns and greater motor difficulties, which affect their independence in daily living skills, such as dressing (Jasmin et

al., 2009). Children who need greater assistance with daily living skills place additional burden and responsibility on caregivers. These increased demands, beyond what is typical for the child's age, can result in increased parenting stress or psychological distress (Estes et al., 2009).

Grooming and Hygiene

Young children need significant caregiver supervision and assistance for bathing, hair care, and oral hygiene for several years before safe independence is achieved. Young toddlers begin to develop interest in assisting with toothbrushing, bathing, and combing or brushing hair around age 2 years. By the time children are age 5 years, they can typically brush their teeth and complete a simple handwashing routine independently. Children should continue to be supported and supervised while bathing until around age 8 years (LaVesser & Hilton, 2010; Shepherd, 2015). Many grooming and hygiene routines are sequential and can be learned in a rote manner with moderate cognitive capacity.

Many children who have difficulty with these personal care routines experience atypical sensory processing patterns and difficulty with self-regulation, which are barriers to engaging in the tasks successfully. The flavors of toothpaste, the textures of different combs or brushes, the scent of shampoos and soaps, and the temperature of bathwater can all contribute to a child's sensitivities to different sensations. A child who does not follow sufficient dental care practices may develop dental decay and pain that affects their eating and nutritional status. From an early age, it is critical that caregivers support the development of good grooming and hygiene habits among children of all abilities to help maintain their physiological health and reduce social ridicule as they get older (Shepherd, 2015).

Sleep and Rest

Regular, uninterrupted *sleep* in infancy and the toddler years is essential to healthy development and overall family quality of life. Sleep includes ceasing active engagement with the environment, achieving a calm arousal state, and sustaining a sleep state without disruption. Infants and toddlers with and without developmental delays can experience challenges with the occupation of sleep. Additional challenges can be present for infants being cared for in a NICU setting. Interruption of the key habits and routines surrounding the occupation of sleep has a profound impact on the health and well-being of children and their caregivers. The recommended amount of sleep for children ages birth to 5 years is presented in Table 27.1. How often and how long a child naps is extremely variable, depending on family schedule, environment, and child temperament.

Sleep challenges at home include difficulty falling asleep, difficulty staying asleep, colic or crying, and issues with negative daytime behaviors (Hauck et al., 2012; Mindell et al., 2011; Price et al., 2012). Sleep disturbances are often one of the primary challenges reported to occupational therapy practitioners by parents of children with developmental delays. Settling down to go to sleep and staying asleep are difficult for children with self-regulation challenges related to modulation of sensory input. Often, children with disabilities or developmental delays more frequently need

TABLE 27.1. Amount of Sleep Needed by Child's Age

AGE	AMOUNT OF DAILY SLEEP NEEDED	NAP FREQUENCY AND DURATION
Newborn–2 months	12–18 hours	Throughout the day
3–11 months	12–16 hours (including naps)	Two to four times daily; 30 minutes–2 hours duration
1–3 years	11–14 hours (including naps)	Once or twice daily; 1–3 hours duration
3–5 years	10–13 hours (including naps)	Once daily

Sources. Information drawn from Paruthi et al. (2016) and Shepherd (2015).

accommodations (e.g., sleep location or position, specific sheets or blankets, music or white noise) to support their sleep habits.

Children who regularly sleep fewer than the recommended hours per day can have difficulties with attention, learning, behavior, and chronic conditions later in life (Paruthi et al., 2016). Sleep disorders affect 10% of typical children and their families (Byars et al., 2012); those with ASD have twice the risk of developing a sleep disorder as typical children (Elrod et al., 2016). Irregular sleep patterns and frequent waking can also lead to changes in parental sleep habits and well-being (Couturier et al., 2005; Hiscock et al., 2007; Touchette et al., 2005).

BEST PRACTICES

As the occupational therapy process is initiated with a new family to address performance limitations in ADLs or sleep routine challenges, the occupational therapist completes a formal evaluation and develops of a plan of care (i.e., intervention plan). The implementation and ongoing review of the intervention strategies by the occupational therapy practitioner is a collaborative process with the child and family in their natural contexts. Through this collaborative and ongoing process, the family and practitioner define what success looks like and begin the conversation about discontinuation of direct services from the very first encounter.

Initiate Evaluation

Evaluation begins with collecting a child's occupational profile through interview with the child (if appropriate) and their caregivers and other important family members. ADLs are an integral component of the occupational profile and an important area of performance to assess. Evaluation of these specific self-care skills in the early childhood population should be done through a multimodal approach that includes proxy report questionnaires, natural context observations, interview, and formal or standardized ADL assessment tools, when they are available and appropriate. Examples of formal assessment tools are described in Table 27.2. A more in-depth listing of assessment tools can be found in Appendix F, "Examples of Assessments for Early Childhood (Birth–5 Years)."

TABLE 27.2. Assessment Tools for ADLs

ASSESSMENT TOOL	AGE RANGE	TYPE
Functional Independence Measure for Children (Msall et al., 1994)	6 months–7 years	▪ Formal ▪ Criterion referenced ▪ Performance based
Pediatric Evaluation of Disability Inventory—Computer Adaptive Test (Haley et al., 2012)	6 months–7 years, 6 months	▪ Formal ▪ Norm referenced ▪ Proxy questionnaire
Preschool Activity Card Sort (Berg & LaVesser, 2006)	3–6 years	▪ Formal ▪ Criterion referenced ▪ Proxy interview and card sort
Roll Evaluation of Activities of Life (Roll & Roll, 2013)	2–18 years, 11 months	▪ Formal ▪ Norm referenced ▪ Proxy questionnaire
Scales of Independent Behavior—Revised Personal Living subscale (Bruininks et al., 1996)	3 months–80 years	▪ Formal ▪ Norm referenced ▪ Proxy questionnaire and interview
Vineland Adaptive Behavior Scales (3rd ed.; Sparrow et al., 2016)	Birth–90 years	▪ Formal ▪ Norm referenced ▪ Proxy questionnaire and interview

It is of critical importance to observe the self-care routine in the natural *context* (e.g., home, child care, preschool). This may include conducting components of the assessment early in the morning or later in the evening, as scheduling allows, or having a parent share a video of the child completing the tasks in the home. By observing the task routine in context, the occupational therapist can analyze the communication, behavioral, physical, sensory, social, temporal, and environmental factors that may be supporting or hindering the child's ADL performance. Self-care skills can be assessed in the child care or preschool natural context during the classroom restroom and handwashing routines, when children don and doff coats for recess, and during nap and rest time routines; classrooms often also implement a toothbrushing expectation after lunch.

When the evaluation process includes interviews and proxy questionnaires for children in preschool programs, it is important to gather information from both the child's family caregivers and their educators. Variations in task performance and independence level across different settings can assist the occupational therapist in analyzing the source of limiting factors. Once the therapist develops a hypothesis about supports and limitations for self-care participation, then they can assess performance patterns and component skills (motor, sensory, cognitive, social, behavioral). By using this top-down evaluation approach, occupational therapist can be sure that goals and intervention plans are client centered and focused on meaningful routines for the child and caregivers.

Develop Positive Partnerships With Families

Collaborative partnership with families in their natural habits, routines, and roles is a critical component of successful intervention to support mastery of self-care and adaptive skills in early childhood. Whenever possible, occupational therapy practitioners should address ADL activity demands and interventions in the location and at the time those daily activities typically occur.

Occupational performance coaching is a strengths-based approach that supports a positive parent–therapist partnership and maximizes parental self-efficacy through problem solving, guided modeling, and reflection (Graham & Rodger, 2010; Graham et al., 2013; Shepherd, 2015). In this approach, occupational therapy practitioners collaborate with parents to set meaningful goals and help them identify ways to promote successful performance of daily living skills. In the context of daily family routines, family-implemented intervention strategies are critical for generalizability and sustainability of outcomes.

Occupational therapy practitioners who view parents as a child's best teacher successfully promote family-directed goals and build parents' capacity to solve occupational performance problems long after the practitioner is no longer involved (Dunn et al., 2012; Dunst et al., 2006; Graham & Rodger, 2010). For more information about family partnerships and contextual interventions, see Chapter 8, "Best Practices in Supporting Family Partnerships," and Chapter 16, "Best Practices in Intervention Under Part C."

Provide Interventions for Toileting

Occupational therapy practitioners can support toileting skills by offering strategies to primary caregivers and educators to promote structured toileting routines and positive toileting reinforcement or by implementing strategies and skill development to improve continence and the adaptive skills related to toileting (e.g., handwashing and lower-extremity dressing).

The most well-known and cited toileting intervention protocol, which dominated the literature in the 1970s, is the *Rapid Toileting Training* (RTT) method (Azrin & Foxx, 1971). RTT is based on operant conditioning principles. Many of the successful components of this method, such as increased fluid intake; positive reinforcement; and scheduled, frequent visits to the bathroom, are still used in contemporary evidence-based approaches. In fact, most current toilet training strategies are derivatives or modifications of RTT (Kroeger & Sorensen-Burnworth, 2009).

Some toilet training strategies require nearly constant attention to a toileting schedule, which may not be feasible for a working parent or an early childhood educator with eight other children in their care. Some strategies require the child to have a certain level of cognition and verbal communication, whereas others can be accessed through visual and nonverbal cues. Selecting and implementing an effective toilet training intervention strategy relies heavily on the identified occupational profile, component skill limitations and strengths, and social and environmental support.

Caregiver coaching

Occupational therapy practitioners can collaborate with parents, early childhood educators, child care providers, and support staff to identify and establish the best communication strategy, environmental set-up, and level of support across settings. As many as 25% of young children go through a period of stool toileting refusal, which includes hiding while having a bowel movement and can lead to other negative outcomes, such as constipation and encopresis (Taubman et al., 2003). It is important to include caregiver education about avoiding negative and punitive language related to toileting.

For severe cases of fecal incontinence and constipation, a medical–behavioral approach is recommended to disimpact the bowels and maintain regular bowel movements, in addition to work with an occupational therapy practitioner to establish positive toileting routines and habits (Law et al., 2016). It is also beneficial for children with language or intellectual delays to use one cue, word, picture, or gesture to indicate that it is time to use the bathroom. Consistency of routine and expectations for management of the toileting tasks is critical to support the development of independence (Shepherd, 2015).

Behavioral modification

When parents and caregivers begin the toilet training process, they sometimes start with an all-or-nothing approach, such as transitioning the child to underwear and hoping for the best outcome. When this strategy is unsuccessful for children with developmental delays or acquired disabilities, occupational therapy practitioners can assist caregivers with developing strategies and routines that will support the toilet training process through evidence-based behavioral approaches. Protocols that use positive reinforcement and rewards for in-toilet elimination, frequent scheduled bathroom visits, increased fluid intake during training, and the exclusion of punitive and negative language result in more frequent in-toilet eliminations, more frequent child-initiated toileting, and earlier achievement of complete dryness (Cicero & Pfadt, 2002; Keen et al., 2007; Law et al., 2016; Rinald & Mirenda, 2012). Practitioners must collaborate with caregivers to assess what prompts and cues are most effective and which types of reinforcement are most motivating across settings.

Wetting alarms

Nocturnal enuresis (i.e., bed-wetting) is often the final stage of toileting independence and frequently the most challenging. The urine alarm was originally developed and described by Mowrer and Mowrer (1938). Contemporary implementation of the device follows a protocol to include setting up the alarm in the child's pajamas, waking the child when the alarm sounds, having the child complete elimination in the toilet, praising the child for use of the toilet and paying minimal attention to bed-wetting, having the child change to dry clothes and linens if needed, and reattaching the alarm before returning to bed. More contemporary versions of these devices with wireless technology allow caregivers to receive notification of wetting through their smartphone (Henriksen & Peterson, 2013). In addition to routine modifications, such as limiting evening fluid intake and toileting at bedtime, this is often a less-invasive intervention strategy to use before pharmaceutical interventions for nocturnal enuresis.

Provide Interventions for Dressing, Grooming, and Hygiene

Teaching adaptive self-care skills can be addressed with various intervention approaches. Occupational therapy practitioners can use graded cueing and prompts generated from behavioral and cognitive learning frames of reference. Compensatory and coaching approaches can be implemented in tandem with formal skill acquisition strategies.

Visual task schedules

Occupational therapy practitioners use a variety of cues and prompts to work with families to establish new daily living skills. Many children benefit from having a visual representation of a new or difficult activity or sequence of tasks. The practitioner starts with a task analysis process to break down the target skill into achievable steps. These steps are then translated into photos, drawings, or graphics and posted sequentially where the child can view them (Hilton & LaVesser, 2010).

Caregivers and the occupational therapy practitioner should introduce the *visual schedule* to the child and model how it can be used before it is initiated in the context of an activity. The visual schedule can have hook-and-loop or dry erase features to assist the child with marking where they are in the process and having a sense of mastery throughout each step in the activity. Other visual strategies that can be used include color coding, video modeling, and visual stories.

Chaining strategies

Dressing and grooming skills are sequential tasks that require supported learning to be completed independently. Children with cognitive impairments or developmental delays may best learn these skills through a behavioral learning approach, such as *chaining.* The occupational therapy practitioner starts by conducting a task analysis to determine the steps of the target dressing or grooming activity. Through the use of behavioral strategies, such as prompts, cues, and reinforcement, each step of the task is mastered and linked to the next in a sequential manner (Anderson et al., 2007; Barnes, 2020; LaVesser & Hilton, 2010).

In *backward chaining,* all of the steps of the task are completed by the caregiver, and the child is prompted to complete the last step and receives reinforcement. The mastery process continues with the adult caregiver completing fewer steps and the child completing more of the task independently to completion. *Forward chaining* allows the child to initiate and master the first step of a task and receive reinforcement for successful completion of that step; then the adult caregiver completes the remainder of the steps. As mastery develops, the child completes more and more steps after task initiation, until they can complete the entire task independently. Both forward and backward chaining are effective to teach dressing, toothbrushing, handwashing, and other sequential hygiene ADLs (Hilton & LaVesser, 2010; Shepherd, 2015).

Task and material modification

Children with complex movement impairments and atypical sensory processing responses may benefit from working with an occupational therapy practitioner to modify the demands and materials used during dressing and grooming routines. Practitioners can work with the family to consider style preferences and cultural practices when selecting garments that will work best with the child's sensory response patterns. Approaches may include moisture-wicking or compression athletic-style shirts or assistance in analyzing the features of waistbands on different shorts and pants. Numerous clothing brands print the sizing information on the inside of the garment rather than using a traditional sewn-in tag. For children with difficulty with body awareness or spatial perception of front and back, tops with a graphic or design on the front can help them learn how to orient the garment before donning it (Barnes, 2020).

Bathing and grooming tasks may be more successful with unscented soaps and shampoos or modified water temperature and pressure. Children who demonstrate tactile or proprioceptive seeking patterns may cooperate and enjoy brushing their teeth with the increased vibratory pressure of an electric toothbrush. The occupational therapy practitioner can demonstrate deep pressure during bathing or hair brushing, which may reduce the maladaptive responses of a child who is defensive to light-touch tactile input.

Children with motor impairments may benefit from elastic waistbands, pullover tops with wide openings, and fabrics with stretch properties. Many mainstream clothing brands and designers have developed clothing lines with adaptive fasteners that require little to no fine motor precision. Occupational therapy practitioners consider adaptations to achieve independence with clothing fasteners for preschoolers; they may recommend these garments.

A variety of adaptive bathing equipment may be necessary for children with motor and postural control limitations that make independence in the bathtub unsafe. Caregivers can collaborate with the occupational therapy practitioner to develop safe and ergonomically sound methods of bathing the child with the use of tub seats or slings, bath mitts, or handheld showerheads (Barnes, 2020; Shepherd, 2015).

Support Sleep and Rest

Occupational therapy practitioners often work closely with families to address the habits and routines of sleep hygiene. Supportive interventions target healthy sleep by developing strategies for caregivers to incorporate into sleep–wake routines in the NICU and manage behavioral issues of infants and toddlers at home (AOTA, 2020; Vergara et al., 2006).

Kangaroo care

Both full-term and premature infants often have difficulty with sleep, state, and temperature regulation. ***Kangaroo care*** is the process of placing an infant in direct chest-to-chest contact with their mother, father, or other caregiver with skin exposed. This process is recommended, regardless of feeding or delivery method, immediately after birth and can continue throughout infancy (Feldman-Winter et al., 2016). Infants who participate in kangaroo care have significantly greater deep sleep time and quiet awake and alert states (Feldman et al., 2002; Kusanagi et al., 2011).

Parent coaching

Occupational therapy practitioners can use in-person ***caregiver education and coaching*** to help parents learn to differentiate infant cries and determine when to assist with soothing, as well as to model controlled comforting and anticipatory guidance to support the development of self-soothing among infants (Hall et al., 2015; Hiscock et al., 2007 ; Kusanagi et al., 2011; Salisbury et al., 2012). Additionally, techniques of bedtime fading and gradual extinction (i.e., gradually delaying parent response to child crying at bedtime) can improve self-soothing, decrease time to fall asleep (sleep latency), and decrease nighttime waking (Gradisar et al., 2016; Hall et al., 2015).

Occupational therapy practitioners can also help parents by educating them on strategies for camping out (i.e., the caregiver staying with a child until they fall asleep), extinction, and setting positive bedtime routines based in sleep hygiene (Blunden, 2011; Johnson et al., 2013; Malow et al., 2014). Through a coaching model, parents and caregivers can examine the sleeping environment in collaboration with the practitioner for temperature, lighting, olfactory, and auditory factors that may need to be modified to create a supportive sleeping environment.

Media use

Evening media use and daytime violent media use are associated with sleep problems among preschool-age children. Children with televisions or other screen devices in their bedroom have a higher rate of sleep difficulty (Garrison et al., 2011). As a part of an overall coaching strategy to help caregivers establish healthy bedtime routines, occupational therapy practitioners should assist parents in setting screen-time limits, particularly in the evening. Caregivers and practitioners can work together to develop replacement bedtime routine activities for screen time, such as reading stories, singing, or quiet play activities for up to an hour before the child is expected to go to sleep. Caregiver education on healthy media use among preschoolers is shown to decrease parent-reported sleep problems across an 18-month period (Garrison & Christakis, 2012).

Monitor Progress

As occupational therapy practitioners implement the intervention plan to address performance of self-care skills and sleep routines, they must continually review the effectiveness of their selected strategies. Formal tools, such as Goal Attainment Scaling (Ottenbacher & Cusick, 1990) and the Canadian Occupational Performance Measure (Law et al., 2019) can be used to quantify progress and aid in clinical decision making. Occupational therapy practitioners should also check in with the child's primary caregivers for perceptions of role competence, parental stress, and overall satisfaction with the therapeutic process and outcomes.

SUMMARY

Participation in ADLs as a part of a home or early childhood education routine is a critical component of healthy child development and engagement in goal-directed behaviors. ADL performance both drives and is supported by cognitive, motor, sensory, emotional, and behavioral performance skills. Through a top-down evaluation process, occupational therapy practitioners can identify occupational performance strengths and limitations. Practitioners partner with families and educators to develop strategies to teach new daily living skills, modify specific tasks and environments, and implement behavioral programs to support independent ADL performance and healthy sleep routines.

REFERENCES

American Occupational Therapy Association. (2020). Occupational therapy practice framework: Domain and process (4th ed.). *American Journal of Occupational Therapy, 74*(Suppl. 2), 7412410010. https://doi.org/10.5014/ajot.2020.74S2001

Anderson, S. R., Jablonski, A. L., Thomeer, M. L., & Knapp, V. M. (2007). *Self-help skills for people with autism: A systematic teaching approach.* Woodbine House.

Azrin, N. H., & Foxx, R. M. (1971). A rapid method of toilet training the institutionalized retarded. *Journal of Applied Behavior Analysis, 4*(2), 89–99. https://doi.org/10.1901/jaba.1971.4-89

Barnes, K. (2020). Children with developmental disabilities. In K. M. Matuska (Ed.), *Ways of living: Intervention strategies to enable participation* (5th ed., pp. 91–106). AOTA Press.

Berg, C., & LaVesser, P. (2006). The Preschool Activity Card Sort. *OTJR: Occupation, Participation and Health, 26,* 143–151. https://doi.org/10.1177/153944920602600404

Blum, N. J., Taubman, B., & Nemeth, N. (2003). Relationship between age at initiation of toilet training and duration of training: A prospective study. *Pediatrics, 111,* 810–814. https://doi.org/10.1542/peds.111.4.810

Blunden, S. (2011). Behavioural treatments to encourage solo sleeping in pre-school children: An alternative to controlled crying. *Journal of Child Health Care, 15,* 107–117. https://doi.org/10.1177/1367493510397623

Bruininks, R. H., Woodcock, R. W., Weatherman, R. F., & Hill, B. K. (1996). *SIB–R: Scales of Independent Behavior—Revised.* Riverside.

Byars, K. C., Yolton, K., Rausch, J., Lanphear, B., & Beebe, D. W. (2012). Prevalence, patterns, and persistence of sleep problems in the first 3 years of life. *Pediatrics, 129,* e276–e284. https://doi.org/10.1542/peds.2011-0372

Cicero, F. R., & Pfadt, A. (2002). Investigation of a reinforcement-based toilet training procedure for children with autism. *Research in Developmental Disabilities, 23,* 319–331. https://doi.org/10.1016/S0891-4222(02)00136-1

Couturier, J. L., Speechley, K. N., Steele, M., Norman, R., Stringer, B., & Nicolson, R. (2005). Parental perception of sleep problems in children of normal intelligence with pervasive developmental disorders: Prevalence, severity, and pattern. *Journal of the American Academy of Child & Adolescent Psychiatry, 44,* 815–822. https://doi.org/10.1097/01.chi.0000166377.22651.87

Dunn, W., Cox, J., Foster, L., Mische-Lawson, L., & Tanquary, J. (2012). Impact of a contextual intervention on child participation and parent competence among children with autism spectrum disorders: A pretest–posttest repeated-measures design. *American Journal of Occupational Therapy, 66,* 520–528. https://doi.org/10.5014/ajot.2012.004119

Dunst, C. J., Bruder, M. B., Trivette, C. M., & Hamby, D. W. (2006). Everyday activity settings, natural learning environments, and early intervention practices. *Journal of Policy and Practice in Intellectual Disabilities, 3,* 3–10. https://doi.org/10.1111/j.1741-1130.2006.00047.x

Elrod, M. G., Nylund, C. M., Susi, A. L., Gorman, G. H., Hisle-Gorman, E., Rogers, D. J., & Erdie-Lalena, C. (2016). Prevalence of diagnosed sleep disorders and related diagnostic and surgical procedures in children with autism spectrum disorders. *Journal of Developmental & Behavioral Pediatrics, 37,* 377–384. https://doi.org/10.1097/DBP.0000000000000248

Estes, A., Munson, J., Dawson, G., Koehler, E., Zhou, X. H., & Abbott, R. (2009). Parenting stress and psychological functioning among mothers of preschool children with autism and developmental delay. *Autism, 13,* 375–387. https://doi.org/10.1177/1362361309105658

Feldman, R., Weller, A., Sirota, L., & Eidelman, A. I. (2002). Skin-to-skin contact (kangaroo care) promotes self-regulation in premature infants: Sleep–wake cyclicity, arousal modulation, and sustained exploration. *Developmental Psychology, 38,* 194–207. https://doi.org/10.1037//0012-1649.38.2.194

Feldman-Winter, L., Goldsmith, J. P., American Academy of Pediatrics Committee on Fetus and Newborn, & American Academy of Pediatrics Task Force on Sudden Infant Death Syndrome.

(2016). Safe sleep and skin-to-skin care in the neonatal period for healthy term newborns. *Pediatrics, 138,* e20161889. https://doi.org/10.1542/pcds.2016-1889

Garfinkel, S. N., Tiley, C., O'Keeffe, S., Harrison, N. A., Seth, A. K., & Critchley, H. D. (2016). Discrepancies between dimensions of interoception in autism: Implications for emotion and anxiety. *Biological Psychology, 114,* 117–126. https://doi.org/10.1016/j.biopsycho.2015.12.003

Garrison, M. M., & Christakis, D. A. (2012). The impact of a healthy media use intervention on sleep in preschool children. *Pediatrics, 130,* 492–499. https://doi.org/10.1542/peds.2011-3153

Garrison, M. M., Liekweg, K., & Christakis, D. A. (2011). Media use and child sleep: The impact of content, timing, and environment. *Pediatrics, 128,* 29–35. https://doi.org/10.1542/peds.2010-3304

Gradisar, M., Jackson, K., Spurrier, N. J., Gibson, J., Whitham, J., Williams, A. S., . . . Kennaway, D. J. (2016). Behavioral interventions for infant sleep problems: A randomized controlled trial. *Pediatrics, 137*(6), e20151486. https://doi.org/10.1542/peds.2015-1486

Graham, F., & Rodger, S. (2010). Occupational performance coaching: Enabling parents' and children's occupational performance. In S. Rodger & A. Kennedy-Behr (Eds.), *Occupation-centred practice with children: A practical guide for occupational therapists* (pp. 203–226). Wiley.

Graham, F., Rodger, S., & Ziviani, J. (2013). Effectiveness of occupational performance coaching in improving children's and mothers' performance and mothers' self-competence. *American Journal of Occupational Therapy, 67*(1), 10–18. https://doi.org/10.5014/ajot.2013.004648

Haley, S. M., Coster, W. J., Dumas, H. M., Fragala-Pinkam, M. A., Moed, R., Kramer, J., ... Ludlow, L. H. (2012). *Pediatric Evaluation of Disability Inventory—Computer Adaptive Test.* https://www.pedicat.com/

Hall, W. A., Hutton, E., Brant, R. F., Collet, J. P., Gregg, K., Saunders, R., . . . Wooldridge, J. (2015). A randomized controlled trial of an intervention for infants' behavioral sleep problems. *BMC Pediatrics, 15,* 181. https://doi.org/10.1186/s12887-015-0492-7

Hauck, Y. L., Hall, W. A., Dhaliwal, S. S., Bennett, E., & Wells, G. (2012). The effectiveness of an early parenting intervention for mothers with infants with sleep and settling concerns: A prospective non-equivalent before–after design. *Journal of Clinical Nursing, 21,* 52–62. https://doi.org/10.1111/j.1365-2702.2011.03734.x

Henriksen, N., & Peterson, S. (2013). Behavioral treatment of bedwetting in an adolescent with autism. *Journal of Developmental and Physical Disabilities, 25,* 313–323. https://doi.org/10.1007/s10882-012-9308-y

Hiscock, H., Canterford, L., Ukoumunne, O. C., & Wake, M. (2007). Adverse associations of sleep problems in Australian preschoolers: National population study. *Pediatrics, 119,* 86–93. https://doi.org/10.1542/pcds.2006-1757

Jasmin, E., Couture, M., McKinley, P., Reid, G., Fombonne, E., & Gisel, E. (2009). Sensori-motor and daily living skills of preschool children with autism spectrum disorders. *Journal of Autism and Developmental Disorders, 39,* 231–241. https://doi.org/10.1007/s10803-008-0617-z

Johnson, C. R., Turner, K. S., Foldes, E., Brooks, M. M., Kronk, R., & Wiggs, L. (2013). Behavioral parent training to address sleep disturbances in young children with autism spectrum disorder: A pilot trial. *Sleep Medicine, 14,* 995–1004. https://doi .org/10.1016/j.sleep.2013.05.013

Joinson, C., Heron, J., Butler, R., VonGontard, A., Butler, U., Emond, A., & Golding, J. (2007). A United Kingdom population-based study of intellectual capacities in children with and without soiling, daytime wetting, and bed-wetting. *Pediatrics, 120,* 308–316. https://doi.org/10.1542/peds.2006-2891

Keen, D., Brannigan, K. L., & Cuskelly, M. (2007). Toilet training for children with autism: The effects of video modeling. *Journal of Developmental and Physical Disabilities, 19,* 291–303. https:// doi.org/10.1007/s10882-007-9044-x

Kroeger, K. A., & Sorensen-Burnworth, R. (2009). Toilet training individuals with autism and other developmental disabilities: A critical review. *Research in Autism Spectrum Disorders, 3,* 607–618. https://doi.org/10.1016/j.rasd.2009.01.005

Kusanagi, M., Hirose, T., Mikuni, K., & Okamitsu, M. (2011). Effect of early intervention using state modulation and cue reading on mother–infant interactions in preterm infants and their mothers in Japan. *Journal of Medical & Dental Sciences, 58,* 89–96. https://doi.org/10.11480/jmds.580301

LaVesser, P., & Hilton, C. (2010). Self-care skills for children with an autism spectrum disorder. In H. Miller-Kuhaneck (Ed.), *Autism: A comprehensive occupational therapy approach* (3rd ed., pp. 427–468). AOTA Press.

Law, E., Yang, J. H., Coit, M. H., & Chan, E. (2016). Toilet school for children with failure to train: Comparing a group therapy model with individual treatment. *Journal of Developmental and Behavioral Pediatrics, 37,* 223–230. https://doi.org/10.1097/ DBP.0000000000000278

Law, M., Baptiste, S., Carswell, A., McColl, M., Polatajko, H., & Pollock, N. (2019). *Canadian occupational performance measure* (5th ed., rev.). COPM Inc.

Lomas Mevers, J., Muething, C., Call, N. A., Scheithauer, M., & Hewett, S. (2018). A consecutive case series analysis of a behavioral intervention for enuresis in children with developmental disabilities. *Developmental Neurorehabilitation, 21,* 336–344. https://doi.org/10.1080/17518423.2018.1462269

Malow, B. A., Adkins, K. W., Reynolds, A., Weiss, S. K., Loh, A., Fawkes, D., . . . Clemons, T. (2014). Parent-based sleep education for children with autism spectrum disorders. *Journal of Autism and Developmental Disorders, 44,* 216–228. https://doi .org/10.1007/s10803-013-1866-z

Mindell, J. A., Du Mond, C. E., Sadeh, A., Telofski, L. S., Kulkarni, N., & Gunn, E. (2011). Efficacy of an Internet-based intervention for infant and toddler sleep disturbances. *Sleep, 34*(4), 451–458B. https://doi.org/10.1093/sleep/34.4.451

Mowrer, O. H., & Mowrer, W. M. (1938). Enuresis—A method for its study and treatment. *American Journal of Orthopsychiatry, 8,* 436–459. https://doi.org/10.1111/j.1939-0025.1938.tb06395.x

Msall, M. E., DiGaudio, K., Rogers, B. T., LaForest, S., Catanzaro, N. L., Campbell, J., & Duffy, L. C. (1994). The Functional Independence Measure for Children (WeeFIM): Conceptual basis and pilot use in children with developmental disabilities. *Clinical Pediatrics, 33,* 421–430. https://doi .org/10.1177/000992289403300708

Ottenbacher, K. J., & Cusick, A. (1990). Goal attainment scaling as a method of clinical service evaluation. *American Journal of Occupational Therapy, 44,* 519–525. https://doi.org/10.5014/ ajot.44.6.519

Paruthi, S., Brooks, L. J., D'Ambrosio, C., Hall, W. A., Kotagal, S., Lloyd, R. M., . . . Wise, M. S. (2016). Recommended amount of sleep for pediatric populations: A consensus statement of the American Academy of Sleep Medicine. *Journal of Clinical Sleep Medicine, 12,* 785–786. https://doi.org/10.5664/jcsm.5866

Price, A. M., Wake, M., Ukoumunne, O. C., & Hiscock, H. (2012). Five-year follow-up of harms and benefits of behavioral infant sleep intervention: Randomized trial. *Pediatrics, 130,* 643–651. https://doi.org/10.1542/peds.2011-3467

Rinald, K., & Mirenda, P. (2012). Effectiveness of a modified rapid toilet training workshop for parents of children with developmental disabilities. *Research in Developmental Disabilities, 33,* 933–943. https://doi.org/10.1016/j.ridd.2012.01.003

Roll, K., & Roll, W. (2013). *The Roll Evaluation of Activities of Life: The evaluation of activities of daily living skills (ADLs) and the instrumental activities of daily living skills (IADLs).* Pearson.

Salisbury, A. L., High, P., Twomey, J. E., Dickstein, S., Chapman, H., Liu, J., & Lester, B. (2012). A randomized control trial of integrated care for families managing infant colic. *Infant Mental Health Journal, 33,* 110–122. https://doi.org/10.1002/imhj.20340

Shepherd, J. (2015). Activities of daily living and sleep and rest. In J. Case-Smith (Ed.), *Occupational therapy for children and adolescents* (pp. 416–460). Elsevier.

Shepherd, J. (2019). Best practices in ADLs to support participation. In G. Frolek Clark, J. E. Rioux, & B. E. Chandler (Eds.), *Best practices for occupational therapy in schools* (2nd ed., pp. 387–394). AOTA Press.

Sparrow, S. S., Cicchetti, D. V., & Saulnier, C. A. (2016). *Vineland Adaptive Behavior Scales, third edition (Vineland-3).* Pearson.

Taubman, B., Blum, N. J., & Nemeth, N. (2003). Stool toileting refusal: A prospective intervention targeting parental behavior. *Archives of Pediatrics & Adolescent Medicine, 157,* 1193–1196. https://doi.org/10.1001/archpedi.157.12.1193

Touchette, É., Petit, D., Paquet, J., Boivin, M., Japel, C., Tremblay, R. E., & Montplaisir, J. Y. (2005). Factors associated with fragmented sleep at night across early childhood. *Archives of Pediatrics & Adolescent Medicine, 159,* 242–249. https://doi .org/10.1001/archpedi.159.3.242

Vergara, E., Anzalone, M., Bigsby, R., & Gorga, D. (2006). Specialized knowledge and skills for occupational therapy practice in the neonatal intensive care unit. *American Journal of Occupational Therapy, 60,* 659–668. https://doi.org/10.5014/ ajot.60.6.659

Best Practices in Supporting Mealtimes and Nutritional Needs (Adaptive Skills)

28

Winifred Schultz-Krohn, PhD, OTR/L, BCP, SWC, FAOTA, and Ashwini Wagle, EdD, MS, RD

KEY TERMS AND CONCEPTS

- Autism spectrum disorder
- Avoidant/restrictive food intake disorder
- Cerebral palsy
- Certified diabetes educator
- Collaborative team model
- Complementary feeding
- Diabetes
- Dietary Reference Intakes
- Digestive diseases and conditions
- Down syndrome
- Dysphagia
- Eating
- Feeding
- Food allergy
- Forced choice
- Interdisciplinary therapeutic feeding team
- Oral–motor interventions
- Phenylketonuria
- Positioning
- Positioning equipment
- Registered dietitian nutritionist
- Self-determination
- Sensory processing disorder
- Texture modifications

OVERVIEW

Early childhood is an important time of growth and learning, and adequate nutrient intake is critical. During this age, children form beliefs about what foods they like and dislike. They notice the foods eaten by people around them and are influenced by these eating choices. Early childhood is also the time to help children form healthy eating habits. Energy (i.e., calories) should be adequate to support growth and development and to reach or maintain desirable body weight.

Eating is the ability to keep food or fluid in the mouth and then swallow (American Occupational Therapy Association [AOTA], 2017). *Feeding* refers to the ability to bring food or fluids to the mouth and is sometimes referred to as *self-feeding*. The skill of eating is essential for infants and young children. The terms *picky eating* and *fussy eating* are not clearly differentiated in the literature and are often used interchangeably to denote feeding difficulties whereby the infant or child exhibits distinct food preferences and rejects specific foods (Taylor & Emmett, 2019; Taylor et al., 2015). The lack of a clear definition makes it problematic to accurately and consistently identify behaviors that are outside the norm for an infant or toddler (Taylor & Emmett, 2019).

ESSENTIAL CONSIDERATIONS

Children grow rapidly from birth to age 5 years; however, the range of normal growth can vary among children because each child is different. Factors affecting growth may be influenced by gender, race, ethnicity, and dietary habits. The Centers for Disease Control and Prevention (CDC; 2017) pediatric growth charts can monitor growth but are not a sole diagnostic tool. On average, children grow around 2.5 inches between the ages of 2 and 5 years and may gain around 4–5 pounds each year (CDC, 2017).

Dietary Reference Intakes

Daily nutritional goals in early childhood have been set by the U.S. Department of Health and Human Services (DHHS) and the U.S. Department of Agriculture (USDA) under the *Dietary Reference Intakes* (DRIs) and Dietary Guidelines (2015–2020; DHHS & USDA, 2015) recommendations. *DRIs* is a term for the nutrient reference values used to plan and assess a person's intake for a healthy diet. The Dietary Guidelines recommend that energy intake (i.e., calories) should be adequate to support growth and development and to reach or maintain desirable body weight. Daily intake must also meet or exceed the recommended dietary allowances for all nutrients for children from birth to age 5 years, including iron and calcium. Estimated dietary intake of 900 kilocalories per day (Kcals/day) for children 1 year of age, 1,000 Kcals/day for children ages 2–3 years, and 1,200 Kcals/day for children ages 4–5 years are recommended for optimal growth and development (Institute of Medicine, 2006).

Food Groups

The DHHS and USDA's (2018) Choose My Plate Program specifies that children from birth to age 5 years should consume a variety of foods from the five major food groups. Each food group supplies important nutrients, including vitamins and minerals. Table 28.1 provides information about foods and serving sizes.

TABLE 28.1. Food Groups

FOOD GROUP	SERVINGS PER DAY	PORTION SIZE FOR AGES 1–3	PORTION SIZES FOR AGES 4–6
Fruits	2–3 servings	¼ cup cooked, frozen or canned ½ piece fresh ¼ cup 100% juice	¼ cup cooked, frozen, or canned ½ piece fresh ⅓ cup 100% juice
Vegetables	2–3 servings	¼ cup cooked	¼ cup cooked ½ cup salad
Grains	6–11 servings	½ slice bread ¼ cup cooked cereal, rice, or pasta ½ cup dry cereal 2–3 crackers	1 slice bread ½ cup cooked cereal, rice, or pasta ½ cup dry cereal 3–4 crackers
Meats and other proteins	2 servings	1 oz meat, fish, chicken, or tofu ¼ cup cooked beans ½ egg	1 oz meat, fish, chicken, or tofu ⅓ cup cooked beans 1 egg
Dairy	2–3 servings	½ cup milk ½ oz cheese ½ cup yogurt	½ cup milk 1 oz cheese ½ cup yogurt

Source. Reprinted from "Portions and Serving Sizes," by HealthyChildren.org, 2015, https://www.healthychildren.org/English/healthy-living/nutrition/Pages/Portions-and-Serving-Sizes.aspx. Copyright © 2015 by the American Academy of Pediatrics. Reprinted with permission.

Children With Special Health Care Needs

Children with special health care needs are examples of high-need, high-risk populations with a wide range of conditions, including chronic diseases; health-related problems, such as prematurity; and congenital defects that require constant monitoring, follow-up, and medical care. The Academy of Nutrition and Dietetics posits that "nutrition services should be provided to children and youth with intellectual and developmental disabilities and special health care needs throughout life in a matter that is interdisciplinary, family centered, community based, and culturally competent" (Ptomey & Wittenbrook, 2015, p. 593). Children with autism spectrum disorder, avoidant/restrictive food intake disorder, cerebral palsy, cystic fibrosis, chromosomal disorders such as Down syndrome, neurological disorders, genetic or inherited metabolic disorders, orofacial cleft, Prader–Willi syndrome, and spina bifida (myelomeningocele) are examples of high-risk populations who have significant nutritional risk factors.

Children with special health care needs may be selective eaters, which may reduce their food acceptance and choices. They may have difficulty with breathing or swallowing or suffer from chronic pain. Other examples include conditions such as failure to thrive, obesity, growth retardation, metabolic disorders, poor feeding skills, drug–nutrient interactions, and sometimes partial or total dependence on enteral or parenteral nutrition (American Academy of Pediatrics, 2019).

The *interdisciplinary therapeutic feeding team,* composed of occupational therapy practitioners, speech therapists, and registered dietitian nutritionists (RDNs), play an important role in nutrition management. (*Note. Occupational therapy practitioner* refers to both occupational therapists and occupational therapy assistants.) Mealtime assistance and support may be needed, such as cutting up food, using adaptive equipment, or setting up a plate, to fully support the child in feeding (oral or enteral).

Educational requirements for occupational therapy practitioners include specific skills in the area of feeding and eating. The external accreditation standards state that entry-level practitioners must be able to "provide interventions for dysphagia and disorders of feeding and eating . . . and train others in precautions and techniques while considering client and contextual factors" (Accreditation Council for Occupational Therapy Education, 2018, p. 6). Practitioners support the complex task of eating by combining the knowledge and skills to foster the biomechanical abilities needed by the child with the cognitive and social–emotional skills that influence eating (AOTA, 2017; Ray, 2015). Additionally, practitioners provide feeding and eating intervention to address positioning of the child, training of parent or caregiver, determination of equipment needs, sensory supports to foster skills, and analysis of environmental factors that affect eating.

RDNs are food and nutrition experts who have completed the Commission on Dietetic Registration's criteria to earn the RDN credential. They help provide enteral and parenteral feeding for children with global developmental delays who may have conditions such as swallowing difficulties, delayed feeding, inadequate consumption, weight loss, and failure to thrive (Ptomey & Wittenbrook, 2015). The interdisciplinary team members, clients, and caregivers work together in the feeding plan of care, including food selection and preparation as part of the intervention plan, texture modifications, positioning, and behavior modifications.

Autism spectrum disorder

Autism spectrum disorder (ASD) is a wide-spectrum neurodevelopmental disorder causing impairments in social interaction, communication, language, and imaginative play, especially in children ages 0–5 years. ASD is influenced by genetic, environmental, and immunologic factors and includes restricted, repetitive, and stereotyped patterns of behavior and activities. Concerns with mealtime behavior and problems eating a variety of foods and eating in various settings are reported at a much higher rate among children with ASD compared with peers and are more often seen among younger children with ASD as compared with school-age children and adolescents with ASD (Gray et al., 2018). Children diagnosed with ASD are often considered "picky eaters" and a nutritionally vulnerable population because they exhibit a selective or picky eating pattern and sensory sensitivity that predisposes them to restricted intake not associated with a lack of appetite (Ranjan & Nasser, 2015).

Studies conducted in the last 2 decades on the commonly used gluten-free/casein-free (GFCF) diet are not conclusive that individuals with ASD have altered metabolism of gluten or casein proteins that may negatively affect behavior (Ranjan & Nasser, 2015). The review completed by Ranjan and Nasser (2015) indicated that the data to assess the effects of GFCF diets were limited, because dietary approaches and outcome measures varied among studies that did control diets and monitoring of adherence to GFCF diets. Additionally, there is little evidence to support the use of omega-3 supplementation to improve core or associated ASD symptoms.

Similarly, evidence was inadequate to assess the effects of short-term digestive enzyme supplements (Peptizyde and Neo-Digestin) in a study conducted by Sathe et al. (2017). The Peptizyde randomized controlled trial reported no significant differences in measures of behavior, sleep quality, or gastrointestinal symptoms. However, the use of Neo-Digestin versus a placebo (Sathe et al., 2017) resulted in significant improvement in symptom severity scores in the treatment group compared with the control group.

Children with ASD often have restricted diets as well as difficulty sitting through mealtimes, so they may not be getting all the nutrients they need. Children with ASD are more likely to accept foods of low texture and higher energy density (Hyman et al., 2012; Sathe et al., 2017). However, a high-fiber diet and physical activity may be more beneficial for positive mealtime behaviors and experiences.

Certain medications, such as methylphenidate (e.g., Ritalin), may cause loss of appetite and reduced food intake, whereas other medications may increase appetite or cause malabsorption of vitamins and minerals (Sturman et al., 2017). Because food selectivity is more common among younger children than among older children, research focused on the role of selective eating and methods of treatment at an earlier age may be needed.

Common feeding concerns for children with ASD may include the following (Hyman et al., 2012; Ranjan & Nasser, 2015):

- Difficulty accepting new foods and resistance to tasting and trying new foods (neophobia);
- Restricted intake based on color, texture, consistency, appearance, taste, smell, brand, packaging, and food temperature (common dislikes include fruits; vegetables; and slippery, soft foods);

- Throwing foods with rejection to textures, especially during infancy, leading to delay introducing solid foods;
- Challenges with how the food may be presented with the plate and cutlery or positioning of food on the plate;
- Increased sensitivity to temperature and texture, which could lead to refusal of foods;
- Disruptive mealtime behaviors and difficulty focusing on the meal;
- Monotonous choice of foods, with repetition of the same foods eaten or insistence that foods be cooked a certain way;
- Constipation and other digestive symptoms, which may be caused by a child's limited food choices; and
- Medication interactions, which may affect appetite and intake among children with ASD.

Avoidant/restrictive food intake disorder

The *Diagnostic and Statistical Manual of Mental Disorders* (5th ed.; American Psychiatric Association [APA], 2013) revised the diagnosis of infant and early childhood–related feeding disorders in the category of eating disorders and created a new designation of **avoidant/restrictive food intake disorder** (ARFID; APA, 2013). The ARFID diagnosis is used with children ages 0–5 years and older and provides increased clarity for the significant problems encountered. Children diagnosed with ARFID present with slowed growth or weight loss, nutritional deficiency, and significant emotional reactions to foods (Zimmerman & Fisher, 2017). The diagnosis of ARFID is differentiated from anorexia and bulimia by the avoidance or restriction of food because of fear or anxiety and not in relation to reducing or limiting physical size.

ARFID can be differentiated from other feeding and eating disorders with the valid and reliable Behavioral Pediatrics Feeding Assessment Scale (Dovey et al., 2016). When children with ARFID were compared with typically developing peers, similar mealtime avoidance behaviors and restlessness were noted, but the frequency of these behaviors between these two groups was significantly different. During meals, children with ARFID were far more restless and demonstrated a greater number of avoidant behaviors (Aldridge et al., 2018).

Phenylketonuria

Phenylketonuria (PKU) is an inherited disorder that is also considered as an inborn error of metabolism in which the body cannot break down an essential amino acid called phenylalanine (Phe). Because Phe is an essential amino acid, it cannot be eliminated entirely from the diet, and it needs to be restricted to maintain adequate levels in the body (Casey, 2013). An RDN must be consulted and needs to manage the meal plans for children with PKU. Studies have indicated that the diet for children from birth to age 5 years may be modified in sources of protein and energy, restricted in Phe, and supplemented with tyrosine (MacLeod & Ney, 2010; Ney et al., 2016). The child's nutrition may be planned around the use of an infant formula, and medical foods with Phe may be removed, but adequate protein and tyrosine must be provided. It is essential that an adequate amount of formula and medical foods be consumed because they are the primary source of daily energy, protein, vitamins, and minerals (Ney et al., 2016).

Frequent monitoring of blood Phe is necessary to ensure adequacy of treatment and to adjust and recalculate the child's meal plan to achieve appropriate blood levels of Phe. Foods high in protein (e.g., dairy foods, meat, fish, poultry, eggs, legumes, nuts) are also high in Phe and are commonly removed from the diet. The amount of total protein that is recommended during infancy and early childhood for patients with PKU is greater than for typical children, about 25%–30% above the DRI for age (MacLeod & Ney, 2010). Effective management of children with PKU requires a team approach; practitioners with expertise in PKU management work closely with the family to achieve and maintain appropriate biochemical control and achieve normal physical and mental growth.

Diabetes

Diabetes is a condition that impairs the body's ability to process blood glucose, also known as blood sugar. Nutritional needs and meal-planning goals for children with diabetes are usually the same as those for nondiabetic children. For children with Type 1 diabetes, carbohydrate intake needs to be balanced with insulin intake and activity levels to keep blood sugar levels under control. The amount of carbohydrates in the child's meals determines their insulin dosage (USDA, 2019).

An RDN or **certified diabetes educator** (CDE) is key in developing a balanced meal plan based on the child's food preferences, nutritional needs, and insulin medication (some insulin medications require a set number of carbohydrates in each meal, whereas others allow for more flexibility). CDEs are diabetes specialists who are medical professionals, such as pharmacists, nurses, dietitians, physicians or social workers who specialize in working with people with diabetes. Eating meals and scheduling insulin injections at the same time every day helps control blood glucose levels.

Epilepsy

Many antiepileptic drugs (AEDs) help manage epileptic attacks (seizures); however, drug–nutrient interactions are common and some medications are known to change metabolism and absorption of many nutrients. Therefore, children with epilepsy may be at high risk of nutrient deficiencies (Stafstrom, 2004). Although research in nutrition therapy for epilepsy is limited, the most common approaches include the ketogenic diet, which contains a high fat (90%), adequate protein, and low carbohydrate balance, along with the Atkins diet (high fat, high protein, low carbohydrate), a diet enriched in polyunsaturated fatty acids, or overall restriction of calorie intake (Esteban-Figuerola et al., 2019; Soltani et al., 2016).

Digestive diseases

Some **digestive diseases and conditions** last a short time (acute), while others are long lasting, even in early childhood years (chronic). Examples of digestive diseases are irritable bowel syndrome (IBS), Crohn's disease, celiac disease, bowel control problems (i.e., fecal incontinence), gas, lactose intolerance, diarrhea, and gastroesophageal reflux disease (GERD).

A nutrition review on digestive health conducted by Korczak and colleagues (2017) suggested that most children with GERD can maintain a healthy lifestyle without medications. An RDN can help a child prevent or relieve their symptoms from GERD by changing their diet. Occupational therapy practitioners provide important information to the family on positioning before, during, and after a meal to minimize GERD.

Sitting upright during the meal is the preferred position for infants and toddlers with GERD (Lightdale & Gremse, 2013; Marcus & Breton, 2013), and avoiding semisupine (reclined) and supine positions after feeding an infant with GERD is recommended. Prone or semiprone positions using a cut-out pillow after a meal have been beneficial for young children with GERD (Ferreira et al., 2014; Lightdale & Gremse, 2013), but monitoring is needed because of risk of sudden infant death syndrome. Positioning an infant in supine is still the recommended position for sleep (Ferreira et al., 2014). Children older than 1 year can be positioned in sitting, semisitting, or prone on a cut-out pillow after a meal. Although 50% of all infants regurgitate or spit up daily (Lightdale & Gremse, 2013), persistent GERD can negatively affect the hunger–satiety cycle as infants develop eating behavior such as arching their backs and refusing to feed, difficulty swallowing due to pain, irritability, weight loss, and vomiting. Positioning is an important part of the intervention services to diminish the negative impact of GERD on eating behaviors.

Food is a common trigger of digestive symptoms among most children in early childhood years. Studies also indicate that certain foods that make the child's symptoms worse may need to be avoided, and dietary changes could help reduce specific symptoms. Nutrition therapy for children with GERD may include decreasing fatty foods and eating small, frequent meals instead of large meals (Moreno, 2014; Rybak et al., 2017).

IBS is a disorder of the gastrointestinal (GI) tract and usually affects the lower GI area such as the small intestine, large intestine, and colon. Irritable bowel disorder (IBD) is inflammation or destruction of the bowel wall, which can lead to sores and narrowing of the intestines. Ulcerative colitis (inflammation of the large intestine causing sores or ulcers) and microscopic colitis (inflammation of the large intestine causing watery diarrhea) are other common types of IBD. Nutrition therapy to control symptoms of IBS may include eating more fiber, avoiding gluten, and following a special diet called the *low-FODMAP diet* (Cozma-Petruț et al., 2017). *FODMAP* stands for *f*ermentable *o*ligosaccharides, *d*isaccharides, *m*onosaccharides, *a*nd *p*olyols, which are all fermentable carbohydrates. Magge and Lembo (2012) have indicated that a diet low in FODMAPs may be clinically recommended for the management of IBS and may be a possible therapeutic approach for decreasing abdominal symptoms and improving quality of life. However, a low-FODMAP diet may not be beneficial to all children.

Neurological disorders

Children with various neurological disorders, such as **cerebral palsy** or **Down syndrome,** exhibit difficulties with eating that can negatively affect nutritional support (Benfer et al., 2014, 2016; Clancy & Hustad, 2011; Dahlseng et al., 2011; Lewis & Kritzinger, 2004). Children diagnosed with cerebral palsy have difficulties with motor control, which often includes the oral musculature. The high incidence of *dysphagia* (swallowing disorder) among children diagnosed with cerebral palsy is well established (Clancy & Hustad, 2011; Dahlseng et al., 2011). The development of oral–motor control is often compromised for children with cerebral palsy and they often have difficulties with drinking thin liquids because of poor lip closure on the nipple and problems coordinating sucking and swallowing. Transitioning to textured and resistive foods can be very challenging, given the problems in developing sufficient oral–motor control. The oral preparatory phase of eating can be compromised, and foods may not be adequately chewed to form a bolus. Once the food has been chewed, prolonged oral transit time places the child with cerebral palsy at risk for aspiration (Benfer et al., 2014, 2016).

Children diagnosed with Down syndrome, a neurodevelopmental disorder, have intellectual disabilities, diminished muscle tone, and problems with coordination that compromise feeding and eating. For children with Down syndrome, their diminished tongue and oral–motor control compromises the oral preparatory and oral phase of eating (Hashimoto et al., 2014; Lewis & Kritzinger, 2004) and choking, gagging, and risk of aspiration are noted (O'Neill & Richter, 2013). The limited tongue control particularly compromises the ability to transition to more textured foods.

Occupational therapy services should be provided to foster proper positioning for eating and help the family and child with food progressions (Wilcox et al., 2009). Food progressions or transitions are systematically provided so the infant or child has an opportunity to explore foods in a safe and supportive environment (Ray, 2015).

Food allergies

In a *food allergy,* the body reacts as though that particular food product is harmful when ingested. The body's immune system creates antibodies to fight the food allergen. As young children are exposed to new foods, there is a higher likelihood that their bodies may manifest allergy symptoms. Every time the child eats (or, in some cases, handles or breathes in) the food, the body releases chemicals such as histamine (Baral & Hourihane, 2005). This triggers allergic symptoms that can affect the respiratory system, gastrointestinal tract, skin, or cardiovascular system. In the case of food allergies, the child must follow a multiple food avoidance diet.

A child could be allergic to any food, but these eight common allergens account for 90% of all reactions among children: (1) milk, (2) eggs, (3) peanuts, (4) soy, (5) wheat, (6) tree nuts (e.g., walnuts, cashews), (7) fish, and (8) shellfish (e.g., shrimp). All food products regulated by the U.S. Food and Drug Administration (2019) must disclose these ingredients on a product label.

In general, most children with food allergies outgrow them. Of those who are allergic to milk, about 80% will eventually outgrow the allergy. About two-thirds of children

with allergies to eggs and about 80% with a wheat or soy allergy will outgrow the allergy by the time they are age 5 years. Other food allergies, such as peanuts, may be harder to outgrow (Waserman & Watson, 2011).

An RDN needs to plan a healthy, allergy-friendly, balanced diet for the child. Nutrients are necessary for proper growth and development during the early childhood years. Removing two or more important foods can result in poor nutrition. Before buying any food product, parents and caregivers must read the entire food label carefully to ensure the product is safe for consumption. It is also important to remember that manufacturers may change ingredients and food preparation methods at any time.

Sensory issues

A *sensory processing disorder* is an abnormal reaction to the sense of touch, smell, taste, movement, sound, or sight; the child may be hypo- or hypersensitive to one or more sensations. Children with sensory processing disorders may negatively react to food odors, taste, texture, and visual appearance. This exaggerated reaction can negatively affect the child's acceptance of common foods and ultimately compromise nutritional intake (Ramos et al., 2017). It may contribute to difficulty with accepting a variety of food textures, frequently seen among children from birth to age 5 years. Although food pickiness is commonly seen around age 18 months, it diminishes by having the child explore foods (Warren, 2018).

Sensory processing issues can compromise a child's willingness to eat a variety of foods and textures (Ramos et al., 2017). In a longitudinal investigation, preschool children displayed picky eating and food refusals or avoidance more frequently, when compared with peers, when the introduction of complementary foods and lumpy foods was delayed past age 9 months. Picky eating behaviors were more frequently noted when children had prolonged bottle feeding (Emmett et al., 2018). Children with ASD exhibit far greater atypical eating behaviors (e.g., limitations in food preferences, hypersensitivity) compared with other diagnostic groups and children of typical development (Mayes & Zickgraf, 2019). When compared with other diagnostic groups and typically developing children, children with ASD accepted far fewer foods with very limited texture variety, preferring breads and chicken nuggets.

Dietary Customs and Practices

Child care providers and caregivers must be aware that some cultures and religions observe customs related to diet and may have sensitivities to certain food products (see Table 28.2). When considering food choices, occupational therapy practitioners should be aware of the dietary practices of the family, including those based on religion, cultures, and ethnicities (Sucher et al., 2016).

BEST PRACTICES

Occupational therapy practitioners have the knowledge and skills to assess and intervene when children's eating and feeding skills are compromised (AOTA, 2017).

TABLE 28.2.   Religion-Based Dietary Practices and Restrictions

RELIGION	COMMON DIETARY PRACTICES	RESTRICTION	OTHER PRACTICES
Buddhism	▪ Refrain from meat ▪ Fish may be consumed ▪ Moderation in all foods ▪ Lacto-ovo vegetarianism is common ▪ Some may be vegan ▪ Most dietary restrictions followed by monks	▪ Meat and poultry, especially beef	▪ Doctrine forbids taking life ▪ Diet varies depending on country of origin ▪ Monks avoid all solid food after noon ▪ Fasting required of monks
Eastern Orthodox Christianity	▪ Selective fasting	▪ Restrictions on meat and fish during fasting	▪ Fasting and restrictions on holy days
Hinduism	▪ Numerous fasting days ▪ Lacto-ovo vegetarianism is common ▪ Some may be vegan ▪ May follow dietary practices according to the Vedic writings or Ayurveda ▪ Goat meat, mutton, and lamb are meats of preference for nonvegetarians ▪ Nonvegetarians eat vegetarian meals on auspicious days or religious occasions ▪ Traditionally, food is eaten with the right hand only	▪ Beef prohibited ▪ Pork, other meats, and fish may be restricted or avoided by some members of this religion	▪ Cows are sacred and cannot be killed or eaten ▪ Products of the sacred cow are pure and desirable, such as butter, ghee, milk, and yogurt ▪ Diet dependent on region of origin and caste ▪ Fasting promotes spiritual growth ▪ Food is to be shared with the poor and hungry
Islam	▪ Coffee, tea, and stimulants are to be avoided, although tea is a common beverage in most Islamic communities ▪ Fasting from all food and drink from sunrise to sunset for the 30-day period during Ramadan ▪ Permitted animals slaughtered according to Muslim law ▪ Traditionally, food is eaten with the right hand only	▪ *Halal:* Permitted foods, such as beef, lamb, poultry, and fish ▪ *Haram:* Prohibited foods, such as pork, birds and animals of prey ▪ Alcohol prohibited ▪ May also exclude gelatin, fats, emulsifiers, stabilizers, and additives from animals	▪ Eating is for good health, and self-indulgence is discouraged ▪ Eating is part of worship, and fasting has a cleansing effect of evil elements ▪ Followers should only eat until two-thirds of their capacity ▪ Food is to be shared with the poor and hungry
Jainism	▪ Followers may be strictly vegetarian or vegan ▪ Fasting is practiced ▪ Traditionally, food is eaten with the right hand only	▪ Only religion that forbids foods that grow under the ground, such as onions, garlic, carrots, roots, and tubers	▪ Wash hands and rinse mouth before and after meals ▪ Products of the sacred cow are pure and desirable, such as butter, ghee, milk, and yogurt ▪ Do not eat after sundown or before the sun rises

(Continued)

TABLE 28.2.   Religion-Based Dietary Practices and Restrictions *(Cont.)*

RELIGION	COMMON DIETARY PRACTICES	RESTRICTION	OTHER PRACTICES
Judaism	• Fasting practiced • Eat only kosher beef, lamb, poultry, and fish (with fins and scales) • Kosher process is based on the laws of Kashruth • Mammals that do not have cloven hooves and that do not chew their cud are forbidden and considered as unclean (e.g., hare, pig, camel) • Animals may only be slaughtered as per Shechitah method • Leavened food may be restricted	• *Kosher* refers to permitted foods that have been selected and prepared according to rules of the Jewish religion • Pork, animals and birds of prey are prohibited • Animals that have hooves and chew their cud are permitted, such as beef, lamb, poultry • Fish with scales and fins are permitted • Shellfish are prohibited • Meat and dairy cannot be consumed together • 1-hour wait applies after consumption of dairy to consume meat and, 6-hour wait applies after the consumption of meat to eat dairy • Separate utensils to cook meat and dairy • *Pareve:* Foods that contain neither meat nor dairy (eggs are pareve but need to be examined for blood spots) • Honey is considered pure • May also exclude gelatin, fats, emulsifiers, stabilizers, and additives from animal origin that are not kosher	• All Orthodox and some Conservative Jews follow the dietary laws, although interpretations may differ
Church of Latter Day Saints or Mormonism	• Moderation in all foods • Encouraged to have 1 year of food in reserve • Fasting 1 day per month recommended	• Alcohol and beverages containing caffeine prohibited	• Caffeine is addictive and leads to poor physical and emotional health • Fasting is the discipline of self-control and honoring to God
Protestant	• Few restrictions of food or fasting observations • Moderation in eating, drinking, and exercise is promoted	• Dietary habits are dictated by ethnicity and country of origin	• God made all animals and natural products for humans' enjoyment • Self-indulgence and drunkenness should be controlled
Roman Catholicism	• Meat restricted on certain days • Fasting practiced	• Meat and animal products may be avoided during Lent or fast days	• Restrictions are consistent with specified days of the church year
Seventh-Day Adventist	• Meat, poultry, and fish are avoided • Most followers are lacto-ovo vegetarians • Fasting during Sabbath practiced from sundown on Friday to sundown on Saturday	• Vegetarian diet is encouraged • Pork prohibited, and meat and fish may be avoided • Alcohol, coffee, and tea prohibited	• Diet satisfies practice to honor God • Health is preserved through eating the right foods, having adequate rest and exercise
Sikhism	• Many followers are vegetarian • Traditionally, food is eaten with the right hand only	• Beef is prohibited • Other meat, poultry, and fish may be consumed • Eggs may be consumed	• Food is to be shared with the poor and hungry • Most Sikhs volunteer for Langar service, where food is given to all visitors at the Sikh temple

Source. Adapted from Sucher et al. (2016).

Evaluate Eating and Feeding Skills

Evaluation of a child's eating and feeding skills can occur for several reasons but is most often sought by a parent when there are struggles in ensuring the child eats a sufficient quantity and variety of foods to be healthy and grow (Nichols et al., 2018). Medical conditions, either acute or chronic, may trigger a referral to evaluate eating and feeding skills, but often the concerns are identified by the parent. Cultural factors influence the decision to seek support and assistance in evaluating a child's eating and feeding skills.

Caregiver report

Parental concerns regarding a child's eating and feeding skills are often the reason the child is seen for an evaluation, unless significant medical issues exist resulting in dysphagia and aspiration (Milano et al., 2019). Reports from parents are an important part of the occupational profile identifying the issues related to the child's eating and feeding behaviors. During the caregiver interview (e.g., parent, child care provider, preschool teacher), variations in the child's eating and feeding behaviors should be identified, particularly if the child's behaviors have recently changed; are long term in nature; or are different depending on environment (home vs. child care or preschool), caregivers present, time of day, foods presented, and medication schedule (Schultz-Krohn, 2006). The parents provide critical information, including health records and previous examinations, in helping identify the complexity of the problem.

Caregivers may have unrealistic goals for the child regarding the quantity and types of foods accepted (Milano et al., 2019), and the occupational therapy practitioner can provide needed information regarding developmental eating and feeding behaviors, including types of foods eaten at specific ages. Important milestones include accepting pureed foods from a spoon between ages 4 and 7 months, eating soft table foods that require minimal chewing and drinking from a cup from ages 8–15 months, and chewing more resistive table foods from ages 10–18 months (Carruth et al., 2004; Cichero, 2017; Morris & Klein, 2000).

Observation

Observing children's feeding and eating skills is an important part of the evaluation process (Marcus & Breton, 2013). During the mealtime, note the following:

- *Posture:* Observe initial posture of head and trunk and changes during the meal.
- *Respiratory:* Observe changes as the meal progresses.
- *Oral–motor control (lips, jaw, tongue):* Observe as the child accepts (or rejects) foods and fluids; lip seal during the eating process to determine liquid loss; tongue ability to move food from the anterior to posterior oral cavity (observed by watching the child's jaw and suprahyoid region); and speed of oral transit with pureed foods from the time the food enters the mouth to the initiation of the swallow (pharyngeal phase).
- *Engagement:* Observe the child's participation or refusal of food, including arching their back and turning their head away from specific foods. Observe the caregiver's

responses to the child's performance (e.g., anxious, abandons food that is spit out).

Assessment tools

Although observations provide helpful information, occupational therapists also may need to use systematic assessment tools to evaluate oral–motor skills and periodically and systematically reassess skills to adjust intervention programs (Barton et al., 2017). A systematic review of oral–motor feeding assessment tools revealed there are very few reliable and valid instruments for infants and children (Barton et al., 2017). Although some assessment tools rely primarily on parental report, most current oral–motor assessment tools use systematic observational skills. The Oral Motor Assessment Scale has been used in various investigations with variable reliability reported (Barton et al., 2017). Likewise, the Dysphagia Disorder Survey, the Functional Feeding Assessment—Modified, and the Schedule for Oral Motor Assessment have all been used in clinical trials, again with limited consistency in reliability. This presents a problem for occupational therapists using standardized assessment tools for initial assessment and periodic reassessments of skills. A listing of assessment tools can be found in Appendix F, "Examples of Assessments for Early Childhood (Birth–5 Years)."

Ongoing and systematic assessment of oral–motor skills, eating, and mealtime behaviors is an important part of the intervention process. Given the complex nature of eating and feeding, it is important for occupational therapists to use a combination of parental report, observation of a mealtime, and standardized assessment when evaluating a child's skills.

Interventions to Support Healthy Eating

This section addresses common interventions used by occupational therapy practitioners to support healthy eating and mealtime participation. Issues and strategies explored include complementary feeding, positioning, adaptive equipment, food modifications, feeding tubes, social participation during mealtimes, mealtime habits and routines, self-determination, pickiness, special diets, and collaboration with other professionals.

Complementary feeding

The introduction of complementary foods at age 6 months is recommended and small amounts can be introduced at age 4 months (Warren, 2018). The term ***complementary feeding*** is used instead of *weaning* because the current recommendations are for introduction of additional liquids and semi-solids for sensory experience, not for nutritional support, between the ages of 4 and 6 months; this introduction should not be delayed past age 6 months and should not be introduced before age 4 months. Restricting the infant's diet to only breastmilk or formula past age 6 months has been associated with a greater likelihood of the child becoming a picky eater as a toddler. Complementary foods provided at age 6 months may include thin baby rice cereal mixed with breastmilk or familiar formula and smooth pureed fruits without added sugar. Lumpy foods should be introduced before age 9 months to avoid later behaviors of picky eating (Emmett et al., 2018) and foster initial chewing skills, which emerge at age 6–9 months.

Infants prefer salty and sweet flavors more than sour or bitter flavors. Fruits may have a combination of sweet and sour, so selecting fruits with a mild and a sweeter flavor is recommended. Complementary foods may be presented to infants and toddlers at different temperatures; the presentation of a new food in a different form may be more enticing (Coulthard et al., 2009; Fries & van der Horst, 2019). For example, offer an infant pureed applesauce at room temperature with a slight lumpiness to encourage more exploration and acceptance. For a toddler, offering easily dissolvable snacks of different colors may be enticing.

Pureed food is introduced in the front of the oral cavity, and tongue mobility is needed to maneuver the food posteriorly to swallow. The oral transit time may be extended because the infant needs to develop the motor skills to maneuver the bolus posteriorly to swallow. Lumpy or textured foods are still soft and easily swallowed. Commercially staged baby foods indicate the lumpiness or texture. As the infant matures and develops more sophisticated chewing patterns, more textured but easy dissolvable foods can be introduced. Because they are still learning to chew and do not have molars until age 3 years, children younger than age 4 years are at the highest risk for choking. They should not be given the following foods because of the risk of choking: whole hot dogs, large chunks of meats and cheese, whole grapes, popcorn, hard candy, gum, hunks of peanut butter, nuts and seeds, and raw vegetables.

When providing new foods, best practice is to introduce one food at a time for up to 7 days to monitor the infant's response for possible allergies. Current recommendations indicate infants at ages 4 to 6 months should be introduced to pureed foods to diminish potential food allergies (Caffarelli et al., 2018; Ferraro et al., 2019). Avoiding potential allergic foods past the age of 6 months is no longer the recommended practice (Waserman & Watson, 2011).

Oral–motor interventions

Oral–motor interventions have successfully advanced sucking and swallowing skills for premature infants (Fucile et al., 2011, 2012). Sensorimotor stimulation to the lips, cheeks, and jaw followed by stimulation to the gums and tongue resulted in improved transition to oral feedings among premature infants when compared with control participants. Additionally, control of sucking and swallowing sequencing was improved with these techniques. An occupational therapy practitioner can provide stimulation to the oral musculature, both extraoral and intraoral, to foster improved sucking and swallowing skills. Sensorimotor oral stimulation for children with spastic cerebral palsy resulted in significant improvements in lip closure, chewing, and control of the bolus (Baghbadorani et al., 2014). Support to oral structures, in particular providing support to the cheeks, while an infant is bottle fed has been shown to significantly improve oral intake (Hwang et al., 2010).

Positioning

Positioning of an infant or child can significantly improve oral–motor skills and the ability to safely eat (Marcus &

Breton, 2013). The preferred position for feeding an infant or child is with slight chin tuck (slight neck flexion) to avoid aspiration. For infants being breastfed, a slight side-lying position is preferred. This allows the infant to latch onto the breast, and the mother can support the infant with their chin slightly tucked. The chin-tuck position is also important when the child has diminished control of the bolus.

As the infant gains motor control and grows, a more upright sitting position should be used during mealtime (Korth & Maune, 2020). This is often suggested for infants at age 6 months. The child should be seated with their head in midline and feet supported during the meal. Although children may eat while in very awkward positions, these positions often require additional energy and effort to safely control the bolus and avoid choking or aspiration. Additionally, specific positioning should be used when an infant or child is suspected of having gastroesophageal reflux (GER) or GERD (Poddar, 2019). When feeding an infant, particularly a premature infant at high risk for GER, it is important to position the infant upright and on their left side after the meal to avoid regurgitation (Corvaglia et al., 2007).

Adaptive equipment

Positioning equipment can provide substantial support when caregivers are feeding an infant or child (Marcus & Breton, 2013). Supportive chairs can assist the child in sitting upright during the meal. A child may tire and begin to slump during a meal because of poor postural control. A tilt-in-space chair, which positions the child in sitting with flexion of the hip, knee, and ankle to 90°, can effectively minimize the impact of gravity and avoid problems in head and trunk control. Simple adaptations can be made to support a child, such as the use of nonslip surfaces under the plate (Korth & Maune, 2020). The same nonslip surface can be placed on the seat of the child's chair to provide additional support during the meal.

Specialized spoons, cups, and plates can help the child with feeding skills. As an example, a child with difficulties maneuvering the spoon may benefit from use of a curved-handled spoon or spoon with a built-up handle. The size of children's spoon bowl should also be considered. Children who have a small jaw or a hyperactive gag would benefit from use of a small-bowl spoon.

Covered cups can be used for a variety of reasons beyond minimizing the potential for spills. Covered cups can regulate the flow of liquid when a child has difficulties controlling the tip action to pour liquid into the mouth. Covered cups may also have a spout that allows the child to control the flow of the liquid.

Food modifications

Factors such as food aversions, dislikes, oral–motor problems, signs of dysphagia, and feeding problems may require alterations in food texture to improve intake and consumption. Texture modifications such as thickened fluids, reducing the lumpiness of foods, or altering the viscosity and stickiness of foods can support feeding and eating skills. Occupational performance indicators for **texture modifications** include prolonged feeding times, lack of chewing, gagging or coughing up the food, not feeding oneself when developmentally expected to, refusal to eat, frequent vomiting, respiratory distress as a meal progresses, and irritability during meals. Thickened liquids have been effective in diminishing episodes of aspiration for children with Down syndrome (Jackson et al., 2016). The interdisciplinary team of occupational therapy practitioners, speech–language pathologists, and registered dietitians works together on an intervention plan (i.e., plan of care) to implement texture modifications, thicken liquids, incorporate nutritional supplements, or add self-feeding equipment.

Nutrition through different types of feeding tubes

Children who have inadequate intake and cannot safely be fed orally are often unable to maintain a healthy weight or hydration status. These children or children who have dysphagia with aspiration may benefit from enteral feedings. Enteral feeding methods vary from nasogastric tube feedings to percutaneous endoscopic gastrostomy tube feedings; they may be used as a supplement to support inadequate intake or may provide for all the caloric needs of the child. RDNs closely monitor the anthropometric measurements and tolerance to the enteral feeding provision and may be required to make adjustments to prevent underfeeding or overfeeding.

The interdisciplinary team composed of the physician, occupational therapy practitioner, speech therapist, and registered dietitian works in collaboration in the plan of care to transition from enteral feeding to oral feeding and provide support in texture modifications, positioning, encouragement, pacing, self-feeding adaptive equipment, and behavior modifications (Marcus & Breton, 2013). Although the nutritional support is provided through nonoral methods, the occupational therapy practitioner should provide oral stimulation and exposure to the smells and textures of foods. This can be done in a nonthreatening manner by having the child tube fed while the caregivers are also eating.

Occupational therapy practitioners have an important role in the scheduling of tube feedings for children who cannot orally consume all of their necessary nutrition. The schedule of their tube feedings can play a large role in the potential transition from tube to oral feedings and affect the child's daily routines. For example, a child who receives all tube feeding overnight may not experience hunger during the day and may not be interested in tasting or eating foods during meals. Likewise, a child who is fed using a continuous drip method may have a disrupted hunger–satiety sequence. The child may never experience hunger and the satisfaction of being full after a meal, which can significantly disrupt the formation of mealtime behaviors and feeding habits.

Although children may need to use a continuous drip tube-feeding schedule for a short period of time, the practitioner should suggest moving to bolus feeds when possible. The transition from tube feedings to oral feedings occurs with input from the interdisciplinary team, including the parent or caregiver. This transition often starts with the sensory experience of foods, with smelling and touching foods before tasting them (Dazeley & Houston-Price, 2015). Sensory aversion can occur when children have limited contact with a variety of foods.

Social implications during feeding

Mealtime is more than a period of time to take in adequate nutrition. Mealtime is often a time of sharing and enjoyment. Children with special needs, particularly children with oral–motor problems or oral hypersensitivity, can disrupt this experience (Provost et al., 2010). The family and preschool or child care habits and routines may be dictated by the needs of the infant or child and not designed to foster family integrity and togetherness (Ray, 2015; Schultz-Krohn, 2006). The occupational therapy practitioner has an important role in supporting social interaction as part of a mealtime routine both at home and in preschool or child care settings. Identifying what habits caregivers would prefer during mealtimes and how to begin to develop those habits creates a positive environment.

Habits and routines to support mealtime

Regularly scheduled mealtimes in a consistent location foster the habit of eating (Fries & van der Horst, 2019). Infants and young children begin to associate a location with the behaviors of eating. This can be beneficial or detrimental, depending on the child's experiences in the location. Creating a supportive environment is important; occupational therapy practitioners and families should provide familiar foods first before introducing the complementary foods, and then return to the familiar foods. Initial refusals of the complementary food may be seen, but with repeated exposure the novel complementary food becomes more familiar. Complementary foods should be eaten by the parents, siblings, and peers because young children imitate behaviors. A child with ASD may be particularly challenged at mealtimes in a busy kitchen with bright lights, cooking smells, and noises. Even the way the furniture is arranged is a potential stressor.

Toddlers and preschoolers can assist with setting the table and selecting a preferred seat at the table to support mealtime routines. At home, families should sit together for a meal to reinforce sitting through a meal and eating foods on the plate. Making meals as predictable and routine as possible can help.

Self-determination and the use of forced choice

Toddlers and preschool-age children can participate in simple meal preparation and make choices regarding foods (Fries & van der Horst, 2019). This option of making choices in food items fosters *self-determination*, the ability to make a choice based on available options and preferences (Carter et al., 2013). For example, allow a child to choose whether they want their banana in thin slices or in strips (Fries & van der Horst, 2019). The choice is present but not the option of refusal, so the child is provided with a *forced choice*. This forced choice is often successful with foods of similar characteristics. Involving the child in creating food pairs is important, such as asking which pairs should be offered (e.g., peaches and nectarines or soft pears and bananas). For a child with ASD, providing a forced choice can help expand the food options and the child's diet.

Be prepared for pickiness

Picky eating is not unique among toddlers and young children (Taylor & Emmett, 2019). Many parents find their child's sensitivity to tastes, colors, smells, and textures the biggest barrier to a balanced diet. Getting the child to try new foods—especially those that are soft and slippery—may be a substantial challenge. A child may avoid certain foods or even entire food groups.

One approach to address the sensory issues related to picky eating is to tackle them outside of the kitchen. Having the child accompany the parent to the supermarket to choose a new food can help with expanding food choices. Once home, the parent and child can work together to decide how to prepare the food. Often children, particularly at preschool age, need repeated opportunities to encounter the food before accepting it (Fries & van der Horst, 2019). Simply becoming familiar with new foods in a low-pressure, positive way eventually can help the child expand the foods accepted.

Obtain a swallow study

Dysphagia is common in many conditions. A referral to other professionals, when appropriate, for further information may be necessary. In medical settings, occupational therapists with specialized formal training and equipment may conduct feeding and swallowing evaluations of children.

Seek guidance and collaborate with a registered dietitian nutritionist

An RDN can identify any nutritional risks on the basis of how the child eats; can provide evidence-based information about diet therapies and supplements advertised as helpful for children, particularly children with ASD; and is a key team member to foster a child's healthy eating habits. A *collaborative team model* that includes all family members, the occupational therapy practitioner, and the RDN is the best approach to support the development of eating skills and healthy eating habits for infants and young children. This approach allows unique family habits and routines to be incorporated into a comprehensive plan.

Proponents of GFCF diets believe people with autism have a "leaky gut," or intestine, which allows parts of gluten and casein to seep into the bloodstream and affect the brain and central nervous system. While this may be effective for certain children (Ghalichi et al., 2016), controlled scientific studies have not confirmed this, and additional research is needed (Piwowarczyk et al., 2018). An RDN should be consulted before any drastic changes are made to a child's diet, because there can be side effects and potential nutrient shortfalls when a GFCF diet is self-prescribed.

SUMMARY

The development of eating and feeding skills for infants and children is a complex process best met through the use of an interdisciplinary team of which the occupational therapy practitioner is a member. Children experience substantial changes in feeding behaviors and skills during the first 5 years of life, and the skills of occupational therapy practitioners are critical in supporting this development. Practitioners possess an understanding of the motor, sensory, social, and developmental demands of feeding and can be instrumental contributors to support the child and family.

RESOURCES

- American Academy of Pediatrics. (2019). *Pediatric nutrition handbook* (8th ed.). Author.
- American Occupational Therapy Association. (2017). The practice of occupational therapy in feeding, eating, and swallowing. *American Journal of Occupational Therapy, 71*, 7112410015. https://doi.org/10.5014/ajot.2017.716S04
- Ernsperger, L., & Stegen-Hanson, T. (2004). *Just take a bite: Easy, effective answers to food aversions and eating challenges!* Future Horizons.
- Grohern, M. E., & Crary, M. A. (2010). *Dysphagia: Clinical management in adults and children.* Mosby Elsevier.
- Marcus, S., & Breton, S. (2013). *Infant and child feeding and swallowing: Occupational therapy assessment and intervention.* AOTA Press.
- Morris, S. E., & Klein, M. D. (2000). *Pre-feeding skills: A comprehensive resource for mealtime development* (2nd ed.). Therapy Skill Builders.

REFERENCES

Accreditation Council for Occupational Therapy Education. (2018). 2018 Accreditation Council for Occupational Therapy Education (ACOTE®) Standards and interpretive guide (effective July 31, 2020). *American Journal of Occupational Therapy, 72*, 7212410005. https://doi.org/10.5014/ajot.2018.72S217

Aldridge, V. K., Dovey, T. M., Hawl, N., Martiniuc, A., Martin, C. L., & Meyer, C. (2018). Observation and comparison of mealtime behaviors in a sample of children with avoidant/restrictive food intake disorders and a control sample of children with typical development. *Infant Mental Health Journal, 39*, 410–422. https://doi.org/10.1002/imhj.21722

American Academy of Pediatrics. (2019). *Pediatric nutrition handbook* (8th ed.). Author.

American Occupational Therapy Association. (2017). The practice of occupational therapy in feeding, eating, and swallowing. *American Journal of Occupational Therapy, 71*(Suppl. 2), 7112410015. https://doi.org/10.5014/ajot.2017.716S04

American Psychiatric Association. (2013). *Diagnostic and statistical manual of mental disorders* (5th ed.). American Psychiatric Publishing.

Baghbadorani, M. K., Soleymani, Z., Dadgar, H., & Salehi, M. (2014). The effect of oral sensorimotor stimulations on feeding performance in children with spastic cerebral palsy. *Acta Medica Iranica, 52*, 899–904.

Baral, V. R., & Hourihane, J. O. (2005). Food allergy in children. *Postgraduate Medical Journal, 81*, 693–701. https://doi.org/10.1136/pgmj.2004.030288

Barton, C., Bickel, M., & Fucile, S. (2017). Pediatric oral motor feeding assessments: A systematic review. *Physical & Occupational Therapy in Pediatrics, 38*, 190–209. https://doi.org/10.1080/01942638.2017.1290734

Benfer, K. A., Weir, K. A., Bell, K. L., Ware, R. S., Davies, P. S. W., & Boyd, R. N. (2014). Oropharyngeal dysphagia in preschool children with cerebral palsy: Oral phase impairments.

Research in Developmental Disabilities, 35, 3469–3481. https://doi.org/10.1016/j.ridd.2014.08.029

Benfer, K. A., Weir, K. A., Bell, K. L., Ware, R. S., Davies, P. S. W., & Boyd, R. N. (2016). Longitudinal study of oropharyngeal dysphagia in preschool children with cerebral palsy. *Archives of Physical Medicine and Rehabilitation, 97,* 552–560. https://doi.org/10.1016/j.apmr.2015.11.016

Caffarelli, C., DiMauro, D., Mastrorilli, C., Bottau, P., Cipriani, F., & Ricci, G. (2018). Solid food introduction and the development of food allergies. *Nutrients, 10,* 1790. https://doi.org/10.3390/nu10111790

Carruth, B. R., Ziegler, P. J., Gordon, A., & Hendricks, K. (2004). Developmental milestones and self-feeding behaviors in infants and toddlers. *Journal of the American Dietary Association, 104,* 51–56. https://doi.org/10.1016/j.jada.2003.10.019

Carter, E. W., Lane, K. L., Cooney, M., Weir, K., Moss, C. K. & Machalicek, W. (2013). Parent assessments of self-determination importance and performance for students with autism or intellectual disability. *American Journal on Intellectual and Developmental Disabilities, 118,* 16–31 https://doi.org/10.1352/1944-7558-118.1.16

Casey, L. (2013). Caring for children with phenylketonuria. *Canadian Family Physician, 59,* 837–840.

Centers for Disease Control and Prevention. (2017). *Clinical growth charts.* Author.

Cichero, J. A. Y. (2017). Unlocking opportunities in food design for infants, children, and the elderly: Understanding milestones in chewing and swallowing across the lifespan for new innovations. *Journal of Texture Studies, 48,* 271–279. https://doi.org/10.1111/jtxs.12236

Clancy, K. J., & Hustad, K. C. (2011). Longitudinal changes in feeding among children with cerebral palsy between the ages of 4 and 7 years. *Developmental Neurorehabilitation, 14,* 191–198. https://doi.org/10.3109/17518423.2011.568467

Corvaglia, L., Rotatori, R., Ferlini, M., Aceti, A., Ancora, G., & Faldella, G. (2007). The effect of body positioning in gastroesophageal reflux in premature infants: Evaluation by combined impedance and pH monitoring. *Journal of Pediatrics, 151,* 591–596. https://doi.org/10.1016/j.jpeds.2007.06.014

Coulthard, H., Harris, G., & Emmett, P. (2009). Delayed introduction of lumpy foods to children during the complementary feeding period affects child's food acceptance and feeding at 7 years of age. *Maternal and Child Nutrition, 5,* 75–85. https://doi.org/10.1111/j.1740-8709.2008.00153.x

Cozma-Petruț, A., Loghin, F., Miere, D., & Dumitrașcu, D. L. (2017). Diet in irritable bowel syndrome: What to recommend, not what to forbid to patients! *World Journal of Gastroenterology, 23,* 3771–3783. https://doi.org/10.3748/wjg.v23.i21.3771

Dahlseng, M. O., Finbraten, A., Juliusson, P. B., Skranes, J., Andersen, G., & Vik, T. (2011). Feeding problems, growth and nutritional status in children with cerebral palsy. *Acta Pediatrica, 101,* 92–98. https://doi.org/10.1111/j.1651-2227.2011.02412.x

Dazeley, P., & Houston-Price, C. (2015). Exposure to foods' non-taste sensory properties. A nursery intervention to increase children's willingness to try fruit and vegetables. *Appetite, 84,* 1–6. https://doi.org/10.1016/j.appet.2014.08.040

Dovey, T. M., Aldridge, V. K., Martin C. L., Wliken, M., & Meyer, C. (2016). Screening avoidant/restrictive food intake disorder (ARFID) in children: Outcomes from utilitarian versus specialist psychometrics. *Eating Behaviors, 23,* 162–167. https://doi.org/10.1016/j.eatbeh.2016.10.004

Emmett, P. M., Hays, N. P., & Taylor, C. M. (2018). Antecedents of picky eating behaviour in young children. *Appetite, 130,* 163–173. https://doi.org/10.1016/j.appet.2018.07.032

Esteban-Figuerola, P., Canals, J., Fernández-Cao, J. C., & Arija Val, V. (2019). Differences in food consumption and nutritional intake between children with autism spectrum disorders and typically developing children: A meta-analysis. *Autism, 23,* 1079–1095. https://doi.org/10.1177/1362361318794179

Ferraro, V., Zanconato, S., & Carraro, S. (2019). Timing of food introduction and the risk of food allergy. *Nutrients, 11,* 1131. https://doi.org/10.3390/nu11051131

Ferreira, C. T., Carvalho, E., Sdepanian, V. L., de Morais, M. B., Vieira, M. C., & Silva, L. R. (2014). Gastroesophageal reflux disease: Exaggerations, evidence and clinical practice. *Jornal de Pediatria, 90,* 105–118. http://doi.org/10.1016/j.jped.2013.05.009

Fries, L. R., & van der Horst, K. (2019). Parental feeding practices and associations with children's food acceptance and picky eating. In C. J. Henry, T. A. Nicklas, & S. Nicklaus (Eds.), *Nestlé Nutrition Institute Workshop Series: Vol. 91. Nurturing a healthy generation of children: Research gaps and opportunities* (pp. 31–39). https://doi.org/10.1159/000493676

Fucile, S., Gisel, E. G., McFarland, D. H., & Lau, C. (2011). Oral and non-oral sensorimotor interventions enhance oral feeding performance in preterm infants. *Developmental Medicine and Child Neurology, 53,* 829–835. https://doi.org/10.1111/j.1469-8749.2011.04023.x

Fucile, S., McFarland, D. H., Gisel, E. G., & Lau, C. (2012). Oral and nonoral sensorimotor interventions facilitate suck–swallow–respiration functions and their coordination in preterm infants. *Early Human Development, 88,* 345–350. https://doi.org/10.1016/j.earlhumdev.2011.09.007

Ghalichi, F., Ghaemmaghami, J., Malek, A., & Ostadrahimi, A. (2016). Effect of gluten free diet on gastrointestinal and behavioral indices for children with autism spectrum disorders: A randomized clinical trial. *World Journal of Pediatrics, 12,* 436–442. https://doi.org/10.1007/s12519-016-0040-z

Gray, K. L., Sinha, S., Buro, A. W., Robinson, C., Berkman, K., Agazzi, H., & Shaffer-Hudkins, E. (2018). Early history, mealtime environment, and parental views on mealtime and eating behaviors among children with ASD in Florida. *Nutrients, 10,* 1867. https://doi.org/10.3390/nu10121867

Hashimoto, M., Igari, K., Hanawa, S., Ito, A., Takahashi, A., Ishida, N., . . . Sasaki, K. (2014). Tongue pressure during swallowing in adults with Down syndrome and its relationship with palatal morphology. *Dysphagia, 29,* 509–518. https://doi.org/10.1007/s00455-014-9538-5

Hwang, Y.-S., Lin, C.-H., Coster, W. J., Bigsby, R., & Vergara, E. (2010). Effectiveness of cheek and jaw support to improve feeding performance of preterm infants. *American Journal of Occupational Therapy, 64,* 886–894. https://doi.org/10.5014/ajot.2010.09031

Hyman, S. L., Stewart, P. A., Schmidt, B., Cain, U., Lemcke, N., Foley, J. T., . . . Ng, P. K. (2012). Nutrient intake from food in children with autism. *Pediatrics, 130,* 145–153. https://doi.org/10.1542/peds.2012-0900L

Institute of Medicine. (2006). *Dietary reference intakes: The essential guide to nutrient requirements.* National Academies Press.

Jackson, A., Maybee, J., Moran, M. K., Wolter-Warmerdam, K., & Hickey, F. (2016). Clinical characteristics of dysphagia in children with Down syndrome. *Dysphagia, 31,* 663–671. https://doi.org/10.1007/s00455-016-9725-7

Korczak, R., Kamil, A., Fleige, L., Donovan, S. M., & Slavin, J. L. (2017). Dietary fiber and digestive health in children. *Nutrition Reviews, 75,* 241–259. https://doi.org/10.1093/nutrit/nuw068

Korth, K., & Maune, N. C. (2020). Assessment and treatment of feeding, eating, and swallowing. In J. C. O'Brien & H. Kuhaneck (Eds.), *Case-Smith's occupational therapy for children and adolescents* (8th ed., pp. 212–238). Elsevier.

Lewis, E., & Kritzinger, A. (2004). Parental experiences of feeding problems in their infants with Down syndrome. *Down Syndrome Research and Practice, 9*(2), 45–52. https://doi.org/10.3104/reports.291

Lightdale, J. R., & Gremse, D. A. (2013). Gastroesophageal reflux: Management guidance for the pediatrician. *Pediatrics, 131,* e1684–e1695. https://doi.org/10.1542/peds.2013-0421

MacLeod, E. L., & Ney, D. M. (2010). Nutritional management of phenylketonuria. *Annales Nestlé, 68,* 58–69. https://doi.org/10.1159/000312813

Magge, S., & Lembo, A. (2012). Low-FODMAP diet for treatment of irritable bowel syndrome. *Gastroenterology & Hepatology, 8,* 739–745.

Marcus, S., & Breton, S. (2013). *Infant and child feeding and swallowing: Occupational therapy assessment and intervention.* AOTA Press.

Mayes, S. D., & Zickgraf, H. (2019). Atypical eating behaviors in children and adolescents with autism, ADHD, other disorders, and typical development. *Research in Autism Spectrum Disorders, 64,* 76–83. https://doi.org/10.1016/j.rasd.2019.04.002

Milano, K., Chatoor, I., & Kerzner, B. (2019). A functional approach to feeding difficulties in children. *Current Gastroenterology Reports, 21,* 51. https://doi.org/10.1007/s11894-019-0719-0

Moreno, M. (2014). Gastroesophageal reflux disease. *JAMA Pediatrics, 168,* 976. https://doi.org/10.1001/jamapediatrics.2013.3373

Morris, S. E., & Klein, M. D. (2000). *Pre-feeding skills: A comprehensive resource for mealtime development.* Academic Press.

Nichols, A., Wasemann, C., Coatie, D., Moon, E., & Weller, J. (2018). Parental perceptions: Raising a child with a feeding and eating disorder. *SIS Quarterly Practice Connections, 3*(2), 2–4.

O'Neill, A. C., & Richter, G. T. (2013). Pharyngeal dysphagia in children with Down syndrome. *Otolaryngology—Head and Neck Surgery, 149,* 146–150. https://doi.org/10.1177/0194599813483445

Piwowarczyk, A., Horvath, A., Łukasik, J., Pisula, E., & Szajewska, H. (2018). Gluten- and casein-free diet and autism spectrum disorders in children: A systematic review. *European Journal of Nutrition, 57,* 433–440. https://doi.org/10.1007/s00394-017-1483-2

Poddar, U. (2019). Gastroesophageal reflux disease (GERD) in children. *Paediatrics and International Child Health, 39,* 7–12. https://doi.org/10.1080/20469047.2018.1489649

Provost, B., Crowe, T. K., Osbourn, P. L., McClain, C., & Skipper, B. J. (2010). Mealtime behaviors of preschool children: Comparison of children with autism spectrum disorder and children with typical development. *Physical & Occupational Therapy in Pediatrics, 30,* 220–233. https://doi.org/10.3109/01942631003757669

Ptomey, L. T., & Wittenbrook, W. (2015). Position of the Academy of Nutrition and Dietetics: Nutrition services for individuals with intellectual and developmental disabilities and special health care needs. *Journal of the Academy of Nutrition and Dietetics, 115,* 593–608. https://doi.org/10.1016/j.jand.2015.02.002

Ramos, C. C., Maximino, P., Machado, R. H. V., Bozzini, A. B., Ribeiro, L. W., & Fisberg, M. (2017). Delayed development of feeding skills in children with feeding difficulties—cross-sectional study in a Brazilian reference center. *Frontiers in Pediatrics, 5,* 229. https://doi.org/10.3389/fped.2017.00229

Ranjan, S., & Nasser, J. A. (2015). Nutritional status of individuals with autism spectrum disorders: Do we know enough? *Advances in Nutrition, 6,* 397–407. https://doi.org/10.3945/an.114.007914

Ray, S. (2015, March). Addressing the relation-based feeding needs of young children. *Early Intervention & School Special Interest Section Quarterly, 22*(1), 1–4.

Rybak, A., Pesce, M., Thapar, N., & Borrelli, O. (2017). Gastroesophageal reflux in children. *International Journal of Molecular Sciences, 18,* 1671. https://doi.org/10.3390/ijms18081671

Sathe, N., Andrews, J. C., McPheeters, M. L., & Warren, Z. E. (2017). Nutritional and dietary interventions for autism spectrum disorder: A systematic review. *Pediatrics, 139,* e20170346. https://doi.org/10.1542/peds.2017-0346

Schultz-Krohn, W. (2006). Feeding and eating for infants and toddlers. *OT Practice, 11*(9), 16–20.

Soltani, D., Ghaffar Pour, M., Tafakhori, A., Sarraf, P., & Bitarafan, S. (2016). Nutritional aspects of treatment in epileptic patients. *Iranian Journal of Child Neurology, 10*(3), 1–12. https://doi.org/10.22037/ijcn.v10i3.9224

Stafstrom, C. E. (2004). Dietary approaches to epilepsy treatment: Old and new options on the menu. *Epilepsy Currents, 4,* 215–222. https://doi.org/10.1111/j.1535-7597.2004.46001.x

Sturman, N., Deckx, L., & van Driel, M. L. (2017). Methylphenidate for children and adolescents with autism spectrum disorder. *Cochrane Database of Systematic Reviews, 11,* CD011144. https://doi.org/10.1002/14651858.CD011144.pub2

Sucher, K., Kittler, P., & Nelms, M. (2016). *Food and culture* (7th ed.). Cengage Learning.

Taylor, C., & Emmett, P. (2019). Picky eating in children: Causes and consequences. *Proceedings of the Nutrition Society, 78,* 161–169. https://doi.org/10.1017/S0029665118002586

Taylor, C. M., Wernimont, S. M., Northstone, K., & Emmett, P. M. (2015). Picky/fussy eating in children: Review of definitions, assessment, prevalence and dietary intakes. *Appetite, 95,* 349–359. https://doi.org/10.1016/j.appet.2015.07.026

U.S. Department of Health and Human Services & U.S. Department of Agriculture. (2015). *2015–2020 dietary guidelines for Americans* (8th ed.). U.S. Government Printing Office.

U.S. Department of Health and Human Services & U.S. Department of Agriculture. (2018). *Choose My Plate program.* U.S. Government Printing Office.

U.S. Food and Drug Administration. (2019). *Food labeling and nutrition.* https://www.fda.gov/food/food-labeling-nutrition

Warren, J. (2018). An update on complementary feeding. *Nursing Children and Young People, 30*(6), 38–47. https://doi.org/10.7748/ncyp.2018.e1032

Waserman, S., & Watson, W. (2011). Food allergy. *Allergy, Asthma & Clinical Immunology, 7*(Suppl. 1), S1–S7. https://doi.org/10.1186/1710-1492-7-S1-S7

Wilcox, D. D., Potvin, M.-C., & Prelock, P. A. (2009, December). Oral motor interventions and cerebral palsy: Using evidence to inform practice. *Early Intervention Special Interest Section Quarterly, 16*(4), 1–4.

Zimmerman, J., & Fisher, M. (2017). Avoidant/restrictive food intake disorder (ARFID). *Current Problems in Pediatric and Adolescent Health Care, 47,* 95–103. https://doi.org/10.1016/j.cppeds.2017.02.005

Best Practices in Supporting Learning and Early Literacy Skills (Cognitive Skills)

29

Gloria Frolek Clark, PhD, OTR/L, BCP; Jayna Niblock, PhD, OTD, OTR/L, BCP; and Taylor Crane Vos, OTD, OTR/L

KEY TERMS AND CONCEPTS

- Attention
- Cognitive skills
- Imitation
- Joint attention
- Language decoding
- Literacy
- Long-term memory
- Memory
- Perceptual functions
- Primary memory
- Problem solving
- Short-term memory
- Temperament
- Working memory

OVERVIEW

Cognitive development in early childhood is strongly associated with exploration of a child's environment and their interactions with caregivers, which may be influenced by the child's temperament. Limitations in a child's cognitive abilities affect their everyday life and ability to engage in a variety of occupations (Wolf & Baum, 2011). Social factors influencing the environments of preschool-age children who were born premature (e.g., low educational level of primary caregiver) have a significant negative impact on their executive functioning (O'Meagher et al., 2017). Children with cognitive difficulties may demonstrate difficulties with learning later in life, behaviors, and social interactions (Frolek Clark & Schlabach, 2013). Between 9.5% and 14.2% of children from birth to age 5 years experience social–emotional problems that cause them difficulties in their general functioning and development as well as their school readiness (Brauner & Stephens, 2006), with boys having greater difficulties than girls (Cooper et al., 2009).

Occupational therapy practitioners can positively influence cognitive development in a variety of early childhood settings. (*Note. Occupational therapy practitioner* refers to both occupational therapists and occupational therapy assistants.) Practitioners may work with children who have genetic conditions or syndromes; developmental delays; or injuries acquired before, during, or after birth. Addressing cognitive concerns in homes, child care settings, preschools, or health care settings can positively influence cognitive development for these children.

One in 10 infants is born prematurely in the United States (Ferré et al., 2016), with an estimated 15 million children born prematurely each year across the world (March of Dimes; Partnership for Maternal, Newborn, & Child Health; Save the Children; & World Health Organization, 2012). Children born prematurely may have cognitive difficulties that can be positively affected through interventions

in the neonatal intensive care unit (NICU) as well as in the home, child care, preschool, or health care settings. Occupational therapy practitioners may educate, collaborate with, and train parents, caregivers, siblings, and peers in activities to promote cognitive development. Children receiving occupational therapy may also have cognitive difficulties that should be addressed, even if the primary focus of the intervention is motor abilities.

ESSENTIAL CONSIDERATIONS

Cognitive skills in young children include temperament; perceptual functions; imitation; attention, including joint attention; memory; and literacy skills. They do not follow a linear, hierarchical development but instead fluctuate on the basis of the activity demands and supports provided in different environments (Kramer & Hinojosa, 2010). Occupational therapy practitioners must understand the influence of these factors and common terminology related to early cognitive skills to engage parents and caregivers in activities that promote cognitive development for the child.

Multiple terms are used in literature to address early cognitive development. Several of them are discussed in this section, including *temperament, perception, attention, memory, imitation, problem solving,* and *early literacy.*

Temperament

Temperament has been increasingly linked to young children's abilities to engage in their environment and learn (Dunn, 2001). In the *International Classification of Functioning, Disability and Health,* the World Health Organization (WHO; 2001, p. b126) defines *temperament* as "general mental functions of constitutional disposition of the individual to react in a particular way to situations, including the set of mental characteristics that makes the individual distinct from others," which means a child is born with innate characteristics that influence their engagement with the world. Children can have temperament risk factors that make them a poor fit to their environment, causing stress and conflict with their early caregivers (Carey & McDevitt, 1995). Poor fit of children's temperament to their environment (e.g., shyness influences the frequency of child-initiated teacher–child interactions), in particular the school environment, has been shown to result in lower academic performance than the child's actual ability level (Al-Hendawi, 2013; Rudasill & Rimm-Kaufman, 2009).

Perceptual Functions

Perceptual functions are a specific mental function (American Occupational Therapy Association, 2020) that is foundational for cognitive development, because children's brains must take in and process the sensory stimuli from various sensory systems to develop an understanding of the world around them (Cronin, 2016b). As children develop, their perception is shaped by their experiences through learning, memory, and expectations (Bernstein, 2010). For example, visual perception is foundational for development of early literacy skills; it requires a child to have developmentally appropriate or corrected visual acuity, visual fields, and oculomotor skills (i.e., tracking, convergence, divergence, scanning) before being able to engage in activities that require attention (Warren, 1993).

Imitation

Imitation is demonstrated by children a few hours after birth as they attend to a variety of sensory stimuli in their environment. Children imitate simple, everyday items and activities they see adults and other children engaging in. Children imitate words for new objects (Jaswal & Hansen, 2006), actions with new tools (Nielsen & Tomaselli, 2010), and complex concepts such as abstract rules (Williamson et al., 2010). As children's attention increases, they develop more mature imitation skills, which continue into adulthood.

Attention

As a central mental function that is foundational for cognition, *attention* involves focus on a specific stimulus, internal or external, for the required length of time to engage in an appropriate response (WHO, 2001). In early childhood, children develop sustained attention skills through play involving *joint attention* (i.e., coordinated engagement of two individuals with each other or an object). Joint attention has been found to enhance memory skills among children and adults (Kim & Mundy, 2012; Kopp & Lindenberger, 2011). Attention supports the development of cognitive skills through social communication, language development, self-regulation, and emotional engagement (Morales et al., 2005; Sheinkopf et al., 2004).

Memory

Memory is another specific mental function; it allows individuals to register and store information to retrieve and use at another time as needed (WHO, 2001). Memory development starts in infancy with unconscious, implicit memory, which is often based on perceptual experiences of the infant (Cronin, 2016b). Perceptual functions influence an infant's immediate memory and how they engage on the basis of a stimulus they perceive as important or unimportant and pleasant or unpleasant. This perceptual filtering is influenced by the infant's physical experiences, cultural context, and social engagement. The memories that develop are intertwined with the perceptual experiences and influence the development of conscious memory as the child grows. In the preschool years, children start to develop explicit, conscious, and intentional memory skills, which they need to advance their cognitive skills (Feldman, 2011).

Short-term memory includes both working memory and primary memory. *Working memory* is the immediate use and recall of memory that is used for following directions and making decisions, and allows children to maintain information for processing to complete verbal and nonverbal tasks (Becker & Morris, 1999). *Primary memory* is a temporary memory that is used for immediate recall requiring cognitive attention and is forgotten if it is not consolidated into long-term memory (WHO, 2001). *Long-term memory* involves both explicit and implicit memories developed throughout a child's lifetime. It allows the storage of information that was originally in short-term memory, for retrieval at a later time (WHO, 2001). Memory is foundational for development of literacy abilities, because children need to remember what words and symbols mean.

Problem Solving

Problem solving is a complex skill that starts with young children engaging in exploratory play and tool use (Keen, 2011). Through varied practice of an action to meet similar but different problems, children develop their ability to effectively problem solve more and more complex difficulties. Problem-solving abilities have been linked to children's spatial understanding (Bates et al., 1980) as well as their ability to understand fundamental aspects of tools that may look different on the surface (Brown, 1990). Children develop the ability to solve a motor problem before the ability to cognitively solve problems (Keen, 2011).

Literacy

Literacy is the ability to read and write a shared language (Bittman et al., 2012). Literacy is built on a foundation of language and communication skills that develop early in life. The National Early Literacy Panel (NELP; 2008) defines *conventional literacy skills* as those that are a part of all literacy practices and easily identifiable components in literacy abilities, including decoding, oral reading fluency, reading comprehension, writing, and spelling. *Language decoding* builds skills needed for early literacy by developing an understanding of letter–sound relationships and an awareness that patterns of letters represent words. Early literacy skills develop between birth and age 5 years and have a clear relationship with the development of conventional literacy skills of reading and writing (NELP, 2008).

The ability to share language begins with communication skills that are developed through imitation in early childhood. Receptive language develops first as children follow directions and understand what adults are communicating to them. Children's language increases in intelligibility throughout early childhood and is not expected to be fully intelligible until age 5 years (Cronin, 2016a). Oral language abilities have been found to have a significant role in later literacy (e.g., listening comprehension, word definitions, grammar; NELP, 2008). Children's written communication skills do not exceed their language comprehension skills, which is why children's writing improves as their reading skills develop. For more information, please read Chapter 13, "Understanding Early Literacy Development."

BEST PRACTICES

Evaluate the Child

Occupational therapists evaluating young children's cognitive skills should begin by gathering an occupational profile through interviews and observations to determine concerns, expectations, supports, and barriers to occupational performance. The child, caregivers, family members, and others are a vital part of the evaluation process because they contribute information about the child's occupational profile (e.g., occupational history, occupations, routines and habitual patterns, areas of strength, areas of weaknesses). This data-gathering process allows the practitioner to understand the child's performance and the environmental demands for identification of appropriate assessments.

The Person–Environment–Occupation Model of Occupational Performance (Law et al., 1996) assists in identifying the dynamic relationships among a person, an environment, and occupations (i.e., activities). This multidomain model enhances identification and analysis of strengths and barriers that affect children's occupational performance and focuses interventions on factors to improve their occupational performance. The model does this by enhancing the congruence of the three domains and adapting to needs. Outcome measures are based on the child's and family's needs. Data should be collected frequently and systematically to continually monitor and assess the child's cognitive abilities and needs and address the needs of their family. Assessment tools are administered when additional information about the child's cognitive skills is needed. Table 29.1 provides some examples. A more in-depth listing of assessment tools can be found in Appendix F, "Examples of Assessments for Early Childhood (Birth–5 Years)."

TABLE 29.1. Examples of Assessment Tools to Identify Cognitive Skills in Early Childhood

ASSESSMENT TOOL	AGES	DESCRIPTION
Bayley Scales of Infant and Toddler Development (4th ed.; Bayley & Alyward, 2019)	16 days–42 months	Standardized measure with a subcategory that emphasizes cognition (e.g., visual preference, attention, memory, sensorimotor, exploration and manipulation, concept formation). Uses caregiver responses to support scoring of certain items.
Behavior Rating Inventory of Executive Function (Preschool Version; Gioia et al., 2000)	2.0–5.11 years	Standardized measures of executive functions, including inhibition, emotional control, working memory, and planning and organizing.
Carolina Curriculum (Johnson-Martin et al., 2004a, 2004b)	▪ Carolina Curriculum for Infants & Toddlers With Special Needs (3rd ed.): Birth–36 months ▪ Carolina Curriculum for Preschoolers With Special Needs (2nd ed.): 24–60 months	Criterion-referenced tool that can be used for evaluation and intervention. Useful in a variety of environments to analyze children's outcomes.
Developmental Assessment of Young Children (2nd ed.; Voress et al., 2012)	Birth–5 years, 11 months	Standardized tool that includes multiple domains, including cognition. Allows examiners to obtain information about a child's abilities through observation, interview of caregivers, and direct assessment.
Early Learning Accomplishment Profile (Hardin & Peisner-Feinburg, 2001)	Birth–36 months	Criterion-referenced assessment instrument that includes skills in six domains of development, including cognition.
Griffiths Mental Development Scales (Griffith, 1996)	Birth–6 years (72 months)	Standardized tool that measures child development across five areas, including foundations of learning. Administration requires specific training.
Miller Assessment for Preschoolers (Miller, 1982)	2 years, 9 months–5 years, 8 months	Standardized tool that includes cognitive abilities. Appropriate for preschool age for mild–moderate developmental delays.

Implement Evidence-Based Intervention to Facilitate Cognitive and Literacy Skills

Collaborating with the family and others to enhance the child's ability to access and participate in their daily routine should be the focus of occupational therapy services. To enhance the cognitive development of young children, occupational therapy practitioners must implement evidence-based practices. During a recent systematic review of cognitive development in early childhood, several evidence-based interventions were identified (Frolek Clark et al., 2019a–d).

Provide interventions with premature infants

Strong evidence (e.g., 13 Level I randomized controlled trials) exists that providing early intervention programs for premature infants increased their cognitive development. In the NICU, the Newborn Individualized Developmental Care and Assessment Program (NIDCAP) was effective for preterm infants with intrauterine growth retardation in both self-regulation and mental development (Als et al., 2011, 2012). A clinic-based intervention program was also effective in increasing cognitive development after 12 months; it focused on parent–child dyad services, which included massage and parent education (Tang et al., 2011). When home activities were added to the clinic-based program, the preterm infants had a higher gain in cognitive outcomes.

Providing interventions at home also had strong evidence. Interventions that provided twice-a-month home visits with emphasis on coaching families in playful learning activities (Wallander, Bann et al., 2014; Wallander, Biasini et al., 2014) and enhancing their preterm child's development during the first 3 years of the child's life were effective, especially for families with low resources (Bann et al., 2016) and for preterm and low-birthweight infants (McManus et al., 2012).

Provide interventions for children with disabilities

Strong evidence exists that cognitive training programs can improve executive function skills among preschoolers with attention deficit hyperactivity disorder (ADHD), autism spectrum disorder (ASD), and developmental delays (Frolek Clark et al., 2019b). Preschoolers with ADHD increased executive functioning skills after 8–11 weeks of executive functioning group interventions (1 hour per week for 8 weeks), with statistically significant improvement in attention, inhibition, memory, and planning (Tamm & Nakonezny, 2015; Tamm et al., 2012). An 11-week community-based cognitive function group resulted in significant improvements in executive functioning among preschoolers with ADHD (Rosenberg et al., 2015).

Occupational therapy practitioners should consider using pivotal response treatment, a play-based approach focused on the child's choice and contingent reinforcement, for preschoolers with ASD (intervention ran for 6–10 months) as a method to increase their cognitive skills (Smith et al., 2015). There is also evidence that training focused on cognitive skills (30 minutes per week for 8 months) resulted in a statistically significant increase in ability to complete complex cognitive tasks for children who had or were at risk for various conditions (Golos et al., 2011). Occupational therapy practitioners may want to use the Interdisciplinary Sensory-Enriched Early Intervention program to increase cognitive scores for preschoolers with and without sensory-processing difficulties (Blanche et al., 2016). Sorensen and colleagues (2016) found cognitive skills increased among preschoolers with cerebral palsy who received Program Intensified Habilitation at a hospital setting for 1 year (inpatient status for 1–2-week phases).

Educate parents to implement interventions

Strong evidence supports occupational therapy practitioners educating parents to implement programs that increase their child's cognitive and literacy skills. These interventions include shared and dialogical reading, play, developmental training, enhanced parental interactions, massage, and caregiver–infant skin-to-skin contact.

Encouraging parents to read to their young child is important. After 6 weeks, toddlers who were read to daily by their mother had statistically significant improvements in attention and comprehension (Cooper et al., 2014). Spanish-speaking children also demonstrated gains in print knowledge and alphabet knowledge after an 8-week home-reading program (Pratt et al., 2015). Preschoolers whose parents read to them using either shared reading or dialogic reading demonstrated an improvement in print and word reading (Pillinger & Wood, 2014).

Educating and modeling for parents the importance of play is an important part of occupational therapy services. Strong evidence exists for increasing cognitive development if the parent's play intervention is focused on the parent–child interaction. Aboud and colleagues (2013) found mothers who played with their infants during a 10-month parenting program (home and group meetings) increased their child's cognitive development. Increased cognitive skills (e.g., working memory, processing speed) were found among preschoolers whose mothers played with them for 3 months (10 minutes daily, 5 days per week; Tachibana et al., 2012). For occupational therapy practitioners working in health care, educating mothers on development and child interactions during routine child health visits also resulted in statistically significant gains in the child's cognitive development (Chang et al., 2015).

Technology may increase cognitive skills, but evidence is mixed. For example, a 5-week nonverbal computer training program for 4-year-olds increased their ability to identify patterns and infer rules, a predictor for academic skills (Bergman Nutley et al., 2011), but other computer programs designed to enhance attention and learning were not effective in enhancing executive functions among preschoolers (Kirk et al., 2016, 2017).

There are three additional evidence-based interventions for young children that occupational therapy practitioners can support on the basis of longitudinal studies. First, encourage parents to feed infants on demand (i.e., when the infant is hungry) rather than on a schedule, because research found higher academic test scores and IQ at age 8 years among participants who were demand-fed as infants (Iacovou & Sevilla, 2013). While in the hospital and at home, parents should be encouraged to massage their premature infant for 10 minutes daily to increase the infant's IQ scores at age 12 months (Abdallah et al., 2013). On the basis of 5- and 10-year follow-up studies, mothers of premature infants should also be encouraged to use kangaroo care (skin to skin) for 14 consecutive days to increase mental development and executive functions (Feldman et al., 2014).

Provide collaborative interventions with the preschool team

Occupational therapy practitioners working in preschools must be knowledgeable about interventions that the team can implement to enhance cognitive development. Strong evidence from multisite studies with large sample sizes indicates that specific programs enhance cognitive and literacy skills among preschoolers at risk for learning delays. The Get Ready intervention enhances the quality of parent–child interactions; a 2-year study of 21 Head Start schools found statistically significant increases in writing, reading, and oral language among the treatment group (Sheridan et al., 2011). The Head Start Research-Based Developmentally Informed intervention, an emergent literacy curriculum studied in 25 Head Start centers, yielded statistically significant positive changes in learning engagement and attention among the treatment group (Nix et al., 2013).

The Read It Again—PreK (RIA) program was studied in 14 schools and showed statistically significant increases among the treatment group on measures of literacy (e.g., rhyme, alliteration, print) but not alphabet knowledge (Justice et al., 2010). Hilbert and Eis (2013) investigated the RIA program in nine preschool classrooms and found statistically significant improvements in vocabulary and print knowledge using 60 lessons over 23 weeks. Adaptations to RIA were studied (20 lessons on DVD, 5 hours of viewing over 5 weeks), resulting in statistically significant improvements for the treatment group on print and word awareness, alphabet knowledge, and rhyme (Schryer et al., 2015).

As preschools implement multitiered systems of supports, occupational therapy practitioners may support preschoolers' learning through knowledge and implementation of Tier II interventions for children at risk for learning difficulties. At-risk 4-year-old readers who received interventions focused on explicit and sequenced developmentally appropriate activities in small groups (30-minute lessons twice a week over a 9-week period) made statistically significant improvements on reading scores in Years 2 and 3 of the study (Level I; Bailet et al., 2011). Another study of preschoolers from Title I preschools who received Tier I or Tier II supports focused on literacy skills found statistically significant increases in print knowledge, letter names, and letter sounds (Level I; Lonigan & Phillips, 2015).

For preschoolers in special education programs, literacy skills can be increased with intensive interventions. Researchers found that preschoolers with developmental delays transitioning to kindergarten had statistically significant positive increases in literacy skills after participating in Kids in Transition to School, an intensive summer readiness program consisting of 2 hours of intervention twice a week for 12 weeks and 8 hours of parent training (Pears et al., 2016). Preschoolers with Down syndrome had statistically significant improvements in letter name, sound

identification, and number of sight words read after participating in the Early Reading Program for 45 weeks (Colozzo et al., 2016).

Pre-kindergarteners who received an intervention focused on working memory, cognitive flexibility, and interference control for 30 minutes over 6 weeks had a statistically significant increase in working memory performance and cognitive flexibility (Röthlisberger et al., 2011). Either alphabet paper books or electronic books should be recommended, given that there was no significant difference between groups (Willoughby et al., 2015).

Occupational therapy practitioners should also encourage movement versus sedentary activities. Palmer et al. (2013) found exercise increased cognitive function for sustained attention among preschoolers who engaged in 30 minutes of movement exercise (e.g., hopping, throwing balls).

SUMMARY

There are a variety of ways occupational therapy practitioners working with children from birth to preschool age can support positive cognitive development. Practitioners can support parents in engaging with their children. In the NICU, practitioners should educate parents about programs such as the NIDCAP, kangaroo care, and infant massage for premature infants. Practitioners working in a home or day care should collaborate with parents and caregivers to engage in active motor activities, shared book reading, and feeding on demand to increase children's cognitive abilities. In preschools, practitioners should support educators in understanding how to incorporate large motor activities to enhance cognitive skills and allow children to develop needed fine motor skills later in life. Practitioners working in health care can support parents' and caregivers' ability to engage in play activities, which improve cognitive outcomes for children later in life. Literature on occupational therapy's role in cognitive development continues to demonstrate the profession's unique contribution to improving this important performance skill in a variety of ways.

REFERENCES

Abdallah, B., Badr, L. K., & Hawwari, M. (2013). The efficacy of massage on short and long term outcomes in preterm infants. *Infant Behavior & Development, 36,* 662–669. https://doi.org/10.1016/j.infbeh.2013.06.009

Aboud, F. E., Singla, D. R., Nahil, M. I., & Borisova, I. (2013). Effectiveness of a parenting program in Bangladesh to address early childhood health, growth and development. *Social Science & Medicine, 97,* 250–258. https://doi.org/10.1016/j.socscimed.2013.06.020

Al-Hendawi, M. (2013). Temperament, school adjustment, and academic achievement: Existing research and future directions. *Educational Review, 65,* 177–205. https://doi.org/10.1080/0013 1911.2011.648371

Als, H., Duffy, F. H., McAnulty, G. B., Butler, S. C., Lightbody, L., Kosta, S., . . . Warfield, S. K. (2012). NIDCAP improves brain function and structure in preterm infants with severe intrauterine growth restrictions. *Journal of Perinatology, 32,* 797–803. https://doi.org/10.1038/jp.2011.201

Als, H., Duffy, F. H., McAnulty, G. B., Fischer, C. B., Kosta, S., Butler, S. C., . . . Ringer, S. A. (2011). Is the Newborn Individualized

Developmental Care and Assessment Program (NIDCAP) effective for preterm infants with intrauterine growth restriction? *Journal of Perinatology, 31,* 130–136. https://doi.org/10.1038/jp.2010.81

American Occupational Therapy Association. (2020). Occupational therapy practice framework: Domain and process (4th ed.). *American Journal of Occupational Therapy, 74*(Suppl. 2), 7412410010. https://doi.org/10.5014/ajot.2020.74S2001

Bailet, L. L., Repper, K., Murphy, S., Piasta, S., & Zettler-Greeley, C. (2011). Emergent literacy intervention for prekindergartners at risk for reading failure: Years 2 and 3 of a multiyear study. *Journal of Learning Disabilities, 46,* 133–153. https://doi.org/10.1177/0022219411407925

Bann, C., Wallander, J. L., Do, B., Thorsten, V., Pasha, O., Biasini, F. J., . . . Carlo, W. A. (2016). Home-based early intervention and the influence of family resources on cognitive development. *Pediatrics, 137,* e20153766. https://doi.org/10.1542/peds.2015-3766

Bates, E., Carlson-Luden, V., & Bretherton, I. (1980). Perceptual aspects of tool using in infancy. *Infant Behavioral Development, 3,* 127–140. https://doi.org/10.1016/S0163-6383(80)80017-8

Bayley, N., & Aylward, G. P. (2019). *Bayley Scales of Infant and Toddler Development administration manual* (4th ed.). Pearson.

Becker, J., & Morris, R. (1999). Working memory(s). *Brain and Cognition, 41,* 1–8. https://doi.org/10.1006/brcg.1998.1092

Bergman Nutley, S. B., Söderqvist, S., Bryde, S., Thorell, L. B., Humphreys, K., & Klingberg, T. (2011). Gains in fluid intelligence after training non-verbal reasoning in 4-year-old children: A controlled, randomized study. *Developmental Science, 14,* 591–601. https://doi.org/10.1111/j.1467-7687.2010.01022.x

Bernstein, D. (2010). *Essentials of psychology* (5th ed.). Wadsworth Publishing.

Bittman, M., Rutherford, L., Brown, J., & Unsworth, L. (2012). Digital natives? New and old media and children's language acquisition. *Family Matters, 91,* 18–26. https://doi.org/10.1177/000494411105500206

Blanche, E. I., Chang, M. C., Gutierrez, J., & Gunter, J. S. (2016). Effectiveness of a sensory-enriched early intervention group program for children with developmental disabilities. *American Journal of Occupational Therapy, 70,* 7005220010. https://doi.org/10.5014/ajot.2016.018481

Brauner, C. B., & Stephens, C. B. (2006). Estimating the prevalence of early childhood serious emotional/behavioral disorders: Challenges and recommendations. *Public Health Reports, 121,* 303–310. https://doi.org/10.1177/003335490612100314

Brown, A. (1990). Domain-specific principles affect learning and transfer in children. *Cognitive Science, 14,* 107–133. https://doi.org/10.1016/0364-0213(90)90028-U

Carey, T., & McDevitt, S. (1995). *Coping with children's temperament: A guide for professionals.* Basic Books.

Chang, S. M., Grantham-McGregor, S. M., Powell, C. A., Vera-Hernandez, M., Lopez-Boo, F., Baker-Henningham, H., & Walker, S. P. (2015). Integrating a parenting intervention with routine primary health care: A cluster randomized trial. *Pediatrics, 136,* 272–280. https://doi.org/10.1542/peds.2015-0119

Colozzo, P., McKeil, L., Petersen, J. M., & Szabo, A. (2016). An early literacy program for young children with Down syndrome: Changes observed over one year. *Journal of Policy and Practice in Intellectual Disabilities, 13,* 102–110. https://doi.org/10.1111/jppi.12160

Cooper, J. L., Masi, R., & Vick, L. (2009). *Social–emotional development in early childhood: What every policymaker should know.* National Center for Children in Poverty.

Cooper, P. J., Vally, Z., Cooper, H., Radford, T., Sharples, A., Tomlinson, M., & Murray, L. (2014). Promoting mother–infant book sharing and infant attention and language development in an impoverished South African population: A pilot study. *Early Childhood Education Journal, 42,* 143–152. https://doi.org/10.1007/s10643-013-0591-8

Cronin, A. (2016a). Life span communication. In A. Cornin & M. B. Mandich (Eds.), *Human development and performance: Throughout the lifespan* (pp. 81–100). Cengage Learning.

Cronin, A. (2016b). Mental functions and learning across the life span. In A. Cornin & M. B. Mandich (Eds.), *Human development and performance: Throughout the lifespan* (pp. 101–122). Cengage Learning.

Dunn, W. (2001). The sensations of everyday life: Empirical, theoretical, and pragmatic considerations (Eleanor Clarke Slagle Lecture). *American Journal of Occupational Therapy, 55,* 608620. https://doi.org/10.5014/ajot.55.6.608

Feldman, R. (2011). *Child development* (6th ed.). Prentice Hall.

Feldman, R., Rosenthal, Z., & Eidelman, A. I. (2014). Maternal–preterm skin-to-skin contact enhances child physiologic organization and cognitive control across the first 10 years of life. *Biological Psychiatry, 75,* 56–64. https://doi.org/10.1016/j.biopsych.2013.08.012

Ferré, C., Callaghan, W., Olson, C., Sharma, A., & Barfield, W. (2016). Effects of maternal age and age-specific preterm birth rates on overall preterm birth rates—United States, 2007 and 2014. *Morbidity and Mortality Weekly Report, 65,* 1181–1184. https://doi.org/10.15585/mmwr.mm6543a1

Frolek Clark, G., Fischbach, J., Crane, T., Nadolny, E., & Corry, J. (2019a). *Cognitive interventions implemented in preschool classrooms for children and youth 0–5 years: Systematic review of related literature from 2010 to 2017* [Critically Appraised Topic]. https://www.aota.org/Practice/Children-Youth/Evidence-based/CAT-CY05-Cognition-Preschool.aspx

Frolek Clark, G., Fischbach, J., Crane, T., Corry, J., & Nadolny, E. (2019b). *Occupational therapy and team-led cognitive development interventions for premature and developmentally delayed infants: Systematic review of related literature from 2010 to 2017* [Critically Appraised Topic]. https://www.aota.org/Practice/Children-Youth/Evidence-based/CAT-CY05-Cognition-Premies.aspx

Frolek Clark, G., Fischbach, J., Crane, T., Nadolny, E., & Corry, J. (2019c). *Occupational therapy and team-led cognitive development interventions for preschool-aged children: Systematic review of related literature from 2010 to 2017* [Critically Appraised Topic]. https://www.aota.org/Practice/Children-Youth/Evidence-based/CAT-CY05-Cognition-Therapist-Led-Preschool.aspx

Frolek Clark, G., Fischbach, J., Crane, T., Corry, J., Nadolny, E. (2019d). *Parent-implemented cognitive development interventions for children and youth 0–5 years: Systematic review of related literature from 2010 to 2017* [Critically Appraised Topic]. https://www.aota.org/Practice/Children-Youth/Evidence-based/CAT-CY05-Cognition-Parent-Implemented.aspx

Frolek Clark, G. J., & Schlabach, T. L. (2013). Systematic review of occupational therapy interventions to improve cognitive development in children ages birth–5 years. *American Journal of Occupational Therapy, 67,* 425–430. https://doi.org/10.5014/ajot.2013.006163

Gioia, G. A., Isquith, P. K., Guy, S., & Kenworthy, L. (2000). *BRIEF: Behavior Rating Inventory of Executive Function professional manual.* Psychological Assessment Resources.

Golos, A., Sarid, M., Weill, M., & Weintraub, N. (2011). Efficacy of an early intervention program for at-risk preschool boys: A two-group control study. *American Journal of Occupational Therapy, 65,* 400–408. https://doi.org/10.5014/ajot.2011.000455

Griffith, R. (1996). *Griffiths Mental Development Scales from Birth to Two Years: Examiners manual.* Association for Research in Infant and Child Development, Test Agency.

Hardin, B. J., & Peisner-Feinberg, E. S. (2001). *The Early Learning Accomplishment Profile (Early Lap) examiner's manual and reliability and validity technical report.* Kaplan Early Learning Company

Hilbert, D. D., & Eis, S. D. (2013). Early intervention for emergent literacy development in a collaborative community pre-kindergarten. *Early Childhood Education Journal, 42,* 105–113. https://doi.org/10.1007/s10643-013-0588-3

Iacovou, M., & Sevilla, A. (2013). Infant feeding: The effects of the scheduled vs. on-demand feeding on mothers' wellbeing and children's cognitive development. *European Journal of Public Health, 23,* 13–19. https://doi.org/10.1093/eurpub/cks012

Jaswal, V. K., & Hansen, M. B. (2006). Learning words: Children disregard some pragmatic information that conflicts with mutual exclusivity. *Developmental Science, 9,* 158–165. https://doi.org/10.1111/j.1467-7687.2006.00475.x

Johnson-Martin, N. M., Attermeier, S. M., & Hacker, B. J. (2004a). *The Carolina Curriculum for Infants & Toddlers With Special Needs (CCITSN)* (3rd ed.). Brookes.

Johnson-Martin, N. M., Attermeier, S. M., & Hacker, B. J. (2004b). *The Carolina Curriculum for Preschoolers With Special Needs (CCPSN)* (2nd ed.). Brookes.

Justice, L. M., McGinty, A. S., Cabell, S. Q., Kilday, C. R., Knighton, K., & Huffman, G. (2010). Language and literacy curriculum supplement for preschoolers who are academically at risk: A feasibility study. *Language Speech & Hearing Services in Schools, 41,* 161–178. https://doi.org/10.1044/0161-1461(2009/08-0058)

Keen, R. (2011). The development of problem solving in young children: A critical cognitive skill. *Annual Review of Psychology, 62,* 1–21. https://doi.org/10.1146/annurev.psych.031809.130730

Kim, K., & Mundy, P. (2012). Joint attention, social-cognition, and recognition memory in adults. *Frontiers in Human Neuroscience, 6,* 172. https://doi.org/10.3389/fnhum.2012.00172

Kirk, H., Gray, K., Ellis, K., Taffe, J., & Cornish, K. (2016). Computerised attention training for children with intellectual and developmental disabilities: A randomised controlled trial. *Journal of Child Psychology and Psychiatry, 57,* 1380–1389. https://doi.org/10.1111/jcpp.12615

Kirk, H., Gray, K., Ellis, K., Taffe, J., & Cornish, K. (2017). Impact of attention training on academic achievement, executive functioning, and behavior: A randomized controlled trial. *American Journal on Intellectual & Developmental Disabilities 122,* 97–117. https://doi.org/10.1352/1944-7558-122.2.97

Kopp, F., & Lindenberger, U. (2011). Effects of joint attention on long-term memory in infants: An event-related potentials study. *Developmental Science, 14,* 660–672. https://doi.org/10.1111/j.1467-7687.2010.01010.x

Kramer, P., & Hinojosa, J. (2010). Developmental perspective: Fundamentals of developmental theory. In P. Kramer & J. Hinojosa (Eds.), *Frames of reference for pediatric occupational therapy* (3rd ed., pp. 23–30). Wolters Kluwer.

Law, M., Cooper, B., Strong, S., Stewart, D., Rigby, P., & Letts, L. (1996). The Person–Environment–Occupation Model: A transactive approach to occupational performance. *Canadian Journal of Occupational Therapy, 63,* 9–23. https://doi.org/10.1177/000841749606300103

Lonigan, C. J., & Phillips, B. M. (2015). Supplemental material for response to instruction in preschool: Results of two randomized studies with children at significant risk of reading difficulties. *Journal of Educational Psychology, 108,* 114–129. https://doi.org/10.1037/edu0000054.supp

March of Dimes; Partnership for Maternal, Newborn, & Child Health; Save the Children; & World Health Organization. (2012). *Born too soon: The global action report on preterm birth.* World Health Organization.

McManus, B. M., Carle, A. C., & Peohlmann, J. (2012). Effectiveness of Part C early intervention physical, occupational, and speech therapy services for preterm or low birth weight infants in Wisconsin, United States. *Academic Pediatrics, 12,* 96–103. https://doi.org/10.1016/j.acap.2011.11.004

Miller, L. J. (1982). *Miller Assessment for Preschoolers: Examiner's manual.* The Foundation for Knowledge in Development.

Morales, M., Mundy, P., Crowson, M., Neal, R., & Delgado, C. (2005). Individual differences in infant attention skills, joint attention, and emotion regulation behaviour. *International Journal of Behavioral Development, 29,* 259–263. https://doi.org/10.1080/01650250444000432

National Early Literacy Panel. (2008). *Developing early literacy: Report of the National Early Literacy Panel.* National Institute for Literacy.

Nielsen, M., & Tomaselli, K. (2010). Overimitation in Kalahari Bushman children and the origins of human cultural cognition. *Psychological Science, 21,* 729–736. https://doi.org/10.1177/0956797610368808

Nix, R. L., Bierman, K. L., Domitrovich, C. E., & Gill, S. (2013). Promoting children's social–emotional skills in preschool can enhance academic and behavioral functioning in kindergarten: Findings from Head Start REDI. *Early Education and Development, 24,* 1000–1019. https://doi.org/10.1080/10409289.2013.825565

O'Meagher, S., Kemp, N., Norris, K., Anderson, P., & Skilbeck, C. (2017). Risk factors for executive function difficulties in preschool and early school-age preterm children. *ACTA Paediatrica, 106,* 1468–1473. https://doi.org/10.1111/apa.13915

Palmer, K. K., Miller, M. W., & Robinson, L. E. (2013). Acute exercise enhances preschoolers' ability to sustain attention. *Journal of Sport and Exercise Psychology, 35,* 433–437. https://doi.org/10.1123/jsep.35.4.433

Pears, K. C., Kim, H. K., Fisher, P. A., & Yoerger, K. (2016). Increasing pre-kindergarten early literacy skills in children with developmental disabilities and delays. *Journal of School Psychology, 57,* 15–27. https://doi.org/10.1016/j.jsp.2016.05.004

Pillinger, C., & Wood, C. (2014). Pilot study evaluating the impact of dialogic reading and shared reading at transition to primary school: Early literacy skills and parental attitudes. *Literacy, 48,* 155–163. https://doi.org/10.1111/lit.12018

Pratt, A. S., Justice, L. M., Perez, A., & Duran, L. K. (2015). Impacts of parent-implemented early-literacy intervention for Spanish-speaking children with language impairment. *International Journal of Language & Communication Disorders, 50,* 569–579. https://doi.org/10.1111/1460-6984.12140

Rosenberg, L., Maeir, A., Tochman, A., Dahan, I., & Hirsch, I. (2015). Effectiveness of a cognitive–functional group intervention among preschoolers with attention deficit hyperactivity disorder: A pilot study. *American Journal of Occupational Therapy, 69,* 6903220040. https://doi.org/10.5014/ajot.2015.014795

Röthlisberger, M., Neuenschwander, R., Cimeli, P., Michel, E., & Roebers, C. M. (2011). Improving executive functions in 5- and 6-year-olds: Evaluation of a small group intervention in prekindergarten and kindergarten children. *Infant and Child Development, 21,* 411–429. https://doi.org/10.1002/icd.752

Rudasill, K. M., & Rimm-Kaufman, S. E. (2009). Teacher–child relationship quality: The roles of child temperament and teacher–child interactions. *Early Childhood Research Quarterly, 24,* 107–120. https://doi.org/10.1016/j.ecresq.2008.12.003

Schryer, E., Sloat, E., & Letourneau, N. (2015). Effects of an animated book reading intervention on emergent literacy skill development. *Journal of Early Intervention, 37,* 155–171. https://doi.org/10.1177/1053815115598842

Sheinkopf, S., Mundy, P., Claussen, A., & Willoughby, J. (2004). Infant joint attention skill and preschool behavioral outcomes in at-risk children. *Development and Psychopathology, 16,* 273–293. https://doi.org/10.1017/S0954579404044517

Sheridan, S. M., Knoche, L. L., Kupzyk, K. A., Edwards, C. P., & Marvin, C. A. (2011). A randomized trial examining the effects of parent engagement on early language and literacy: The Getting Ready intervention. *Journal of School Psychology, 49,* 361–383. https://doi.org/10.1016/j.jsp.2011.03.001

Smith, I. M., Flanagan, H. E., Garon, N., & Bryson, S. E. (2015). Effectiveness of community-based early intervention based on pivotal response treatment. *Journal of Autism & Developmental Disorders, 45,* 1858–1872. https://doi.org/10.1007/s10803-014-2345-x

Sorensen, K., Liverod, J. R., Lerdal, B., Vestrheim, I. E., & Skranes, J. (2016). Executive functions in preschool children with cerebral palsy–assessment and early intervention: A pilot study *Developmental Neurorehabilitation, 19*(2), 111–116. https://doi.org/10.3109/17518423.2014.916761

Tachibana, Y., Fukushima, A., Saito, H., Yoneyama, S., Ushida, K., & Kawashima, R. (2012). A new mother–child play activity program to decrease parenting stress and improve child cognitive abilities: A cluster randomized controlled trial. *PLoS ONE, 7*(7), e38238. https://doi.org/10.1371/journal.pone.0038238

Tamm, L., & Nakonezny, P. A. (2015). Metacognitive executive function training for young children with ADHD: A proof-of-concept study. *Attention Deficit and Hyperactivity Disorders, 7*(3), 183–190. https://doi.org/10.1177/1087054712445782

Tamm, L., Nakonezny, P. A., & Hughes, C. W. (2012). An open trial of a metacognitive executive function training for young children with ADHD. *Journal of Attention Disorders, 18,* 551–559. https://doi.org/10.1177/1087054712445782

Tang, M. H., Lin. C. K., Lin, W. H., Chen, C. H., Tsai, S. W., & Chang, Y. Y. (2011). The effect of adding a home program to weekly institutional-based therapy for children with undefined developmental delay: A pilot randomized clinical trial. *Journal of the Chinese Medical Association, 74,* 259–266. https://doi.org/10.1016/j.jcma.2011.04.005

Wallander, J. L., Bann, C. M., Biasini, F. J., Goudar, S. S., Pasha, O., Chomba, E., . . . Carlo, W. A. (2014). Development of children at risk for adverse outcomes participating in early intervention in developing countries: A randomized controlled trial. *Journal of Child Psychology & Psychiatry & Allied Disciplines, 55,* 1251–1259. https://doi.org/10.1111/jcpp.12247

Wallander, J. L., Biasini, F. J., Thorsten, V., Dhaded, S. M., Jong, D. M., Chomba, E., . . . Carlo, W. A. (2014). Dose of early intervention treatment during children's first 36 months of life is associated with developmental outcomes: An observational cohort study in three low/low-middle income countries. *BMC Pediatrics, 14,* 281–281. https://doi.org/10.1186/1471-2431-14-281

Warren, M. (1993). A hierarchical model for evaluation and treatment of visual perceptual dysfunction in adult acquired brain injury, Part 1. *American Journal of Occupational Therapy, 47,* 42–54. https://doi.org/10.5014/ajot.47.1.42

Williamson, R. A., Jaswal, V. K., & Meltzoff, A. N. (2010). Learning the rules: Observation and imitation of a sorting strategy by 36-month-old children. *Developmental Psychology, 46,* 57–65. https://doi.org/10.1037/a0017473

Willoughby, D., Evans, M. A., & Nowak, S. (2015). Do ABC eBooks boost engagement and learning in preschoolers? An experimental study comparing eBooks with paper ABC and storybook controls. *Computers and Education, 82,* 107–117. https://doi.org/10.1016/j.compedu.2014.11.008

Wolf, T., & Baum, C. (2011). Impact of mild cognitive impairments on participation: Importance of early identification of cognitive loss. In N. Katz (Ed.), *Cognition, occupation, and participation across the life span* (pp. 41–50). Bethesda, MD: AOTA Press.

World Health Organization. (2001). *International classification of functioning.* Geneva: Author.

Voress, J. K., Maddox, T., & Hammill, D. D. (2012). *Developmental Assessment of Young Children examiner manual* (2nd ed.). Pearson.

Best Practices in Supporting Development of Fine and Visual–Motor Coordination (Physical Skills)

30

Elizabeth Koss Schmidt, MOT, OTR/L; Kristen Martin, MOT, OTR/L; Margaret Bassi, OTD, OTR/L; and Kelly Tanner, PhD, OTR/L, BCP

KEY TERMS AND CONCEPTS

- Bimanual intensive therapy
- CareToy
- Constraint-induced movement therapy
- Fine motor
- Fine motor development

- Home-based parent coaching
- Mother–infant transaction program
- Supporting Play, Exploration, and Early Developmental Intervention
- Visual acuity

- Visual–motor activities
- Visual–motor integration
- Visual–motor skills
- Visual perception
- Visual processing

OVERVIEW

An important area of development for occupational therapy practitioners to focus on children from birth to age 5 years is their fine and visual–motor skills. (*Note. Occupational therapy practitioner* refers to both occupational therapists and occupational therapy assistants.) *Fine motor* refers to the small muscle movements, typically in the hands and fingers, that are used as children engage in their daily life skills (occupations), including play and learning (e.g., manipulating objects, cutting, coloring), ADLs such as dressing (e.g., fastening clothing), self-feeding (e.g., opening containers, finger feeding, using utensils), and hygiene (e.g., opening toothpaste tube, manipulating tools such as a toothbrush or hairbrush). *Visual–motor skills* refer to the ability to control the muscle movements of the eyes, *visual acuity* refers to clarity of vision, and *visual processing* refers to the ability to process the information one is seeing. *Visual–motor integration* includes the ability to integrate visual processing and visual–motor skills. Visual motor integration is necessary for children to incorporate what they are seeing with their fine and large motor movements to perform various occupations.

ESSENTIAL CONSIDERATIONS

Fine and visual–motor development occurs in phases and can be dependent on the child's unique experiences. When the acquisition of age-appropriate fine and visual–motor milestones is impeded, this may be referred to as a *fine and visual–motor delay*. Average timing of fine and visual–motor milestones varies, but occupational therapy practitioners need to be aware of these average ranges to identify delays that indicate treatment. A brief summary is provided in this section regarding the identification of fine and visual–motor delays, goal development, and treatment planning.

Fine motor development refers to the growth and refinement of small, intricate muscle movements (see Table 30.1). Fine motor skill development also occurs through children's interaction with their environment, through a process of trial and error. When children see one motor pattern is successful to achieve their goal, they practice that movement pattern again and again so that it can be further refined. Children begin to develop a hand preference between ages 2 and 4 years (Sheridan et al., 2008). Early handedness may be an indicator of neurological abnormality, including cerebral palsy (Sheridan et al., 2008). Children develop prewriting skills (e.g., imitating vertical and horizontal strokes; imitating circular strokes; copying a cross, triangle, and square) before they learn to copy uppercase and lowercase letters. Grasp also develops gradually and specifically develops from the ulnar to radial sides and proximally to distally (Case-Smith & O'Brien, 2010). See Table 30.2 for more information.

There are many components to visual and visual–motor skills. *Visual acuity* refers to the clarity of a child's vision and can be tested during an eye examination by an optometrist, ophthalmologist, or optician. Children who have poor visual acuity may squint, rub their eyes, or position their head closer to the task (e.g., closer to paper). Visual processing of visual skills includes visual tracking, convergence, saccades, visual fixation, and visual attention. *Visual perception* is the process of understanding visual input. Visual–motor integration includes visual movements to collect visual information, ability to process that information, and ability to coordinate motor movement to complete the task.

Visual–motor development occurs through children's experiences with vision and with other senses, including hearing, touch, taste, smell, proprioception, and vestibular input (Sheridan et al., 2008). As children explore their environment through sensory exploration and play, their

TABLE 30.1.   Phases of Fine and Visual–Motor Development

AGE	FINE AND VISUAL–MOTOR MILESTONES
2–4 months	▪ Begins reaching and swiping for items of interest ▪ Holds a toy (e.g., rattle) and shakes it ▪ Begins to recognize familiar people and objects from farther away ▪ Exhibits primitive reflex integration
6 months	▪ Tries to reach for things farther away ▪ Brings items to mouth ▪ Likes to look at self in mirror
9 months	▪ Isolates index finger to point or poke ▪ Passes items from one hand to another ▪ Watches an item as it falls
12 months	▪ Bangs items together ▪ Releases and removes item into open container
2 years	▪ Starts to develop hand preference (early stages) ▪ Builds towers of four or more blocks ▪ Copies horizontal and vertical lines
3 years	▪ Copies a circle ▪ Unscrews lids ▪ Completes a puzzle with three pieces ▪ Builds a tower of six or more blocks
4 years	▪ Copies simple shapes (e.g., square, triangle) ▪ Begins to use scissors (to snip or cut in a straight line) ▪ Draws a person with two to four body parts
5 years	▪ Draws a person with six body parts ▪ Starts to copy some capital letters ▪ Begins to cut more complex shapes with scissors

Sources. Information drawn from Bayley (2006), Case-Smith & O'Brien (2010), Centers for Disease Control and Prevention (2019), Folio & Fewell (2000), and Sheridan et al. (2008).

visual perception improves. They also begin integrating their visual and motor systems as their fine and large motor skills develop. Children use their experiences to help refine their visual–motor integration and develop motor planning skills, which are necessary for functional activities (Sheridan et al., 2008).

BEST PRACTICES

During an evaluation, occupational therapists should include the whole family and other caregivers, when possible and as appropriate, to identify what is meaningful to the child and their family and what should be addressed during treatment. Additionally, occupational therapists may collect information from a variety of sources involved in the child's life through interview, screening and assessment tools, and skilled observations to determine areas of needed intervention to promote independence in the identified meaningful occupations.

Conduct an Interview to Gather Occupational Profile Data

Occupational therapists typically begin the evaluation by gathering occupational profile data from the parents or caregivers, the child, and sometimes other individuals actively involved in the child's life such as the child's preschool teachers. The occupational profile informs the therapist about what the family and child want to do or need to do and assists in understanding current strengths and barriers to participation. The therapist should inquire about all occupations to identify those that support or limit participation.

Occupational therapists should assess and intervene in performance skills, including motor skills, that affect children's ability to independently participate in their meaningful occupations (American Occupational Therapy Association [AOTA], 2020b). These performance skills include motor skills (e.g., stabilizes, reaches, grips, manipulates, coordinates) and process skills (e.g., attends, notices, searches and locates, sequences, adjusts; AOTA, 2020b). Although this chapter specifically focuses on fine and visual–motor skills, occupational therapists should consider multiple factors during the evaluation process, including cognition (e.g., attention, problem solving), social factors (e.g., interactions, regulation), and sensory progressing (e.g., responses to environmental stimuli, self-regulation).

TABLE 30.2.   Grasp Pattern Development

AGE	GRASP PATTERN
2 months	Palmar grasps object that an adult places in hand (using whole hand to hold item)
5–6 months	Grasps smaller objects (e.g., small cube) with the whole hand or the ulnar side of the hand
7–8 months	Starts to grab items with the radial side of the hand
8–9 months	Grasps small items using a raking motion
11 months	Pincer grasp develops, using pad of index finger and thumb
1–1.5 years	Uses whole hand to pick up writing instrument
2–3 years	Uses extended fingertips hold writing instrument
4–5 years	Develops tripod grasp patterns

Sources. Information drawn from Centers for Disease Control and Prevention (2019) and Folio & Fewell (2000).

Skilled observations are often essential to understanding which components support and challenge a child's occupational performance. Occupational therapists can observe a child engaging in ADLs in their natural environments, or they can simulate an activity to analyze which fine and visual–motor skills may be affecting the child's independence. For example, a child may have difficulty self-feeding at mealtime because of difficulties with both fine motor skills (e.g., dexterity for opening a container, pincer grasp to pick up a piece of cereal) and visual–motor skills (e.g., coordinating bringing the spoon to the mouth).

Similarly, occupational therapists should consider fine and visual–motor skills associated with play and prewriting skills for young children. For example, a child may have difficulty stacking blocks when building a tower for play, attending to the task, identifying where a puzzle piece goes, or drawing or copying shapes. In addition to analyzing fine and visual–motor skills, occupational therapists assess the impact of other sensory processing skills (e.g., visual, auditory, vestibular, tactile, proprioceptive) on the child's success in these activities. All observations should include the collection of data so that the occupational therapy practitioner can monitor progress of these occupations after intervention.

Standardized assessments that focus on occupational performance can assist occupational therapists in analyzing an area of occupation, identifying goals, and measuring progress (Kreutzer et al., 2011). There are also specific assessments that measure performance skills (e.g., hand function, fine or visual–motor skills). See Table 30.3 for examples. A more in-depth listing of assessment tools can be found in Appendix F, "Examples of Assessments for Early Childhood (Birth–5 Years)."

Provide Evidence-Based Interventions

A recent systematic review (Tanner et al., 2020) reported on the strength of evidence for interventions to promote motor development among children from birth to age 5 years (Frolek Clark & Kingsley, 2020). Three themes were identified, including (1) early interventions for children from birth to age 3 years, (2) preschool interventions for children ages 3–5 years, and (3) interventions for children with or at high risk of cerebral palsy. Of these themes, few studies analyzed fine and visual–motor interventions specifically. There were no interventions for preschool-age children targeting fine and visual–motor skills that were rated as having strong evidence, as defined by support from at least two Level I studies with consistent results (AOTA, 2020a; U.S. Preventive Services Task Force, 2018). However, there were some interventions with moderate evidence that targeted fine and visual–motor interventions for children ages 3–5 years. There was also strong evidence identified within the theme for children with or at high risk for cerebral palsy.

Early intervention for children from birth to age 3 years

Many studies analyzed early intervention for children from birth to age 3 years, but few reported on fine or visual–motor skill development at this age. Among the few that reported on fine and visual–motor skill development were

---

TABLE 30.3. Examples of Assessment Tools Used for Occupational Performance and Fine and Visual–Motor Skills

CONSTRUCT	TEST (AUTHOR, YEAR PUBLISHED)	AGES	DESCRIPTION
Occupational performance	Canadian Occupational Performance Measure (Law et al., 2019)	Children or adults	Measure of client's self-perception of problems encountered in occupational performance
	Goal Attainment Scaling (McDougall & King, 2007)	Any	Individualized, criterion-referenced measure of change based on unique goals and outcomes for the client
	Pediatric Functional Independence Measure (Kreutzer et al., 2011)	6 months–8 years	Documents and tracks functional performance for individuals with acquired or congenital disabilities
Fine and visual–motor skills	Assisting Hand Assessment (Krumlinde-Sundholm & Eliasson, 2003)	18 months–12 years	Includes hand function for children with hemiparesis
	Bayley Scales of Infant and Toddler Motor Development (4th ed.; Bayley & Aylward, 2019).	1–42 months	Includes a fine motor subtest
	Beery–Buktenica Developmental Test of Visual Motor Integration (Beery et al., 2010)	2–99 years	Includes ability to integrate visual and motor skills
	Peabody Developmental Motor Scales (2nd ed.; Folio & Fewell, 2000)	Birth–5 years	Includes a fine motor section
	Quality of Upper Extremity Skills Test (DeMatteo et al., 1992)	18 months–8 years	Includes motor skills and hand function for children with cerebral palsy

interdisciplinary home-based, parent-implemented early intervention programs: Supporting Play, Exploration, and Early Developmental Intervention (SPEEDI); a mother–infant transaction program; and CareToy.

There is moderate evidence that **home-based parent coaching** can improve motor development for infants from birth to age 3 years, inclusive of both gross and fine motor outcomes. Home-based parent coaching is an inter-active, collaborative approach that includes five key characteristics: (1) joint planning, (2) observation, (3) action/practice, (4) reflection, and (5) feedback (Rush & Shelden, 2019). One study found home-based, parent-implemented early intervention demonstrated improvements for overall motor development but did not demonstrate differences between the intervention and control group on the Ages and Stages Questionnaire, which included parent report of fine motor skills (Carlo et al., 2013). Another study used home-based parent coaching and analyzed the effects on fine motor development. This intervention consisted of daily movement experiences in an enriched environment to provide increased opportunities for the infant to initiate movements (Dusing et al., 2015). This intervention also involved a collaborative effort among the therapist, parent, and infant. In fact, **Supporting Play, Exploration, and Early Developmental Intervention (SPEEDI)** was initially led by a health care professional in the neonatal intensive care unit (NICU) and then was implemented by the parent at home. This intervention is focused on coaching parents to identify ways to enrich their environments to enhance development by encouraging infants to initiate movements (Dusing et al., 2015). One study found SPEEDI demonstrated significant improvements in motor outcomes, including prereaching and reaching behaviors (Dusing et al., 2015).

Similarly, a modified **mother–infant transaction program** included daily 1-hour sessions for 7 days before discharge from the NICU and four home visits that focused on self-regulation and interactions, including signs of distress and signs of the infant's emotional states (Nordhov et al., 2010). Children in this modified mother–infant transaction program demonstrated improvements in fine and visual–motor skills, as seen on the grooved pegboard test, in particular in placing the right keys in a box with their nondominant hand at age 5 years (Nordhov et al., 2010).

There is moderate evidence supporting CareToy for improving motor skills among infants born prematurely. Infants exposed to **CareToy,** an intelligent baby gym used to provide intensive home-based early intervention through telerehabilitation sessions, showed improvements in visual acuity and overall motor skills (Sgandura et al., 2016, 2017).

Overall, occupational therapy practitioners can play a significant role for children from birth to age 3 years in promoting fine and visual–motor development. Practitioners may consider collaborative approaches to working with parents through parent coaching and home programs and should support parents in incorporating opportunities for fine and visual–motor development into their routines.

Preschool-age interventions for children ages 3–5 years

Preschool programs that address handwriting and visual–motor skills have moderate evidence to support their use in practice (Lust & Donica, 2011; Ohl et al., 2013). Fine and visual–motor programs may include both individual and group or consultative services and can incorporate the use of a manualized curriculum (Lust & Donica, 2011). Often, these programs can be delivered in a classroom setting by a trained interventionist.

In one study, a manualized handwriting intervention was provided to children in a Head Start program for 20 minutes, three times per week, from October to March, resulting in statistically significant increases in both fine motor precision and fine motor integration in comparison with the control group (Lust & Donica, 2011). Another study provided fine and visual–motor instruction to kindergarteners using a Tier 1 response-to-intervention model over a 10-week period. The intervention included both direct and consultative occupational therapy services in combination with general education classroom activities and resulted in statistically significant increases in visual–motor integration and fine motor scores in comparison with the control group (Ohl et al., 2013).

Interventions for children with or at risk for cerebral palsy

There is strong evidence supporting early intervention for improving motor outcomes for children at risk for cerebral palsy; however, most of these studies did not distinguish between fine and large motor skill development and looked instead at scores on standardized assessments that combine these domains (Morgan et al., 2015, 2016). More information regarding the results of these studies is available in Chapter 31, "Best Practices in Supporting Large Motor Coordination (Physical Skills)."

Similarly, there is strong evidence to support the use of child-focused and context-focused interventions to improve motor outcomes for children with cerebral palsy (Kruijsen-Terpstra et al., 2016; Law et al., 2011). Although these studies did not explicitly analyze fine motor outcomes independently of overall motor outcomes, occupational therapy practitioners can still use these components when addressing fine and visual–motor skill development, similar to the Person–Environment–Occupation model (Law et al., 1996). For example, a practitioner working in a preschool setting with a child with cerebral palsy may use adaptive scissors such as spring scissors (context or environment focused) while working to improve grip strength (child or person focused) to snip paper.

Finally, **constraint-induced movement therapy** (CIMT) and **bimanual intensive therapy** (BIT) also have strong evidence supporting their use in improving motor skills and function for children with unilateral cerebral palsy. Both CIMT and BIT focus on improving hemiparetic function using intensive therapy and motor learning principles; CIMT constrains the non-affected arm to encourage use of the affected arm while BIT utilizes a bimanual approach to encourage use of the affected arm. Studies on CIMT and BIT analyzed the impact specifically on hand function of the affected upper extremity, including fine motor skills, and found improvements after participants engaged with each intervention (Hoare et al., 2013). CIMT and BIT, as well as components of motor learning, are suggested for improving fine motor skills of the affected arm among children with unilateral cerebral palsy (Ramey et al., 2013).

Additional Interventions to Enhance Fine and Visual–Motor Development

Occupational therapy practitioners may engage in a variety of other interventions that have limited evidence to support them to address performance skill areas that may be affecting a child's participation in daily activities. Specific fine motor activities to address dexterity, rotation, distal finger use, bilateral coordination, and tool use can be found in Table 30.4.

Visual–motor activities can also address visual–motor control and integration. Activities may include dot-to-dot books and activities, tracing activities, maze activities, puzzles or pattern games, stringing beads or pieces of cereal, sewing or lacing boards, imitating and copying shapes and letters in a variety of media, and block designs. Occupational therapy practitioners may also include activities that will lead to independence in ADLs, such as practicing fasteners on the child's clothing, opening containers for their snack, and playing games that require attention and dexterity (see Table 30.4). When using interventions that have limited evidence available, practitioners should carefully collect quantifiable data to monitor progress and ensure the intervention is addressing the child's needs. In addition, practitioners can use principles of motor learning (see Chapter 31) to support the development of treatment activities.

To promote functional grasp and use of writing utensils and scissors, occupational therapy practitioners may consider the use of vertical surfaces, tweezer games, manipulation of nuts and bolts, lacing activities, or activities using an

TABLE 30.4.   Fine Motor and Visual–Motor Activities

SKILL	ACTIVITY
Dexterity	*Promoting dissociation of the radial and ulnar sides of the hand:* ▪ Picking up small objects between the tips of the thumb and index finger, one at a time, and placing into small containers ▪ Picking up small objects with tweezers, using the index finger and thumb ▪ Pulling small pieces of dough, clay, or putty with the thumb and index finger and rolling into little balls ▪ Holding a marker or pen with the last two fingers while removing or placing the cap ▪ Holding play dough or a cotton ball in the palm with the last two fingers while writing, coloring, or picking up small objects with the thumb side of the hand ▪ Picking up objects one at a time with the first three fingers and holding them in the palm with the last two fingers ▪ Holding multiple coins in one hand and then placing them one at a time into a "piggy" bank by moving them out to the fingertips *Promoting finger shift and rotation:* ▪ Spinning tops ▪ Opening screw-top containers for play items such as bubbles ▪ Picking up pegs, puzzle pieces, construction set pieces, or small objects and rotating to position them for use ▪ Turning knobs to operate a toy or musical device *Promoting distal finger use:* ▪ Tracing around and coloring in small areas in drawings or coloring books ▪ Drawing small circles ▪ Practicing buttoning and unbuttoning small buttons ▪ Using a small eyedropper to drip water into bottles or on paper
Bilateral coordination	▪ Practicing throwing and catching a ball with two hands ▪ Pushing and pulling large rolling toys with two hands ▪ Playing clapping games ▪ Playing with items that connect and pull apart ▪ Opening different types of containers; pulling caps off markers ▪ Playing with construction and building kits ▪ Stringing beads and using lacing cards ▪ Practicing using fasteners ▪ Engaging in cooking tasks (e.g., stirring while holding the mixing bowl, using a rolling pin with two hands) ▪ Participating in sports and playground activities, including climbing, monkey bars, jump rope, wheelbarrow walking, and ball games
Tool use	▪ Practicing tapping and banging with one item on another (e.g., drum toys, hammer sets) ▪ Practicing scooping with a large spoon or small shovel (e.g., using water, sand, rice, noodles) ▪ Playing with clothespins and other pinch clips that open and close ▪ Using tongs to transfer soft items from one container to another ▪ Using spray bottles ▪ Making designs in shaving cream with an isolated finger, stick, or dowel ▪ Scribbling, coloring within boundaries, and imitating prewriting strokes and shapes with crayons ▪ Practicing scissors skills (e.g., snipping, cutting across a sheet of paper, cutting along a line, cutting out shapes)

eye dropper or clothespin. Furthermore, practitioners may consider compensatory strategies, such as pencil grips, having a child hold something small on the ulnar side of their palm (e.g., penny, paper clip), or adaptive scissors to help promote independence.

SUMMARY

Fine and visual–motor development are foundational components of voluntary motor movements that support participation in a variety of meaningful occupations. Occupational therapists should assess performance skills associated with fine and visual–motor skills, analyze how they affect children's performance of meaningful occupations, and use evidence-based interventions to address these deficits. A recent systematic review identified research with strong or moderate evidence for interventions that address fine or visual–motor skills for children in early intervention (children from birth to age 3 years), children in the preschool setting (children ages 3–5 years), and children with or at risk of cerebral palsy. These interventions include home-based parent coaching during early intervention, CareToy, fine and visual–motor interventions in a preschool setting, CIMT, BIT, and context- or child-focused therapies using principles of motor learning.

Other interventions may be used to target fine and visual–motor development that have limited evidence available at this time, but when interventions with low strength of evidence are used, occupational therapy practitioners should carefully document the child's progress to confirm effects of the intervention. All assessment, goal setting, and intervention planning should be conducted with the input of the child, parent or caregiver, and other key stakeholders identified as important to the child and family, such as other family members or teachers.

REFERENCES

American Occupational Therapy Association. (2020a). *Guidelines for systematic reviews.* https://ajot.submit2aota.org/journals/ajot/forms/systematic_reviews.pdf

American Occupational Therapy Association. (2020b). Occupational therapy practice framework: Domain and process (4th ed.). *American Journal of Occupational Therapy, 74*(Suppl. 2), 7412410010. https://doi.org/10.5014/ajot.2020.74S2001

Bayley, N., & Aylward, G. (2019). *Bayley Scales of Infant and Toddler Motor Development* (4th ed.). Pearson.

Beery, K. E., Buktenica, N., & Beery, N. A. (2010). *Beery–Buktenica Developmental Test of Visual–Motor Integration* (6th ed.). Pearson.

Carlo, W. A., Goudar, S. S., Pasha, O., Chomba, E., Wallander, J. L., Biasini, F. J., . . . National Institute of Child Health and Human Development Global Network for Women's and Children's Health Research Investigators. (2013). Randomized trial of early developmental intervention on outcomes in children after birth asphyxia in developing countries. *Journal of Pediatrics, 162,* 705–712.e3. https://doi.org/10.1016/j.jpeds.2012.09.052

Case-Smith, J., & O'Brien, J. C. (2010). *Occupational therapy for children.* Mosby.

Centers for Disease Control and Prevention. (2019). *Important milestones: Your child by 5 years.* https://www.cdc.gov/ncbddd/actearly/milestones/milestones-5yr.html

DeMatteo, C., Law, M., Russell, D., Pollock, N., Rosenbaum, P., & Walter, S. (1992). *QUEST: Quality of Upper Extermity Skills Test.* McMaster University, CanChild Centre for Childhood Disability Research.

Dusing, S. C., Brown, S. E., Van Drew, C. M., Thacker, L. R. & Hendricks-Munoz, K. D. (2015). Supporting play exploration and early development intervention from NICU to home: A feasibility study. *Pediatric Physical Therapy, 27,* 267–274. https://doi.org/10.1097/PEP.0000000000000161

Folio, M. R., & Fewell, R. R. (2000). *Peabody Developmental Motor Scales (2nd ed.) examiner's manual.* PRO-ED.

Frolek Clark, G., & Kingsley, K. (2020). Occupational therapy practice guidelines for early childhood: Birth–5 years. *American Journal of Occupational Therapy, 74,* 7403397010. https://doi.org/10.5014/ajot.2020.743001

Hoare, B., Imms, C., Villanueva, E., Rawicki, H. B., Matyas, T., & Carey, L. (2013). Intensive therapy following upper limb botulinum toxin A injection in young children with unilateral cerebral palsy: A randomized trial. *Developmental Medicine & Child Neurology, 55,* 238–247. https://doi.org/10.1111/dmcn.12054

Kreutzer, J. S., DeLuca, J., & Caplan, B. (Eds.). (2011). WeeFIM II®. In *Encyclopedia of clinical neuropsychology.* Springer. https://doi.org/10.1007/978-0-387-79948-3_4889

Kruijsen-Terpstra, A. J. A., Ketelaar, M., Verschuren, O., Gorter, J. W., Vos, R. C., Verheijden, J., . . . Visser-Meily, A. (2016). Efficacy of three therapy approaches in preschool children with cerebral palsy: A randomized controlled trial. *Developmental Medicine & Child Neurology, 58,* 758–766. https://doi.org/10.1111/dmcn.12966

Krumlinde-Sundholm, L., & Eliasson, A. (2003). Development of the Assisting Hand Assessment: A Rasch-built measure intended for children with unilateral upper limb impairments. *Scandinavian Journal of Occupational Therapy, 10,* 16–26. https://doi.org/10.1080/11038120310004529

Law, M., Baptiste, S., Carswell, A., McColl, M. A., Polatajko, H., & Pollock, N. (2019). *Canadian Occupational Performance Measure* (5th ed., rev.). COPM, Inc.

Law, M., Cooper, B. A., Strong, S., Stewart, D., Rigby, P., & Letts, L. (1996). The Person–Environment–Occupation model: A transactive approach to occupational performance. *Canadian Journal of Occupational Therapy, 63,* 9–23. https://doi.org/10.1177/000841749606300103

Law, M. C., Darrah, J., Pollock, N., Wilson, B., Russell, D. J., Walter, S. D., . . . Galuppi, B. (2011). Focus on function: A cluster, randomized controlled trial comparing child- versus context-focused intervention for young children with cerebral palsy. *Developmental Medicine & Child Neurology, 53,* 621–629. https://doi.org/10.1111/j.1469-8749.2011.03962.x

Lust, C. A., & Donica, D. K. (2011). Effectiveness of a handwriting readiness program in Head Start: A two-group controlled trial. *American Journal of Occupational Therapy, 65,* 560–568. https://doi.org/10.5014/ajot.2011.000612

McDougall, J., & King, G. (2007). *Goal attainment scaling: Description, utility, and applications in pediatric therapy services* (2nd ed.). https://mississaugahalton.rehabcareontario.ca/Uploads/ContentDocuments/gasmanual_.pdf

Morgan, C., Darrah, J., Gordon, A. M., Harbourne, R., Spittle, A., Johnson, R., & Fetters, L. (2016). Effectiveness of motor interventions in infants with cerebral palsy: A systematic review. *Developmental Medicine & Child Neurology, 58,* 900–909. https://doi.org/10.1111/dmcn.13105

Morgan, C., Novak, I., Dale, R. C., & Badawi, N. (2015). Optimising motor learning in infants at high risk of cerebral palsy: A pilot study. *BMC Pediatrics, 15,* 30. https://doi.org/10.1186/s12887-015-0347-2

Nordhov, S. M., Ronning, J. A., Dahl, L. B., Ulvund, S. E., Tunby, J., & Kaaresen, P. I. (2010). Early intervention improves cognitive outcomes for preterm infants: Randomized controlled trial. *Pediatrics, 126,* e1088–e1094. https://doi.org/10.1542/peds.2010-0778

Ohl, A. M., Graze, H., Weber, K., Kenny, S., Salvatore, C., & Wagreich, S. (2013). Effectiveness of a 10-week Tier-1 response to intervention program in improving fine motor and visual–motor skills in general education kindergarten students. *American Journal of Occupational Therapy, 67,* 507–514. https://doi.org/10.5014/ajot.2013.008110

Ramey, S. L., Coker-Bolt., P., & DeLuca, S. C. (Eds.). (2013). *Handbook of pediatric constraint-induced movement therapy (CIMT): A guide for occupational therapy and health care clinicians, researchers, and educators.* AOTA Press.

Rush, D., & Shelden, M. (2020). *The early childhood coaching handbook* (2nd ed.). Brookes.

Sgandura, G., Bartalena, L., Cecchi, F., Cioni, G., Giampietri, M., Greisen, G., . . . CareToy Consortium. (2016). A pilot study on early home-based intervention through an intelligent baby gym (CareToy) in preterm infants. *Research in Developmental Disabilities, 53–54,* 32–42. https://doi.org/10.1016/j.ridd.2016.01.013

Sgandura, G., Lorentzen, J., Inguaggiato, E., Bartalena, L., Beani, E., Cecchi, F., . . . CareToy Consortium. (2017). A randomized clinical trial in preterm infants on the effects of a home-based early intervention with the "CareToy System." *PLoS One, 12,* e0173521. https://doi.org/10.1371/journal.pone.0173521

Sheridan, M., Sharma, A., & Cockerill, H. (2008). *From birth to five years: Children's developmental progress* (4th ed.). Routledge.

Tanner, K., Schmidt, E. K., Martin, K., & Bassi, M. (2020). Systematic review of interventions within the scope of occupational therapy practice to improve motor performance for children ages 0–5 years. *American Journal of Occupational Therapy, 74,* 7402180060. https://doi.org/10.5014/ajot.2020.039644

U.S. Preventive Services Task Force. (2018). *Grade definitions.* https://www.uspreventiveservicestaskforce.org/Page/Name/grade-definitions

Best Practices in Supporting Large Motor Coordination (Physical Skills)

31

Elizabeth Koss Schmidt, MOT, OTR/L; Kristen Martin, MOT, OTR/L; Margaret Bassi, OTD, OTR/L; and Kelly Tanner, PhD, OTR/L, BCP

KEY TERMS AND CONCEPTS

- Balance
- Coordination
- Feedback
- Implicit learning
- Large motor delay
- Large motor skills
- Manual guidance
- Meaningful activities
- Motor development
- Person–Environment–Occupation model
- Praxis and motor planning
- Primitive reflexive movements
- Repetition
- Strength
- Transfer of learning

OVERVIEW

One of the primary areas that pediatric occupational therapy practitioners focus on is motor skill development. (*Note. Occupational therapy practitioner* refers to both occupational therapists and occupational therapy assistants.) *Large motor skills* allow a child to move from simple engagement with their environment to imitation of others' movement patterns and actions and then independent practice and mastery of these skills. Examples of large motor skills include crawling, walking, and running. When the acquisition of age-appropriate large motor milestones is impeded, this is referred to as *large motor delay.* Slowed development of motor functions may inhibit exploration of one's environment, creating additional delays in other areas of development, such as cognition and social–emotional skills (Case-Smith et al., 2013). In the United States, the incidence of developmental delay or disability is one in six children (Centers for Disease Control and Prevention [CDC], 2019).

This chapter describes overall motor development from birth to age 5 years and best practices for motor evaluations and intervention for occupational therapy practitioners.

ESSENTIAL CONSIDERATIONS

Motor development occurs in phases and can largely depend on the child's experiences. The average time frame for children to develop specific motor milestones is fairly wide, so it is important for occupational therapy practitioners to understand the general progression of motor development for screening and assessment, goal writing, and intervention planning. Fine motor and large motor are very closely related for infants and young children. As children start to reach, they roll, and upper-extremity strength is required for other large motor skills, such as sitting and crawling. A brief summary is provided in this section.

Infants first demonstrate *primitive reflexive movements,* which are involuntary reactions that occur in response to an external stimulus (Gallahue, 1989). These primitive reflexive movements are typically integrated, or are no longer present, by ages 4–12 months, depending on the specific reflex and the child (Sheridan et al., 2008).

Newborns require support of their head at an early age. They also primarily maintain midline positioning in supine and their head face down or down and to the side in prone. In prone, newborn infants may lift their face off the surface for 1–2 seconds at a time during the first month of life. As infants begin developing their cervical muscles, their head control also improves. Infants gradually begin exploring their hands with their mouth (birth–3 months) and may begin reaching up toward toys or people around age 3 months. In supine, infants may demonstrate individual finger and ankle movements, and they may engage in reciprocal kicking as well (Campbell et al., 2002). As they get older and grow, they bring their hands to their knees or feet and begin bringing their feet toward their mouth (Campbell et al., 2002). In prone, infants gradually develop the strength to lift their head to 45 degrees and then to 90 degrees (Campbell et al., 2002). Additionally, they should begin visually tracking objects and people in prone, supine, and supported sitting.

Children's control, balance, coordination, and strength improve as they further refine each motor skill through experiences and repetition (see Table 31.1; Sheridan et al., 2008). For example, infants typically roll from prone to supine first, and as they become stronger and their motor skills more refined, they may begin rolling from supine to prone. Similarly, children may start moving by pivoting while in prone, then crawling on their stomach, and then creeping in a quadruped position.

A child's large motor skills also become more refined with more experience and specific practice of each skill. For example, toddlers begin to walk with a large gait and seem

TABLE 31.1.   Movement and Large Motor Development Milestones

AGE	MOVEMENT AND LARGE MOTOR DEVELOPMENT MILESTONES
2 months	▪ Can hold head up and begins to push up when lying on stomach ▪ Makes smoother movements with arms and legs ▪ Exhibits primitive reflex integration
4 months	▪ Holds head steady, unsupported ▪ Pushes down on legs when feet are on a hard surface ▪ May be able to roll over from stomach to back ▪ Brings hands to mouth ▪ When lying on stomach, pushes up to elbows
6 months	▪ Rolls over in both directions (front to back, back to front) ▪ Begins to sit without support ▪ When standing, supports weight on legs and might bounce ▪ Rocks back and forth, sometimes crawling backward before moving forward
9 months	▪ Stands, holding on ▪ Can get into sitting position ▪ Sits without support ▪ Pulls to stand ▪ Crawls
1 year	▪ Gets to a sitting position without help ▪ Pulls up to stand, walks holding on to furniture ("cruising") ▪ May take a few steps without holding on ▪ May stand alone
18 months	▪ Walks alone ▪ May walk up steps and run ▪ Pulls toys while walking ▪ Can participate in undressing as balance improves
2 years	▪ Stands on tiptoe ▪ Kicks a ball ▪ Begins to run ▪ Climbs onto and down from furniture without help ▪ Walks up and down stairs holding on ▪ Throws ball overhand
3 years	▪ Climbs well ▪ Runs easily ▪ Pedals a tricycle (three-wheel bike) ▪ Walks up and down stairs, one foot on each step
4 years	▪ Hops stands on one foot up to 2 seconds ▪ Catches a bounced ball most of the time
5 years	▪ Stands on one foot for 10 seconds or longer ▪ Hops; may be able to skip ▪ Swings and climbs

Source. Adapted from CDC (n.d.).

more clumsy initially. As they refine this skill, they begin walking with more coordination, and running, skipping, and galloping. Additionally, they require less and less support as these skills become more coordinated. For example, children may begin by creeping up and down the stairs, progress to walking with support and placing both feet on each step, then move on to walking with support but alternating their feet on each step, and finally achieve a mature pattern of walking up and down the stairs without support and alternating their feet on each step.

Children with certain conditions, such as Down syndrome, may have slightly different norms for their developmental milestones. Children with abnormal development or delays in reaching these milestones may have developmental delay or other specific conditions.

BEST PRACTICES

Occupational therapists should include the child's family and any other caregivers during the evaluation process when identifying meaningful occupational goals and when intervention planning. This ensures that the family and caregivers are able to successfully implement intervention strategies across settings, which is central to achieving desired outcomes.

Conduct an Evaluation

The *Occupational Therapy Practice Framework: Domain and process* (4th ed.; American Occupational Therapy Association [AOTA], 2020b) includes motor as a performance skill, which represents "small, observable actions related to moving oneself or moving and interacting with tangible task objects . . . in the context of performing . . . a relevant daily life task" (p. 87). Fine and large motor skills are involved in daily activities (occupations; e.g., play, toileting, education). All occupational therapy evaluations should include aspects related to the child's daily life activities (occupations). Evaluations often include an interview, record review, skilled professional observations, and assessment tools, as needed.

Occupational therapists typically begin the evaluation with an occupational profile to collect data from the child, their parents or caregivers, and sometimes other key informants identified by the parent or caregiver. The data from this interview inform the occupational therapist of specific occupations that may need further assessment through skilled observation.

After the interview, the occupational therapist then observes the child participating in self-care activities or occupations that are reported as challenging. In natural settings (e.g., home, preschool, community), the occupational therapist observes the child in their daily routines to observe what aspects of occupations are strengths or challenges and how motor skills may affect the child's independence in these occupations. In a health care setting, these occupations may need to be simulated for the therapist to observe them. Parents may also share videos or describe their child performing the task at home or in the community.

The occupational therapist analyzes the motor skills the child uses to participate in age-appropriate occupations, including play, school, and ADLs such as feeding, dressing, and toileting. The child's independence in these occupations may be affected by a combination of movement skills, including large motor skills (e.g., getting into and out of a chair, walking around the room). These skilled observations should include the collection and reporting of quantitative data (e.g., "Requires more than 3 minutes and four verbal prompts to put on one shoe due to balance issues during sitting").

Standardized assessments can identify area of occupations, help determine goals, and measure progress. Examples include the Pediatric Functional Independence Measure (Kreutzer et al., 2011), Goal Attainment Scaling (McDougall & King, 2007), and the Canadian Occupational Performance Measure (Law et al., 2019). Additionally, the Gross Motor Function Measure (Russell et al., 2013) can be used to identify how children with cerebral palsy (CP) or Down syndrome are performing compared with other children. The Gross Motor Function Classification System levels can be used to monitor progress (Palisano et al., 1997, 2008). There are also specific assessments that can analyze gross motor skills and offer a way to monitor changes in this area

after intervention (see Table 31.2). A more in-depth listing of assessment tools can be found in Appendix F, "Examples of Assessments for Early Childhood (Birth–5 Years)."

In addition, the occupational therapist may assess the child's neuromusculoskeletal and movement-related functions (joint mobility, joint stability), muscle functions (strength, postural tone), and movement functions (motor reflexes, involuntary movement reactions, voluntary movements, gait and mobility during daily living activities). Pain should also be screened to determine whether this is interfering with sleep or other occupations. Depending on the results of the evaluation and the context, the occupational therapist may also refer the child to another professional, such as a physical therapist.

Provide Evidence-Based Interventions

A recent systematic review (Tanner et al., 2020) investigated the current evidence for interventions to promote motor development and prevent further delay among children from birth to age 5 years (Frolek Clark & Kingsley, 2020). Three themes were identified: (1) early interventions for children from birth to age 3 years, (2) preschool interventions for children age 3–5 years, and (3) interventions for children with or at high risk of CP. The strength of evidence for each intervention was rated according to guidelines from AOTA (2020a), modified from the U.S. Preventive Services Task Force (2018). According to these guidelines, interventions are given a rating of *strong* if they are supported by at least two Level I studies (i.e., systematic reviews, meta-analyses, randomized controlled trials) with consistent results between studies. The best practices identified through this review are described further for each theme.

Theme 1: Early intervention

For children from birth through age 3 years, there is strong evidence that early intervention programs can improve motor performance and perhaps prevent further delay (Spittle et al., 2012), including for premature children and those with low birthweight (Park et al., 2014). However, it is worth noting that these improvements are only seen in the short term (i.e., postintervention) and not necessarily maintained at follow-up.

Some early interventions are hospital based and begin as early as during a newborn's stay in the neonatal intensive care unit (NICU). Moderate evidence exists that the Newborn Individualized Developmental Care and Assessment Program improved short-term motor function for premature infants and significantly enhanced motor functioning for preterm infants with severe intrauterine growth restrictions (Als et al., 2011).

Home-based and parent-implemented early intervention programs have moderate evidence for improving motor development (Dusing et al., 2015; Nordhov et al., 2010; Van Hus et al., 2016; Wallander et al., 2014). These programs use a coaching model to teach parents how to support their child's development. Programming can begin while infants are still in the NICU and continues at regular intervals, such as weekly (Dusing et al., 2015; Nordhov et al., 2010). Although a variety of professionals have implemented these types of programs, occupational therapy

TABLE 31.2.   Examples of Assessment Tools Used for Large Motor Skills

TEST	AGES	DESCRIPTION
Alberta Infant Motor Scale (Piper et al., 1992)	Birth–18 months	Assesses motor skills for infants
Bayley Scales of Infant and Toddler Motor Development (4th ed.; Bayley & Aylward, 2019)	1–42 months	Includes large motor section
Bruininks–Oseretsky Test of Motor Proficiency (2nd ed.; Bruininks & Bruininks, 2005)	4–21 years, 11 months	Includes bilateral coordination, balance, running speed, and agility
Goal Attainment Scaling (McDougall & King, 2007)	Any	Individualized, criterion-referenced measure of change based on unique goals and outcomes for child
Gross Motor Function Classification System (Palisano et al., 1997, 2008)	2–18 years	For children with cerebral palsy, measure is based on self-initiated movement, with emphasis on sitting, transfers, and mobility
Gross Motor Function Measure (Russell et al., 2013)	5 months–16 years; items are appropriate for motor skills at or below the developmental milestones for a 5-year-old	Large motor skills: lying and rolling, sitting, crawling and kneeling, standing, walking, running, and jumping
Peabody Developmental Motor Scales (2nd ed.; Folio & Fewell, 2000)	Birth–5 years	Includes large motor function
Pediatric Evaluation of Disability Inventory: Computerized Adaptive Test (Haley et al., 2012)	Birth–21 years	Electronic interview; includes self-care, mobility, and social skills
Test of Infant Motor Performance (Campbell et al., 2002)	34 weeks–4 months postterm	Includes motor function and reflexes for premature infants
Pediatric Functional Independence Measure II (WeeFIM II® System; Kreutzer et al., 2011)	6 months–7 years	Includes functional mobility

practitioners are well positioned to use this model of care to address meaningful daily activities in natural settings. It is important to note that although there are other benefits to home-based and parent-implemented early intervention models, studies have found that the impact on motor skills seems to be small and only lasts for a short period of time (i.e., months rather than years).

Moderate strength of evidence exists that Qigong massage improved large motor skills among children with Down syndrome or CP (Silva et al., 2012). Research did not indicate statistically significant differences for children with prematurity (Abdallah et al., 2013). Moderate strength of evidence exists that CareToy, a "smart" infant gym, improved motor skills among children with prematurity (Sgandurra et al., 2013, 2016).

Interventions such as powered mobility, tummy time, swimming programs, and sensory-enhanced center-based early intervention have been researched; however, the results of the review indicated that each of these was supported by only one article, and therefore the current evidence is low that any of these interventions can improve motor skills (Blanche et al., 2016; Dias et al., 2013; Jones et al., 2012; Wentz, 2017). Occupational therapy practitioners who use these interventions should collect their own data on outcomes to determine whether the child is making progress. Also of note, safe sleep practices (i.e., babies younger than age 1 year should sleep alone, on their back, in a crib without blankets) lead to infants spending much

of their time in supine. It is important for practitioners to work with families and other stakeholders to implement safe prone time throughout the day while continuing to reinforce principles of safe sleep (i.e., "Back to sleep, tummy to play").

Theme 2: Interventions for preschool-aged children

Occupational therapy practitioners may work with children at home, at a child care center, or even in a center-based program and may address participation in many different occupations, including participation in play and self-care skills. For children ages 3–5 years, there is strong evidence that video game interventions are effective for improving large motor skills (Hsieh et al., 2015, 2016; Salem et al., 2012). Research has examined pairing traditional rehabilitation with 30 minutes of video game playing, with positive results (Hsieh et al., 2016). Therefore, practitioners may try using a commercial gaming system that incorporates balance and coordination skills for half of children's weekly 60-minute session for 4 weeks. A practitioner may collaborate with a teacher to use a low-cost virtual reality gaming system in a classroom of children with developmental disabilities who experience difficulty with balance (Salem et al., 2012).

There is moderate evidence to support the use of physical movement breaks for preschool-age children (Bellows et al., 2013; Monsalves-Alvarez et al., 2015). The strength of evidence is low that sensory-based therapy can improve large motor skills for children ages 3–5 years (Iwanaga et al., 2014).

Theme 3: Interventions for children with or at risk for cerebral palsy

There is strong evidence that early intervention improves motor outcomes for children at risk for CP. Children who participated in the Goals–Activity–Motor Enrichment program (using principles of goal-directed therapy, motor learning principles, and environmental modification) demonstrated improved motor outcomes compared with children who received standard care (Morgan et al., 2015, 2016). Occupational therapy practitioners may use motor learning principles as well as positioning when working with a child in their natural environment (see Table 31.3). The Coping With and Caring for Infants With Special Needs Program is an intervention approach focusing on infant positioning (Dirks et al., 2016) that can improve the amount of time a child spends in positions challenging core strength, leading to improved functional mobility.

Occupational therapy practitioners can address both the specific body structures and the functions of the child (e.g., targeting strength, range of motion, and specific movement patterns) and modify the environment they are in to improve accessibility and motor outcomes for children with CP. There is strong evidence for both child-focused and context-focused interventions to improve motor outcomes for children with CP, and this closely aligns with the *Person–Environment–Occupation (PEO) model* (Kruijsen-Terpstra et al., 2016; Law et al., 2011). The PEO model outlines the importance of examining the person, their environment, and the occupations they are performing to maximize outcomes. For example, a practitioner working in a preschool setting with a child with CP may provide adaptive seating (context or environment focused) as well as work to improve core strength (child or person focused) to improve participation in seated, tabletop activities for the student.

Constraint-induced movement therapy (CIMT) and bilateral intensive therapy (BIT) seek to improve movement and function for children with unilateral CP through intensive therapy (3–6 hours per day up to 5 days per week) using principles of motor learning and encouraging bilateral use or forced use of the more affected side (Hoare et al., 2013). There is strong evidence that both BIT and CIMT improve motor outcomes for children with unilateral CP with little difference between the interventions (Hoare et al., 2013).

Hippotherapy is a therapeutic intervention in which the child engages in horseback riding specifically to address trunk strength, control, and balance (Kwon et al., 2015). Hippotherapy has moderate evidence in improving motor outcomes for children with CP (Tanner et al., 2020).

Additional Large Motor Interventions

Additional factors that underlie motor skill development and use include coordination, strength, praxis and motor planning, and balance (see Table 31.4). These play an important role from the most basic step of environmental exploration all the way to independent occupational performance (see Exhibit 31.1).

SUMMARY

Large motor development is foundational for participation in meaningful occupations; therefore, occupational therapy practitioners must address children's motor skills when they are delayed. Typical large motor development varies across individuals, yet practitioners should be cognizant of typical motor trajectories and age ranges for the development of foundational large motor skills. Occupational therapists should evaluate large motor skills to determine appropriate goals and interventions to improve independence in ADLs and increase participation across environments. Therapists may gather data about large motor skills through interviews, skilled observations, and record review, and they may use standardized assessments to identify the child's

TABLE 31.3. Motor Learning Principles

PRINCIPLE	DESCRIPTION
Meaningful activities	Activities that are important to and preferred by the child should be presented. The activity must be sufficiently salient for the child to want to perform the action and to direct their attention to the task.
Feedback	Careful provision of feedback is important to encourage motor development. Children with more receptive language and cognitive skills can be provided with more feedback and with more specific feedback on performance. More feedback should be provided earlier when the child is learning a new skill, with feedback reduced as the child becomes more proficient. Timing of feedback should be such that the child is able to easily determine what they are receiving feedback for.
Implicit learning	The child plays a role in learning a new skill, including monitoring their own movement patterns to determine whether they are effective in achieving a specific movement pattern to accomplish a goal.
Repetition	The child requires a high level of repetition to gain a new skill. The caregivers and occupational therapy practitioners should provide enough opportunities for practice for the child to develop a new skill.
Manual guidance	The child must be able to know whether their attempt to perform a motor skill is successful, so minimal manual support should be provided, and support should be removed as soon as the child begins to initiate action on their own.
Transfer of learning	The child must have an opportunity to practice a new motor skill in a variety of environments and situations.

Sources. Case-Smith & O'Brien (2013); Case-Smith et al. (2013); Kleim & Jones (2008); Morgan et al. (2014).

TABLE 31.4. Motor Components

COMPONENTS	EXAMPLES
Coordination	• Coordination of the two sides of the body • Coordination of the upper and lower body • Smooth, fluid coordination while moving through space
Strength	• Maintaining body position against gravity • Adapting movement against resistance or weight • Postural control • Shoulder stability • Grip and pinch strength, sustained grasp
Praxis and motor planning	• Correctly sequencing steps for a task • Completing a familiar task in a novel environment • Completing a familiar task with additional steps • Completing a familiar task using novel materials
Balance	• Completing a task on a dynamic surface • Completing a task requiring reaching away from body or base of support • Completing a task requiring functional mobility around or over obstacles

EXHIBIT 31.1.   Influence of Underlying Factors on Children's Occupations

Occupational performance is influenced by the context and environment, performance skills, performance patterns, and client factors (AOTA, 2020b). The child's interactions must be carefully analyzed for effective intervention. For example, a young child who is attempting to complete lower body dressing must have the strength, coordination, and balance as well as focus, problem-solving skills, and upper-body coordination to hold the pants. The child may need to balance on one foot momentarily and coordinate where their leg is compared with the hole of their pants to thread their legs into the pants. The child then needs to be able to pull their pants up over their hips and fasten the button and zipper with sufficient force, using fine motor skills such as dexterity, grasp, and release. As the child ages, they will need to be able to generalize this process to novel clothing items in new environments or among other occupations (e.g., clothing management for toileting).

For this one ADL, a child must use all of these factors in combination to be successful. Regardless of the intervention used, using motor learning principles is important. The activity should be meaningful, and initial practice should incorporate a variety of feedback. Repetitive practice, fading cues and guidance, and the opportunity to practice in novel environments will support the child's successful acquisition of the targeted skill.

Note. ADL = activity of daily living.

strengths and needs. Occupational therapy practitioners should address large motor development in the context of natural routines to improve the child's participation in their school, home, or community.

A recent systematic review identified interventions with strong evidence to support their use in early intervention, in preschool settings, and for children with or at risk of CP. These included early intervention for children from birth to age 3 years; physical movement breaks during preschool for children ages 3–5 years; and CIMT, BIT, and context- or child-focused therapies using principles of motor learning for children with or at risk of CP. When using interventions with low strength of evidence, practitioners should carefully document the child's progress.

Occupational therapy practitioners in health care should collaborate with the family when identifying and prioritizing goals, planning treatment, selecting interventions, and developing a home program. Practitioners working in early intervention (home) and preschool settings must work with their team, which includes the family, to set child goals or child and family outcomes. It is vital to the child's success that the practitioners understand the family's priorities and concerns, their schedule, and what may or may not work for their family unit.

REFERENCES

Abdallah, B., Badr, L. K., & Hawwari, M. (2013). The efficacy of massage on short and long term outcomes in preterm infants. *Infant Behavior and Development, 36,* 662–669. https://doi.org/10.1016/j.infbeh.2013.06.009

Als, H., Duffy, F. H., McAnulty, G. B., Fischer, C. B., Kosta, S., Butler, S. C., . . . Ringer, S. A. (2011). Is the Newborn Individualized Developmental Care and Assessment Program (NIDCAP) effective for preterm infants with intrauterine growth restriction? *Journal of Perinatology, 31,* 130–136. https://doi.org/10.1038/jp.2010.81

American Occupational Therapy Association. (2020a). *Guidelines for systematic reviews.* https://ajot.submit2aota.org/journals/ajot/forms/systematic_reviews.pdf

American Occupational Therapy Association. (2020). Occupational therapy practice framework: Domain and process (4th ed.). *American Journal of Occupational Therapy, 74*(Suppl. 2), 7412410010. https://doi.org/10.5014/ajot.2020.74S2001

Bayley, N., & Aylward, G. P. (2019). *Bayley Scales of Infant and Toddler Development* (4th ed.; Bayley-4). NCS Pearson.

Bellows, L. L., Davies, P. L., Anderson, J., & Kennedy, C. (2013). Effectiveness of a physical activity intervention for Head Start preschoolers: A randomized intervention study.

American Journal of Occupational Therapy, 67, 28–36. https://doi.org/10.5014/ajot.2013.005777

Blanche, E. I., Chang, M. C., Gutierrez, J., & Gunter, J. S. (2016). Effectiveness of a sensory-enriched early intervention group program for children with developmental disabilities. *American Journal of Occupational Therapy, 70,* 7005220010. https://dx.doi.org/10.5014/ajot.2016.018481

Bruininks, R., & Bruininks, B. (2005). *Bruininks–Oseretsky Test of Motor Proficiency* (2nd ed.). NCS Pearson.

Campbell, S. K., Wright, B. D., & Linacre, J. M. (2002). Development of a functional movement scale for infants. *Journal of Applied Measurement, 3*(2), 190–204. https://www.winsteps.com/a/JAM-Infants.pdf

Case-Smith, J., Frolek Clark, G. J., & Schlabach, T. L. (2013). Systematic review of interventions used in occupational therapy to promote motor performance for children ages birth–5 years. *American Journal of Occupational Therapy, 67,* 413–424. https://doi.org/10.5014/ajot.2013.005959

Case-Smith, J., & O'Brien, J. C. (2013). Applying occupation and motor learning principles in pediatric CIMT: Theoretical foundations and conceptual framework. In S. L. Ramey, P. Coker-Bolt, & S. C. DeLuca (Eds.), *Handbook of pediatric constraint-induced movement therapy (CIMT): A guide for occupational therapy and health care clinicians, researchers, and educators* (pp. 41–54). AOTA Press.

Centers for Disease Control and Prevention. (n.d.). *CDC's developmental milestones.* https://www.cdc.gov/ncbddd/actearly/milestones/index.html

Centers for Disease Control and Prevention. (2019). *Important milestones: Your child by five years.* https://www.cdc.gov/ncbddd/actearly/milestones/milestones-5yr.html

Dias, J. A. B. S., Manoel, E. J., Dias, R. B. M., & Okazaki, V. H. A. (2013). Pilot study on infant swimming classes and early motor development. *Perceptual and Motor Skills, 117,* 950–955. https://doi.org/10.2466/10.25.PMS.117x30z2

Dirks, T., Hielkema, T., Hamer, E. G., Reinders-Messelink, H. A., & Hadders-Algra, M. (2016). Infant positioning in daily life may mediate associations between physiotherapy and child development—video-analysis of an early intervention RCT. *Research in Developmental Disabilities, 53–54,* 147–157. https://doi.org/10.1016/j.ridd.2016.02.006

Dusing, S. C., Brown, S. E., Van Drew, C. M., Thacker, L. R., & Hendricks-Muñoz, K. D. (2015). Supporting play exploration and early development intervention from NICU to home: A feasibility study. *Pediatric Physical Therapy, 27,* 267–274. https://doi.org/10.1097/PEP.0000000000000161

Folio, M. R., & Fewell, R. R. (2000). *Peabody Developmental Motor Scales (2nd ed.): Examiner's manual.* PRO-ED.

Frolek Clark, G., & Kingsley, K. (2020). Occupational therapy practice guidelines for early childhood: Birth–5 years. *American Journal of Occupational Therapy, 74,* 7403397010. https://doi.org/10.5014/ajot.2020.743001

Gallahue, D. L. (1989). *Understanding motor development: Infants, children, adolescents* (2nd ed.). McGraw-Hill Higher Education.

Haley, S. M., Coster, W. J., Ludlow, L. H., Haltiwanger, J., & Andrellos, P. (2012). *Pediatric Evaluation of Disability Inventory: Computerized Adaptive Test.* www.pedicat.com

Hoare, B., Imms, C., Villanueva, E., Rawicki, H. B., Matyas, T., & Carey, L. (2013). Intensive therapy following upper limb botulinum toxin A injection in young children with unilateral

cerebral palsy: A randomized trial. *Developmental Medicine & Child Neurology, 55,* 238–247. https://doi.org/10.1111/dmcn.12054

Hsieh, H. C., Lin, H. Y., Chiu, W. H., Meng, L. F., & Liu, C. K. (2015). Upper-limb rehabilitation with adaptive video games for preschool children with developmental disabilities. *American Journal of Occupational Therapy, 69,* 6904290020. https://doi.org/10.5014/ajot.2015.014480

Hsieh, R. L., Lee, W. C., & Lin, J. H. (2016). The impact of short-term video games on performance among children with developmental delays: A randomized controlled trial. *PLoS ONE, 11,* e0149714. https://doi.org/10.1371/journal.pone.0149714

Iwanaga, R., Honda, S., Nakane, H., Tanaka, K., Toeda, H., & Tanaka, G. (2014). Pilot study: Efficacy of sensory integration therapy for Japanese children with high-functioning autism spectrum disorder: Sensory integration therapy for ASD. *Occupational Therapy International, 21*(1), 4–11. https://doi.org/10.1002/oti.1357

Jones, L., Bellis, M. A., Wood, S., Hughes, K., McCoy, E., Eckley, L., . . . Officer, A. (2012). Prevalence and risk of violence against children with disabilities: A systematic review and meta-analysis of observational studies. *Lancet, 380,* 899–907. https://doi.org/10.1016/S0140-6736(12)60692-8

Kleim, J. A., & Jones, T. A. (2008). Principles of experience-dependent neural plasticity: Implications for rehabilitation after brain damage. *Journal of Speech, Language, and Hearing Research, 51*(1). https://doi.org/10.1044/1092-4388(2008/018)

Kreutzer, J. S., DeLuca, J., & Caplan, B. (2011). WeeFIM II. In *Encyclopedia of clinical neuropsychology.* Springer.

Kruijsen-Terpstra, A. J. A., Ketelaar, M., Verschuren, O., Gorter, J. W., Vos, R. C., Verheijden, J., . . . Visser-Meily, A. (2016). Efficacy of three therapy approaches in preschool children with cerebral palsy: A randomized controlled trial. *Developmental Medicine & Child Neurology, 5,* 758–766. https://doi.org/10.1111/dmcn.12966

Kwon, J.-Y., Chang, H. J., Yi, S.-H., Lee, J. Y., Shin, H.-Y., & Kim, Y.-H. (2015). Effect of hippotherapy on gross motor function in children with cerebral palsy: A randomized controlled trial. *Journal of Alternative and Complementary Medicine, 21,* 15–21. https://doi.org/10.1089/acm.2014.0021

Law, M., Baptiste, S., Carswell, A., McColl, M. A., Polatajko, H., & Pollock, N. (2019). *Canadian Occupational Performance Measure* (5th ed., rev.). COPM, Inc.

Law, M. C., Darrah, J., Pollock, N., Wilson, B., Russell, D. J., Walter, S. D., . . . Galuppi, B. (2011). Focus on function: A cluster, randomized controlled trial comparing child- versus context-focused intervention for young children with cerebral palsy. *Developmental Medicine & Child Neurology, 53,* 621–629. https://doi.org/10.1111/j.1469-8749.2011.03962.x

McDougall, J., & King, G. (2007). *Goal Attainment Scaling: Description, utility, and applications in pediatric therapy services* (2nd ed.). Thames Valley Children's Center.

Monsalves-Alvarez, M., Castro-Sepulveda, M., Zapata-Lamana, R., Rosales-Soto, G., & Salazar, G. (2015). Motor skills and nutritional status outcomes from a physical activity intervention in short breaks on preschool children conducted by their educators: A pilot study. *Nutrición Hospitalaria, 32,* 1576–1581. https://doi.org/10.3305/nh.2015.32.4.9514

Morgan, C., Darrah, J., Gordon, A. M., Harbourne, R., Spittle, A., Johnson, R., & Fetters, L. (2016). Effectiveness of motor interventions in infants with cerebral palsy: A systematic review.

Developmental Medicine & Child Neurology, 58, 900–909. https://doi.org/10.1111/dmcn.13105

Morgan, C., Novak, I., Dale, R. C., & Badawi, N. (2015). Optimising motor learning in infants at high risk of cerebral palsy: A pilot study. *BMC Pediatrics, 15,* 30. https://doi.org/10.1186/s12887-015-0347-2

Morgan, C., Novak, I., Dale, R. C., Guzzetta, A., & Badawi, N. (2014). GAME (Goals–Activity–Motor Enrichment): Protocol of a single blind randomised controlled trial of motor training, parent education and environmental enrichment for infants at high risk of cerebral palsy. *BMC Neurology, 14,* 203. https://doi.org/10.1186/s12883-014-0203-2

Nordhov, S. M., Ronning, J. A., Dahl, L. B., Ulvund, S. E., Tunby, J., & Kaaresen, P. I. (2010). Early intervention improves cognitive outcomes for preterm infants: Randomized controlled trial. *Pediatrics, 126,* e1088–e1094. https://doi.org/10.1542/peds.2010-0778

Palisano, R., Rosenbaum, P., Bartlett, D., & Livingston, M. (2008). Content validity of the expanded and revised Gross Motor Function Classification System. *Developmental Medicine & Child Neurology, 50,* 744–750. https://doi.org/10.1111/j.1469-8749.2008.03089.x

Palisano, R., Rosenbaum, P., Walter, S., Russell, D., Wood, E., & Galuppi, B. (1997). Development and reliability of a system to classify gross motor function in children with cerebral palsy. *Developmental Medicine and Child Neurology, 39,* 214–223. https://doi.org/10.1111/j.1469-8749.1997.tb07414.x

Park, H. Y., Maitra, K., Achon, J., Loyola, E., & Rincón, M. (2014). Effects of early intervention on mental or neuromusculoskeletal and movement-related functions in children born low birthweight or preterm: A meta-analysis. *American Journal of Occupational Therapy, 68,* 268–276. https://doi.org/10.5014/ajot.2014.010371

Piper, M. C., Pinnell, L. E., Darrah, J., Maguire, T., & Byrne, P. J. (1992). Construction and validation of the Alberta Infant Motor Scale (AIMS). *Canadian Journal of Public Health, 83,* S46–S50.

Russell, D. J., Rosenbaum, P. L., Wright, M., & Avery, L. M. (2013). *Gross Motor Function Measure (GMFM-66 & GMFM-88) user's manual* (2nd ed.). Mac Keith Press.

Salem, Y., Gropack, S. J., Coffin, D., & Godwin, E. M. (2012). Effectiveness of a low-cost virtual reality system for children with developmental delay: A preliminary randomised single-blind controlled trial. *Physiotherapy, 98,* 189–195. https://doi.org/10.1016/j.physio.2012.06.003

Sgandurra, G., Bartalena, L., Cecchi, F., Cioni, G., Giampietri, M., Greisen, G., . . . Dario, P. (2016). A pilot study on early home-based intervention through an intelligent baby gym (CareToy) in preterm infants. *Research in Developmental Disabilities, 53–54,* 32–42. https://doi.org/10.1016/j.ridd.2016.01.013

Sgandurra, G., Ferrari, A., Cossu, G., Guzzetta, A., Fogassi, L., & Cioni, G. (2013). Randomized trial of observation and execution of upper extremity actions versus action alone in children with unilateral cerebral palsy. *Neurorehabilitation and Neural Repair, 27,* 808–815. https://doi.org/10.1177/1545968313497101

Sheridan, M., Sharma, A., & Cockerill, H. (2008). *From birth to five years: Children's developmental progress* (4th ed.). Routledge.

Silva, L. M., Schalock, M., Garberg, J., & Smith, C. L. (2012). Qigong massage for motor skills in young children with cerebral palsy and Down syndrome. *American Journal of Occupational Therapy, 66,* 348–355. https://doi.org/10.5014/ajot.2012.003541

Spittle, A., Orton, J., Anderson, P., Boyd, R., & Doyle, L. W. (2012). Early developmental intervention programmes post-hospital discharge to prevent motor and cognitive impairments in preterm infants. *Cochrane Database of Systematic Reviews, 12,* CD005495. https://doi.org/10.1002/14651858.CD005495.pub3

Tanner, K., Schmidt, E. K., Martin, K., & Bassi, M. (2020). Interventions within the scope of occupational therapy practice to improve motor performance for children ages 0–5 years: A systematic review. *American Journal of Occupational Therapy, 74,* 7402180060. https://doi.org/10.5014/ajot.2020.039644

U.S. Preventive Services Task Force. (2018). *Grade definitions.* https://www.uspreventiveservicestaskforce.org/Page/Name/grade-definitions

Van Hus, J., Jeukens-Visser, M., Koldewijn, K., Holman, R., Kok, J. H., Nollet, F., & Van Wassenaer-Leemhuis, A. G. (2016). Early intervention leads to long-term developmental improvements in very preterm infants, especially infants with bronchopulmonary dysplasia. *Acta Paediatrica, 105,* 773–781. https://doi.org/10.1111/apa.13387

Wallander, J. L., Bann, C. M., Biasini, F. J., Goudar, S. S., Pasha, O., Chomba, E., . . . Carlo, W. A. (2014). Development of children at risk for adverse outcomes participating in early intervention in developing countries: A randomized controlled trial. *Journal of Child Psychology & Psychiatry & Allied Disciplines, 55,* 1251–1259. https://doi.org/10.1111/jcpp.12247

Wentz, E. E. (2017). Importance of initiating a "tummy time" intervention early in infants with Down syndrome. *Pediatric Physical Therapy, 29,* 68–75. https://doi.org/10.1097/PEP.0000000000000335

Best Practices in Supporting Social Participation (Communication)

32

Kris Pedersen, SLPD, CCC-SLP, and Stephanie Parks, PhD, OT/L

KEY TERMS AND CONCEPTS

- Augmentative or alternative communication (AAC)
- Choice boards
- Choice making
- Emergent literacy
- Expressive language
- Functional communication training
- Gestures
- Language
- Modeling
- Peer-mediated interventions
- Pragmatic language
- Procedural visual supports
- Receptive language
- Scaffolding
- Social–emotional reciprocity
- Social participation
- Social routines
- Spatial visual supports
- Speech production
- Temporal visual supports
- Visual supports

OVERVIEW

In occupational therapy, *social participation* interweaves occupations to support the child's desired engagement in social situations with family, peers, and friends (Gillen & Boyt Schell, 2014). The development of interpersonal communication and social interdependence involves basic social interaction (performance) skills closely linked to communication and cognition, including initiating interactions, using and understanding nonverbal gestures or looks, producing speech fluently (e.g., spoken, signed, computer generated), requesting, responding to questions, taking turns, expressing feelings and emotions in a way that is socially appropriate, expressing empathy, and what in early childhood settings is often called using friendship skills (e.g., offering thanks, compliments; American Occupational Therapy Association [AOTA], 2020; Crabtree & Watson, 2019).

Essential to a young child's social participation is the ability to communicate. Young children at risk of, or identified with, a variety of delays and disabilities have difficulty with social communication skills, which often significantly affects their social participation. One in 12 children have identified challenges with communication. According to the National Health Interview Survey in 2012, nearly 8% of children ages 3–17 years have a communication disorder, with the highest prevalence among children ages 3–6 years (11%; Black et al., 2015). Occupational therapy practitioners work in close partnership with parents as well as other team members (e.g., speech–language pathologists, educators, social workers) to support children with social and communication challenges as they access and learn from their environment and participate in the social world. (*Note. Occupational therapy practitioner* refers to both occupational therapists and occupational therapy assistants.)

ESSENTIAL CONSIDERATIONS

Communication is often broken down into *speech production,* or the sounds made to form words, and *language,* which involves the use of words spoken, written, signed, or expressed through augmentative or alternative communication (AAC) to interact with others (American Speech-Language-Hearing Association [ASHA], n.d.-c). Speech sound disorders include both articulation and phonological disorders. Some children have difficulty making certain sounds and have errors in their speech (e.g., distortions, substitutions), whereas other children experience errors that follow a certain pattern, such as leaving off sounds at the ends of words. For example, young children with articulation disorders may experience neurological issues, such as childhood apraxia of speech, or structural abnormalities, such as cleft palate. Children with Down syndrome or cerebral palsy can experience speech sound disorders because of the motoric nature of their disability.

Language can be divided into several components: receptive, expressive, and pragmatic or social language. *Receptive language* is how one understands the words and sentences one hears. *Expressive language* is how one puts one's thoughts into words and sentences. Expressive language can take various forms; it can be verbal, gestural, or communicated through AAC. Important to expressive language is understanding how children communicate and why, or the functions of communications, which include such things as protesting, commenting, and social interaction. *Pragmatic language* refers to the social use of language—taking turns, adjusting language depending on the listener or situation, and following conversational rules such as staying on topic (ASHA, n.d.-c).

The following section outlines the development of social communication skills. Although all children attain social and communication skills that affect social participation at varying rates, occupational therapy practitioners need to be aware of the stages and process of social interactions and communication development. See Table 32.1

TABLE 32.1.   Social Communication Development Milestones

AGE	SOCIAL COMMUNICATION MILESTONES
2 months	▪ Begins to smile at people ▪ Can briefly calm self (may bring hands to mouth) ▪ Coos, makes gurgling sounds ▪ Turns head toward sound
4 months	▪ Copies some movements and facial expressions ▪ Begins to babble ▪ Cries in different ways to show hunger, pain, or tiredness
6 months	▪ Likes to play with others, especially parents ▪ Strings together vowel sounds and takes turns when making sounds ▪ Responds to name ▪ Begins to say consonant sounds (e.g., jabbering with *m, b*)
9 months	▪ Has favorite toys ▪ Understands *no* ▪ Copies sounds and gestures of others ▪ Points to things
1 year	▪ Plays peekaboo and patty-cake ▪ Responds to simple requests ▪ Says "mama" and "dada" and exclamations such as "uh-oh"
2 years	▪ Copies others, especially adults and older children ▪ Plays mainly beside other children ▪ Points to things or pictures when named ▪ Uses two- to four-word phrases ▪ Repeats words overheard in conversation
3 years	▪ Shows affection for friends without prompting ▪ Takes turns in games ▪ Shows wide range of emotions ▪ Names a friend ▪ Says first name, age, and gender ▪ Carries on a simple conversation using two to three sentences
4 years	▪ Pretends in play ▪ Would rather play with other children than by themselves ▪ Talks about what they like and are interested in ▪ Tells stories ▪ Sings songs or rhymes from memory, such as "Itsy Bitsy Spider"
5 years	▪ Wants to please and be like friends ▪ Likes to sing, dance, and act ▪ Likely to agree with rules ▪ Tells a simple story using full sentences ▪ Sometimes demanding and sometimes very cooperative

Source. Adapted from Centers for Disease Control and Prevention (2019).

for information on social communication development milestones. This section also addresses the need for moving beyond the developmental model and recommends evaluating and holistically addressing social participation using an occupation-centered approach.

Development of Early Vocalization and Social–Emotional Reciprocity (Birth–12 Months)

Early social communication skills are marked by stages of vocalizations and changes in oral–motor development (e.g., touch, lips). Infants' crying and vegetative sounds express their basic feelings of hunger, pleasure or displeasure, and need for comfort. As the infant begins to explore how their mouth moves, cooing behavior develops that sounds like open-mouthed and "throaty" sounds. As they explore how their lips move, they begin making "raspberries," and changes in the rise and fall of their voice are noted. Infants then begin to make sounds that are adultlike, repeating them in a consonant–vowel pattern called *reduplicated and variegated babbling.*

This vocal play that unfolds in the first year of life is critical to a baby's ability to produce speech sounds later that form words and combinations of words. Not only does the oral exploration provide practice coordinating fine movements among consonants, vowels, and syllables, but caregiver responsiveness to an infant's sounds positively affects later language and social interaction. When caregivers respond to the sounds of infants, infants learn their sounds are important for social interaction (Franklin et al., 2014; Goldstein et al., 2009).

Social–emotional reciprocity is the back and forth or dance of communication between adult and child that develops in this first year and leads to co-occupation (Pierce, 2011). It begins with a sharing of interests, affect, and emotions. Infants learn to attend to adults, objects, and, eventually, experiences in a social context. As adults respond to an infant's behaviors, the infant learns to shift their attentional focus and change their behaviors to affect the responses of others. A key component of social–emotional reciprocity is joint attention. This sharing and coordinating of attention with a social partner is a critical skill in understanding the perspective of others and the development of intentional communication (Adamson & Chance, 1998). In unstable relationships or if the child has a developmental disability, the social communications may not be reinforced, and development in this area can be delayed.

Initially, adults do most of the work of communication by attaching meaning to the behaviors of the infant and interpreting their looks, reaches, and expressions as communicative. An infant looks at their caregiver, and the caregiver responds with an "ooh" or "ahh" or phrases such as, "You like that ball," or, "You want to be picked up." Over time, this back and forth exchange leads to the infant developing intentional communication by understanding that their actions and expressions have meaning and can provoke a response. The infant learns that when they fuss in a certain way or make a particular sound or gesture, an adult will typically pick them up, feed them, or play with them. Through adults' responsiveness to these early behaviors, children learn the many ways and many reasons they can communicate. Children's use of eye gaze, facial expressions, body language, and gestures is the foundation for experiencing their environment and interacting with caregivers (Adamson & Chance, 1998; Yoder et al., 1998).

Development of Social Communication (12–24 Months)

As children make the transition to symbolic or intentional communication, word use and gestures play an important role. Young children use gestures before they begin to speak, and these gestures predominate until age 18 months or when the child exhibits a spurt in word use. The development of motor skills for communication dominates the first year of life.

Gestures carry various meanings and allow infants to develop the complexities of language early on. Infants use gestures, a movement of their body to communicate, to show objects to caregivers in play and to point to or reach for what they want. They refer to objects and actions that are close and far away. Infants also develop symbolic or referential gestures, which shows their learning of representation. As children communicate with intent, they develop a range of purposes or functions, including requesting or protesting objects and actions and sharing experiences by showing, commenting, and engaging in joint attention and interaction (Acredolo & Goodwyn, 1988; Bates et al., 1987, 1989).

Later Social Communication Development (2–5 Years)

The toddler years are characterized by rapid growth in vocabulary size, types of words (e.g., nouns, verbs, adjectives), and ways of combining those words to form short phrases and eventually sentences. Children learn to put together words in different ways, have conversations with others, and tell stories. The language skills that have developed over the early years are put to work in social situations and environments. Children refine their social communication skills as they develop friendships and encounter new social situations. They learn to understand the perspective of others and how different situations call for different uses of language. They learn to initiate and respond in play and in conversations; they also learn about social rules and how to repair breakdowns. The preschool years also find children learning about the written form of communication and developing early literacy skills.

During these early years, children not only learn to listen and express themselves, they also learn skills needed for later reading and writing. This period of *emergent literacy,* knowledge of reading and writing skills, involves interacting with and learning from print. Children experience print in books, in magazines, on signs, and on everyday household items. They learn how to orient a book, attend to alphabet letters, rhyme, and scribble with writing instruments. An important early skill is phonological awareness, or the connection among the sounds in a word. Activities that expose children to letters and the sounds they make enhance later reading skills. The development of early language skills is critical for a child's literacy development (Roth et al., 2006; Terrell & Watson, 2018).

Early Indicators of Social Communication Delays and Disorders

Beyond developmental milestones such as the first word and word combinations, early signs or indicators that children need intervention or additional supports include how often they socially communicate, whether it be through vocalizations, gestures, or verbal words (McCathren et al., 1999), and the variety of things they communicate about (e.g., protesting, requesting, commenting). Children should have a range of types of words and sentence structures. They should understand words and directions with increasing complexity and produce more sounds and be more understood as they grow (Paul et al., 2018).

Key indicators of social communication impairment include skills typically developed in the first year (e.g., social–emotional reciprocity, including joint attention and imitation). These skills are particularly challenging for children with autism (Charmon et al., 1997; Dawson et al., 2004). Later in early childhood, young children who interact more with adults than peers and have fewer initiations during play and conversations are also at risk (Brady et al., 2004).

Moving Toward Occupation-Centered Practice With Young Children

Throughout the last decade, occupational therapy leaders and researchers working in early childhood have called for a better understanding of the essence of children's occupations, the social co-construction of occupation, and ultimately young children's optimal social participation (O'Brien & Kuhaneck, 2020; Olson, 2009). Coster (1998) proposed that the dominance of the developmental model has become one of the largest obstacles to practitioners becoming more occupation centered. Likewise, Humphry (2002) argued that there has been an overreliance on other disciplines in understanding child development without appreciating the impact of context and the child's natural social partners, both of which influence skill acquisition and occupational performance.

Occupational therapy practitioners using a developmental perspective predominately will base their evaluation and interventions for young children on biologic maturation and development patterns. However, the developmental model and frame of reference alone, although beneficial, lack consideration of environmental barriers, the significance of relationships, and routines and habits needed for social participation. This traditional emphasis on developmental sequences (i.e., milestones) as the organizing framework may lead to "splinter skills," as opposed to addressing the young child and family's role expectations, social routines, and co-constructed regulation, which contribute to social participation (Rodger & Kennedy-Behr, 2017). Hence, the significance of context and social interactions is critical to children's learning and social participation.

BEST PRACTICES

Interventions should be based on contextually mediated practices whereby everyday activities and interests are used to promote the child's participation and learning (Dunst,

2006). Opportunities for practicing existing social and communication skills and learning new ones must be provided. Effective intervention strategies should be included in everyday routine activities to promote opportunities for the child to be successfully engaged. This section explores evaluation and intervention planning related to supporting social participation in everyday occupations for young children and their families.

Use Occupation-Based Assessment Practices and Authentic Assessment Strategies

First, occupational therapists use family and caregiver interviews and authentic assessment strategies to gather information on the child's performance across natural environments and everyday routines to develop an occupational profile (AOTA, 2020). Caregivers' goals for their young children with social communication challenges may involve expanding how and why they socially communicate, increasing the frequency and effectiveness of their social communication, and engaging them in social interactions with others so they can more fully participate in daily activities and routines.

As discussed in the previous section, occupational therapy practitioners use occupation-based assessment and intervention practices to support the social participation and communication of young children during their everyday social interactions. The Person–Environment–Occupation model (Law et al., 1996), for example, guides practitioners to consider not only the child's social and communication skills and abilities but also the tasks and activities that are meaningful as well as the environments in which engagement and participation in occupations occur.

This requires authentic assessment strategies to assess the child, in their natural environment, as well as note the barriers and facilitators to occupational performance and participation (Law & Dunbar, 2007). A more in-depth listing of assessment tools can be found in Appendix F, "Examples of Assessments for Early Childhood (Birth–5 Years)."

Develop an Intervention Plan or Plan of Care (Health Care Settings)

When possible, interventions and supports should be provided in the natural context of everyday activities to maximize children's engagement and participation. Occupational therapists should complete the intervention plan (or plan of care) identifying goals and strategies in partnership with families and other team members.

Implement Effective Interventions

Occupational therapy practitioners provide interventions to promote participation in occupations through increased social communication skills. Several strategies are described in this section. Table 32.2 provides a list of common strategies to promote young children's interest and engagement in communication in any setting.

Promote social communication and participation through routines

Routines help a child learn to understand and make sense of their world. Routines provide structure, comfort, and confidence while freeing "space" to process and develop skills in the social context of learning (Olson, 2009). *Social routines* are complex sequences of behavior that provide

TABLE 32.2. Strategies to Promote Social Participation and Examples

STRATEGIES TO PROMOTE SOCIAL PARTICIPATION AND COMMUNICATION	EXAMPLES
Use interest-based materials, activities, routines	▪ Follow along with what the child likes to do ▪ Imitate the child so they become interested in what is being taught ▪ Provide caregivers with support and assistance to develop and facilitate daily routines
Create and use natural opportunities for social communication	▪ Offer choices in activities and materials ▪ Consider accessibility of materials (e.g., are they out of reach or in a container with a lid?) ▪ Consider whether multiple or additional items are needed; do not offer all items at once ▪ Use pauses and wait time to create opportunities, give time to process and generate responses
Acknowledge attempts to communicate	▪ Observe how and why the child socially communicates ▪ Use breakdowns and challenges as a teaching and learning opportunity
Model communication and social participation	▪ Provide the verbal or visual cue so the child can imitate ▪ Use a variety of types of words (e.g., nouns, verbs, descriptive words, location words) ▪ Model social play interactions ▪ Use different ways to enter and maintain an interaction ▪ Use different ways to communicate (e.g., gesture, sign, verbal word, picture) ▪ Build or scaffold by modeling more complex or varied communication or play skills
Use supports to enhance participation	▪ Use visual supports to help children understand and as a way to communicate ▪ Use props during shared book reading ▪ Use peers and caregivers to model ▪ Use augmentative or alternative communication to offer easily accessible ways to communicate

a context for social engagement among children, parents, siblings, peers, and caregivers. Young children learn social routines through consistent exposure to and observations of others as well as direct instruction. For children and families receiving early intervention services, the use of naturally occurring routines is the preferred vehicle for intervention and considered best practice (Division for Early Childhood, 2014).

Lack of routines may result in physical and temporal disarray or disorganization, increased stress, and dysfunction, which can affect well-being. Occupational therapy practitioners often support early childhood educators and families with young children in developing and incorporating predictable routines within their daily life to strengthen relationships and promote successful participation. For example, bedtime routines and rituals provide comfort and reassurance before sleep. Children with delays and disabilities may resist participation in preschool and family routines (e.g., avoidance, exhibiting challenging behaviors). Families, teachers, and caregivers may find that when routines are disrupted or are unsuccessful, there is heightened anxiety and distress for the family or preschool classroom.

When social games and activities are repetitive and have a predictable sequence, children are afforded many opportunities to hear and see social communication. They anticipate how the game, activity, or interaction will go. When parents and occupational therapy practitioners interrupt the sequence by pausing, waiting excitedly, or doing something unexpected or silly, they provide opportunities for children to practice the social interaction or communication modeled. Adults can entice children to communicate by engaging with them, being face to face, and offering ideas for how to play and interact. Adults can create opportunities for communication and social participation by arranging the environment, placing items out of reach or in containers so the child needs to request the items, or changing up an activity by responding in an unpredictable way, such as giving them the wrong item (Owens, 2018; Paul et al., 2018).

Prevent challenging behaviors with functional communication supports

Young children with language delays or communication challenges may also have an increase in challenging behavior (e.g., tantrums, aggression, self-injury). *Functional communication training* (FCT; Carr & Durand, 1985) is a common function-based behavioral intervention used to decrease or prevent challenging behavior by using a functional behavior assessment to identify the function of the child's challenging behavior and then teaching a replacement behavior. In FCT, the replacement behavior is a new, more appropriate form of communication, such as pointing, gesturing, signs, pictures, or speech.

Respond, model, and scaffold

Following a child's lead and *scaffolding* (i.e., building on existing skills by providing the right level and type of input) support can enhance engagement and promote social participation in daily routines. How adults interact with children affects how they develop and use social

communication performance skills to participate in daily activities and routines. The language and interactions that are modeled support successful interactions with others. Responding positively to a child's cues to interact and communicate acknowledges the child's attempts and encourages them to continue to interact with others. Responding to a child's communicative attempts leads to better language outcomes (Halle et al., 2004). Caregivers and occupational therapy practitioners should observe and document how a young child communicates using traditional means (i.e., using words or word approximations) as well as nontraditional communication attempts and should be ready to respond by interpreting and scaffolding in these moments. A child's nontraditional communication attempts might include vocalizations, movements, facial expressions, eye movements, and other behaviors.

The focus should be on reciprocal interactions or the back and forth interactions in play and in communicating. Adults stimulate communication by modeling, whether using words, sharing a book, or having a conversation. *Modeling* to enhance social communication may involve demonstrating the back and forth of communication or turn taking that occurs both in conversation and in play. Turn taking may include playing social games such as peekaboo, putting toys in a bucket or activating a toy, or it can involve language by saying a word or sentence after a child does.

Scaffolding play and communication allows adults to model more complex forms within a child's zone of proximal development. For example, for a child using single words, the adult models two-word phrases. When a child points to request, caregivers acknowledge the request by modeling a verbal word. Adults should talk about what they and the child are doing and seeing, adding ideas and vocabulary to what the child offers to expand or extend their learning. Adults also fill in the gaps by modeling language that was missing or in error by repeating back what was said in the correct form (Owens, 2018; Paul et al., 2018).

Facilitate choice making

Teaching children to make choices is a critical aspect of social communication and leads to the development of self-determination (Palmer et al., 2013). *Choice making* increases the opportunities for children with disabilities to communicate their wants and needs, leading to increased participation. Some, but not all children, begin to communicate to express their choices, first in pointing to objects and then in naming the objects. However, choice making is often facilitated by the adults who set up the young child's environment. Wehmeyer (1996) noted that choice making is "a process of selecting between alternatives based on individual preferences" (p. 14) and recognized that children with disabilities are sometimes less likely to be offered choices because people may perceive they have limited capacity. Occupational therapy practitioners can be instrumental in facilitating and encouraging choice making throughout the child's everyday routines to promote participation.

Use visual supports

Visual supports help children understand the world around them, give them a way to communicate, and give them control and flexibility in accessing and participating in their environment. They can help children prepare for social situations and teach skills needed in those social situations (Quill, 2000). Using visual supports such as photos of objects; picture symbols that represent materials, activities, or tasks; and even written words for older preschoolers incorporated into daily routines and schedules has been found to be an effective strategy to assist young children in comprehending rules, expectations, and transitions in the home or classroom (Meadan et al., 2011).

In a study comparing two naturalistic interventions, the Picture Exchange Communication System (PECS) and Pivotal Response Training (PRT), in an early intervention context, the researchers found PECS was just as effective as PRT in increasing the verbal communication skills of young children with autism spectrum disorder when implemented in a natural context (Schriebman & Stahmer, 2014). Using visual support interventions such as PECS early in children's life may assist them in building social communication skills and promote social participation.

Several types of visual supports can be used with children. *Temporal visual supports,* such as an individualized visual schedule, help a child understand the time and sequence of an activity and help with task completion and waiting. *Procedural visual supports* help children to understand and follow routines, rules, and expectations of everyday activities. *Spatial visual supports,* such as visual boundaries marking pathways or work areas on the floor or wall, can help children understand environmental set-ups and the relationship between materials and people. Finally, visual supports such as *choice boards* can be used to help children express control over their environment and advocate for their needs, feelings, and preferences (Dalrymple, 1995). Examples of visual supports include choice boards with options displayed, visual schedules of steps or sequence of activities, transitional objects to hold, first–then sequence cards, and timers. Social Stories™ and scripts are also helpful to learn how to navigate social situations (Gray, 2004; Quill, 2000). Visual supports can also be used as a way for children to enter into play with peers, express preferences at mealtime or playtime, and express how they are feeling.

Occupational therapy practitioners and other team members supporting the child and family need to assess the level of symbolic understanding of the child when designing and creating visual supports and can consider use of real objects, pictures of real objects, picture symbols, and written words. Collaboration with a speech–language pathologist is recommended.

Use peer-mediated social strategies

When children do not socially communicate often, do not have the words to express themselves, or communicate in idiosyncratic ways, they can experience communication breakdowns in which others do not receive their message. Often these breakdowns or unsuccessful moments can result in the child not communicating or participating and exhibiting increasing negative responses. Interventions to bridge this communication breakdown involve practicing social communication strategies, often while providing visual supports to help the child engage and practice in social situations.

At times, setting up natural situations and providing prompts to practice new social communication skills can be successful. In an approach often referred to as *incidental teaching of social behavior,* the occupational therapy practitioner positively reinforces desired social behavior (e.g., "I like how you helped Jose"). In addition to incidental instruction, practitioners also may use explicit, direct instruction of friendship and social skills in groups. With this strategy, structured group activities are implemented to teach social scripts, play organization, and emotional literacy and to reinforce friendship skills, such as problem solving strategies or how to give thanks or compliments (Chandler, 2010).

Peer-mediated interventions include social play opportunities between peers and the child with disabilities that occur in the natural environments (O'Brien & Kuhaneck, 2020). These strategies have been shown to be effective in teaching social communication skills, thus promoting social participation (McMaster et al., 2006). For example, occupational therapy practitioners might use peer-mediated strategies to teach how to initiate or enter into play or a conversation, how to respond appropriately, and how to use turn taking to keep an interaction going. Adults can encourage the responsivity of social partners by giving examples and prompts for responses. Giving evaluative feedback is critical, whether it be positive encouragement or explicit comments on the effectiveness of an interaction.

Advocate for inclusive services for children with social communication challenges

For children with delays and disabilities, natural and inclusive environments are essential to developing performance skills needed for social participation. To develop friendships, young children with disabilities need opportunities and supports to interact and play with peers. Often, children with disabilities have difficulties with appropriate social skills and have not yet developed problem-solving or conflict resolution strategies. Instead of segregating children with these challenging behaviors and fewer adaptive social communication skills, occupational therapy practitioners can advocate for high-quality inclusive environments that offer role models with the adaptive social communication skills children with disabilities need to learn friendship skills and social participation.

Work collaboratively to provide augmentative and alternative communication interventions

Young children with communication impairments and developmental delays benefit from AAC. Working closely with speech–language pathologists and other team members, including families, occupational therapy practitioners can support the planning and implementation of AAC interventions. *AAC* systems may include unaided systems, such as sign language and gestures, or aided systems, such as use of pictures, symbols, and speech-generating devices. Practitioners can help assess the most efficient way for young children to access communication systems, including using switches, eye gaze, or direct access. It is important to note that research has shown that AAC interventions have not hindered language development for children with disabilities but improve overall communication (Millar et al., 2006). Additional information on assistive technology, including AAC, can be found in Chapter 7, "Best Practices in the Use of Assistive Technology to Enhance Participation."

Support early literacy development

When homes and preschools are filled with literacy-rich information and experiences, children have better success in reading and writing when they get into school (Terrell & Watson, 2018). Sharing books or spending time looking at and talking about books together is important for young children. Adults should be encouraged to share books rather than simply reading the text on a page. Sharing the experience involves talking about what is happening on a page, repeating common words, posing thoughtful questions about what has happened or what might happen, and pointing out similarities or differences. Other activities include drawing attention to labels and text in the environment, signs on the road, menus in a restaurant, and labels on household products. Singing and rhyming activities also encourage play with sounds in words (Roth et al., 2006; Terrell & Watson, 2018).

As children spend time interacting with books, adults can encourage them to tell stories about books. Dialogic book reading offers children opportunities to engage in a dialogue about the book and has been shown to enhance language outcomes (Grygas Coogle et al., 2018). In this approach, the adult asks questions and responds to the child's comments or questions so the child learns to tell a story. Adults scaffold or expand the child's language by adding information, asking more complex questions, and prompting for more information (Whitehurst et al., 1994; Zevenbergen & Whitehurst, 2003). See Chapter 13, "Understanding Early Literacy Development," for more information on literacy.

SUMMARY

By understanding the breadth of social communication development and the influence of environment, occupational therapy practitioners can serve as a substantial support for young children and their family's social participation. Children need to be able to access their environment and fully participate by expressing wants, needs, and preferences; sharing ideas and thoughts; reading; writing; and engaging in shared conversations. Early experiences of joint attention, social reciprocity, and development of intentional communication can be enhanced during everyday social experiences. Practitioners can encourage and support caregivers to recognize and appropriately respond to social communication attempts, model ways to have successful interactions, and support language and literacy skills. In addition, using the environment and routines increases the frequency of learning opportunities and makes learning contextually relevant.

For children to fully participate in the social world, it is imperative to support their social communication abilities for more meaningful occupational participation. The work of occupational therapy practitioners can support a child's development of communication and can positively affect the child and family's social participation.

RESOURCES

AOTA resources
- Autism Spectrum Disorder Critically Appraised Topic: https://bit.ly/3izzhY0
- Children and Youth 5–21 Years: A Systematic Literature Review: https://bit.ly/3mdoJA6

ASHA resources
- *Language in Brief* (ASHA, n.d.-a): https://bit.ly/2Zx6DPX
- *Social Communication Disorder* (ASHA, n.d.-b): https://bit.ly/2GTQg9J

REFERENCES

Acredolo, L. P., & Goodwyn, S. W. (1988). Symbolic gesturing in normal infants. *Child Development, 59,* 450–466. https://doi.org/10.2307/1130324

Adamson, L. A., & Chance, S. E. (1998). Coordinating attention to people, objects and language. In A. Wetherby, S. Warren, & J. Reichle (Eds.), *Transitions in prelinguistic communication* (Vol. 7, pp. 15–37). Brookes.

American Occupational Therapy Association. (2020). Occupational therapy practice framework: Domain and process (4th ed.). *American Journal of Occupational Therapy, 74*(Suppl. 2), 7412410010. https://doi.org/10.5014/ajot.2020.74S2001

American Speech-Language-Hearing Association. (n.d.-a). *Language in brief.* https://www.asha.org/Practice-Portal/Clinical-Topics/Spoken-Language-Disorders/Language-In--Brief/

American Speech-Language-Hearing Association. (n.d.-b). *Social communication disorder.* https://www.asha.org/Practice-Portal/Clinical-Topics/Social-Communication-Disorder/

American Speech-Language-Hearing Association. (n.d.-c). *What is speech? What is language?* Retrieved from https://www.asha.org/public/speech/development/Speech-and-Language/

Bates, E., O'Connell, B., & Shore, C. (1987). Language and communication in infancy. In J. Osofsky (Ed.), *Handbook of infant development* (pp. 149–203). Wiley.

Bates, E., Thal, D., Fenson, L., Whitesell, K., & Oakes, L. (1989). Integrating language and gesture in infancy. *Developmental Psychology, 25,* 1004–1019. https://doi.org/10.1037/0012-1649.25.6.1004

Black, L. I., Vahratian, A., & Hoffman, H. J. (2015). *Communication disorders and use of intervention services among children aged 3–17 years: United States, 2012* (NCHS Data Brief No. 205). National Center for Health Statistics.

Brady, N., Marquis, J., Fleming, K., & McLean, L. (2004). Prelinguistic predictors of language growth in children with developmental disabilities. *Journal of Speech, Language, and Hearing Research, 47,* 663–677. https://doi.org/10.1044/1092-4388(2004/051)

Carr, E. G., & Durand, V. M. (1985). Reducing behavior problems through functional communication training. *Journal of Applied Behavior Analysis, 18,* 111–126. https://doi.org/10.1901/jaba.1985.18-111

Centers for Disease Control and Prevention. (2019). *CDC's developmental milestones.* https://www.cdc.gov/ncbddd/actearly/milestones/index.html

Chandler, B. E. (Ed.). (2010). *Early childhood: Occupational therapy services for children birth to five.* AOTA Press.

Charmon, T., Swettenham, J., Baron-Cohen, S., Cox, A., Baird, G., & Drew, A. (1997). Infants and autism: An investigation of empathy, pretend play, joint attention, and imitation. *Developmental Psychology, 22,* 781–789. https://doi.org/10.1037//0012-1649.33.5.781

Coster, W. (1998). Occupation-centered assessment of children. *American Journal of Occupational Therapy, 52,* 337–344. https://doi.org/10.5014/ajot.52.5.337

Crabtree, L., & Watson, L. (2019). Best practices in enhancing social participation. In G. Frolek Clark, J. Rioux, & B. Chandler (Eds.), *Best practices for occupational therapy in schools* (2nd ed., pp. 447–453). AOTA Press.

Dalrymple, N. J. (1995). Environmental supports to develop flexibility and independence. In K. A. Quill (Ed.), *Teaching children with autism: Strategies to enhance communication and socialization* (pp. 243–264). Delmar.

Dawson, G., Toth, K., Abbott, R., Osterling, J., Munson, J., Estes, A., & Liaw, J. (2004). Early social attention impairments in autism: Social orienting, joint attention, and attention to distress. *Developmental Psychology, 40,* 271–283. https://doi.org/10.1037/0012-1649.40.2.271

Division for Early Childhood. (2014). *DEC recommended practices in early intervention/early childhood special education* 2014. https://www.dec-sped.org/dec-recommended-practices

Dunst, C. (2006). Parent-mediated everyday child learning opportunities: I. Foundations and operationalization. *CASEinPoint, 2*(2).

Franklin, B., Warlaumont, A. S., Messinger, D., Bene, E., Iyer, S. N., Lee, C., . . . Oller, D. K. (2014). Effects of parental interaction on infant vocalization rate, variability and vocal type. *Language Learning and Development, 10,* 279–296. https://doi.org/10.1080/15475441.2013.849176

Gillen, G., & Boyt Schell, B. (2014). Introduction to evaluation, intervention, and outcomes for occupations. In B. A. Boyt Schell, G. Gillen, & M. Scaffa (Eds.), *Willard and Spackman's occupational therapy* (12th ed., pp. 606–609). Lippincott Williams & Wilkins.

Goldstein, M. H., Schwade, J. A., & Bornstein, M. H. (2009). The value of vocalizing: Five month–old infants associate their own noncry vocalizations with responses from caregivers. *Child Development, 80,* 636–644. https://doi.org/10.1111/j.1467-8624.2009.01287.x

Gray, C. (2004). Social Stories™ 10.0: The new defining criteria and guidelines. *Jenison Autism Journal, 15,* 2–21.

Grygas Coogle, C., Floyd, K. K., & Rahn, N. L. (2018). Dialogic reading and adapted dialogic reading with preschoolers with autism spectrum disorder. *Journal of Early Intervention, 40,* 363–379. https://doi.org/10.1177/1053815118797887

Halle, J., Brady, N., & Drasgow, E. (2004). Enhancing socially adaptive communicative repairs of beginning communicators with disabilities. *American Journal of Speech–Language Pathology, 13,* 43–54. https://doi.org/10.1044/1058-0360(2004/006)

Humphry, R. (2002). Young children's occupations: Explicating the dynamics of developmental processes. *American Journal of Occupational Therapy, 56,* 171–179. https://doi.org/10.5014/ajot.56.2.171

Law, M., Cooper, B., Strong, S., Stewart, D., Rigby, P., & Letts, L. (1996). The Person–Environment–Occupation model: A transactive approach to occupational performance. *Canadian Journal of Occupational Therapy, 63,* 9–23. https://doi.org/10.1177/000841749606300103

Law, M., & Dunbar, S. (2007). Person–Environment–Occupation model. In S. Dunbar (Ed.), *Occupational therapy models for intervention with children and families* (pp. 27–50). SLACK.

McCathren, R. B., Yoder, P. J., & Warren, S. F. (1999). The relationship between prelinguistic vocalization and later expressive vocabulary in young children with developmental delay. *Journal of Speech, Language, and Hearing Research, 42,* 915–924. https://doi.org/10.1044/jslhr.4204.915

McMaster, K. L., Fuchs, D., & Fuchs, L. S. (2006). Research on peer-assisted learning strategies: The promise and limitations of peer-mediated instruction. *Reading & Writing Quarterly, 22,* 5–25. https://doi.org/10.1080/10573560500203491

Meadan, H., Ostrosky, M., Triplett, B., Michna, A., & Fettig, A. (2011). Using visual supports with young children with autism spectrum disorder. *Teaching Exceptional Children, 43*(6), 28–35. https://doi.org/10.1177/004005991104300603

Millar, D., Light, J., & Schlosser, R. (2006). The impact of augmentative and alternative communication intervention on the speech production of individuals with developmental disabilities: A research review. *Journal of Speech, Language, and Hearing Research, 49,* 248–264. https://doi.org/10.1044/1092-4388(2006/021)

O'Brien, J., & Kuhaneck, H. (Eds.). (2020). *Case-Smith's occupational therapy for children and adolescents* (8th ed.). Elsevier.

Olson, L. J. (2009). A frame of reference to enhance social participation. In P. Kramer & J. Hinojosa (Eds.), *Frames of reference for pediatric occupational therapy* (2nd ed., pp. 306–348). Lippincott Williams, & Wilkins.

Owens, R. E. (2018). *Early language intervention for infants, toddlers and preschoolers.* Pearson.

Palmer, S. B., Summers, J. A., Brotherson, M. J., Erwin, E. J., Maude, S. P., Stroup-Rentier, V., & Chu, S. Y. (2013). Foundations for self-determination in early childhood: An inclusive model for children with disabilities. *Topics in Early Childhood Special Education, 33*(1), 38–47. https://doi.org/10.1177/0271121412445288

Paul, R., Norbury, C., & Gosse, C. (2018). *Language disorders from infancy through adolescence* (5th ed.). Elsevier.

Pierce, D. (2011). Co-occupation: The challenges of defining concepts original to occupational science. *Journal of Occupational Science, 16,* 203–207. https://doi.org/10.1080/14427591.2009.9686663

Quill, K. A. (2000). *Do–watch–listen–say: Social and communication intervention for children with autism.* Brookes.

Rodger, S., & Kennedy-Behr, A. (Eds.). (2017). *Occupation-centered practice with children: A practical guide for occupational therapists.* Wiley.

Roth, F., Paul, D., & Pierotti, A. (2006). *Let's talk: for people with special communication needs.* American Speech–Language–Hearing Association.

Schriebman, L., & Stahmer, A. (2014). A randomized trial comparison of the effects of verbal and pictorial naturalistic communication strategies on spoken language for young children with autism. *Journal of Autism and Developmental Disorders, 44,* 1244–1251. https://doi.org/10.1007/s10803-013-1972-y

Terrell, P., & Watson, M. (2018). Laying a firm foundation: Embedding evidence-based emergent literacy practices into early intervention and preschool environments. *Language, Speech and Hearing Services in Schools, 49,* 148–164. https://doi.org/10.1044/2017_LSHSS-17-0053

Wehmeyer, M. L. (1996). Self-determination as an educational outcome: Why is it important to children, youth, and adults with disabilities? In D. J. Sands & M. L. Wehmeyer (Eds.), *Self-determination across the lifespan: Independence and choice for people with disabilities* (pp. 13–36). Brookes.

Whitehurst, G. J., Arnold, D. S., Epstein, J. N., Angell, A. L., Smith, M., & Fischel, J. E. (1994). A picture book reading intervention in day care and home for children from low-income families. *Developmental Psychology, 30,* 679–689. https://doi.org/10.1037/0012-1649.30.5.679

Yoder, P. J., Warren, S. F., McCathren, R., & Leew, S. (1998). Does adult responsivity to child behavior facilitate communication development? In A. Wetherby, S. Warren, & J. Reichle (Eds.), *Transitions in prelinguistic communication* (Vol. 7, pp. 39–58). Brookes.

Zevenbergen, A. A., & Whitehurst, G. J. (2003). Dialogic reading: A shared picture book reading intervention for preschoolers. In A. van Kleeck, S. A. Stahl, & E. B. Bauer (Eds.), *On reading books to children: Parents and teachers* (pp. 177–200). Erlbaum.

Best Practices in Supporting Social, Emotional, and Self-Regulation Skills (Social–Emotional Skills)

33

Karrie Kingsley, OTD, OTR/L

KEY TERMS AND CONCEPTS

- Alert Program
- Co-regulation
- DIR/Floortime™
- Emotional and behavioral regulation
- Emotional skills
- Massage
- Mindfulness
- Parent–child interaction therapy
- Schoolwide positive behavior support
- Self-regulation
- Sensory strategies
- Skin-to-skin contact
- Social behaviors
- Social cognition
- Social knowledge
- Social skills
- Social Stories™

OVERVIEW

This chapter includes definitions of and best practices for self-regulation and social–emotional development in children from birth to age 5 years. Occupational therapy practitioners must recognize the complexity and interrelatedness of development for infants and young children and acknowledge that some of these developmental areas may overlap. (*Note. Occupational therapy practitioner* refers to both occupational therapists and occupational therapy assistants.) In the Individuals with Disabilities Education Improvement Act (IDEA, 2004), Part C early intervention combines social development and emotional development as one of the five developmental domains. Therefore, to capture the best practices as exhaustively as possible, evidence regarding social skills, behavior, and attachment are included in this chapter. Contexts explored include home, community, health care, and preschool settings.

Social skills are most simply defined as skills a child needs to successfully interact with others for a variety of purposes (Griswold & Townsend, 2012). Generalizing social skills across a variety of settings is referred to as *social competence* (Kauffman & Kinnealey, 2015). According to the Council for Exceptional Children (CEC; 2003), social skills include **social behaviors, emotional and behavioral regulation, social cognition,** and **social knowledge**.

- *Social behaviors* include actions that facilitate engagement with others, including initiating and responding to others (Marrus et al., 2015).
- *Emotional and behavioral regulation* includes the ability to manage emotions and behavior and grade them appropriately for a situation, such as inhibiting disruptive behavior after losing a game.
- *Social cognition* is the ability to perceive and process social information and includes skills such as emotion recognition, theory of mind, and reading body language (Sasson et al., 2013).
- *Social knowledge* is understanding broad social constructs and expectations, such as what it means to be a friend (Kauffman & Kinnealey, 2015).

The *Occupational Therapy Practice Framework: Domain and Process* (4th ed.; *OTPF*) lists 27 contributing performance skills under the larger concept of *social interaction skills* (e.g., approaches, regulates, expresses emotion, takes turn, empathizes; American Occupational Therapy Association [AOTA], 2020).

Social skills increase in complexity with age. Social skills during infancy include serve and return interactions with caregivers (e.g., the infant gestures or cries and the adult responds with eye contact or a hug), social referencing caregivers (e.g., the infant reads facial expressions to help them understand a situation and make decisions), and joint attention (e.g., shared attention), while preschool introduces the concepts of friendships, and schools require children to interact with a variety of social partners. Having deficits in social skills or interaction is not a diagnosis but an associated feature for many children with developmental disabilities or traumatic experiences.

Emotional skills include understanding one's own emotions, understanding the emotions of others, emotional regulation and control, and behavioral control to engage in healthy relationships with other children and adults (Missouri Department of Mental Health, n.d.). Based on the definition provided by the CEC (2003), emotional skills overlap and are integral to social skills and social competence. As with social skills, emotional skills improve with age and development. Infants learn to regulate initially through co-regulation with caregivers and then to self-soothe. *Co-regulation* is defined as warm, responsive interactions that provide the support children need to modulate their feelings and behaviors (Gillespie, 2015). Toddlers begin to learn concepts of emotions, and behavioral control emerges with adult support. Preschool children learn more about the emotions of others and continue to refine their ability to control their behavior.

Self-regulation is a term used within many professions, including psychology and education, in addition to occupational therapy. It is not always clear how occupational therapy practitioners operationally define self-regulation in the literature (Martini et al., 2016). For the purposes of this chapter, **self-regulation** is defined as

> the ability to establish and maintain an optimal state for a given situation. This includes regulating one's sensory needs, emotions, and impulses to meet the demands of the environment, reach one's goals, and behave in a socially appropriate way. (Kuypers, 2013, p. 1)

Additionally, a child needs to use emotional regulation and executive functioning to maintain self-regulation (Kuypers, 2013); children need to be able to modulate sensation, regulate emotions, and use inhibition and metacognitive aspects of executive functioning to self-regulate. Furthermore, for a young child to successfully interact with adults and peers socially, they need to integrate their emotional skills and self-regulation skills. Self-regulation grows with age and development. Initially, infants and young children rely on caregivers to support their ability to self-regulate; as they gain metacognition and executive functioning skills, children improve their ability to regulate in novel and stressful situations.

ESSENTIAL CONSIDERATIONS

A variety of diagnoses and risk factors are associated with young children experiencing delays in the areas of social skills, emotional development, and self-regulation.

Etiology

Common risk factors and associated diagnoses include children born preterm or with low birthweight, autism spectrum disorder (ASD), fetal alcohol spectrum disorders (FASD), or attention deficit hyperactivity disorder (ADHD); and children exposed to maltreatment (Biederman et al., 2012; Gill et al., 2018; Hoffman et al., 2016; Martin et al., 2018). The incidence of low birthweight in the U.S. is 8%; the prevalence of premature birth in the U.S. is 10%, with disparity in the Black community, where prevalence is 14% (Martin et al., 2018). Infants who have stayed in the neonatal intensive care unit (NICU) after birth were found to be at risk for over-responsiveness to sensory stimuli, which can influence their ability to self–regulate (Mitchell et al., 2015). The prevalence of ASD in the United States is 1 in 59 children, and male children are four times more likely than female children to be diagnosed (CDC, 2018). The number of children with FASD is challenging to capture; however, a recent study reported a conservative estimate of 1%–5% of children and a weighted prevalence of 3%–10% of children in the United States (May et al., 2018). A total of 388,000 children between the ages of 2 and 5 years were diagnosed with ADHD in the United States in 2016 (Danielson et al., 2018). Infants from birth to age 1 year are at the

highest risk for maltreatment, with a 2.5% prevalence rate; the rate overall for children in the United States in 2017 was 5.6% (U.S. Department of Health and Human Services, 2018). Further complicating the developmental trajectory for infants and young children with developmental delays is their increased risk for maltreatment compared to typically developing infants and children (CDC, 2017).

A large number of children in early childhood are likely to experience delays in social, emotional, and self-regulation skill development. Many of the associated diagnoses are not given to children under the ages of 2 to 5 years, potentially increasing the delay in access to intervention.

Associated Long-Term Outcomes

Children who have difficulties or delays in the areas of social, emotional, and self-regulation skills are at risk for poorer outcomes throughout childhood. Researchers have identified interrelated mechanisms among these skill areas. Studies have repeatedly found correlation between early social, emotional, and self-regulation skills and future academic achievement (Denham et al., 2012; Montroy et al., 2014; Skibbe et al., 2019). Children with better behavioral self-regulation tend to have better social skills (Montroy et al., 2014); emotionally negative or aggressive behavior was predictive of problems in early school adjustment and academics in kindergarten (Denham et al., 2012). Specifically, children with early development of self-regulation are more likely to have higher scores in math and literacy (Hubert et al., 2015; Montroy et al., 2014; Skibbe et al., 2019). Children rated by their parents to have higher levels of self-regulation at age 4 years had fewer problem behaviors at age 6 years based on parent and teacher reports (Sawyer et al., 2015).

There are several theories as to how self-regulation, emotional development, behavior, and social skills interact to promote success in school. One theory suggests children with better behavioral and emotional regulation have stronger social skills, which results in positive classroom relationships (Denham et al., 2012; Montroy et al., 2014). Another theory suggests children who struggle to regulate their emotions and behavior have more disruptive behavior, which creates a negative classroom relationship, leads to poorer relationships with teachers, and decreases the child's ability to learn (Montroy et al., 2014).

Preschool and child care expulsion rates are frequently associated with externalized child behaviors (Carlson et al., 2012). Additional factors contributing to preschool expulsion include the level of disruption of the learning environment, teachers fearing accountability should harm or injury occur, and the teacher's perceived stress level (Gilliam & Reyes, 2018). Unfortunately, although Black preschool children represent only 19% of enrollment, they represent 47% of suspensions, even though they were "not necessarily misbehaving more frequently than peers" (Wesley & Ellis, 2017, p. 23). Social and emotional skills provide the foundation for child success in child care, preschool, and kindergarten environments (Denham et al., 2012).

When looking at a specific diagnosis or experience, the relationship between self-regulation, social skills, emotional development, and academic and social performance is strong. As secondary disabilities associated with FASD include deficits in self-regulation and social–emotional development, children with all subtypes of FASD are more likely to have a disruption in their school experience, engage in criminal activity, demonstrate sexually inappropriate behaviors, and abuse substances (Kodituwakku, 2009; Moilanen et al., 2010). Children with ASD face barriers across their lifespan often related to differences in their self-regulation and social skills (Tanner et al., 2015). Social skills of preschool children with ASD were associated with later school achievement in all domains (Miller et al., 2017). Children who experience maltreatment are more likely to exhibit difficulties with executive function, behavior, and academic achievement early in life and struggle with depression, substance abuse, and suicidal behavior across their lifespan (Hong et al., 2018). Researchers further found poverty to be a confounding variable in determining the cognitive impact of maltreatment. Research has established that children growing up in socioeconomically disadvantaged families are at risk for poorer academic achievement and less developed self-regulation skills (Schmitt et al., 2014).

There is general consensus that early intervention for children living in low socioeconomic status families is extremely important to offset the impact of the social and environmental stress on development. To best serve their clients, occupational therapy practitioners need to be mindful of the larger contexts of the families they serve in early childhood beyond the developmental trajectories of the children (Whitcomb et al., 2015).

BEST PRACTICES

The first step in formulating the best interventions to use with a child is to complete the evaluation process. In addition to the interview, formal observation, and record review, occupational therapists must use standardized measures to evaluate social–emotional development, self-regulation, and behavior, and link results to occupational performance. After the areas of strength and concerns are identified through a thorough evaluation process, an intervention plan can be formulated incorporating evidence-based intervention practices.

Conduct a Thorough Evaluation

The evaluation process can differ based on funding source or setting, but the process will begin by gathering data for the occupational profile (AOTA, 2020). Evaluation methods may include record review, caregiver interview, naturalistic and structured observations of the child, and standardized assessment tools. Which tools occupational therapists select for an assessment are commonly linked to suspected areas of concern, the reason for referral, and funding agency criteria for eligibility for occupational therapy services (see Table 33.1 for commonly used tools). For a list of assessment tools that are frequently used to evaluate child development and participation, see Appendix F, "Examples of Assessments for Early Childhood (Birth–5 Years)."

Evaluation by occupational therapists under IDEA Part C and B

IDEA Part C (for children birth age 3 years) outlines the requirements for initial occupational therapy assessment.

The Part C regulations differentiate the terms *evaluation,* which refers to the eligibility process in identifying whether an infant or toddler qualifies as having a disability, and *assessment,* where the strengths and needs in all areas of development are analyzed by an appropriately trained interventionist to establish specific service recommendations (IDEA, 2004, §303.21). When completing an assessment, the occupational therapist, as part of the multidisciplinary team, must review the evaluation results, personally observe the child, and identify the strengths and needs across the five developmental areas (cognitive, physical, communication, social or emotional, and adaptive; IDEA, 2004, §303.21). Therefore, when selecting assessment tools, it would be most efficient to use one or two that capture all five areas of development as outlined by IDEA Part C.

Part B of IDEA has regulations regarding the evaluation and reevaluation process for children who are ages 3–5 years. Key elements include ensuring the assessment tools are not racially or culturally biased, assessing a child in all areas of suspected disability, and being sufficient to determine all of the child's related service needs (§300.304). The individualized education program (IEP) team must review existing evaluation data and evaluate the child to determine their eligibility for special education services and related services (§300.305). Best practices for evaluations include record review, parent or caregiver and teacher interviews, formal observations of the child during natural routines and context, and, if needed, valid and reliable assessment tool data. All occupations should be discussed to determine the child's strengths and needs in occupational performance (AOTA, 2020).

The IEP team must determine whether the child's behavior is impeding their or others' learning. If the answer is yes, then the team is required to "consider the use of positive behavior interventions and supports (PBIS), and other strategies to address that behavior" (IDEA, 2004, §300.324(a)(2)(i)). When a child's conduct is a manifestation of the child's disability, the IEP team is required to conduct a functional behavioral assessment (FBA), which identifies the function of the negative behavior (e.g., gain or avoid something) and the environmental conditions that affect the occurrence and reinforce the behavior. After the FBA is completed, the data are used to develop an individualized written plan called the behavioral intervention plan that describes the positive behavioral interventions, strategies, and supports for the child (IDEA, 2004, §300.530(f)(1)).

Data from all sources should be used to inform priorities and write individualized family service plan (IFSP) outcomes and IEP goals for improving social–emotional development and self-regulation skills. Outcomes written to meet IDEA Part C criteria should be free from professional jargon and reflect the child's skill performance in the context of a natural routine occurring in a natural environment. Goals written for preschoolers according to the IDEA must be measurable and reflect the child's performance in the least restrictive environment.

Evaluations by occupational therapists in health care

When evaluating a young child in the health care setting, occupational therapists should consider screening for social–emotional development, self-regulation, and behavior as part

TABLE 33.1. Commonly Used Assessments for Social–Emotional Skills in Early Childhood

TOOLS	AGE RANGE	SOCIAL SKILLS	EMOTIONAL BEHAVIOR	SELF-REGULATION
Ages and Stages Questionnaire, 3rd Edition (Squires et al., 2009)*	1–66 months	X		
Ages and Stages Questionnaire—Social Emotional (Squires et al., 2009)*	1–72 months	X	X	X
Bayley Scales of Infant and Toddler Development-4 (Bayley & Aylward, 2019)	16 days–42 months	X	X	X
Brigance Early Childhood Screens III (French, 2013)*	0–35 months; 3–5 years; K–First grade	Social–emotional skills		
Child Behavioral Checklist—Preschool (Achenbach & Rescoria, 2000)	1½ –5 years	X	X	X
Developmental Assessment of Young Children, 2nd Edition (Voress & Maddox, 2013)	Birth to 5 years, 11 months	Social–emotional domain		
Miller Function & Participation Scales (Miller, 2006)	2½–7 years, 11 months	X		X
Pediatric Evaluation of Disability Inventory Computer Adaptive Test (Haley et al., 2012)	6 months to 7 years	X		
Preschool and Kindergarten Behavior Scales, 2nd Edition (Merrell, 2003)	3–6 years	X	X	
Social-Emotional Assessment Measure (Squires et al., 2014)	2–66 months	X	X	X
Sensory Processing Measure—Preschool (Parham et al., 2007).	2–5 years	X		X
Sensory Profile 2—Infant (Dunn, 2014)	Birth to 6 months			X
Sensory Profile 2—Toddler (Dunn, 2014)	7–35 months			X
Social Skills Improvement System (Preschool; Gresham & Elliot, 2008)	3–18 years	X	X	

*Screening tool

of their process. While medical insurance companies differ in how they define medical necessity, most will fund occupational therapy intervention to improve outcomes related to ADLs. An infant's or child's social–emotional development, self-regulation, or behavior may be an underlying barrier that affects ADL performance. However, if during the evaluation process concerns are raised about the child's social–emotional development, self-regulation, and behavior that are not billable to a health insurance provider, occupational therapists must refer families to appropriate funders to address these concerns. Other funders may include the local department of mental health or IDEA.

Provide Evidence-Based Interventions

Many different evidence-based practices address the development of social, emotional, and self-regulation skills in early childhood. This section presents evidence-based interventions commonly used in occupational therapy. Interventions have been organized by the following themes: touch-based, parent-mediated/coaching, teacher-mediated/preschool, and other popular interventions used in occupational therapy practice.

Touch-based interventions

Kangaroo care and massage are evidence-based interventions used with infants and young children.

Kangaroo care, skin-to-skin contact. In infancy, emotional development is discussed initially around attachments with caregivers. Many interventions focus on caregiver–child bonding and are caregiver mediated. Research supports the use of kangaroo care or **skin-to-skin contact** to promote maternal–infant attachment with effectiveness seen with dosing as little as 30 minutes at a time (Ahn et al., 2010; Cho et al., 2016; Feldman et al., 2014). Kangaroo care and skin-to-skin interventions provide direct skin contact between an infant and a caregiver. Occupational therapy practitioners working in NICUs or clinics or providing home-based early intervention should recommend the use of skin-to-skin interventions to improve caregiver and infant attachment. This is particularly important with children who did not receive natural touch opportunities because of complex medical needs, institutionalization, or removal from their biological parent.

Massage. Several forms of *massage* can be used with children. The most supported in the literature is qigong massage, a manual therapy technique based on the principles of Chinese medicine (Silva et al., 2011) that requires training to be a competent provider. Several studies have found that qigong massage improves child behavior and increases self-regulation in children with and without ASD in early childhood (Bodison & Parham, 2018; Silva et al., 2011). Other manualized forms of massage (e.g., Babies First Massage, therapist-designed protocols) have been shown to improve child behavior, social behavior, and parent–child interactions (Bennett et al., 2013; Juneau et al., 2015; Oswalt & Biasini, 2011). Occupational therapy practitioners can recommend manualized massage programs to improve self-regulation and child behavior. The use of massage can also be used to improve caregiver and child interaction for toddlers and infants who are too big for skin-to-skin interventions.

Parent-mediated interventions and coaching interventions

Interventions that provide parent training have positively changed child behaviors.

Parent–child interaction therapy. **Parent–child interaction therapy** (PCIT) is a manualized approach that trains parents how to interact with their children through the use of a one-way mirror while parents receive real-time guidance via an earpiece (Ros et al., 2016). PCIT is typically used to address parenting behavior and externalized child behaviors (Bagner et al., 2016) and requires training to implement. After families participated in PCIT, researchers found a large reduction in challenging behavior, aggression, and defiance and improved social behavior and emotional regulation (Bagner et al., 2016; Fung et al., 2014; Rodríguez et al., 2014). Occupational therapy practitioners can become trained in PCIT, or they can refer families who are at risk for problems with parenting behavior and child externalized behavior to a trained provider.

Developmental, individual-difference, relationship-based DIR/Floortime. The **DIR/Floortime**™ intervention model is a commonly used approach for children with ASD. DIR/Floortime is a six-stage framework used to develop functional and symbolic ways of thinking and relating to others (Wieder & Greenspan, 2003). Occupational therapy practitioners may obtain pre- or post-professional training to learn how to use this approach. Two studies examined parent-delivered DIR/Floortime with preschool-age children and found significantly improved child attention and initiation with a caregiver, improved socio-emotional behavior, and better engagement (Pajareya & Nopmaneejumruslers, 2011; Solomon et al., 2014). A randomized controlled trial found parent training using the DIR/Floortime model had a large effect on how well the parents were able to interpret and reason about their own and their child's behavior and mental states, which is a mediating factor in attachment (Sealy & Glovinsky, 2016). The use of DIR/Floortime is effective for home-based early childhood services to address a variety of social–emotional and self-regulation outcomes.

Teacher-mediated and preschool interventions

Research in preschools has found mindfulness and PBIS can greatly affect positive performance.

Mindfulness. Mindfulness has become an increasingly popular approach to address child behavior and self-regulation. **Mindfulness** emerged out of Buddhist meditative practices and involves being attentive and aware of the present moment free of judgment (Moreno-Gómez & Cejudo, 2018). A wealth of research is available regarding the effectiveness of mindfulness in early childhood educational settings. Mindfulness delivered in preschool classrooms was found to have significant effects on attention, externalized behaviors (Moreno-Gómez & Cejudo, 2018), social–emotional development, social competence (Flook et al., 2015), self-regulation, self-reliance, and behavioral control (Lemberger-Truelove et al., 2018). The populations researched included children who are identified as at risk as a result of living in low socioeconomic status households.

Positive behavioral interventions and supports. Schoolwide positive behavior support (SWPBS) has been widely adopted in pre-kindergarten–12 education and is considered a best practice to prevent problem behaviors and promote positive behaviors and social skills in children (Stanton-Chapman et al., 2016). **SWPBS** includes praising and reinforcing desired behaviors, teaching social skills and replacement behaviors in the natural context, and using research to support intervention. SWPBS uses a three-tiered approach to increase the supports as needed for children who do not respond to the integrated tier one approaches in their classrooms. It is best to individualize PBIS strategies using data collected through functional behavioral assessments and incorporate the expertise of the entire IEP team. The use of PBIS has been shown to improve social skills and reduce problem and externalized behaviors in a variety of populations, including preschool programs in community-based Head Start programs (Dunlap et al., 2018; Stanton-Chapman et al., 2016).

As a member of the IEP team, occupational therapy practitioners need to contribute to the functional behavioral assessment and assist in the generation of the individualized positive behavior support plan for children. An occupational therapist must review the IEP and ensure implementation of the positive behavior support plan during the occupational therapy evaluation process and intervention. Not doing so would violate the child's educational rights.

Other common occupational therapy interventions

Several highly popular interventions frequently used by occupational therapy practitioners in early childhood settings may not have research evidence supporting their efficacy at this time. Practitioners may choose to use these interventions based on practice-based evidence.

Social Stories. **Social Stories**™ provide children with individualized stories that provide social cognition for an anticipated situation that may change routines or an unfamiliar social situation (Gray & Garand, 1993). Social Stories are typically used with children with ASD. A low level of research evidence supports the use of Social Stories with preschool children. The use of Social Stories in combination with sensory strategies reduced the number of incidences of problem behaviors in the classroom (Thompson & Johnston, 2013). During the phase where Social Stories were read daily, a reduction in aggression was observed in typically developing Head Start preschoolers (Benish & Bramlett, 2011).

Sensory integration and sensory-based interventions. A limited amount of research exists regarding the effectiveness of sensory integration treatment and sensory-based interventions (i.e., sensory strategies), and it is even more limited for children from birth to age 5 years. Sensory integration treatment is one of the most used approaches for children with ASD. **Sensory strategies** are frequently used by occupational therapy practitioners in homes and school environments to address self-regulation in children. Sensory strategies are ways of providing sensory experiences throughout a child's environments and activities as a compensation for sensory processing differences to support participation in occupations (Bodison & Parham, 2018). Practitioners should collect data to determine the effectiveness of these interventions on a case-by-case basis.

Two studies examined the use of therapy balls for seating (Bagatell et al., 2010; Schilling & Schwartz, 2004). One found qualitative data suggesting increased task engagement during seated work on the ball (Schilling & Schwartz, 2004); the other study found low levels of evidence for in-seat behavior for kindergarten students who were identified as having vestibular and proprioception-seeking behaviors (Bagatell et al., 2010).

Two studies have examined the use of weighted vests with 2- to 5-year-olds, providing low levels of evidence (Fertel-Daly et al., 2001; Reichow et al., 2010). Research on the use of weighted vests in 2- to 4-year-olds identified as having pervasive developmental disorder-not otherwise specified (PDD-NOS) found increases in attention to task and decreased self-stimulatory behavior (Fertel-Daly et al., 2001). Another study found no impact on task engagement (Reichow et al., 2010).

The Alert Program. Many occupational therapy practitioners use the cognitive self-regulation program called the *Alert Program*, which teaches children to recognize their level of alertness and identify strategies for maintaining a "just right" level of alertness (Williams & Shellenberger, 1996). One study that measured effectiveness in 3- to 5-year-olds found improvements in the children's ability to use self-regulation vocabulary and recognize feelings with no statistically significant results (Blackwell et al., 2014). Some very rigorous studies using the Alert Program have shown statistically significant improvements with older children diagnosed with FASD, including one study that showed an increase in gray matter growth in brain areas associated with emotional regulation and inhibitory control in 8- to 12-year-olds with FASD post-intervention compared to controls (Soh et al., 2015).

When providing intervention, occupational therapy practitioners must document thoroughly. There are multiple purposes of documentation, including data collection to monitor progress. Data regarding a child's response to intervention and their progress are important for many intervention decisions, including continuation of service, frequency of service, duration of service, and service delivery models. Additionally, recognizing that some interventions commonly used in early childhood occupational therapy practice have limited evidence in the literature, occupational therapy providers need to use data collection as a method to inform their practice-based evidence. See Chapter 6, "Best Practices in Data-Based Decision Making."

Outcomes

Payment sources often drive the types of outcomes or goals used when working with infants and young children. IDEA Part C requires jargon-free outcomes based on routines in the natural environment. IDEA Part B services require professionals to write goals specific to how the child will access their educational program in the least restrictive environment. Health care–related goals require measuring a child's progress in terms of medical necessity and ADL performance. See Exhibit 33.1 for sample outcome and goal language.

SUMMARY

Occupational therapy practitioners working in early childhood have many choices and decisions to make when evaluating and formulating treatment plans for their clients, and no single piece of evidence should dominate the decision-making process. Practitioners are trained to

---

EXHIBIT 33.1.	Example Language for Addressing Social–Emotional Development and Self-Regulation
OUTCOME LANGUAGE (IFSP)	**GOAL LANGUAGE (IEP)**
▪ Self-soothe	▪ Complete teacher-directed task
▪ Seek caregiver for comfort	▪ Identify their level of alertness and emotional state
▪ Follow 1-step directions	▪ Follow 2-step directions
▪ Ask for access to self-regulation strategies	▪ Identify others' emotions
▪ Express feelings	▪ Select a self-regulation strategy
▪ Comfort others	▪ Comfort friends
	▪ Seek an adult for help

Note. IEP = individualized education program; IFSP = individualized family service plan.

consider the child and family system, the environments the child engages in, and the desired occupational participation. The art and skill are to use professional reasoning to ensure the child and family participate in the therapeutic process with consistent progress.

REFERENCES

Achenbach, T., & Rescoria, L. (2000). *Child behavior checklist preschool (Preschool CBCL)*. ASEBA.

Ahn, H. Y., Lee, J., & Shin, H. J. (2010). Kangaroo care on premature infant growth and maternal attachment and post-partum depression in South Korea. *Journal of Tropical Pediatrics, 56*(5), 342–344. https://doi.org/10.1093/tropej/fmq063

American Occupational Therapy Association. (2020). Occupational therapy practice framework: Domain and process (4th ed.). *American Journal of Occupational Therapy, 74*(Suppl. 2), 7412410010. https://doi.org/10.5014/ajot.2020.74S2001

Bagatell, N., Mirigliani, G., Patterson, C., Reyes, Y., & Test, L. (2010). Effectiveness of therapy ball chairs on classroom participation in children with autism spectrum disorders. *American Journal of Occupational Therapy, 64*, 895–903. https://doi.org/10.5014/ajot.2010.09149

Bagner, D. M., Coxe, S., Hungerford, G. M., Garcia, D., Barroso, N. E., Hernandez, J., & Rosa-Olivares, J. (2016). Behavioral parent training in infancy: A window of opportunity for high-risk families. *Journal of Abnormal Child Psychology, 44*, 901–912. https://doi.org/10.1007/s10802-015-0089-5

Bayley, N., & Aylward, G. P. (2019). *Bayley Scales of Infant and Toddler Development* (4th ed.). NCS Pearson.

Benish, T. M., & Bramlett, R. K. (2011). Using Social Stories to decrease aggression and increase positive peer interactions in normally developing preschool children. *Educational Psychology in Practice, 27*, 1–17. https://doi.org/10.1080/02667363.2011.549350

Bennett, C., Underdown, A., & Barlow, J. (2013). Massage for promoting mental and physical health in typically developing infants under the age of six months. *Cochrane Database of Systematic Reviews, 4*, CD005038. https://doi.org/10.1002/14651858.CD005038.pub3

Biederman, J., Spencer, T. J., Petty, C., Hyder, L. L., O'Connor, K. B., Surman, C. B. H., & Faraone, S. V. (2012). Longitudinal course of deficient emotional self-regulation CBCL profile in youth with ADHD: Prospective controlled study. *Neuropsychiatric Disease and Treatment, 8*, 267–276. https://doi.org/10.2147/NDT.S29670

Blackwell, A. L., Yeager, D. C., Mische-Lawson, L., Bird, R. J., & Cook, D. M. (2014). Teaching children self-regulation skills within the early childhood education environment: A feasibility study. *Journal of Occupational Therapy, Schools, & Early Intervention, 7*(3–4), 204–224. https://doi.org/10.1080/19411243.2014.966013

Bodison, S. C., & Parham, L. D. (2018). Specific sensory techniques and sensory environmental modifications for children and youth with sensory integration difficulties: A systematic review. *American Journal of Occupational Therapy, 72*, 7201190040. https://doi.org/10.5014/ajot.2018.029413

Carlson, J. S., Mackrain, M. A., Van Egeren, L. A., Brophy-Herb, H., Kirk, R. H., Marciniak, D., . . . Tableman, B. (2012). Implementing a statewide early childhood mental health consultation approach to preventing childcare expulsion. *Infant Mental Health Journal, 33*(3), 265–273. https://doi.org/10.1002/imhj.21336

Centers for Disease Control and Prevention. (2017). *Childhood maltreatment among children with disabilities.* https://www.cdc.gov/ncbddd/disabilityandsafety/abuse.html

Centers for Disease Control and Prevention. (2018). *Facts about developmental disabilities.* https://www.cdc.gov/ncbddd/developmentaldisabilities/facts.html

Cho, E., Kim, S., Kwon, M., Cho, H., Kim, E., Jun, E., & Lee, S. (2016). The effects of kangaroo care in the neonatal intensive care unit on the physiological functions of preterm infants, maternal–infant attachment, and maternal stress. *Journal of Pediatric Nursing, 31*, 430–438. https://doi.org/10.1016/j.pedn.2016.02.007

Council for Exceptional Children, Division for Learning Disabilities and Division for Research. (2003, Fall). Social skills instruction for students with learning disabilities. *Current Practice Alerts,* Issue 9, pp. 1–4.

Danielson, M. L., Bitsko, R. H., Ghandour, R. M., Holbrook, J. R., Kogan, M. D., & Blumberg, S. J. (2018). Prevalence of parent-reported ADHD diagnosis and associated treatment among U.S. children and adolescents, 2016. *Journal of Clinical Child & Adolescent Psychology, 47*(2), 199–212. https://doi.org/10.1080/15374416.2017.1417860

Denham, S. A., Bassett, H. H., Thayer, S. K., Mincic, M. S., Sirotkin, Y. S., & Zinsser, K. (2012). Observing preschoolers' social-emotional behavior: Structure, foundations, and prediction of early school success. *Journal of Genetic Psychology, 173*, 246–278. https://doi.org/10.1080/00221325.2011.597457

Dunlap, G., Strain, P., Lee, J. K., Joseph, J., & Leech, N. (2018). A randomized controlled evaluation of prevent-teach-reinforce for young children. *Topics in Early Childhood Special Education, 37*(4), 195–205. https://doi.org/10.1177/0271121417724874

Dunn, W. (2014). *Sensory profile 2 manual* (2nd ed.). Pearson.

Feldman, R., Rosenthal, Z., & Eidelman, A. (2014). Maternal-preterm skin-to-skin contact enhances child physiologic organization and cognitive control across the first 10 years of life. *Biological Psychiatry, 75*, 56–64. https://doi.org/10.1016/j.biopsych.2013.08.012

Fertel-Daly, D., Bedell, G., & Hinojosa, J. (2001). Effects of a weighted vest on attention to task and self-stimulatory behaviors in preschoolers with pervasive developmental disorders. *American Journal of Occupational Therapy, 55*, 629–640. https://doi.org/10.5014/ajot.55.6.629

Flook, L., Goldberg, S. B., Pinger, L., & Davidson, R. J. (2015). Promoting prosocial behavior and self-regulatory skills in preschool children through a mindfulness-based kindness curriculum. *Developmental Psychology, 51*(1), 44–51. https://doi.org/10.1037/a0038256

French, B. (2013). *Brigance Early Childhood Screens III*. Curriculum Associates.

Fung, M. P., Fox, R. A., & Harris, S. E. (2014). Treatment outcomes for at-risk young children with behavior problems: Toward a new definition of success. *Journal of Social Service Research, 40*, 623–641. https://doi.org/10.1080/01488376.2014.915283

Gill, K., Thompson-Hodgetts, S., & Rasmussen, C. (2018). A critical review of research on the Alert Program. *Journal of Occupational Therapy, Schools & Early Intervention, 11*, 212–228. https://doi.org/10.1080/19411243.2018.1432445

Gillespie, L. (2015). Rocking and rolling—It takes two: The role of co-regulation in building self-regulation skills. *Young Children, 70*(3), 94–96.

Gilliam, W. S., & Reyes, C. R. (2018). Teacher decision factors that lead to preschool expulsion: Scale development and preliminary validation of the preschool expulsion risk measure. *Infants & Young Children, 31*(2), 93–108. https://doi.org/10.1097/IYC.0000000000000113

Gray, C. A., & Garand, J. D. (1993). Social stories: Improving responses of students with autism with accurate social information. *Focus on Autistic Behavior, 8*(1), 1–10. https://doi.org/10.1177/108835769300800101

Griswold, L. A., & Townsend, S. (2012). Assessing the sensitivity or the evaluation of social interaction: Comparing social skills in children with and without disabilities. *American Journal of Occupational Therapy, 66,* 709–717. https://doi.org/10.5014/ajot.2012.004051

Gresham, R., & Elliot, S. N. (2008). *Social Skills Improvement System (SSIS) Rating Scales.* NCS Pearson.

Haley, S. M., Coster, W. J., Dumas, H. M., Fragala-Pinkham, M. A., & Moed, R. (2012). *Pediatric Evaluation of Disability Inventory Computer Adaptive Test (PEDI-CAT).* CRE Care.

Hoffman, J. A., Bunger, A. C., Roberstson, H. A., Cao, Y., & West, K. Y. (2016). Child welfare caseworker's perspectives on the challenges of addressing mental health problems in early childhood. *Children and Youth Services Review, 65,* 148–155. https://doi.org/10.1016/j.childyouth.2016.04.003

Hong, S., Rhee, T. G., & Piescher, K. N. (2018). Longitudinal association of child maltreatment and cognitive functioning: Implications for child development. *Child Abuse & Neglect, 84,* 64–73. https://doi.org/10.1016/j.chiabu.2018.07.026

Hubert, B., Guimard, P., Florin, A., & Tracy, A. (2015). Indirect and direct relationships between self-regulation and academic achievement during the nursery/elementary school transition of French students, *Early Education and Development, 26,* 5–6, 685–707. https://doi.org/10.1080/10409289.2015.1037624

Individuals with Disabilities Education Improvement Act of 2004, Pub. L. 108–446, 20 U.S.C. §§ 1400-1482.

Juneau, A. L., Aita, M., & Héon, M. (2015). Review and critical analysis of massage studies for term and preterm infants. *Neonatal Network, 34,* 165–177. https://doi.org/10.1891/0730-0832.34.3.165

Kauffman, N. A., & Kinnealey, M. (2015). Comprehensive social skills taxonomy: Development and application. *American Journal of Occupational Therapy, 69,* 6902220030. https://doi.org/10.5014/ajot.2015.013151

Kodituwakku, P. W. (2009). Neurocognitive profile in children with fetal alcohol spectrum disorders. *Developmental Disabilities Research Reviews, 15*(3), 218–224. https://doi.org/10.1002/ddrr.73

Kuypers, L. (2013). The zones of regulation: A framework to foster self-regulation. *Sensory Integration Special Interest Section Quarterly, 36*(4), 1–4.

Lemberger-Truelove, M. E., Carbonneau, K. J., Atencio, D. J., Zieher, A. K., & Palacios, A. F. (2018). Self-regulatory growth effects for young children participating in a combined social and emotional learning and mindfulness-based intervention. *Journal of Counseling & Development, 96,* 289–302. https://doi.org/10.1002/jcad.12203

Marrus, N., Glowinski, A. L., Jacob, T., Klin, A., Jones, W., Drain, C. E., . . . Constantino, J. N. (2015). Rapid video-referenced ratings of reciprocal social behavior in toddlers: A twin study. *Journal of Child Psychology and Psychiatry, and Allied Disciplines, 56,* 1338–1346. https://doi.org/10.1111/jcpp.12391

Martin, J. A., Hamilton, B. E., Osterman, M. J. K., Driscoll, A. K., & Drake, P. (2018). Births: Final data for 2017. *National Vital Statistics Reports, 67*(8), 1–50. https://www.cdc.gov/nchs/data/nvsr/nvsr67/nvsr67_08-508.pdf

Martini, R., Cramm, H., Egan, M., & Sikora, L. (2016). Scoping review of self-regulation: What are occupational therapists talking about? *American Journal of Occupational Therapy, 70,* 7006290010. https://doi.org/10.5014/ajot.2016.020362

May, P., Chambers, C., Kalberg, W., Zellner, J., Feldman, H., Buckley, D., . . . Hoyme, H. (2018). Prevalence of fetal alcohol spectrum disorders in 4 U.S. communities. *JAMA, 319*(5), 474–482. https://doi.org/10.1001/jama.2017.21896

Merrell, K. W. (2003). *Preschool and Kindergarten Behavior Scales* (2nd ed.). Pro-Ed.

Miller, L. J. (2006). *Miller Function and Participation Scales examiner's manual.* Psychological Corp.

Miller, L. E., Burke, J. D., Troyb, E., Knoch, K., Herlihy, L. E., & Fein, D. A. (2017). Preschool predictors of school-age academic achievement in autism spectrum disorder. *Clinical Neuropsychology, 31*(2), 382–403. https://doi.org/10.1080/13854046.2016.1225665

Missouri Department of Mental Health. (n.d.). *Early childhood mental health: What is social and emotional development.* https://dmh.mo.gov/healthykids/parents/social-emotional-development

Mitchell, A. W., Moore, E. M., Roberts, E. J., Hachtel, K. W., & Brown, M. S. (2015). Sensory processing disorder in children ages birth–3 years born prematurely: A systematic review. *American Journal of Occupational Therapy, 69,* 6901220030. https://doi.org/10.5014/ajot.2015.013755

Moilanen, K., Shaw, D., & Fitzpatrick, A. (2010). Self-regulation in early adolescence: Relations with mother-son relationship quality and maternal regulatory support and antagonism. *Journal of Youth and Adolescence, 39*(11), 1357–1367. https://doi.org/10.1007/s10964-009-9485-x

Montroy, J. J., Bowles, R. P., Skibbe, L. E., & Foster, T. D. (2014). Social skills and problem behaviors as mediators of the relationship between behavioral self-regulation and academic achievement. *Early Childhood Research Quarterly, 29,* 298–309. https://doi.org/10.1016/j.ecresq.2014.03.002

Moreno-Gómez, A.-J., & Cejudo, J. (2018). Effectiveness of a mindfulness-based social-emotional learning program on psychosocial adjustment and neuropsychological maturity in kindergarten children. *Mindfulness, 10,* 111–121. https://doi.org/10.1007/s12671-018-0956-6

Oswalt, K., & Biasini, F. (2011). Effects of infant massage on HIV-infected mothers and their infants. *Journal for Specialists in Pediatric Nursing, 16,* 169–178. https://doi.org/10.1111/j.1744-6155.2011.00291.x

Pajareya, K., & Nopmaneejumruslers, K. (2011). A pilot randomized controlled trial of DIR/Floortime™ parent training intervention for pre-school children with autistic spectrum disorders. *Autism, 15*(5), 563–577. https://doi.org/10.1177/1362361310386502

Parham, D., Ecker, C., Miller-Kuhaneck, H., Henry, D. A., & Glennon, T. J. (2007). *Sensory Processing Measure–Preschool: Manual.* Western Psychological Services.

Reichow, B., Barton, E. E., Sewell, J. N., Good, L., & Wolery, M. (2010). Effects of weighted vests on the engagement of children with developmental delays and autism. *Focus on Autism and Other Developmental Disabilities, 25*(1), 3–11. https://doi.org/10.1177/1088357609353751

Rodríguez, G. M., Bagner, D. M., & Graziano, P. A. (2014). Parent training for children born premature: A pilot study examining the moderating role of emotion regulation. *Child Psychiatry and Human Development, 45*, 143–152. https://doi.org/10.1007/s10578-013-0385-7

Ros, R., Hernandez, J., Graziano, P. A., & Bagner, D. M. (2016). Parent training for children with or at risk for developmental delay: The role of parental homework completion. *Behavior Therapy, 47*(1), 1–13. https://doi.org/10.1016/j.beth.2015.08.004

Sasson, N., Nowlin, R., & Pinkham, A. (2013). Social cognition, social skill, and the broad autism phenotype. *Autism, 17*(6), 655–667. https://doi.org/10.1177/1362361312455704

Sawyer, A., Chittleborough, C., Mittinty, M., Miller-Lewis, L., Sawyer, M., Sullivan, T., & Lynch, J. (2015). Are trajectories of self-regulation abilities from ages 2–3 to 6–7 associated with academic achievement in the early school years?: Self-regulation and early academic achievement. *Child: Care, Health and Development, 41*(5), 744–754. https://doi.org/10.1111/cch.12208

Schilling, D. L., & Schwartz, I. S. (2004). Alternative seating for young children with autism spectrum disorder: Effects on classroom behavior. *Journal of Autism and Developmental Disorders, 34*(4), 423–432. https://doi.org/10.1023/B:JADD.0000037418.48587.f4

Schmitt, S. A., McClellan, M. M., Tominey, S. L., & Acock, A. C. (2014) Strengthening school readiness for Head Start children: Evaluation of a self-regulation intervention. *Early Childhood Research Quarterly, 30*, 20–31. https://doi.org/10.1016/j.ecresq.2014.08.001

Sealy, J., & Glovinsky, I. P. (2016). Strengthening the reflective functioning capacities of parents who have a child with a neurodevelopmental disability through a brief, relationship-focused intervention. *Infant Mental Health Journal, 37*(2), 115–124. https://doi.org/10.1002/imhj.21557

Silva, L. M., Schalock, M., & Gabrielsen, K. (2011). Early intervention for autism with a parent-delivered Qigong massage program: A randomized controlled trial. *American Journal of Occupational Therapy, 65*, 550–559. https://doi.org/10.5014/ajot.2011.000661

Skibbe, L. E., Montroy, J. J., Bowles, R. P., & Morrison, F. J. (2019). Self-regulation and the development of literacy and language achievement from preschool through second grade. *Early Childhood Research Quarterly, 46*, 240–251. https://doi.org/10.1016/j.ecresq.2018.02.005

Soh, D. W., Skocic, J., Nash, K., Stevens, S., Turner, G. R., & Rovet, J. (2015). Self-regulation therapy increases frontal gray matter in children with fetal alcohol spectrum disorder: Evaluation by voxel-based morphometry. *Frontiers in Human Neuroscience, 9*(108), 1–12. https://doi.org/10.3389/fnhum.2015.00108

Solomon, R., Van Egeren, L. A., Mahoney, G., Quon Huber, M. S., & Zimmerman, P. (2014). PLAY Project Home Consultation intervention program for young children with autism spectrum disorders: A randomized controlled trial. *Journal of Developmental & Behavioral Pediatrics, 35*(8), 475–485. https://doi.org/10.1097/dbp.0000000000000096

Squires, J., Bricker, D., Waddell, M., Funk, K., Clifford, J., & Hoselton, R. (2014). *Social Emotional Assessment/Evaluation Measure (SEAM)* (research ed.). Brookes.

Squires, J., Twombly, E., Bricker, D., & Potter, L. (2009). *Ages and Stages Questionnaires* (3rd ed.) *(ASQ-3)*. Brookes.

Stanton-Chapman, T. L., Walker, V. L., Voorhees, M. D., & Snell, M. E. (2016). The evaluation of a three-tier model of positive behavior interventions and supports for preschoolers in Head Start. *Remedial and Special Education, 37*(6), 333–344. https://doi.org/10.1177/0741932516629650

Tanner, K., Hand, B. N., O'Toole, G., & Lane, A. E. (2015). Effectiveness of interventions to improve social participation, play, leisure, and restricted and repetitive behaviors in people with autism spectrum disorder: A systematic review. *American Journal of Occupational Therapy, 69*, 6905180010. https://doi.org/10.5014/ajot.2015.017806

Thompson, R., & Johnston, S. (2013). Use of Social Stories to improve self-regulation in children with autism spectrum disorders. *Physical & Occupational Therapy in Pediatrics, 33*(3), 271–284. https://doi.org/10.3109/01942638.2013.768322

U.S. Department of Health and Human Services, Administration for Children and Families, Children's Bureau. (2018). *Child maltreatment 2017.* https://www.acf.hhs.gov/cb/research-data-technology/statistics-research/child-maltreatment

Voress, J. K., & Maddox, T. (2013). *Developmental Assessment of Young Children* (2nd ed.). Pro-Ed.

Wesley, L., & Ellis, A. L. (2017). Exclusionary discipline in preschool: Young black boys' lives matter. *Journal of African American Males in Education, 8*(2), 22–29. http://journalofafricanamericanmales.com/wp-content/uploads/2017/12/3-Wesley-Ellis-2017-ExclusionaryDiscipline-in-PreSchool.pdf

Whitcomb, D. A., Carrasco, R. C., Neuman, A., & Kloos, H. (2015). Correlational research to examine the relation between attachment and sensory modulation in young children. *American Journal of Occupational Therapy, 69*, 6904220020. https://doi.org/10.5014/ajot.2015.015503

Wieder, S., & Greenspan, S. I. (2003). Climbing the symbolic ladder in the DIR model through floor time/interactive play. *Autism, 7*(4), 425–435, https://doi.org/10.1177/1362361303007004008

Williams, M. S., & Shellenberger, S. (1996). *"How does your engine run?": A leader's guide to the Alert Program for self-regulation.* TherapyWorks.

Best Practices in Supporting Play and Leisure Activities

34

Bonnie Riley, OTD, OTR/L

KEY TERMS AND CONCEPTS

- Associative play
- Constructive play
- Contextual influences
- Co-occupations
- Cooperative play
- Exploratory play
- Functional play
- Materials
- Meaningfulness
- Modeling
- Natural contexts and routines
- Onlooker play
- Parallel play
- Play
- Play outcomes
- Prompting
- Social skill interventions
- Solitary play
- Symbolic play

OVERVIEW

Play is a meaningful childhood occupation, a desired outcome of occupational therapy intervention, and should be prioritized as an occupational therapy outcome for children (Miller Kuhaneck et al., 2013). The *Occupational Therapy Practice Framework: Domain and Process* (4th ed.; American Occupational Therapy Association [AOTA], 2020), which identifies play and leisure as occupations, defines **play** as "an activity which is intrinsically motivated, internally controlled, freely chosen, and may include the suspension of reality" (p. 90; Skard & Bundy, 2008) and defines *leisure* as "nonobligatory activity that is intrinsically motivated and engaged in during discretionary time, that is, time not committed to obligatory occupations such as work, self-care, or sleep" (as quoted in Parham & Fazio, 1997, p. 250).

Play is undeniably an important childhood occupation; it promotes personal well-being as well as cognitive, motor, and social development (Parham & Fazio, 2008; Yogman et al., 2018). Preschool children who are given the opportunity to play for a single 15-minute session are two times more likely to feel a reduction in stress than children not offered the same opportunity (Yogman et al., 2018). The American Academy of Pediatrics emphasizes the importance of play as a tool for stress reduction and as essential for healthy child development, including promotion of executive function skills and healthy parent–child bonds, through its Power of Play initiative (Yogman et al., 2018).

As children's cognitive, motor, and social capacities develop during play, their leisure pursuits also develop and change. Children pursue leisure activities for recreation and rejuvenation, depending on their interests. From a functionalist perspective, leisure activities are vital for well-being and prepare the child for work (Parham & Fazio, 2008).

This chapter addresses the benefits of play as well as unique concerns children with delays or disabilities may experience when participating in play. The social and family contexts for play are emphasized, and tools for authentic play assessment and evaluation are introduced. Intervention considerations and strategies are described to promote play as a valuable childhood occupation.

ESSENTIAL CONSIDERATIONS

To support opportunities for inclusive play, a child's physical and cognitive needs must be considered (Law et al., 2015). *Meaningfulness* during play should be determined by individual children or amongst individual groups and families; the meaning will vary from child to child and family to family and should be emphasized by promoting freedom of choice within play.

Benefits of Play and Leisure

Play is an important protective factor for children who may be at risk for poor health outcomes (McDonald et al., 2016), and leisure shared between the child and family is important for family well-being. Promoting play initiated by the child and encouraging child playfulness can improve the child's mental health, which can have long-lasting implications for a child with a disability. Parents of children with a disability value their child's ability to independently play (Childress, 2011); however, a child with a developmental delay may participate differently in play and experience play both positively and negatively (Graham et al., 2018).

Play during leisure is an important opportunity for healthy family **co-occupations,** or activities shared between child and parent or caregiver. Leisure is important for family health as well as parent well-being and competency (Hodge et al., 2015).

Play creates learning opportunities

Play promotes the development of many skills important for lifelong learning, including executive functioning. When play is flexible and children have the opportunity to make decisions during play, they begin to develop cognitive processing skills. As a child explores during play, a foundation for higher learning develops. For example, a child building a fort with blankets must explore the physical qualities of the objects being used to meet their goal of making a place to hide. Additionally, play may support a child's readiness for learning and ability to retain learning. For instance, a child carrying letters on a toy train to match with letters on an alphabet rug is promoting learning through letter recognition during play.

Play improves mental health

Play fosters positive well-being while offering the opportunity to discover self-awareness and develop social relationships. Activities pursued as play and leisure are selected because they are fun and exciting, and happiness will result. The experience of play itself is motivating to the child, which supports resiliency and positive self-esteem (Parham & Fazio, 2008). As a child distinguishes their play interests and expands their play behaviors, opportunities to share their interests with others can expand their social interactions.

Play during caregiving routines

Opportunities to play throughout the day are important. Integrating play as household tasks are addressed and caregiving routines are initiated by the adult offer an increased opportunity for children and their families to play. In the home, play may occur most frequently while the parent is engaged in other activities and as a support during caregiving routines (Childress, 2011).

Impact of Delays and Disabilities on Children's Play

For a child with a disability, "collaborative play is beneficial . . . regardless of their disability" (Childress, 2011, p. 112). Children with a disability may require parent support to realize increasing competency with play. Parents tend to scaffold and provide opportunities for play in which they know their child can be successful and use play to help the child adjust to daily situations in which they must engage (Childress, 2011).

Play may demand motor skills, social interaction skills (e.g., turn taking, coping skills or frustration tolerance, perseverance), and process skills (e.g., imitation, problem solving, sequence, planning). Play is positive for a child with a disability when they can play on their own and a negative experience when they feel excluded from play with limited choices in their play (Graham et al., 2018). When a child with a developmental disability is playing, their play patterns may vary from those of typically developing children. Preschool children with a disability present with unique play patterns, preferring to engage with a limited number of toys that provide sensorimotor input for relatively short periods of time and spending as much as 20% of their time watching others in the room (Fallon & MacCobb, 2013). A child with a disability may engage in play by watching a game, and when they participate in play, they often require adult support or follow the lead of others (Graham et al., 2018).

The presence of a developmental delay influences the development of play. For example, the severity of motor impairments negatively affects the ability of a child with cerebral palsy to engage in pretend play (Pfeifer et al., 2011). A child with sensory processing challenges will likely demonstrate play influenced by sensory preferences and miss social cues when playing with others, which leads to an increase in the likelihood of conflict during play with others (Cosbey et al., 2012). A child with autism spectrum disorder may have expressive and receptive language challenges, difficulty with fine motor skills, and differential visual perception abilities; the severity of all these symptoms influence the child's play (Pierucci et al., 2014). The higher a child's intelligence or mental age the more likely it is that the child will demonstrate self-regulation during play and engage in pretend play.

When an occupational therapy practitioner promotes play as an outcome of intervention, contextual influences on play must be considered and optimized (King et al., 2018). (*Note. Occupational therapy practitioner* refers to both occupational therapists and occupational therapy assistants.) ***Contextual influences*** on play can promote the abilities of a child with a disability and include the presence of others, the time of day the play is occurring, as well as the ability to physically access where play is occurring and to adapt to the sensory aspects of the play. Additionally, children with a developmental disability value social interaction during play (Graham et al., 2018); therefore, the context should be structured to promote the opportunity for socialization.

BEST PRACTICES

Play is a meaningful childhood occupation with many implications for overall health and well-being. When play is included in an occupational therapy evaluation, the individual's perception of the activity as play as well as their play skills should be considered. Occupational therapy practitioners may use play as the outcome of intervention and as an intervention tool to build skills.

Initiate Evaluation: Complete an Occupational Profile

Capturing the complexity of play during an occupational therapy evaluation or as part of a multidisciplinary team begins with interviewing persons (e.g., parents, grandparents, child care provider, preschool teacher) with knowledge about the child's occupations. Gathering the occupational profile provides the occupational therapist with information about the supports and barriers to the child's performance in all occupations while also providing insight into the child's strengths and interests in play. Some questions and prompts to promote discussion about the child's play include the following:

- "What fun activities do you and your child like to do together (e.g., going for a walk, swinging at the playground, blowing bubbles)?"
- "Describe your child's play with other children."
- "What are your child's interests? What things does your child enjoy, and what holds their attention (e.g., people, places, toys, pet, being outside)?"
- "What makes your child happy, laugh, or smile?"

- "Describe the routines and activities your child does not like or does not choose. What makes the routine or activity difficult and uncomfortable?"
- "Who are key family members, other caregivers, and important people who play with your child, and in what settings does this occur?"
- "Describe new play opportunities or activities that you would like your child to try to expand their play repertoire."

Observe Young Children's Play

In addition to interviews and record reviews gathered by the occupational therapist, the occupational therapy practitioner uses observations of the child playing with peers, siblings, and parents or caregivers in natural contexts (e.g., home, preschool, community) and within their natural routines to support the authentic assessment of play. Practitioners in health care settings should use observation of the child in the clinic while using parent report or videos to augment their assessment.

Assessing play requires the occupational therapist to make inferences about intrinsic factors to play through observed behavior (Parham & Fazio, 2008). The child's playfulness, play preferences, and social behaviors and skills in play patterns should also be noted (Mulligan, 2014). Formal observation should occur within **natural contexts and routines.** These contexts greatly expand and rapidly change in early childhood. An infant's play may occur during skin-to-skin contact while they listen to their parent's voice and gentle rocking is provided. In comparison, a preschooler's play frequently occurs in community spaces, such as a playground, with family and strangers present while they engage in numerous play behaviors and interactions. Understanding the development of play behaviors and social interactions supports the practitioner's authentic assessment when they observe a child playing.

Observe play with toys and objects

Occupational therapy practitioners may describe play by observing the child interact with objects (see Exhibit 34.1). **Exploratory play** occurs when a child engages with an object mainly to understand the possible uses of the object.

> **EXHIBIT 34.1.** Key Features and Qualitative Aspects of Play to Note During Authentic Observations of Play
>
> - Note the kinds of play materials the child frequently selects.
> - Analyze the flexibility in the child's play engagement. For example, do they get "stuck" and engage in repetitive, restrictive play activities?
> - Document the child's focus on actions with objects (e.g., bang, shake, put in and take out) and how they explore the characteristics of objects.
> - Does the child use materials to construct or create? If so, what materials do they use?
> - Observe how the child uses objects in symbolic or pretend ways.
> - Does the child use toys and materials to create meaningful sequences and stories in their play? For example, the child pretends to put toothpaste on a toothbrush, puts the cap on the tube, brushes the baby's teeth, and puts the baby to bed.
> - For preschoolers, note whether the child is able to assume a role and use props while playing. If not, what are the barriers to participation in role-play?

Functional play occurs when a child uses objects in manners imitating others who have used the object. **Symbolic play** is when the child applies their imagination to the manipulation of the object. **Constructive play** occurs as rules are applied and new uses of the object are created.

Observe social play participation

Play may occur individually or with others, and the interactions with others may become increasingly complex. The social behaviors of play (identified in Table 34.1) describe a child's interaction with others during play activities.

Supplement Authentic Assessment Using Assessment Tools

Occupational therapists may support observations of authentic play with an assessment tool. Examples of

TABLE 34.1. Social Behaviors of Play and Strategies to Promote Social Interaction

SOCIAL PLAY BEHAVIORS	PLAY DESCRIPTION	STRATEGIES TO PROMOTE PLAY
Solitary play	Child plays alone; is aware only of their own play	Provide context supports to promote self-discovery and sensory play; scaffold opportunities for observation to mimic child or imitate adult or peer
Onlooker play	Child watches another child playing from a periphery	Provide opportunities to observe play that is meaningful to the child and play in which the child may engage
Parallel play	Child plays alongside other child and may use similar toys; however, children do not interact	Provide context supports to promote self-regulation and interaction; scaffold opportunities to take turns
Associative play	Child begins share things or join in other play while playing alongside other children	Provide variety of popular ideas and items during play; scaffold play by emphasizing structured opportunities to join play
Cooperative play	Child plays and interacts with other children for a common purpose or goal	Provide opportunity for each child to have similar task to achieve a goal or finish an activity; scaffold play with simple, easy-to-follow rules

Source. Adapted from Movahedazarhouligh (2018).

TABLE 34.2. Play Assessments Commonly Used by Occupational Therapists

PLAY ASSESSMENT TOOL	DESCRIPTION
Pediatric Interest Profiles (Henry, 2000)	Kid Play Profile surveys child's interest and participation in specific play and leisure activities
Play Assessment Scale (Fewell, 1986)	Examines skills demonstrated during play with specified set of toys and one adult examiner providing verbal interaction
Revised Knox Preschool Play Scale (Knox, 2008)	Evaluates play behaviors (categorized as space management, gross motor play, materials management, symbolic play, and social participation) during 15-minute observation using rating scale in two different natural play settings
Test of Playfulness (Skard & Bundy, 2008)	Evaluates playfulness (intrinsic motivation, suspension of reality, and internal locus of control) during free play using observational tool

assessment tools are described in Table 34.2. For a list of assessment tools that are frequently used to evaluate child development and participation, see Appendix F, "Examples of Assessments for Early Childhood (Birth–5 Years)."

Identify Desired Play Outcomes

The focus of *play outcomes* varies by the child's age, the context in which the play is occurring, and the priorities of the child's family. Additionally, the setting in which services are being provided influences the desired play outcomes. When a child receives early intervention services, outcomes focus on the child's development of play skills with their family in their daily contexts. The occupational therapy practitioner uses evaluation results to identify or modify toys and play activities that are safe, developmentally appropriate, fun, and environmentally matched for the child and family (AOTA, 2012).

When the child is age 3 years or older, the occupational therapy practitioner may work with the preschool, child care, or community on environmental modification and object adaptation to promote the child's ability to successfully play. A child's ability to participate in social interactions during play with others and their ability to access play for learning are important to promote their success in academic or education settings. When providing services in a health care organization or community clinic, the practitioner addresses play skills and participation to support the child's leisure development, facilitate participation in

family routines, and promote occupational performance. Table 34.3 provides examples of outcomes or goals for various settings.

Enhance Child's Play as Occupation

Occupational therapy intervention should prioritize play as a valuable occupation for children. When addressing play, occupational therapy practitioners may address motor, cognitive, and social interaction skills to promote the child's success. To increase a child's ability to participate in play activities, the practitioner relies on task analysis to identify opportunities and challenges in play activities. Activity simplification strategies may also be beneficial to emphasize what is ultimately needed for the child to participate in play. Structured learning opportunities may be necessary to overcome behaviors limiting play participation and social interaction. Although the practitioner may direct to facilitate the child's play, it is important for the play to remain child centered.

Adapt the context

To promote participation and engagement, occupational therapy practitioners may need to adapt (e.g., modify task, method, and materials) the context (e.g., environmental factors) to enhance a child's play skills. As modifications are considered, it is important to emphasize the child's freedom of choice in prioritizing adaptations (Kolehmainen et al.,

TABLE 34.3. Play Outcomes in Early Childhood Settings

PRACTICE SETTING	PROFESSIONAL COLLABORATION	EXAMPLE OUTCOME OR GOALS
Early intervention	Occupational therapy practitioner may be primary service provider to address outcomes as part of transdisciplinary team	Cassandra will play with her "music and light-up toys" (cause-and-effect toys) so Grandma can get the older kids off to school in the morning.
Preschool services	Occupational therapy practitioner works on multidisciplinary team to address goals shared by all professionals on team	During outside play on the playground, Jack will independently use at least two pieces of equipment (e.g., slide, swing, climber, balls) on 4/5 consecutive days.
Health care and community services	Occupational therapy practitioner will address specific goals on interprofessional team	While sitting independently, Jose will use his hands to play with toys with his family for 5 minutes on 4/5 consecutive days.

2015; O'Connor & Stagnitti, 2011). Implementing sensory strategies to minimize negative sensory aspects of the environment or negative behavior responses to sensory factors can be important for enabling play participation for some children (Pfeiffer et al., 2017). Accommodations, such as providing a picture schedule, may help children initiate play during unstructured play periods (Case-Smith, 2013).

Additionally, the social context can be modified to include peers who are developmentally more mature and have higher cognitive levels to encourage play initiation and responses among children with developmental disabilities (Case-Smith, 2013; Lang et al., 2011). The occupational therapy practitioner can be instrumental in supporting the child's play development in natural community contexts with peers by adapting the physical and social environment for play and coaching the caregiver in play behaviors (Fabrizi et al., 2016).

Adapt play materials

The *materials* and toys used during play may be adapted to promote the child's ability to participate in play. The tangible objects or toys available for play may be modified to promote play. For instance, increasing the availability of social and unstructured toys (e.g., puppets, dolls, trucks, blocks, balls) over isolate or structured toys (e.g., puzzles, books) helps children with developmental disabilities demonstrate more positive social interactions (Case-Smith, 2013).

Additionally, introducing technology during play can support play participation for children with physical disabilities; LEGO robots have been shown to increase playfulness during free play when motor abilities are compromised (Ríos-Rincón et al., 2016). Technology may also include using switch-access toys, which allow the child to produce more complex motor sequences during play by activating the cause-and-effect switch. When the occupational therapy practitioner uses technology or switch access to facilitate play, the child needs to be able to learn how to access the switch while the practitioner supports successful movement patterns and positioning (Beauchamp et al., 2018).

Enhance social interactions through play

Relationship-based interventions promote the play behaviors of children with a developmental disability. When occupational therapy practitioners focus on strategies to improve positive adult–child interactions, children demonstrate an increase in social behaviors at more advanced play levels (Case-Smith, 2013).

Instruction may be necessary for children with developmental disabilities to gain social competence during play. Instruction interventions may include social scripts, Social Stories™, or video models (Case-Smith, 2013). Two teaching strategies used during social skill instruction are *modeling* the desired skill through use of a peer, adult, or video model and *prompting* (i.e., verbal, gestures, physical, visual) to encourage the desired response. In peer-mediated interventions, practitioners may use a video model to review teaching moments from previous play sessions with the peer before the new play session begins and to introduce prompts to be used during the session (Kent et al., 2018).

Social skill interventions, including directly teaching social skills, facilitating interactions with modeling and praise, and encouraging activities with peers without disabilities, can help promote social interactions during play (Lang et al., 2011). In addition to instruction of techniques, play activities may be structured to promote turn taking and problem solving. Additionally, selection of certain types of activities may help promote social interactions; playground play providing proprioceptive input has been associated with increased social interactions (Miller et al., 2017).

The occupational therapy practitioner should work with the child and their family to develop play strategies to expand social interactions and promote healthy relationships. The practitioner may coach the caregiver for sensitive responses to the child's cues, emphasize positive affect, and provide strategies to scaffold and encourage interactive play through imitation, modeling, and flexible responses. Parent-mediated interventions must be implemented with careful consideration of the context of the family as well as attention to the parents' skills, interaction style, and personality and the child's developmental levels and behaviors (Case-Smith, 2013).

Enhance mental health through play

Play, structured and unstructured, has been shown to promote positive mental health outcomes and reduce stress; 30 minutes of daily play for children who were hospitalized resulted in decreased anxiety and negative emotions (Li et al., 2016). As the occupational therapy provider offers opportunities for play during intervention and promotes participation in play and leisure, they are also promoting the child's mental health. The opportunity to make choices during play promotes a child's self-awareness and positive self-regard. Additionally, providing opportunities for motor planning during play and supports for a child to access play increases the child's self-esteem (Miller et al., 2017). Furthermore, when play is facilitated between parents or caregivers and the child, play provides the opportunity for adults to anticipate their child's needs, and the child recognizes a social context responsive to their individual needs (Childress, 2011).

Enhance symbolic or pretend play

Occupational therapy practitioners may provide interventions for symbolic or pretend play. The ability to imitate during play is important for play development and elaboration during symbolic and pretend play. Encouraging the ability to imitate play actions is a strategy that can help a child learn how to initiate their own play and increase their understanding of how to use toys in play, how to substitute objects during play, or how to elaborate play sequences (Pfeifer et al., 2011). Once a child is able to imitate during play, addressing pretend play is a priority for supporting their problem solving, language and communication, and emotional regulation. It is also important for practitioners to promote meaningful, authentic experiences before expecting young children to pretend or take on a role representing these experiences. Children imitate what they have experienced; therefore, background knowledge including authentic experiences is critical to the occupational performance of symbolic play.

Promote motor skills through play

Specific toys may be introduced during play to support motor skill development. Features and functions of toys can promote sensory exploration, grasp development, and gross motor skill coordination. Aspects of toys should provide the "just-right challenge," to promote and also challenge the child's strengths while ensuring the child is having fun. Toys and play materials should support an optimal fit between the child's abilities and the sensory and motor demands of play. It is important that toys and materials available during play offer flexibility to be integrated during play in many manners.

Enhance self-care skills through play

Occupational therapy practitioners should understand and consider family routines and priorities when exploring opportunities to increase play. Often, play is most valuable to the child and the family when embedded into caregiving routines; for example, bathtime is more fun with a plastic cup "submarine," and a healthy snack time is more successful when the caregiver and child host a tea party for stuffed animals. Play increases success with caregiving routines while also promoting independence in self-care activities. As children develop play skills, their independence in self-care activities likewise increases. For example, as a child gains balance to jump on one foot during play, the child is able to balance on one foot when donning pants to support the caregiving routine of dressing.

Gather Data for Ongoing Progress Monitoring

To monitor the effectiveness of intervention in developing play skills, it is important that measurable outcomes or goals be written that reflect the child and family's priorities for play as well as promote participation in play experiences in preschool or child care settings. The child and family's priorities may range from sharing with siblings to accessing play opportunities in the community to initiating play with a toy. The desired progress through intervention should be discussed so that the vision is shared among team members. For example, progress may be viewed as increased repertoire through use of toys and materials in a creative, novel, or imaginative manner; increased ability to make choices and problem solve during play; increased time engaged in play; increased joint attention and responsiveness to nonverbal communication; or increased expressions of playfulness (Miller Kuhaneck et al., 2013). Goal Attainment Scaling is also a tool that is sensitive for measuring progress and can be used for monitoring progress toward play participation outcomes (Harpster et al., 2018). See Chapter 6, "Best Practices in Data-Based Decision Making," for more information on monitoring progress.

SUMMARY

Daily play is important for a child's well-being as well as cognitive, motor, and social development and may occur throughout their daily routines. Children with disabilities may be limited in how they access, initiate, and engage in play and leisure activities. A child with a disability is likely to engage in play for shorter periods of time, is less likely to engage in pretend play, and demonstrates limited social behaviors during play than their typical peers. The family, caregiver, or educator of a child with a disability provides a consistent opportunity to scaffold and support social play for the child.

In partnership with the family and team, the occupational therapy practitioner has the opportunity to improve meaningful play engagement. To emphasize play as an occupation, authentic assessments should be used, and play as an outcome should be prioritized. During intervention, the practitioner may adapt the play environment or the play objects to enhance engagement in play. Additionally, the practitioner may select toys and materials and purposefully include peers to support the child's development and ability to participate in the occupation of play.

REFERENCES

American Occupational Therapy Association. (2012). *Learning through play.* https://www.aota.org/About-Occupational-Therapy/Patients-Clients/ChildrenAndYouth/Play.aspx

American Occupational Therapy Association. (2020). Occupational therapy practice framework: Domain and process (4th ed.). *American Journal of Occupational Therapy, 74*(Suppl. 2), 7412410010. https://doi.org/10.5014/ajot.2020.74S2001

Beauchamp, F., Bourke-Taylor, H., & Brown, T. (2018). Therapists' perspectives: Supporting children to use switches and technology for accessing their environment, leisure, and communication. *Journal of Occupational Therapy, Schools, & Early Intervention, 11,* 133–147. https://doi.org/10.1080/19411243.2018.1432443

Case-Smith, J. (2013). Systematic review of interventions to promote social–emotional development in young children with or at risk for disability. *American Journal of Occupational Therapy, 67,* 395–404. https://doi.org/10.5014/ajot.2013.004713

Childress, D. C. (2011). Play behaviors of parents and their young children with disabilities. *Topics in Early Childhood Special Education, 31,* 112–120. https://doi.org/10.1177/0271121410390526

Cosbey, J., Johnston, S., Dunn, L., & Bauman, M. (2012). Playground behaviors of children with and without sensory processing disorders. *OTJR: Occupation, Participation and Health, 32*(2), 39–47. https://doi.org/10.3928/15394492-20110930-01

Fabrizi, S., Ito, M., & Winston, K. (2016). Effect of occupational therapy–led playgroups in early intervention on child playfulness and caregiver responsiveness: A repeated-measures design. *American Journal of Occupational Therapy, 70,* 700220020. https://doi.org/10.5014/ajot.2016.017012

Fallon, J., & MacCobb, S. (2013). Free play time of children with learning disabilities in a noninclusive preschool setting: An analysis of play and nonplay behaviours. *British Journal of Learning Disabilities, 41,* 212–219. https://doi.org/10.1111/bld.12052

Fewell, R. (1986). *Play Assessment Scale* (5th ed.). University of Washington.

Graham, N., Nye, C., Mandy, A., Clarke, C., & Morriss-Roberts, C. (2018). The meaning of play for children and young people with physical disabilities: A systematic thematic synthesis. *Child: Care, Health and Development, 44,* 173–182. https://doi.org/10.1111/cch.12509

Harpster, K., Sheehan, A., Foster, E., Leffler, E., Schwab, S., & Angeli, J. (2018). The methodological application of Goal

Attainment Scaling in pediatric rehabilitation research: A systematic review. *Disability and Rehabilitation*, 2855–2864. https://doi.org/10.1080/09638288.2018.1474952

Henry, A. (2000). *Pediatric Interest Profiles: Surveys of play for children and adolescents, Kid Play Profile, Preteen Play Profile, Adolescent Leisure Interest Profile.* Psychological Corporation.

Hodge, C., Bocarro, J. N., Henderson, K. A., Zabriskie, R., Parcel, T. L., & Kanters, M. A. (2015). Family leisure: An integrative review of research from select journals. *Journal of Leisure Research, 47,* 577–600. https://doi.org/10.18666/jlr-2015-v47-i5-5705

Kent, C., Cordier, R., Joosten, A., Wilkes-Gillan, S., & Bundy, A. (2018). Peer-mediated intervention to improve play skills in children with autism spectrum disorder: A feasibility study. *Australian Occupational Therapy Journal, 65,* 176–186. https://doi.org/10.1111/1440-1630.12459

King, G., Imms, C., Stewart, D., Freeman, M., & Nguyen, T. (2018). A transactional framework for pediatric rehabilitation: Shifting the focus to situated contexts, transactional processes, and adaptive developmental outcomes. *Disability and Rehabilitation, 40,* 1829–1841. https://doi.org/10.1080/09638288.2017.1309583

Knox, S. (2008). Development and current use of the Revised Knox Preschool Play Scale. In L. Parham & L. Fazio (Eds.), *Play in occupational therapy for children* (2nd ed., pp. 55–70). Elsevier.

Kolehmainen, N., Ramsay, C., McKee, L., Missiuna, C., Owen, C., & Francis, J. (2015). Participation in physical play and leisure in children with motor impairments: Mixed-methods study to generate evidence for developing an intervention. *Physical Therapy, 95,* 1374–1386. https://doi.org/10.2522/ptj.20140404

Lang, R., Kuriakose, S., Lyons, G., Mulloy, A., Boutot, A., Britt, C., . . . Lancioni, G. (2011). Use of school recess time in the education and treatment of children with autism spectrum disorders: A systematic review. *Research in Autism Spectrum Disorders, 5,* 1296–1305. https://doi.org/10.1016/j.rasd.2011.02.012

Law, M., Anaby, D., Imms, C., Teplicky, R., & Turner, L. (2015). Improving the participation of youth with physical disabilities in community activities: An interrupted time series design. *Australian Occupational Therapy Journal, 62,* 105–115. https://doi.org/10.1111/1440-1630.12177

Li, W., Kwan, J., Ka, Y., & Blondi Ming, C. (2016). Play interventions to reduce anxiety and negative emotions in hospitalized children. *BMC Pediatrics, 16,* Article 36. https://doi.org/10.1186/s12887-016-0570-5

McDonald, S., Kehler, H., Bayrampour, H., Fraser-Lee, N., & Tough, S. (2016). Risk and protective factors in early child development: Results from the All Our Babies (AOB) pregnancy cohort. *Research in Developmental Disabilities, 58,* 20–30. https://doi.org/10.1016/j.ridd.2016.08.010

Miller, L., Schoen, S., Camarata, S., McConkey, J., Kanics, I. Valdez, A., & Hampton, S. (2017). Play in natural environments: A pilot study quantifying the behavior of children on playground equipment. *Journal of Occupational Therapy, Schools, & Early Intervention, 10,* 213–231. https://doi.org/10.1080/19411243.2017.1325818

Miller Kuhaneck, H., Tanta, K. J., Coombs, A. K., & Pannone, H. (2013). A survey of pediatric occupational therapists' use of play. *Journal of Occupational Therapy, Schools, & Early Intervention, 6,* 213–227. https://doi.org/10.1080/19411243.2013.850940

Movahedazarhoulighi, S. (2018). Teaching play skills to children with disabilities: Research-based interventions and practices. *Early Childhood Education Journal, 46,* 587–599. https://doi.org/10.1007/s10643-018-0917-7

Mulligan, S. (2014). *Occupational therapy evaluation for children: A pocket guide* (2nd ed.). Lippincott Williams & Wilkins.

O'Connor, C., & Stagnitti, K. (2011). Play, behaviour, language and social skills: The comparison of a play and a non-play intervention within a specialist school setting. *Research in Developmental Disabilities, 32,* 1205–1211. https://doi.org/10.1016/j.ridd.2010.12.037

Parham, D., & Fazio, L. (Eds.). (1997). *Play in occupational therapy for children.* Mosby.

Parham, D., & Fazio, L. (Eds.). (2008). *Play in occupational therapy for children* (2nd ed.). Elsevier.

Pfeifer, L., Pacciulio, A., Santos, C., Santos, J., & Stagnitti, K. (2011). Pretend play of children with cerebral palsy. *Physical & Occupational Therapy in Pediatrics, 31,* 390–402. https://doi.org/10.3109/01942638.2011.572149

Pfeiffer, B., Coster, W., Snethen, G., Derstine, M., Piller, A., & Tucker, C. (2017). Caregivers' perspectives on the sensory environment and participation in daily activities of children with autism spectrum disorder. *American Journal of Occupational Therapy, 71,* 7104220020. https://doi.org/10.5014/ajot.2017.021360

Pierucci, J., Barber, A., Gilpin, A., Crisler, M., & Klinger, L. (2014). Play assessments and developmental skills in young children with autism spectrum disorders. *Focus on Autism and Other Developmental Disabilities, 30,* 35–43. https://doi.org/10.1177/1088357614539837

Ríos-Rincón, A., Adams, K., Magill-Evans, J., & Cook, A. (2016). Playfulness in children with limited motor abilities when using a robot. *Physical & Occupational Therapy in Pediatrics, 36,* 232–246. https://doi.org/10.3109/01942638.2015.1076559

Skard, G., & Bundy, A. (2008). Test of Playfulness. In L. Parham & L. Fazio (Eds.), *Play in occupational therapy for children* (2nd ed., pp. 71–94). Elsevier.

Yogman, M., Garner, A., Hutchinson, J., Hirsh-Pasek, K., & Golinkoff, R. (2018). The power of play: A pediatric role in enhancing development in young children. *Pediatrics, 142*(3), e20182058. https://doi.org/10.1542/peds.2018-2058

Best Practices in Supporting Children Who Are Deaf and Hard of Hearing

35

Meredith Gronski, OTD, OTR/L, CLA

KEY TERMS AND CONCEPTS

- Acquired hearing loss
- Auditory neuropathy spectrum disorder
- Bone-anchored hearing aid
- Cochlear implant
- Conductive hearing loss
- Congenital hearing loss
- Deaf culture
- Fluctuating and stable hearing loss
- Hearing aids
- Mild hearing loss
- Mixed hearing loss
- Moderate hearing loss
- Personal frequency modulation
- Postlingual hearing loss
- Prelingual hearing loss
- Profound hearing loss
- Sensorineural hearing loss
- Severe hearing loss
- Sudden and progressive hearing loss
- Symmetrical and asymmetrical hearing loss
- Unilateral and bilateral hearing loss

OVERVIEW

Almost every newborn infant in the United States (98%) is screened for hearing loss. Of those children, almost 10% are diagnosed with hearing loss by age 3 months (Centers for Disease Control and Prevention, 2016). Newborn hearing screening plays a critical role in identifying and supporting the development and quality of life (QoL) of young children who are deaf and hard of hearing (d/hh). Each year, around 65% of children with a diagnosed hearing loss are enrolled in Part C early intervention services under the Individuals With Disabilities Education Improvement Act of 2004 (P. L. 108-446). The majority of these children receive service coordination and communication interventions.

However, a significant portion of children with hearing loss have additional documented disabilities or delays (Cupples et al., 2014; Picard, 2004). It is rare for a child who is d/hh to have a documented hearing loss in isolation, with no additional occupational performance deficits. Often, a child with a significant hearing loss has experienced prematurity, meningitis, or cytomegalovirus infection (CMV), all of which frequently have a secondary impact on neurologic development. Additionally, hearing loss can be associated with a genetic syndrome, which may also include a mosaic of impairments that contribute to occupational performance limitations.

Occupational therapy practitioners can provide interventions for children who are d/hh in the context of early intervention, inpatient hospital programs, pediatric outpatient clinics, mainstream early childhood education programs (e.g., child care, preschool, Early or Head Start), and specialized public or private schools for the deaf. (*Note. Occupational therapy practitioner* refers to both occupational therapists and occupational therapy assistants.) The scope of occupational therapy practice in this area includes addressing impairments related to social skills, sensory processing, self-regulation behaviors, executive function skills, and motor skills to facilitate a child's skillful occupational performance in social, learning, play, and self-care routines. Practitioners can educate teachers, families, and health professionals that maladaptive behaviors, sensorimotor deficits, academic delays, and social struggles of children who are d/hh are not always directly related to the hearing loss; rather, each child who is d/hh has unique strengths and functional impairments that limit occupational performance and social participation.

ESSENTIAL CONSIDERATIONS

One of the most critical factors to consider when working with families of children who are d/hh is the nuance of terminology used to characterize hearing loss, communication approaches, and audiological devices. Often, occupational performance deficits are linked to the type or cause of hearing loss or the configuration of hearing devices used by the child. The family's chosen communication approach is fundamental to how the occupational therapy practitioner should approach evaluation and intervention strategies.

Types and Causes of Hearing Loss

Hearing loss can be described as ***congenital*** (present at birth) or ***acquired*** (occurring after birth). When hearing loss occurs later in childhood, audiology and otolaryngology practitioners note whether the acquired hearing loss developed ***prelingually*** (before acquisition of spoken language) or ***postlingually*** (after acquisition of spoken language). This is often an integral factor in speech–language

---

TABLE 35.1.   Definitions of Hearing Loss

TYPE	
TYPE OF HEARING LOSS	**DEFINITION**
Conductive hearing loss	Hearing loss caused by something that stops sounds from getting through the outer or middle ear. This type of hearing loss can often be treated with medicine or surgery.
Sensorineural hearing loss	Hearing loss that occurs when there is a problem in the way the inner ear or hearing nerve works.
Mixed hearing loss	Hearing loss that includes both a conductive and a sensorineural hearing loss.
Auditory neuropathy spectrum disorder	Hearing loss that occurs when sound enters the ear normally, but, because of damage to the inner ear or the hearing nerve, sound is not organized in a way that the brain can understand.
DEGREE	
DEGREE OF HEARING LOSS	**DEFINITION**
Mild hearing loss	A person with a mild hearing loss may hear some speech sounds, but soft sounds are hard to hear.
Moderate hearing loss	A person with a moderate hearing loss may hear almost no speech when another person is talking at a normal level.
Severe hearing loss	A person with severe hearing loss hears no speech when a person is talking at a normal level and only some loud sounds.
Profound hearing loss	A person with a profound hearing loss does not hear any speech and hears only very loud sounds.
CONFIGURATION	
TYPE OF HEARING LOSS CONFIGURATION	**DEFINITION**
Unilateral and bilateral	Hearing loss is in one ear (unilateral) or both ears (bilateral).
Symmetrical and asymmetrical hearing loss	Hearing loss is the same in both ears (symmetrical) or is different in each ear (asymmetrical).
Sudden and progressive hearing loss	Hearing loss worsens over time (progressive) or happens quickly (sudden).
Fluctuating and stable hearing loss	Hearing loss gets either better or worse over time (fluctuating) or stays the same over time (stable).

Note. Adapted from Centers for Disease Control and Prevention (2019).

intervention approach and significantly influences selection of a communication style by the child's family.

Genetic factors account for more than 50% of children with hearing loss, and about 20% of those children have a hearing loss associated with a diagnosed syndrome (Morton & Nance, 2006). Aside from genetic factors, some other leading causes of hearing loss among children are maternal infection (including CMV), prematurity, and other prenatal environmental causes. Children may have a congenital, conductive hearing loss caused by a physical anomaly of the ear, such as microtia or atresia. Acquired hearing loss can most often be attributed to chronic ear infections and treatment with ototoxic antibiotics (e.g., gentamicin) for an acquired infection, such as meningitis or measles.

Each child who is d/hh has a unique configuration of access to sound and loss (see Table 35.1 for types and degrees of loss). To diagnose a hearing loss, an audiologist performs a hearing test that measures whether the child is able to respond to tones at a variety of pitches and volumes. Volume levels are measured in decibels, and pitches are measured in frequencies. The results of a hearing test are mapped onto an audiogram, with decibels on the y-axis and frequencies on the x-axis. The most common environmental sounds, including articulated speech sounds, are presented in Figure 35.1.

Types of Hearing Devices and Technology

When an infant or young child is diagnosed with a permanent hearing loss that cannot be reversed by medication or surgical repair, an audiologist recommends a hearing device or assistive technology system to enhance or replicate the child's access to sound. These devices have small components and often require maintenance and care by the family as the child develops independence in caring for their own device. It is also important for occupational therapy practitioners to be familiar with basic functioning of devices and how to identify malfunction in each.

Hearing aids act as a microphone and amplifier to make sounds louder for the listener. Hearing aids are programmable to amplify certain frequencies of sound and not others as well as dampen background noise. Hearing aids can be beneficial for both conductive and sensorineural hearing loss; however, they have an effectiveness ceiling for severe and profound losses. Most young children are fitted with custom ear molds that hold the device in place on the outer ear, and the body of the device hooks behind the ear (National Institute on Deafness and Other Communication Disorders [NIDCD], 2016b). Children are fitted for new ear molds as they grow. Children begin to learn to independently and skillfully don and doff their hearing aid at around age 3 years, depending on fine motor skill development. Children

FIGURE 35.1. Familiar sounds audiogram.

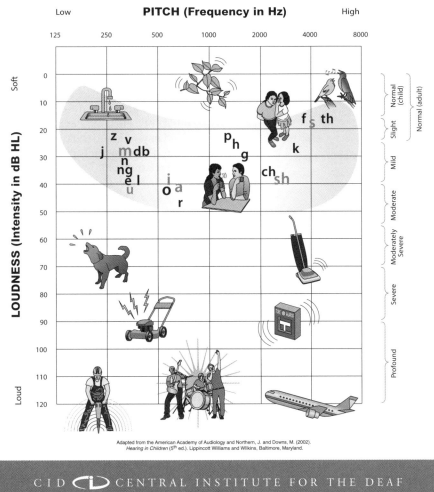

Source. Reprinted from *Familiar sound audiogram*, by the Central Institute for the Deaf, 2019, retrieved from https://cid.edu/wp-content/uploads/2016/05/CID-AUDIOGRAM-ENGLISH.pdf. Copyright © 2019 by the Central Institute for the Deaf. Reprinted with permission.

typically need an adult to assist them with changing the battery in the device until around age 7 years.

A *cochlear implant* (CI) is a surgically implanted device that bypasses the middle ear acoustic conduction physiology to conduct an electrical sound signal directly to the auditory nerve. An electrode array is implanted into the cochlea and connected to a processor that receives environmental sound from a microphone. A transmitter and stimulator attach to a magnet just below the skin over the mastoid bone; they receive signals from a speech processor and convert them to electric impulses onto the auditory nerve (see Figure 35.2). A child is eligible for a CI if they have a severe to profound sensorineural hearing loss that is no longer benefitted by a hearing aid. Children who receive a CI require intensive therapy to acquire effective listening and spoken language skills. With early implantation before age 18 months, CI users are better able to hear sounds, speech, and music, and they develop language skills at a rate comparable to children with typical hearing. Many children with CIs succeed in community-based preschool classrooms (NIDCD, 2017a).

A *bone-anchored hearing aid* is a hearing aid that amplifies and conducts sound through vibrations directly to the skull, bypassing the middle ear. This device is typically used by children who have a unilateral hearing loss,

FIGURE 35.2.   Ear with a cochlear implant.

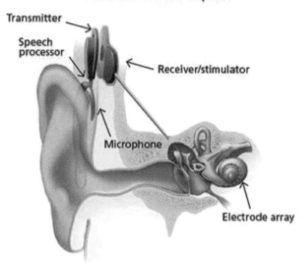

Ear with cochlear implant

Source. Reprinted from *What Are Cochlear Implants?* (NIH Publication No. 00-4798) by the National Institute on Deafness and Other Communication Disorders, https://www.nidcd.nih.gov/health/cochlear-implants.

atresia, or a middle ear disorder. The anchor for the device is surgically implanted, and insurance coverage is limited, because this is considered a prosthetic device, not a hearing aid (NIDCD, 2017b).

A *personal frequency modulation* system can be used as an assistive technology system to amplify speech and environmental sounds directly to hearing aids using radio waves. This device reduces background noise and improves clarity for listeners. A speaker, such as a parent or preschool teacher, uses a microphone that transmits the signal to the receiver, which is integrated into the listener's hearing aids (Mroz, 2019). Occupational therapy practitoners collaborate with audiologists and teachers of the deaf to maximize the person–environment fit of this technology at home and in early childhood education settings.

Types of Communication Approaches

Several communication approaches are available for a family of a child who is d/hh to use. They range from completely visual to completely spoken (see Table 35.2). An audiologist, speech–language pathologist (SLP), and teacher of the deaf work together to support a family in selecting their chosen communication approach. An occupational therapy practitioner can assist the team in support of communication skills through the development of fine motor skills and praxis for sign language fluency or strategies for visual attention needed for following cues and prompts.

Cultural Considerations

Occupational therapy practitioners should strive to understand and consider the unique perspectives, values, and influences of a family's own culture as well as the culture of their chosen community and communication approach.

Some families, health care professionals, and educational teams view hearing loss as a medical condition to be remediated. However, a significant number of individuals who are d/hh do not believe that being deaf is a disability or impairment. These individuals identify as members of ***Deaf culture*** and prefer to be referred to with identity-first language (e.g., "a Deaf child") and always capitalize the word *Deaf*.

Throughout this chapter, we use the phrase "who is deaf or hard of hearing (d/hh)" because it is inclusive of all perspectives and cultures. The terms *hearing loss* and *impairment* are only used to refer to the audiological configuration and not to describe an individual. A person who is hard of hearing has some level of residual hearing. A person who is deaf (lowercase *d*) has little to no residual hearing. A person who identifies as Deaf (uppercase *D*) generally has minimal or no residual hearing, communicates primarily with sign language, and prefers to socialize with others who are Deaf as a part of a close-knit community (Fain, 2019).

Understanding each family member's identity relative to Deaf and hearing culture is critical for a successful therapeutic relationship. This perspective may vary depending on whether the child who is d/hh has hearing parents or whether the child has Deaf parents and relatives. Occupational therapy practitioners need to be able to respectfully engage with a family through a sign language interpreter (if appropriate), repair communication breakdowns, and be open to learning the chosen communication style of the family. Most important, practitioners should always face and speak directly to an individual who is d/hh (Fain, 2019).

BEST PRACTICES

As the occupational therapy process is initiated to address the occupational performance needs of a child who is d/hh, the occupational therapist uses a top-down approach to formal evaluation and development of an intervention plan. The implementation and ongoing review of the intervention strategies by the occupational therapy practitioner is a collaborative process with the child, primary caregivers, and educational team. Through this collaborative and ongoing process, the family, team, and occupational therapy practitioner work together to define what success looks like for the child in the least restrictive environment.

Conduct an Evaluation

Evaluation of children who are d/hh has traditionally focused on a single domain: communication. Occupational therapy can improve the outcomes of children who are d/hh by focusing on the performance of functional skills and the quality of participation in everyday occupations. This translates what team members already know about the impact of hearing loss into functional daily life intervention priorities and strategies that will improve the QoL of children who are d/hh and their families.

The occupational therapy evaluation should start with an occupational profile that includes the integral family members and early childhood educators, when appropriate. The occupational therapist should discuss daily habits, routines, and roles with the family and observe performance skills and patterns in context to identify barriers and supports. When the occupational therapist begins to analyze

TABLE 35.2. **Communication Approaches**

COMMUNICATION METHOD	APPROACH DESCRIPTION	HEARING AND AMPLIFICATION REQUIREMENTS	FAMILY OR CAREGIVER INVOLVEMENT	OCCUPATIONAL THERAPY ROLE
American Sign Language (ASL), Signed Exact English (SEE), Pidgin Signed English (PSE)	A hand-based language approach that has its own grammar and linguistic principles. *Sensory mode:* Visual	Individual decision about amplification and access to sound is supported.	Family must make a commitment to learning sign language consistently and giving opportunities for social interaction with Deaf community.	▪ Fine motor range, dexterity, and coordination support ▪ Fluency of movement ▪ Bilateral/bimanual coordination ▪ Visual attention ▪ Caregiver coaching, education. ▪ Environmental modification for clear sight lines and proximity to speaker/interpreter ▪ Self-advocacy skills ▪ Visual supports for ADL/IADL task completion
Total Communication (TC)	An approach that uses both spoken language and sign language concurrently. It may also include gestures, finger spelling, or lip reading. *Sensory mode:* Visual and auditory	Consistent use of amplification devices and technology is strongly encouraged.	Family must make a commitment to learn and use the selected sign language system and collaborate with teachers and therapists to promote language expansion.	▪ Fine motor range, dexterity, and coordination support ▪ Fluency of movement ▪ Bilateral/bimanual coordination ▪ Visual attention ▪ Caregiver coaching, education. ▪ Environmental modification for clear sight lines and proximity to speaker or interpreter ▪ Self-advocacy skills ▪ Amplification device care/use/ management, if applicable ▪ Visual supports for ADL/IADL task completion
Auditory Verbal (AV), Listening and Spoken Language (LSL)	An approach that emphasizes spoken language development through listening without the use of visual cues. *Sensory mode:* Auditory	Early, consistent, and appropriate use of hearing devices is critical.	Family must establish an optimal listening environment and actively carryover strategies to promote listening and language development in all contexts.	▪ Visual attention ▪ Caregiver coaching and education; family routines ▪ Environmental modification for clear sight lines and proximity to speaker/interpreter ▪ Self-advocacy skills ▪ Amplification device care/use/ management
Cued Speech (CS)	An approach that combines hand cues with natural mouth positions used to cue each syllable or phoneme of speech. *Sensory mode:* Visual and auditory	Early, consistent, and appropriate use of hearing devices is important.	Family must learn to and use speak-and-cue prompts at all times in all play and daily routine activities.	▪ Visual attention ▪ Caregiver coaching and education; family routines ▪ Environmental modification for clear sight lines and proximity to speaker/interpreter ▪ Self-advocacy skills ▪ Amplification device care/use/ management ▪ Visual supports for ADL/IADL task completion

Note. ADL = activities of daily living; IADL = instrumental activities of daily living.

the child's specific client factors and performance skills, they should make special considerations to accommodate the child's access to sound, mode of communication, and receptive and expressive language skills. Occupational therapists should fully understand the family's cultural perspective on hearing loss and use an interpreter, if needed (Fain, 2019). Standardized assessment tools that rely on verbal prompts may need to be modified, and the occupational therapist must consider these modifications when interpreting and reporting assessment results. An in-depth listing of assessment tools can be found in Appendix F, "Examples of Assessments for Early Childhood (Birth–5 Years)."

Finally, whenever possible, occupational therapists should use nonverbal methods of assessment, contextual observations, and proxy report measures to complete a thorough and valid evaluation process.

Provide Interventions

Occupational therapy practitioners often provide interventions for children who are d/hh in the context of early intervention when families are first learning about their child's hearing status, learning to manage hearing devices, and negotiating evolving family culture. Many children who are d/hh have motor skill delays and atypical sensory processing patterns that prompt their family to seek services at pediatric outpatient clinics. Given the myriad genetic and developmental conditions associated with hearing loss that can also contribute to low muscle tone or dyspraxia, occupational therapy practitioners have a unique role in supporting fine motor development and dexterity for accurate and fluent sign language communication. As a child reaches preschool age, they may be identified for occupational therapy services in community-based early childhood education programs (e.g., day care, preschool, Early or Head Start) and in specialized public or private schools for the deaf. An overview of intervention activity examples across occupational performance areas is highlighted in Exhibit 35.1.

Social and play skills

Children who are d/hh engage in limited interactions with hearing peers (Fain, 2019; Hintermair, 2010). Without these interactions, children who are d/hh do not experience the same levels of social participation or the emotional and scholastic benefits that such participation provides. Although opportunities for free and unstructured play have been limited in many early childhood programs in exchange for structured literacy skill instruction, engaging in play builds the capacity to problem solve, make friends, develop fine and large motor skills, and foster appropriate emotional understanding and expression.

Traditionally, occupational therapy practitioners have focused on developing these individual capacities in an effort to support overall play skill development. However, using play as the therapeutic modality directly facilitates the acquisition of delayed skills while providing opportunity for a child to participate in their role as a player with peers, regardless of hearing status.

Occupational therapy practitioners can partner with SLPs to support peer relationship development of children who are d/hh. SLPs support the development of pragmatic language skills, and occupational therapy practitioners support a child's social–emotional skill development and engage these developing skills in the context of spontaneous play scenarios with natural peer interactions. The practitioner may facilitate fine motor skill and praxis development for cooperative block construction, game piece manipulation, or effortless use of dramatic play materials. Children who are d/hh often feel socially isolated because of their communication differences and may demonstrate more advanced play skills, emotional regulation, and prosocial behaviors in smaller groups (Fain, 2019). Occupational therapy interventions can also support social advocacy skills to help children develop strategies to let peers and adults know when they did not understand what was said, want to initiate or terminate a play interaction, need assistance with hearing devices, or need to safely share personal information if lost or in danger.

Vestibular dysfunction and sensory processing

The auditory and vestibular anatomical structures are continuous and linked in physiology and organization. As a result, congenital anomaly or insult in the inner ear that leads to sensorineural hearing loss may also disrupt peripheral vestibular function (Cushing et al., 2008; DeKegel et al., 2012). The vestibular system affects body and head orientation, muscle tone, and multisensory integration, which can result in delayed development of motor skills. Delays in the area of vestibular control and motor development have widely been reported among children with congenital or acquired sensorineural hearing loss (Phillips & Backous,

---

EXHIBIT 35.1. Examples of Intervention and Supports for Children Who Are Deaf or Hard of Hearing

- Observe and offer behavioral consultation and self-regulation strategies during an audiology mapping or auditory–verbal training session.
- Provide in-service workshops to early childhood educators and other professionals on the impact of vestibular hypofunction on motor development, play skills, and behavior regulation.
- Suggest play-based activities with parents that foster motor skills and complement language-rich activities to carry over to goals across home, speech therapy sessions, and preschool.
- Organize weekly individual or group sessions to develop balance-based large motor skills at home, a neighborhood park, or a community play group.
- Encourage early childhood educators and parents to use playground equipment and community participation (e.g., gymnastics, swimming, martial arts) to ensure appropriate movement and sensory input throughout the day.
- Use a language-rich structured routine (e.g., snack time) to facilitate initiation, organizational, turn taking, and memory skills.
- Organize a social skills scavenger hunt (e.g., say "hi" to a family member, hold the door for someone else, ask someone their favorite animal).
- Conduct a co-treatment activity with an SLP to support sign language dexterity and fluency.
- Use forward and backward chaining for independent donning and doffing of hearing aids and cochlear implants.
- Create a visual schedule for device management and self-care during morning and bedtime routines.

Note. SLP = speech-language pathologist.

2002; Rine et al., 2000, 2004; Schlumberger et al., 2004). Children who are d/hh have an increased risk of developing balance and large motor deficits compared with children with typical hearing, and start walking an average of 2.5 months later than their peers with typical hearing (Cushing et al., 2008; De Kegel et al., 2012; Livingstone & McPhillips, 2011; Schlumberger et al., 2004).

It is common for a family of an infant or toddler with a newly identified hearing loss to be coached to "bombard" their child with verbal interactions to facilitate access to and learning of language. Parents and caregivers may feel it is necessary to interact with their child face to face and more often place them in a high chair, swing, or car seat to accomplish this. Occupational therapy practitioners can collaborate with families and SLPs to determine play positions that include prone (e.g., tummy time) and opportunities for large motor development, while still allowing language-rich interactions.

In addition to the motor and postural implications of vestibular hypofunction, atypical sensory processing patterns are present at varying levels among 50%–70% of children with cochlear implants (Bharadwaj et al., 2009; Koester et al., 2014). Children who are consistently overstimulated by the feel of a clothing tag and the proximity of peers on the playground or those who crave movement and deep pressure to recognize where their body is in space tend to have difficulty paying attention, act impulsively, and resist many task demands. Using knowledge of environmental adaptation and evidence-based self-regulation and sensory integration approaches, occupational therapy interventions should focus on the development of strategies that support occupational participation in natural contexts by harnessing sensory inputs that support functioning and reduce challenging sensory inputs (Dunn et al., 2012; Dunst et al., 2006).

Occupational therapy practitioners should be aware of the relationship between hearing loss and vestibular hypofunction to identify when a child who is d/hh may be exhibiting additional deficits that may delay motor development and contribute to occupational performance barriers and a reduction in participation. Practitioners can also contribute this knowledge to otolaryngology team members to support cochlear implantation candidacy decisions.

In addition to using developmental and habilitative approaches, occupational therapy practitioners have a role to educate caregivers and community center staff that children with hypofunctioning vestibular systems should always swim with a minimum of contact guard supervision. Once the child is underwater, there is no mechanism for internal awareness of which way is up, which places the child at a greater risk for drowning. In addition, children who use CIs are at risk of mild electric shock and damage to device components when exposed to static, such as when sliding on a plastic playground slide, when removing a winter hat, or when getting up from a plastic preschool chair.

Cognition and executive functioning

Postlingual hearing loss identification can result in barriers to developmental skills, cognitive performance, and functional status. Any period of auditory deprivation causes changes in cognitive processes (Watson et al., 2007). Despite advances in hearing aid and CI technologies, many children who are d/hh continue to lag behind typically hearing peers in language, literacy, and cognitive abilities (Marschark et al., 2007). Although children with typical hearing and those who are d/hh both use memory and task attention strategies at an early age, implementation of verbal rehearsal methods (self-talk) are delayed among children who are d/hh (Burkholder-Juhasz et al., 2007; Figueras et al., 2008; Remine et al., 2008).

Occupational therapy practitioners have essential knowledge and skills to teach cognitive memory and attention strategies that can support turn taking in play, family and self-care routines, and daily preschool activities. Practitioners can provide graduated support and teach cueing strategies to parents and early childhood educators to ensure task success. Strategies can be developed for remembering where shoes and favorite toys are stored, regulating behavior during transitions, and self-monitoring during multistep chore activities and grooming tasks. Rather than cognition and learning being only provided by an early childhood educator or neuropsychologist, occupational therapy practitioners can intervene to support performance in all contexts of early childhood.

Ongoing data collection

As occupational therapy practitioners implement the intervention plan to address occupational performance, they must continually review the effectiveness of their selected strategies. Formal tools, such as Goal Attainment Scaling (Ottenbacher & Cusick, 1990), can be used to quantify progress and aid in clinical decision making. The tracking of early childhood individualized education program goals through work samples, data logs, and session notes is critical to adhere to regulations and to keep the educational team informed of progress being made or adjustments that may be necessary. Occupational therapy practitioners should also check in with the child's primary caregivers for feelings of self-efficacy with parenting roles, stress levels, and overall satisfaction with routines-based strategies.

SUMMARY

Deficits in communication and verbal capacity are the most frequently noted challenges for children who are d/hh, and intervention often focuses on these areas. It is essential for occupational therapy practitioners to broaden their sense of professional relatedness to build a new team of collaborators to best provide services for these children, including audiologists, otolaryngologists, teachers of the deaf, and SLPs. Case Example 35.1 provides an example of a collaborative approach to intervention. The scope of occupational therapy in early childhood settings is constantly growing and developing. Practitioners must continue to broaden their focus to capture the unique concerns of children who are d/hh and shift practice to more directly address participation in home preschool and community activities and routines.

CASE EXAMPLE 35.1. NICHOLAS: A COLLABORATIVE APPROACH TO INTERVENTION IN AN EARLY CHILDHOOD SCHOOL FOR THE DEAF

Nicholas was a 4-year-old preschooler with a bilateral profound hearing loss. He had had bilateral cochlear implants since age 18 months. In addition, he had vestibular hypofunctioning, as documented by his otolaryngologist and audiologist. His strengths included his near-average receptive and expressive language skills; however, he sometimes had difficulty with the pragmatics of language with peers. He would talk loudly and in a high-pitched voice when he was excited to share a story, and he generally did not have a good perception of conversational turn taking.

Nicholas had poor large motor and balance skills because of his vestibular hypofunction, which affected his attention for conversations, classroom learning activities, and play. He was constantly in motion to maintain his balance. He had a tendency to seek out movement (e.g., spinning, rocking) because his brain was not registering information from his dysfunctional vestibular structures. Nicholas benefitted from supported seating so that he was better able to attend, converse, and answer questions, as opposed to focusing on managing his large motor stability.

Occupational therapy services had been a part of Nicholas's service plan from birth. When he enrolled in this inclusive deaf education early childhood program, the occupational therapy team's priorities were to (1) improve Nicholas's large motor skills and balance for play, ADLs (including toileting), and safety in the school; (2) improve his social skills and conversational appropriateness; and (3) improve his sensory processing behaviors and attention.

The occupational therapist was first in contact with Nicholas's otolaryngologist, who diagnosed him with vestibular areflexia. It was important for the occupational therapist to understand whether Nicholas had some vestibular function or whether his system was not functioning at all. It was discovered that although all his structures were formed normally according to a magnetic resonance imaging scan, his vestibular ocular reflex was not responsive to rotary chair testing. This indicated that his system was *areflexic*, or not functioning at all. The occupational therapist and otolaryngologist together determined that Nicholas was relying on visual and proprioceptive inputs to maintain balance and perform the motor skills at which he was proficient.

On the basis of this information, the therapist devised an intervention plan to add movement activities to Nicholas's day to satisfy his sensory-craving behaviors and developed strategies to support him in more difficult large motor challenges of daily activities. Throughout his preschool day, Nicholas added the following strategies:

- He stabilized himself by leaning his upper back against the wall while donning and doffing his pants for toileting.
- He sat on the floor to don and doff his jacket at recess and to unpack and pack his backpack at the beginning and end of the day.

- He spun in the early childhood educator's desk chair when arriving at school (before circle time), before conversational snack time, and before 1:1 speech sessions. The occupational therapist asked the early childhood educators to spin Nicholas 10 times in both directions to stimulate his vestibular system bilaterally. This was a quick activity that was performed without disruption to the daily schedule. Early childhood educators were informed about signs of overarousal and how to handle it, and classroom rules were established so that the other children did not freely engage in this activity without supervision.
- He was encouraged by early childhood educators to use the playground equipment during morning and afternoon recess to ensure he was maximizing his vestibular input during this part of his school day.

By obtaining a stable position in which to complete the ADLs of preschool, Nicholas was able to complete them with near independence and in a more organized way. He no longer became frustrated when his classmates lined up and departed before he was ready, and the early childhood educator reported less frustration with having to redirect or assist him. His early childhood educators also reported anecdotally that immediately after the rotary movement activities and after recess, his attention was better and he was better able to sit still.

To address Nicholas's social skills and conversational pragmatics, the occupational therapist worked closely with Nicholas's early childhood educator and speech-language pathologist (SLP). Eye contact was often difficult for Nicholas because of his instability, but the occupational therapist learned from Nicholas's classroom early childhood educator that he was primarily an auditory learner. The occupational therapist, SLP, and deaf education early childhood educator together developed cues to give Nicholas when he needed to make eye contact in social situations. Behavioral and visual cues were developed for Nicholas and used consistently across settings and disciplines when he needed to lower the volume and pitch of his voice. Also, because Nicholas's parents worked full time, he enrolled in the after-school program developed by the occupational therapist, which focused on social skills development.

Throughout the year, Nicholas was better able to converse with his classmates, notice the feelings of his early childhood educators or friends, and respond appropriately. He continued to need external cues from adults to support his eye contact and remember to lower his voice when he was excited. Overall, his play skills blossomed, and his parents reported better play at home with his siblings.

Note. Adapted from "Team Efforts to Serve Children Who Are Deaf or Hard of Hearing," by M. Gronski, 2012, *OT Practice, 17*(17), 15–18. Copyright © 2012 by the American Occupational Therapy Association. Adapted with permission.

REFERENCES

Bharadwaj, S. V., Daniel, L. L., & Matzke, P. L. (2009). Sensory-processing disorder in children with cochlear implants. *American Journal of Occupational Therapy, 63,* 208–213. https://doi.org/10.5014/ajot.63.2.208

Burkholder-Juhasz, R. A., Levi, S. V., Dillon, C. M., & Pisoni, D. B. (2007). Nonword repetition with spectrally reduced speech: Some developmental and clinical findings from pediatric cochlear implantation. *Journal of Deaf Studies and Deaf Education, 12,* 472–485. https://doi.org/10.1093/deafed/enm031

Centers for Disease Control and Prevention. (2016). *EHDI Hearing Screening & Follow-Up Survey (HSFS).* https://www.cdc.gov/ncbddd/hearingloss/2016-data/13-2016-HSFS-Explanations-508.pdf

Centers for Disease Control and Prevention. (2019). *Types of hearing loss.* https://www.cdc.gov/ncbddd/hearingloss/types.html

Central Institute for the Deaf. (2019). *Familiar sounds audiogram.* https://cid.edu/wp-content/uploads/2016/05/CID-AUDIOGRAM-ENGLISH.pdf

Cupples, L., Ching, T. Y. C., Crowe, K., Seeto, M., Leigh, G., Street, L., . . . Thomson, J. (2014). Outcomes of 3-year-old children with hearing loss and different types of additional disabilities. *Journal of Deaf Studies and Deaf Education, 19,* 20–39. https://doi.org/10.1093/deafed/ent039

Cushing, S. L., Papsin, B. C., Rutka, J. A., James, A. L., & Gordon, K. A. (2008). Evidence of vestibular and balance dysfunction in children with profound sensorineural hearing loss using cochlear implants. *Laryngoscope, 118,* 1814–1823. https://doi.org/10.1097/MLG.0b013e31817fadfa

De Kegel, A., Maes, L., Baetens, T., Dhooge, I., & Van Waelvelde, H. (2012). The influence of a vestibular dysfunction on the motor development of hearing-impaired children. *The Laryngoscope, 122,* 2837–2843. https://doi.org/10.1002/lary.23529

Dunn, W., Cox, J., Foster, L., Mische-Lawson, L., & Tanquary, J. (2012). Impact of a contextual intervention on child participation and parent competence among children with autism spectrum disorders: A pretest–posttest repeated-measures design. *American Journal of Occupational Therapy, 66,* 520–528. https://doi.org/10.5014/ajot.2012.004119

Dunst, C. J., Bruder, M. B., Trivette, C. M., & Hamby, D. W. (2006). Everyday activity settings, natural learning environments, and early intervention practices. *Journal of Policy and Practice in Intellectual Disabilities, 3,* 3–10. https://doi.org/10.1111/j.1741-1130.2006.00047.x

Fain, B. (2019). Best practices in supporting students with hearing impairments or deafness. In G. Frolek Clark, J. Rioux, & B. Chandler (Eds.), *Best practices for occupational therapy in schools* (2nd ed., pp. 263–270). AOTA Press.

Figueras, B., Edwards, L., & Langdon, D. (2008). Executive function and language in deaf children. *Journal of Deaf Studies and Deaf Education, 13,* 362–377. https://doi.org/10.1093/deafed/enm067

Gronski, M. (2012). Team efforts to serve children who are deaf or hard of hearing. *OT Practice, 17*(17), 15–18.

Hintermair, M. (2010). Quality of life of mainstreamed hearing-impaired children: Results of a study with the Inventory of Life Quality of Children and Youth (ILC). *Zeitschrift fur Kinder-und Jugendpsychiatrie und Psychotherapie, 38,* 189–199. https://doi.org/10.1024/1422-4917/a000032

Individuals With Disabilities Education Improvement Act of 2004, Pub. L. 108–446, 20 U.S.C. §§ 1400–1482.

Koester, A. C., Mailloux, Z., Coleman, G. G., Mori, A. B., Paul, S. M., Blanche, E., . . . Cermak, S. A. (2014). Sensory integration functions of children with cochlear implants. *American Journal of Occupational Therapy, 68,* 562–569. https://doi.org/10.5014/ajot.2014.012187

Livingstone, N., & McPhillips, M. (2011). Motor skill deficits in children with partial hearing. *Developmental Medicine & Child Neurology, 53,* 836–842. https://doi.org/10.111/j/1469-8749.2011.04001.x

Marschark, M., Rhoten, C., & Fabich, M. (2007). Effects of cochlear implants on children's reading and academic achievement. *Journal of Deaf Studies and Deaf Education, 12,* 269–282. https://doi.org/10.1093/deafed/enm013

Morton, C. C., & Nance, W. E. (2006). Newborn hearing screening—A silent revolution. *New England Journal of Medicine, 345,* 2151–2164. https://doi.org/10.1056/NEJMra050700

Mroz, M. (2019). *FM systems for people with hearing loss.* https://www.healthyhearing.com/help/assistive-listening-devices/fm-systems

National Institute on Deafness and Other Communication Disorders. (2017a). *Cochlear implants* (NIH Publication No. 00-4798). https://www.nidcd.nih.gov/health/cochlear-implants

National Institute on Deafness and Other Communication Disorders. (2017b). *Hearing aids* (NIH Pub. No. 13-4340). https://www.nidcd.nih.gov/health/hearing-aids

Ottenbacher, K. J., & Cusick, A. (1990). Goal Attainment Scaling as a method of clinical service evaluation. *American Journal of Occupational Therapy, 44,* 519–525. https://doi.org/10.5014/ajot.44.6.519

Phillips, J. O., & Backous, D. D. (2002). Evaluation of vestibular function in young children. *Otolaryngologic Clinics of North America, 35,* 765–790. https://doi.org/10.1016/s0030-6665(02)00062-2

Picard, M. (2004). Children with permanent hearing loss and associated disabilities: Revisiting current epidemiological data and causes of deafness. *Volta Review, 104,* 221–236.

Remine, M. D., Care, E., & Brown, P. M. (2008). Language ability and verbal and nonverbal executive functioning in deaf students communicating in spoken English. *Journal of Deaf Studies and Deaf Education, 13,* 531–545. https://doi.org/10.1093/deafed/enn010

Rine, R. M., Braswell, J., Fisher, D., Joyce, K., Kalar, K., & Shaffer, M. (2004). Improvement of motor development and postural control following intervention in children with sensorineural hearing loss and vestibular impairment. *International Journal of Pediatric Otorhinolaryngology, 68,* 1141–1148. https://doi.org/10.1016/j.ijporl.2004.04.007

Rine, R. M., Cornwall, G., Gan, K., LoCascio, C., O'Hare, T., Robinson, E., & Rice, M. (2000). Evidence of progressive delay of motor development in children with sensorineural hearing loss and concurrent vestibular dysfunction. *Perceptual and Motor Skills, 90,* 1101–1112. https://doi.org/10.2466/pms.2000.90.3c.1101

Schlumberger, E., Narbona, J., & Manrique, M. (2004). Nonverbal development of children with deafness with and without cochlear implants. *Developmental Medicine and Child Neurology, 46,* 599–606. https://doi.org/10.1111/j.1469-8749.2004.tb01023.x

Watson, D. R., Titterington, J., Henry, A., & Toner, J. G. (2007). Auditory sensory memory and working memory processes in children with normal hearing and cochlear implants. *Audiology and Neurotology, 12,* 65–76. https://doi.org/10.1159/000097793

Best Practices in Supporting Children With Visual Impairments

36

Tammy Bruegger, OTD, MSE, OTR/L, ATP

KEY TERMS AND CONCEPTS

- Albinism
- Amblyopia
- Categorization
- Cortical or cerebral visual impairment
- De Morsier's syndrome
- Deaf-blindness
- Function object use
- Hemianopsia
- Learning Media Assessment
- Leber's congenital amaurosis
- Legal blindness
- Low vision
- Microphthalmia
- Nystagmus
- Object constancy
- Object permanence
- Ocular visual impairment
- Optic nerve hypoplasia or atrophy
- Orientation
- Orientation and mobility instructor
- Retinitis pigmentosa
- Retinopathy of prematurity
- Spatial relationships
- Strabismus
- Sturge–Weber syndrome
- Teacher of the Visually Impaired
- Usher syndrome
- Visual scanning

OVERVIEW

Low vision and blindness is one of the leading causes of disability in the United States and most developed and developing countries, whether from ocular or neurological causes (Bourne et al., 2017; Chan et al., 2018). In a recent study, 12.4% of children and adults had low vision or blindness (Varma et al., 2017). The American Printing House for the Blind (2017) reported that in 2017, 63,357 children from birth to age 21 years had low vision or blindness. Varma et al. (2017) reported that in 2015, 69% of children's visual impairments were due to uncorrected refraction errors. They also predicted a 26% increase in visual impairment by 2060. This is significant in that children who have uncorrected refraction errors or neurological visual impairment are affected developmentally over their lifetime, so there will be an increased number of persons with visual impairment of all ages.

In a review of the literature on statistics of blindness and low vision, researchers reported that there was no significant difference in the incidence of blindness by race or ethnicity. However, women and people with lower socioeconomic, education, and literacy levels have an increase in visual impairment, possibly because of lack of access to health care and vision services for conditions that affect vision (Ulldemolins et al., 2012).

Vision greatly affects development and learning for all children and even more so for children who have low vision and blindness (Brémond-Gignac et al., 2011; Fazzi et al., 2015; Merabet et al., 2017). Most resources state that more than 80% of learning occurs through vision (Project Ideal, 2013). Therefore, anything that affects vision either prenatally or postnatally may affect development in all other areas. Early identification, accurate assessment, and intervention are critical to provide a developmental foundation for occupational performance throughout childhood and adult life.

As a foundation for discussion of vision in early childhood, it is important to define the common terms:
- ***Low vision*** is a reduction in visual acuity no better than 20/60 but better than 20/200 in the better eye with correction (American Printing House for the Blind, 2017).
- ***Legal blindness*** is visual acuity no better than 20/200 in the better eye with the best correction and a central visual field that is no greater than 20 degrees (American Foundation for the Blind, 2020).

There are several types of visual conditions. Children with visual impairment may have an ocular-based visual condition, a neurological condition, or a combination of ocular and neurological conditions, in addition to other neurological conditions. ***Cortical or cerebral visual impairment*** (CVI) is a neurological visual impairment that occurs because of damage to the brain and visual pathways (Lueck & Dutton, 2015; Roman-Lantzy, 2007), as opposed to an ***ocular visual impairment,*** which occurs in the structures of the eye to the optic chiasm. CVI involves not only the eye but also the optic nerve; dorsal and ventral optic pathways; lateral geniculate body; and brain, including the occipital, temporal, parietal, and frontal lobes (Lueck & Dutton, 2015). Of the children reported to have low vision or blindness, more than 22% are diagnosed with CVI.

CVI is the leading cause of low vision and blindness among children worldwide, but it is often misidentified or not identified at all (Chokron & Dutton, 2016; Kong et al., 2014; Merabet et al., 2017; Roman-Lantzy, 2018). It may be seen in conjunction with or caused by other neurological or brain-based conditions, such as cerebral palsy, periventricular leukomalacia, traumatic brain injury, hydrocephalus, and anoxia. Ocular conditions may also occur with neurological visual impairment, such as *hemianopsia* (i.e., visual field deficit), *strabismus* (i.e., misalignment of the eyes), or *amblyopia* (i.e., loss of vision in one eye), further clouding the appropriate diagnosis, assessment, and intervention. CVI, retinopathy of prematurity, and optic nerve hypoplasia are the most common diagnoses seen among children besides general acuity issues (Fazzi et al., 2012).

ESSENTIAL CONSIDERATIONS

Visual impairment affects the child's overall development and participation in daily occupations. In turn, occupational performance skills are affected, resulting in subtle issues that produce additional barriers to participation. It is important to consider these foundation skills in planning assessment and intervention. Interprofessional collaboration is critical to address all of these important foundation skills for successful outcomes and participation in life activities and occupations.

Impact on Participation and Development

Occupational therapy practitioners address occupations, the daily life activities in which people engage (American Occupational Therapy Association [AOTA], 2020). (*Note. Occupational therapy practitioner* refers to both occupational therapists and occupational therapy assistants.) Children's early occupations include self-help, rest and sleep, social participation, play and leisure, communication, learning, and literacy. These occupations occur in context and are influenced by the child's performance skills (e.g., motor, process, and social interactions) and performance patterns (e.g., routines, roles, habits) as well as the context (e.g., cultural, temporal) and environment (e.g., physical, social). Without intact vision, all of these areas are affected (Lueck & Dutton, 2015; Roman-Lantzy, 2018).

The timing of the condition that affects vision is important; if it occurs during a critical time in development, it affects not only vision but also other areas of development. Studies in neuroplasticity and vision show that many other areas of the brain are involved in visual development (Lueck & Dutton, 2015; Merabet et al., 2017). Visual impairment affects typical development, including motor skills, ADLs, play, cognition, and communication (Fazzi et al., 2015; Lueck & Dutton, 2015; Merebet et al., 2017; Oluonye & Sargent, 2018; Salavati et al., 2014). In addition, because 80% of what is learned is from visual input, future development is affected because of the child's inability to learn incidentally and their disadvantage from loss of visual learning.

Social skills

Without eye contact, emotional bonding may be difficult. Not only does the child not receive input from the mother or caregiver, but the caregiver does not receive the reciprocal input and reinforcement from the child that helps establish a bond (Brémond-Gignac et al., 2011; Lueck & Dutton, 2015). Vision allows anticipation of movement. If the child sees the caregiver walking toward them when they are crying, they may anticipate being picked up or touched. If they do not see the person, they may startle if suddenly picked up or touched. It is important to speak before touching and give touch cues before picking up or providing care to the child.

Learning

Cognitive development depends on a child's early sensory experiences from vision, hearing, movement, and tactile exploration. Typically, the ability to localize and explore visually develops before the ability to localize sound, to move, and to explore tactilely. Without the full use of vision to connect the various sensory inputs, it is more difficult for the child to perceive objects or situations that may be more apparent to sighted children.

Children who have a visual impairment may have different patterns of development related to attention and exploration, awareness of objects with which they have no tactile experience, *object permanence* (i.e., knowing that objects exist when they are not immediately available), *object constancy* (i.e., recognizing similarities in objects), *categorization* (i.e., identifying similarities and differences in objects and events), *spatial relationships* (i.e., understanding where objects are in relation to one another), and *orientation* (i.e., understanding where objects are in relation to other people and objects in the environment; Baladron et al., 2016; Lueck & Dutton, 2015). Development of these concepts must be through the other senses—tactile, auditory, smell, kinesthetic, proprioceptive, and vestibular (movement)—as well as use of any available vision.

Motor skills

A child's vision greatly affects the development of fine and large motor skills (Bakke et al., 2019). Vision affects the child's ability to move around in their environment. Children also are motivated by visual input to sit up, get on all fours, crawl, pull to stand, and walk (Bakke et al., 2019; Lueck & Dutton, 2015). Vision is critical in development of cause and effect, object permanence, and *function object use* (i.e., understanding the use and purpose of objects, such as that a comb is used to comb hair; Lueck & Dutton, 2015). Visually guided reach (using vision to locate while reaching for an object) in all positions is affected when a child's vision is impaired. In addition, because of lack of movement and play in a variety of positions, children with visual impairment may have decreased strength in their arms, shoulders, and trunk as well as decreased trunk rotation during ambulation or other movements (Bakke et al., 2019; Chokron & Dutton, 2016). This affects development of reach, grasp, and fine motor and manipulation skills.

Play skills

Children develop imitation and play skills through incidental learning and observation. Without vision, it is difficult for a child to learn through incidental means, so it is important to provide other ways of learning through tactile, auditory, and kinesthetic sensory modes by touching, manipulating, and helping the child experience play and functional skills.

Collaborative Teaming to Support Children With Visual Impairments

Children with special needs in early childhood may receive services from occupational therapy, physical therapy, speech pathology, early childhood education, special education, ophthalmology or optometry, and other medical or educational services. Other professionals who may be part of the team with children who have visual impairment include the *teacher of the visually impaired* (TVI; i.e., a teacher who specializes in instruction and strategies for low vision and blindness) and the *orientation and mobility instructor* (O & M; i.e., a teacher trained in cane use and other vision-related mobility skills).

Early intervention services are provided in the natural environment, such as the home, preschool, or child care center. Therefore, communication and collaboration with parents and caregivers is important and helps ensure that any intervention is carried out in all settings in which the child participates. Research suggests that early intervention services should follow a delivery model of services that is family centered (Hatton et al., 2002; Pletcher & Younggren, 2013). As the child grows, services may be provided in preschools and in community settings, such as the park, restaurants, and playgrounds. This allows the child with a visual impairment to experience learning in real settings (experiential learning) through interaction with real materials and objects in real settings. Practitioners should collaborate and work as a team with other professionals to increase effectiveness of services to the family and child (Welp et al., 2016; Workman et al., 2016).

Conditions and Diagnoses

Vision can be affected by a variety of ocular and neurological conditions, resulting in many different visual conditions, as described in Table 36.1.

Early Signs of Visual Impairments

Identification of visual impairment is reliant on observations from parents, physicians, and other caregivers in infancy. These observations may be obtained from observing the child or interviewing the parent regarding their concerns. Signs of a visual impairment are listed in Exhibit 36.1. Observation of several of these signs warrants a referral to a vision professional (American Association for Pediatric Ophthalmology and Strabismus, 2019).

BEST PRACTICES

Assessing children with visual impairment involves review of medical records, structured or semistructured parent interview, assessment of occupational performance, and other assessment tools to develop an occupational profile of the child. This is an ongoing assessment that continues to be developed as the child receives other medical and educational services and with continued development (AOTA, 2020; Bruegger, 2019).

Evaluate Occupational Performance

Evaluation includes gathering the occupational profile and analyzing occupational performance.

Occupational profile

The occupational therapist may interview the parent or other caregiver using semiformal questions or various assessment tools to develop the child's occupational profile. The Canadian Occupational Performance Measure (Law et al., 2019) and AOTA's (2017) occupational profile template are semistructured interview tools that are useful in developing an occupational profile for the child through interviewing the parent. This is important to determine the child's strengths and needs in occupations and occupational performance skills affected by visual impairment.

Medical records, including assessments from ophthalmology, neurology, developmental medicine, and other physicians, should be reviewed at the beginning of the process to determine diagnoses and other medical issues affecting the child's vision and development. Neurological tests, such as magnetic resonance imaging, may show evidence of lesions that may affect vision, especially CVI (visual processing). Although this diagnosis is not identified until later, there is a negative impact on development (Baladron et al., 2016; Bruegger, 2019; Jackel, 2019). Review of records is an ongoing process as the child receives additional medical or educational interventions.

Observe in natural environments

Gathering authentic, formal data through formal observations of the child is essential. In the natural environment, the occupational therapist observes the child's exploration and reaction to toys and materials. By structuring the environment, the therapist can promote the child's active exploration. Therapists should be sure the child has proper positioning and support to facilitate motor activity. The therapist should also consider the environment (e.g., reduce background clutter, adjust lighting for the child; McDowell & Budd, 2018) and materials (e.g., use objects with various sensory features, e.g., sound, taste, texture, smell, size, colored lights).

Contrasts between the background and test object are important. High-contrast materials are easier for the child to see. Present objects at different distances and in different areas of the visual field while encouraging the child to touch objects with their hand. Occupational therapists should observe performance in a variety of environments to determine supports and limitations in the physical and social aspects of the environment.

Augment observations with assessment tools

Children with visual impairment often achieve developmental milestones at a different time, order, and rate than sighted children (Lueck & Dutton, 2015). Because most standardized tools do not include normative samples of children with low vision or blindness and most of the items are vision dependent, these tools usually underestimate the child's abilities. See Table 36.2 for a list of assessment tools specifically designed for children with visual impairment.

In addition, a functional vision assessment can be conducted by an occupational therapist or in collaboration with a TVI. This ecological assessment includes observation of the eyes; acuity; oculomotor skills; viewing of objects

TABLE 36.1.   Visual Conditions and Interventions (General, Medical, and Occupational Therapy)

CONDITION AND DEFINITION	INTERVENTIONS
Albinism: Lack of pigment in the eyes, skin, or hair; sensitive to bright light and glare; may have nystagmus, low vision, or blindness	Bifocals, magnifiers, tinted sunglasses, and other optical devices
Amblyopia: Reduced vision in one eye because the brain is favoring the other eye	Eyeglasses, eye patching, exercises
Cortical or cerebral visual impairment (CVI): A neurological visual impairment; decreased visual processing in the brain	Visual simplification, use of color preference, movement, highlight salient features, other CVI strategies
De Morsier's syndrome (septo-optic dysplasia): Optic nerve is underdeveloped; may cause blindness in one or both eyes	Strategies for low vision or blindness; use of AT
Leber's congenital amaurosis: Inherited condition caused by degeneration of the retina; infant is born blind or develops severe vision loss	Experimental treatment with gene therapy (medical); strategies for low vision or blindness
Microphthalmia: Rare inherited disease in which one or both eyes are abnormally small; varies from reduced vision to blindness	Artificial eyeball used to maintain eye socket. OT may help with low vision or blind strategies
Nystagmus: Involuntary, rapid, repetitive horizontal, vertical, or circular movements of one or both eyes; child may lose their place when reading	OT may help with strategies for access to learning such as placing a cut-out reading window over words or using a card to "underline" text
Optic nerve hypoplasia or atrophy: Underdevelopment or degeneration of the optic nerve may cause permanently dimmed or blurred vision, reduced field of vision, difficulty with contrast and fine detail	Use of appropriate lighting, high contrast, and bold colors may help children with optic nerve atrophy see more clearly
Retinitis pigmentosa: Degeneration of the retina, resulting in decreased night vision, gradual loss of peripheral vision, and sometimes loss of central vision resulting in blindness	Depending on the degree of vision loss, use of electronic magnifiers, night-vision scopes, and other assistive technology. OT may help with training to use AT.
Retinopathy of prematurity: Growth of abnormal blood vessels in the eye because of premature birth; increased risk of retinal detachment, reduced vision, and blindness	Laser therapy (medical) and use of low vision AT (OT)
Strabismus: Eyes are not aligned because the ocular muscles do not work together; may be inherited or caused by disease or injury	May be corrected with eyeglasses, eye-muscle exercises, surgery, or patching the stronger eye (medical)
Sturge–Weber syndrome: Genetic condition with facial birthmark; seizures; and neurological, visual (glaucoma, field deficit), and developmental symptoms	Treatment includes laser treatment for the port-wine stain (i.e., birthmark), anticonvulsants, and medical or surgical treatment for glaucoma (medical); low vision and blind adaptations and AT (OT)
Usher syndrome: Partial or total hearing loss with gradual vision loss resulting from retinitis pigmentosa; may have balance issues	Hearing aids, training in sign language and lip reading, devices for impaired vision, and counseling to prepare for the future

Note. AT = assistive technology; OT = occupational therapy.

Sources. American Association for Pediatric Ophthalmology and Strabismus (2019); American Foundation for the Blind (2020); Boston Children's Hospital (2019); Higueros et al. (2017); Texas School for the Blind (2019); Zallmann et al. (2018).

EXHIBIT 36.1.   Early Signs of a Visual Impairment

- Avoids bright light or squints in bright light and prefers dim light (i.e., photophobia)
- Gazes at bright lights
- Closes one eye
- Nondirected or roving eye movements
- Lack of response to parent's face in absence of voice or sound
- Decreased imitation of facial expression
- Decreased following of moving objects or people
- Decreased reach for or interest in bottle, toys, or objects when presented without sound
- Limited interest in television, books, and toys
- Decreased identification of colors, objects, or shapes when older
- Bumps into objects when moving
- Presses or pokes the eyes.

in near, middle, and distant space; visual scanning; saccadic eye movements; eye alignment; contrast sensitivity; eye–hand coordination; color preference; and complexity of materials. If a child has CVI, the occupational therapist may use the CVI Range to determine visual processing, especially if the child has known neurological conditions, such as cerebral palsy, anoxia, or traumatic brain injury (Roman-Lantzy, 2007, 2019). In order to provide comprehensive assessment of a child with CVI, it may be necessary to use a variety of formal and informal assessments (Bruegger, 2019; Law & Canadian Association of Occupational Therapists, 1991; Lueck et al., 2019).

As the child nears school age, a ***Learning Media Assessment*** may be conducted by the teacher of the visually impaired and the educational team to determine the child's optimum learning style, such as print size, braille or tactile

TABLE 36.2. Assessment Tools Designed or Adapted for Children With Visual Impairments

ASSESSMENT TOOL	FORMAT AND AGE RANGE
Battelle Developmental Inventory (3rd ed.; Newborg, 2020)	▪ Standardized (birth–8 years) ▪ Adapted for children with vision impairment
Callier–Azusa Scale (for children with deaf-blindness; Callier Center for Communication Disorders, 1978)	▪ Criterion referenced (birth–10 years)
Cortical Visual Impairment Range (Roman-Lantzy, 2007, 2018)	▪ Interview, observation, checklist (all ages)
Developmental Assessment for Individuals With Severe Disabilities (Dykes & Murzek, 2018)	▪ Criterion referenced (birth–6 years)
Functional Scheme: Functional Skills Assessment (Nielsen, 1974)	▪ Observation (birth–48 months developmental level)
Functional Vision and Learning Media Assessment Kit (American Printing House for the Blind, n.d.)	▪ Observational (preschool to adult) ▪ Individualized assessment based on visual function and academic needs.
Hawaii Early Learning Profile (VORT Corporation, 2019; adapted for children with visual impairment and multiple disabilities)	▪ Criterion referenced and curriculum based (birth–6 years)
Oregon Project for Preschool Children Who Are Blind or Visually Impaired (Southern Oregon Education Service District, 2019)	▪ Criterion referenced and curriculum based (birth–6 years)

Sources: American Printing House for the Blind (n.d.); Willings (2017).

print, or auditory and other sensory means. The occupational therapist is a vital member of the team for comprehensive assessment. For a list of assessment tools that are frequently used to evaluate child development and participation, see Appendix F, "Examples of Assessments for Early Childhood (Birth–5 Years)."

Provide Evidence-Based Interventions

Interventions may improve vision skills and development, building on these skills because of the brain's neuroplasticity, including use of residual vision or compensatory techniques to aid development in motor, sensory, and social skills; communication; play; literacy; and ADLs (Lueck & Dutton, 2015). There are many strategies that may be effectively used by occupational therapy practitioners working with children with visual impairments.

Use assistive technology and adapt the environment and objects

For children who have low vision, magnification of materials and enlargement of print font or pictures may be used to optimize viewing of books and materials. Magnification should not be so great that it affects viewing area and makes it difficult for the child to navigate materials. Determining the print and symbol size that is most easily seen over time and in the context of written sentences and books, as opposed to letters in isolation, is important. Often a child may see a smaller size print in isolation, but in a book, sentence, or paragraph, they may have more difficulty seeing for reading because of crowding of letters. Visual components should be easier so that the child can focus on the cognitive aspects of the task (e.g., reading, writing, concept development).

Lighting is extremely important for children who have low vision and blindness. Use of lighted materials often aids in localization to materials or objects. In addition, environments with low lighting may affect the child's ability to use residual vision; therefore, it is imperative to provide natural, indirect lighting and to reduce glare from excessive lighting. Additional lamps may need to be used at the desk or table for viewing and placed over the child's shoulder, not directly in their eyes. This is also important when choosing magnifiers to use for visual tasks. Collaboration with others regarding devices (e.g., magnifiers, glasses, other visual aids) and other assistive technology from an optometrist or low vision specialist is important to facilitate incorporation into daily routines. Occupational therapy practitioners can assist in training the child in use of these devices during functional tasks.

Provide effective strategies

Teaching *visual scanning* (i.e., the ability to use vision to look in a systematic manner, top to bottom, left to right) is important during self-help skills to locate the spoon during feeding, hygiene items around the sink, or clothing in a closet or in a drawer. Visual scanning is also important while moving to locate obstacles or objects during play. Visual scanning is critical during movements, classroom work, and other ADLs.

Other strategies include using verbal cues or tactile cues to inform the child what is happening in the environment and tell them when you are going to touch them. Ask permission to help if possible. Use hand-under-hand interactions with the child instead of "grabbing" their hands and taking them through actions or activities. Allow them to feel your hands doing the activity with them and touch the materials as they feel comfortable.

Expanding the visual field or attention to that field through visual stimulation with lighted toys, wands, adaptive switches, video or computerized games, and placement of materials and objects in the affected visual field may be useful. This has been shown to increase the visual field for children and adults with field deficits (Waddington & Hodgson, 2017). Nielsen (n.d.) created the Little Room, a five-sided small space with superior acoustics for young children with visual impairments to explore objects that are suspended or attached to the sides. This has encouraged independent exploration, movement, and vocalization.

Provide appropriate intervention based on type of visual impairment

Interventions for ocular visual impairment are different than interventions for neurologically based CVI (see Table 36.3).

Support Participation for Children With Deaf-Blindness

When a child has ***deaf-blindness*** (i.e., the combination of hearing and visual impairment that causes such severe communication and other developmental and educational needs that they cannot be accommodated in special education programs solely for children with deafness or children with blindness; Individuals with Disabilities Education Act, 2004), they need many different learning and communication options. Strategies should encourage use of any residual vision and hearing during daily routines. Communications adaptations should support natural social interactions and conversations through symbolic and nonsymbolic methods.

TABLE 36.3.   Comparing Strategies for Ocular Visual Impairment and Cortical Visual Impairment

TYPE OF IMPAIRMENT	STRATEGIES FOR THERAPY
Ocular low vision	▪ Wear corrective lenses if prescribed to optimize residual vision. ▪ Explore the use of magnification or magnifiers with functional activities and play. ▪ Use high-contrast materials, such as bold print; dark lines on paper; dark pencil, marker, or crayons on light background. ▪ Use adequate lighting to optimize residual vision and reduce fatigue. ▪ Use adaptations and visual skills during play, ADLs, and literacy to optimize use of vision. Notice fatigue and need for visual breaks. ▪ Select toys and other materials using light, contrast, and texture to aid with learning and play. ▪ Use a cut-out tactile signature or writing guides to aid in writing skills. ▪ Use assistive technology to optimize function in play; leisure; communication; and cognitive, preacademic, and academic activities.
Ocular blindness	▪ Develop tactile skills, particularly tactile discrimination. ▪ Develop auditory skills for common environmental sounds and digital text to speech (voice or sound output). ▪ Develop orientation and mobility skills (e.g., orientation in space during movement, use of an ambulation mobility device or white cane) through collaboration with an orientation and mobility professional. ▪ Develop fine and gross motor skills or compensatory strategies. ▪ Use tactile search pattern techniques. ▪ Develop independence in self-help skills using other sensory systems. ▪ Use assistive technology to support literacy and function.
Cortical visual impairment	▪ Use visual simplification, color, and light preferences to highlight salient features of materials for increased visual localization, fixation, attention, and interaction. ▪ Use a shield to block out extraneous visual input to increase focus on salient features or localization to visual stimuli. ▪ Develop visually guided reach first through visual localization, motor coordination and strength, and integration of vision with motor skills for reaching. Grading the amount of reach and time of visual localization increases success and motivation (i.e., starting with smaller range of movement and increasing range of movement and time localizing on the visual target). ▪ Use ocular motility skills (visual localization, fixation, saccades and gaze shifting, convergence and divergence, visual tracking and scanning) as a foundation for functional abilities. ▪ Control visual input to avoid overstimulation; eliminate extraneous noise or visual distractions by using a black feltboard or foamboard shield, or shadow box with materials; and limit additional visual stimulation by assessing the environment for visual distractors or barriers. ▪ Use touch or movement cues to aid in locating objects (e.g., bring spoon to mouth by moving the spoon before bringing it to mouth; use contrasting color to aid in seeing the spoon). ▪ Use color highlighting with salient features (e.g., bubbling or outline of objects, letters, pictures, symbols). Outline openings of containers and inset puzzles with red or yellow duct tape, paint, wax covered string, and so on, to assist in location of opening. Use color coding or matching for puzzles. ▪ Use assistive technology to support literacy and function. ▪ Consider visual needs when designing and addressing literacy and other occupational performance areas.

Note. ADLs = activities of daily living.
Sources. Baker-Nobles & Rutherford (1995); Baladron et al. (2016); Bruegger (2019); Hatlen (1996); Lueck & Dutton (2015); McDowell & Budd (2018); Roman-Lantzy (2007, 2019); Texas School for the Blind (2019); Waddington & Hodgson (2017).

| EXHIBIT 36.2. | Strategies for Working With Children With Deaf-Blindness |

- Greet the child by touching the back of their hand or shoulder, and introduce yourself by saying your name and presenting your name sign or tactile symbol. Pause and wait for the child's response while maintaining touch to their hand or shoulder (touch cue).
- Offer your hands to the child; place your hands beside or slightly underneath the child's hands.
- Encourage the child to explore the materials and the environment tactilely. Place your hands under child's hands to assist with exploration (hand-under-hand assistance).
- Encourage a variety of communicative functions (e.g., request, reject).
- At the end of an activity, use tactile sign by placing your hands under the child's hands, and sign *finish* with coactive movement with the child for the sign. Tactilely model for the child how to put objects in a *finish* box or push them away to signal the end of the activity.
- Say goodbye by using a goodbye gesture (e.g., wave, high five, touch cue on shoulder) and having the child tactilely attend to this signal.
- Determine the child's preferences by observation, and use those actions or objects in your interactions and in your development of conversations.
- Provide time for the child to process information, and observe the child for an anticipatory response. Wait to give them time to respond.
- Teach concepts using "real" objects through touch and exploration and use physical demonstration with hand under hand exploration or describing actions.
- Use verbal description, tactile sign language (a method of receiving sign language or fingerspelling by placing one's hands over a communication partner's hands to feel their shape and movement), tactile objects or color, and high-contrast pictures if the child has residual vision.
- Attend to, interpret, and respond immediately to the child's communication behaviors, allowing the child to respond using the most natural means (e.g., point, touch a symbol, reach for an object, use hand-under-hand sign language).

Sources. American Foundation for the Blind (n.d.); Moss & Hagood (1995); National Center on Deaf-Blindness (n.d.); Nelson et al. (2009); Van Dijk (2019).

Communication adaptations include the use of selected tactile symbols (e.g., objects, tangible symbols, textured items, signs) to meet the child's communication needs.

Children with deaf-blindness need extensive experience with objects, signs, and other symbols during natural everyday situations. Tactile strategies help the child to anticipate familiar events and direct their attention to ongoing activity through tactile schedules, transition schedules, and communication options with tactile symbols. This increases the child's opportunity for social interactions, supports participation in activities, supports receptive and expressive communication, and helps the child learn. Providing real objects in routines is important for development of ADLs, fine and large motor skills, and other areas of occupational performance. Using assistive technology as a tool may further reduce barriers to function. Exhibit 36.2 provides intervention strategies for children with deaf-blindness.

SUMMARY

Children with visual impairment have specialized needs that require consideration of their sensory needs; present and future visual abilities; and development of motor, self-help, communication, play, and social–emotional skills. Occupational therapy practitioners are vital members of the team to help visually impaired children develop occupational performance skills for successful participation in occupations and life.

RESOURCES

- **Ablenet, Inc.: www.ablenetinc.com**
  Resource for assistive technology devices and toys
- **American Foundation for the Blind: www.afb.org**
  National organization dedicated to advocacy; provides information, research, and resources for people with low vision and blindness

- **American Printing House for the Blind: www.aph.org**
  National organization that produces braille, written materials, and products for people who have low vision and blindness
- **Developmental Guidelines for Infants With Visual Impairments (Lueck et al., 2008)**
  Resource on development of children with visual impairment
- **Enabling Devices, Inc.: www.enablingdevices.com**
  Resource for assistive technology devices and toys
- **Hadley Institute for the Blind: www.hadley.edu**
  School that provides education for individuals with visual impairment, parents, and professionals
- **Little Bear Sees: www.littlebearsees.org**
  Organization that promotes information and develops iPad applications for people with CVI
- **National Center on Deaf-Blindness: www.nationaldb.org**
  Resources for supporting and educating children and adults with deaf-blindness
- **National Federation of the Blind's Early Childhood Initiatives: https://nfb.org/programs-services/early-childhood-initiatives**
  Resource on early childhood from organization that provides information and research on blindness
- **Paths to Literacy: www.pathstoliteracy.org**
  Resources and information on CVI, visual impairment, and blindness
- **Perkins School for the Blind: www.perkins.org**
  School for children with visual impairment; provides information and education on visual impairment
- **Start Seeing CVI: www.startseeingcvi.com**
  Advocacy group that provides information and support on CVI
- **Texas School for the Blind and Visually Impaired: www.tsbvi.edu**
  School for the blind that provides information and education on visual impairment

- **University of North Carolina Center for Literacy and Disability Studies: https://unc.live/2ZOpeav**
  Resources for literacy for children with multiple disabilities, including blindness
- **Wonderbaby: www.wonderbaby.org/**
  Online resource on children with visual impairment

REFERENCES

American Association for Pediatric Ophthalmology and Strabismus. (2019). *Vision screening guidelines.* https://aapos.org/patients/patient-resources/vision-screening-patients

American Foundation for the Blind. (n.d.). *Resources for parents of children who are blind or visually impaired.* https://www.afb.org/blindness-and-low-vision/familyconnect-8160

American Foundation for the Blind. (2020). *Glossary of eye conditions.* https://www.afb.org/blindness-and-low-vision/eye-conditions#lowvision

American Occupational Therapy Association. (2017). Occupational profile template. *American Journal of Occupational Therapy, 71,* 7112420030. https://doi.org/10.5014/ajot.2017.716S12

American Occupational Therapy Association. (2020). Occupational therapy practice framework: Domain and process (4th ed.). *American Journal of Occupational Therapy, 74,* 7412410010. https://doi.org/10.5014/ajot.2020.74S2001

American Printing House for the Blind. (n.d.). *Functional Vision and Learning Media Assessment.* Author.

American Printing House for the Blind. (2017). *Annual report 2017: Distribution of eligible students based on the federal quota census of January 4, 2016 (Fiscal Year 2016).* Author.

Baker-Nobles, L., & Rutherford, A. (1995). Understanding cortical visual impairment in children. *American Journal of Occupational Therapy, 49,* 899–903. https://doi.org/10.5014/ajot.49.9.899

Bakke, H. A., Cavalcante, W. A., de Oliveira, I. S., Sarinho, S. W., & Cattuzzo, M. T. (2019). Assessment of motor skills in children with visual impairment: A systematic and integrative review. *Clinical Medicine Insights: Pediatrics, 13.* https://doi.org/10.1177/1179556519838287

Baladron, C., Bauer, C., & Merabet, L. (2016). Cerebral versus ocular visual impairment: The impact on developmental plasticity. *Frontiers in Psychology, 7, 1958,* https://doi.org/10.3389/fpsyg.2016.01958

Boston Children's Hospital. (2019). *Vision therapy services: Frequently asked questions.* Author.

Bourne, R., Flaxman, S., Braithwaite, T., Cicinelli, M., Das, A., Jonas, J., . . . Taylor, H. R. (2017). Magnitude, temporal trends, and projections of the global prevalence of blindness and distance and near vision impairment: A systematic review and meta-analysis. *Lancet Global Health, 5,* E888–E897. https://doi.org/10.1016/S2214-109X(17)30293-0

Brémond-Gignac, D., Copin, H., Lapillonne, A., & Milazzo, S. (2011). Visual development in infants: Physiological and pathological mechanisms. *Current Opinion in Ophthalmology, 22,* S1–S8. https://doi.org/10.1097/01.icu.0000397180.37316.5d

Bruegger, T. (2019). *A descriptive case series on the occupational performance of children with cerebral (cortical) visual impairment* [Unpublished doctoral dissertation]. University of Kansas.

Callier Center for Communication Disorders. (1978). *Callier-Azusa Scale.* https://calliercenter.utdallas.edu/evaluation-treatment/callier-azusa-scale/

Chan, T., Friedman, D. S., Bradley, C., & Massof, R. (2018). Estimates of incidence and prevalence of visual impairment, low vision, and blindness in the United States. *Journal of the American Medical Association: Ophthalmology, 136,* 12–19. https://doi.org/10.1001/jamaophthalmol.2017.4655

Chokron, S., & Dutton, G. N. (2016). Impact of cerebral visual impairments on motor skills: Implications for developmental coordination disorders. *Frontiers in Psychology, 7.* https://doi.org/10.3389/fpsyg.2016.01471

Dykes, M. K., & Murzek, D. W. (2018). *Developmental Assessment for Individuals With Severe Disabilities* (3rd ed.). Western Psychological Services.

Fazzi, E., Molinaro, A., & Hartmann, E. (2015). The potential impact of visual impairment and CVI on child development. In A. Lueck & G. Dutton (Eds.), *Vision and the brain: Understanding cerebral visual impairment in children* (pp. 83–104). AFB Press.

Fazzi, E., Signorini, S. G., La Piana, R., Bertone, C., Misefari, W., Galli, J., . . . Bianchi, P. E. (2012). Neuro-ophthalmological disorders in cerebral palsy: Ophthalmological, oculomotor, and visual aspects. *Developmental Medicine and Child Neurology, 54,* 730–736. https://doi.org/10.1111/j.1469-8749.2012.04324.x

Hatlen, P. (1996). *The core curriculum for blind and visually impaired students, including those with additional disabilities.* RE:view, 28, 25–32.

Hatton, D. D., McWilliam, R. A., & Winton, P. J. (2002). *Infants and toddlers with visual impairments: Suggestion for early interventionists.* https://www.ericdigests.org/2003-5/infants.htm

Higueros, E., Roe, E., Granell, E., & Baselga, E. (2017). Sturge–Weber syndrome: A review. *Actas Dermosifiliographicas, 108,* 407–417. https://doi.org/10.1016/j.ad.2016.09.022

Individuals With Disabilities Education Improvement Act of 2004, Pub. L. 108-446, 20 U.S.C. §1400-1482.

Jackel, B. (2019). A survey of parents of children with cortical or cerebral visual impairment: 2018 follow-up. *Seminars in Pediatric Neurology, 31,* 3–4. https://doi.org/10.1016/j.spen.2019.05.002

Law, M., Baptiste, S., Carswell, A., McColl, M., Polatajko, H. & Pollock, N. (2019). *Canadian Occupational Performance Measure* (5th ed., rev.). COPM, Inc.

Law, M., & Canadian Association of Occupational Therapists. (1991). *Canadian Occupational Performance Measure.* Canadian Association of Occupational Therapists.

Lueck, A., Chen, D., Kekelis, L., & Hartmann, E. (2008). *Developmental guidelines for infants with visual impairments* (2nd ed.). American Printing House.

Lueck, A., & Dutton, G. (Eds.). (2015). *Vision and the brain: Understanding cerebral visual impairment in children.* New York: AFB Press.

Lueck, A., Dutton, D., & Chokron, S. (2019). Profiling children with cerebral visual impairment using multiple methods of assessment to aid in differential diagnosis. *Seminars in Pediatric Neurology, 31,* 5–14. https://doi.org/10.1016/j.spen.2019.05.003

McDowell, N., & Budd, J. (2018). The perspectives of teachers and paraeducators on the relationship between classroom clutter and learning experiences for students with cerebral visual impairment. *Journal of Visual Impairment & Blindness, 112,* 248–260. https://doi.org/10.1177/0145482X1811200304

Merabet, L. B., Mayer, D. L., Bauer, C. M., Wright, D., & Kran, B. S. (2017). Disentangling how the brain is "wired" in cortical (cerebral) visual impairment. *Seminars in Pediatric Neurology, 24*(2), 83–91. https://doi.org/10.1016/j.spen.2017.04.005

Moss, K., & Hagood, L. (1995). *Teaching strategies and content modifications for the child with deaf-blindness.* https://www.tsbvi.edu/deafblindness/203-resources/4250-teaching-strategies-and-content-modifications-for-the-child-with-deaf-blindness

National Center on Deaf-Blindness. (n.d.). *Educational practices.* https://www.nationaldb.org/info-center/educational-practices/

Nelson, C., van Dijk, J., Oster, T., & McDonnell, A. (2009). *Child-guided strategies: The Van Dijk approach to assessment.* American Printing House for the Blind.

Newborg, J. (2020). *Battelle Developmental Inventory* (3rd ed.). Riverside.

Nielsen, L. (1974). *Functional Scheme Assessment.* https://active-learningspace.org/assessment

Nielsen, L. (n.d.). *The Little Room.* http://activelearningspace.org/equipment/purchase-equipment/little-room

Oluonye, N., & Sargent, J. (2018). Severe visual impairment: Practical guidance for paediatricians. *Paediatrics & Child Health, 28,* 379–383. https://doi.org/10.1016/j.paed.2018.06.007

Pletcher, L., & Younggren, N. (2013). *The early intervention workbook: Essential practices for quality services.* Brookes.

Project Ideal. (2013). *Visual impairments.* http://www.projectidealonline.org/v/visual-impairments/

Roman-Lantzy, C. (2007). *Cortical visual impairment: An approach to assessment and intervention.* AFB Press.

Roman-Lantzy, C. (2018). *Cortical visual impairment: An approach to assessment and intervention* (2nd ed.). AFB Press.

Roman-Lantzy, C. (Ed.). (2019). *Cortical visual impairment: Advanced principles.* APH Press.

Southern Oregon Education Service District. (2019). *Oregon Project Curriculum and Skills Inventory.* Author.

Ulldemolins, A. R., Lansingh, V. C., Valencia, L. G., Carter, M. J., & Eckert, K. A. (2012). Social inequalities in blindness and visual impairment: A review of social determinants. *Indian Journal of Ophthalmology, 60,* 368–375. https://doi.org/10.4103/0301-4738.100529

Van Dijk, J. (2019). *Child guided assessment.* https://www.perkinselearning.org/videos/webcast/child-guided-assessment

Varma, R., Tarczy-Hornoch, K., & Jiang, X. (2017). Visual impairment in preschool children in the United States: Demographic and geographic variations from 2015 to 2060. *Journal of the American Medical Association: Ophthalmology, 135,* 610–616. https://doi.org/10.1001/jamaophthalmol.2017.1021

VORT Corporation. (2019). *Hawaii Early Learning Profile (HELP).* Menlo Park, CA: Author.

Waddington, J., & Hodgson, T. (2017). Review of rehabilitation and habilitation strategies for children and young people with homonymous visual field loss caused by cerebral vision impairment. *British Journal of Visual Impairment, 35,* 197–210. https://doi.org/10.1177/0264619617706100

Welp, A., Woodbury, R., & McCoy, M. (2016). *Making eye health a population health imperative: Vision for tomorrow.* https://www.ncbi.nlm.nih.gov/books/NBK402380/

Willings, C. (2017). *Educational assessments.* https://www.teachingvisuallyimpaired.com/educational-assessments.html

Workman, M., Vogtle, L., & Yuen, H. K. (2016). Factors associated with comfort level of school-based occupational therapists in providing low-vision services. *Occupational Therapy in Health Care, 30,* 152–165. https://doi.org/10.3109/07380577.2015.1101793

Zallmann, M., Leventer, R. J., Mackay, M. T., Ditchfield, M., Bekhor, P. S., & Su, J. C. (2018). Screening for Sturge–Weber syndrome: A state-of-the-art review. *Pediatric Dermatology, 35,* 30–42. https://doi.org/10.1111/pde.13304

Best Practices in Supporting Children With Health Needs

Julie Jones, OTD, OTR/L, BCP

37

KEY TERMS AND CONCEPTS

- Assistive technology
- Children with special health care needs
- Data-driven decision making
- Gastric or gastrostomy tube
- Gastrojejunal or transjejunal tube
- Health literacy
- Home nursing
- Individualized health plan
- Jejunal tube
- Nasoduodenal tube
- Nasogastric tube
- Nasojejunal tube
- Participation-focused, authentic, collaborative, and explicit
- School nurses

OVERVIEW

According to the Health Resources and Services Administration of the U.S. Department of Health and Human Services (DHHS, 2019), 1 in 5 families have children with special health care needs (CSHCN). *CSHCN* are defined as "those who have or are at increased risk for a chronic physical, developmental, or emotional condition and who also require health and related services of a type or amount beyond that required by children generally" (McPherson et al., 1998, p. 138). In 2013, the DHHS reported that 23% of households have at least one CSHCN, and many of these children have multiple medical diagnoses. The cause of their special health care needs is multifactorial and may occur during the prenatal, perinatal, or postnatal stages as a result of chromosomal abnormalities, infections, lack of oxygen, medication reactions, or physical trauma (Bobzien et al., 2015).

Occupational therapy services can help promote the health and well-being of CSHCN and their families. Occupational therapy practitioners provide a variety of services to promote the child's access to and engagement in everyday routines. (*Note. Occupational therapy practitioner* refers to both occupational therapists and occupational therapy assistants.) When working with a young child with special health care needs, a practitioner may provide services in the health care, preschool, community, or home setting (American Occupational Therapy Association [AOTA], 2015).

ESSENTIAL CONSIDERATIONS

A relationship exists between the health condition of CSHCN and the functional skill development that the child may experience (Lollar et al., 2012). Some children experience problems with breathing, circulation, attention, anxiety, pain, and motor coordination, with 85% experiencing at least one functional difficulty (Lollar et al., 2012). This section reviews support for the family, importance of coordination between teams, functional difficulties that have the potential to affect a child's occupational engagement, and medical equipment.

Support for the Family

Families of CSHCN may have different values and belief systems that affect how occupational therapy services are provided and delivered. Acknowledging that some families may have stronger cultural influences on the basis of their origin, heritage, or socioeconomic status is essential (Lowry & Shaw, 2013). For example, cultural influences regarding feeding practices are important when delivering family-centered services that are sensitive to the family's needs (Howe et al., 2019). The most successful interventions are implemented by professionals with strong cultural awareness, which may include race, ethnicity, socioeconomic status, gender, or sexual orientation (Eddy, 2013).

Home nursing care

CSHCN have many medical challenges and require an abundance of resources and services after they have been discharged home after birth or subsequent admissions (Elias et al., 2012). When the child's needs outweigh the parent's capacity, *home nursing* is often prescribed. Some children with intensive health needs may be technology dependent and require respiratory support such as a tracheostomy and ventilators, and will need home nursing services (Elias et al., 2012). Additionally, some CSHCN may need other supports related to intravenous lines, enteral feeding devices, colostomy bags, and urinary catheters (Elias et al., 2012). This creates an overall system of health care where providers need to coordinate and collaborate on services to meet the complex needs of CSHCN and their families (Elias et al., 2012).

Diversity among families

When working with families with a language barrier, an interpreter is essential for effective communication. The occupational therapy practitioner must schedule extra time for visits to successfully communicate with the family (Lowry & Shaw, 2013). Families of CSHCN come from a variety of socioeconomic levels, and support may be needed in the form of **health literacy,** a person's ability to read, listen, and interpret health information and apply these skills in everyday health situations (National Network of Libraries of Medicine, n.d.). Health literacy "affects individuals' ability to make health decisions and actively participate in health-related activities" (AOTA, 2017a, para. 1). As our health care system becomes more and more fast paced and complex, low health literacy knowledge may become more of an obstacle for many families. This creates an increased need for occupational therapy practitioners to educate families and increase awareness to promote health literacy in families who struggle with understanding their child's medical needs (AOTA, 2017a).

Family well-being

Families of CSHCN must quickly learn to navigate the complex world of the health care system (Pizur-Barnekow et al., 2011). A study found that 12% of families with CSHCN receive regular counseling to address the daily stress of having a CSHCN (DHHS, 2013). Factors such as medical expenses, the amount of time required to care for their child, and chronic uncertainty about their child's future all contribute to higher than average stress (Brehaut et al., 2009). Other factors that contribute to a family's overall well-being include employment loss, underemployment, and significant financial challenges (Kuo et al., 2011). Along with daily stressors, parents of CSHCN reported poor sleep, which in turn affected their memory and overall health (McBean & Schlosnagle, 2015).

Occupational therapy practitioners should understand that family well-being may influence child well-being.

Parents often experience feelings of inadequacy and isolation along with feelings of unmet needs for both the child and family. Being aware of the many challenges families face with a CSHCN helps to build a trusting and collaborative relationship with service providers (Lowry & Shaw, 2013). Because their background is rooted in mental health, occupational therapy practitioners can address the mental health needs of children, families, and other caregivers in a variety of practice settings (AOTA, 2016b). Providing easily accessible resources to aid with their overall well-being is important (see Table 37.1).

Coordinating With Health Care Providers

Coordinated and consistent communication with health care providers is an excellent way to build interprofessional partnerships and broaden professional practice (Leinwand et al., 2018). Families reported that communication difficulties among their child's professionals are a barrier to effectively managing their child's care (Pizur-Barnekow et al., 2011). Some health care team members may be unsure how to best meet the family's needs, but occupational therapy practitioners can bridge that gap. Team members with knowledge of one another's roles, responsibilities, and expertise support successful collaboration (Leinwand et al., 2018).

Impact on Daily Occupations

CSHCN often have more challenges engaging in their occupations because of their medical needs and, for some, the development of subsequent musculoskeletal or sensory impairments. Impairments may present as muscle stiffness, muscle shortening, body fatigue, or pain. Along with these impairments, sensory impairments related to proprioception and neuropathies may also affect a child. These complexities can potentially influence a child's performance skills such as motor, processing, and social interaction. Play, feeding, sleep, social participation, self-help, learning activities, and social participation can be affected (see Table 37.2).

TABLE 37.1. Resources for Families

RESOURCE	DESCRIPTION
Child Care Aware of America https://www.childcareaware.org/resources/map/	Nonprofit organization that advocates child care policies. Provides state-specific resources related to child care, health and social services, financial assistance, and resources for children with special needs (Child Care Aware, n.d.)
Complex Child https://complexchild.org/	Monthly online magazine that provides resources and personal experience information in family-friendly language (Complex Child, n.d.)
Parent to Parent USA https://www.p2pusa.org	Nonprofit organization that connects parents of special needs children with other parents of children with similar disabilities (Parent to Parent, USA, n.d.)
The Arc https://www.thearc.org/	Nonprofit organization that promotes the rights of individuals with disabilities. Offers state-by-state resources related to family support, employment programs, and leisure/recreation activities (The Arc, n.d.)
PACER Center https://www.pacer.org	Nonprofit organization that provides resources to individuals with disabilities, families, and professionals working with individuals with special health care needs. Livestream events and workshops are offered (PACER Center, n.d.)
Understood https://www.understood.org	Nonprofit organization that provides tools and support for families regarding educational challenges, friendships, family issues, and community support (Understood, n.d.)

TABLE 37.2. Diagnoses and Health Care Considerations and Impact on Participation

CONDITION	INCIDENCE	ACUTE AND CHRONIC HEALTH CARE NEEDS	PRIMARY IMPACT ON PARTICIPATION	SOURCES
Autism spectrum disorder	1 in 59	Sleep disorders, gastrointestinal, behavior	Play, feeding, mealtime participation, social skills, sleep, self-help, pre-academic skills	CDC (2019); Mayo Clinic (2018)
Cerebral palsy	1 in 323	Difficulty breathing, swallowing, and talking; seizures, pain, and constipation; muscle tone disorders	Play, feeding, mealtime participation, social skills, sleep, self-help, pre-academic skills	CDC (2018a)
Cleft lip and palate	1 in 940	Surgery, difficulty with speech and feeding, dental issues, ear infections and hearing problems.	Feeding and social participation	March of Dimes (2017); Parker et al. (2010)
Critical congenital heart defects	1 in 100	Surgery, oxygen supplementation, difficulty with weight gain and oral intake	Sleep, reduced activity tolerance	March of Dimes (2013); CDC (2018b)
Down syndrome	1 in 700	Potential congenital heart defects, hearing loss, intellectual and developmental disabilities, sleep disorders, vision issues	Play, feeding, mealtime participation, social skills, sleep, self-help, pre-academic skills	CDC (2018c)
Fetal alcohol spectrum disorders	1 in 20	Difficulty with growth; vision or hearing problems, intellectual or developmental disabilities, central nervous system issues, congenital heart defects	Play, feeding, mealtime participation, social skills, sleep, self-help, pre-academic skills	March of Dimes (2016)
Seizure/epilepsy disorders	1 in 693	Potential problems with learning and motor development	Play, feeding, mealtime participation, social skills, sleep, self-help, pre-academic skills	Zack & Kobau (2017)

Note. CDC = Centers for Disease Control and Prevention.

Play and leisure

CSHCN often experience difficulties engaging in play and leisure routines as a result of delays in their overall development. When a CSHCN struggles to engage in play, families often advocate for their child by seeking play opportunities and changing the environment to meet their child's individualized play needs (Fabrizi et al., 2016). A high prevalence of CSHCN have cognitive impairments and learning disabilities. This may be the result of missed opportunities to explore and learn about their environment because of their medical complexities.

Eating and feeding

Along with difficulties with play and learning, CSHCN may demonstrate inconsistent feeding patterns because of fluctuations in muscle tone, low functional activity tolerance, and respiratory or digestive issues (Fraker & Walbert, 2003). Feeding is a complex skill, and many premature infants struggle to feed because of comorbid diagnoses related to neurology, cardiology, or pulmonology (Park et al., 2018).

CSHCN often experience poor oral intake and inadequate nutrition to support their growth and overall health (Lowry & Shaw, 2013). They may have oral aversion resulting in emesis before, during, or after meals. Because of difficulties with oral feeding, enteral or parenteral support may be necessary (Elias et al., 2012). Sometimes temporary or permanent feeding tubes are placed to meet the child's nutritional needs. The type of tube inserted is dependent on the child's short- and long-term nutritional needs as well as other medical factors (see Table 37.3).

Feeding challenges can create stress in caregivers before, during, and after meals. Caregivers often experience feelings of guilt and may blame themselves when their child has feeding difficulties. Sometimes the caregiver–child relationship is affected as well as the overall family function at mealtime, resulting in a negative cycle of feeding behaviors (Estrem et al., 2017).

Social participation

The child's overall health condition and functional limitations affect their ability to participate in social activities (Houtrow et al., 2012). When in the community (e.g., parks, restaurant, library), CSHCN often encounter environmental barriers related to access, safety, technology, support systems, public attitudes, and general policies related to community participation (Kramer et al., 2018). Along with navigating community barriers, parents of CSHCN must spend more time preparing to go out into the community than parents of typical children. They often need an adaptive car seat and supplies such as oxygen tanks, apnea monitors, medications, or other medical necessities (Bobzien et al., 2015). Because of limited community experiences, CSHCN often have unmet social needs, which can have long-term consequences.

Sleep and rest

A child with special health care needs may struggle to engage in healthy sleep habits and routines. They often have comorbid diagnoses or medical conditions that result in behavior problems, anxiety, attention difficulties,

TABLE 37.3.   Types of Feeding Tubes

TYPE OF TUBE	DESCRIPTION
Nasogastric (NG) tube	NG tubes are typically used short term (i.e., 1–6 months). NG tubes enter through the nose and feed into the stomach. In some circumstances, children with malformations to anatomical structures will need an NG tube long term.
Nasoduodenal (ND) tube	ND tubes enter through the nose but extend past the stomach and into the initial part of the small intestine called the duodenum. Typically used short term (i.e., 1–6 months) for children who cannot tolerate stomach feedings. Feedings must be delivered very slowly over 18–24 hours.
Nasojejunal (NJ) tube	NJ tubes are similar to ND tubes, but extend a little farther into the small intestine so feedings are into the jejunum. Used for a short period of time (i.e., 1–6 months) for children who cannot tolerate stomach feedings. Feedings must be delivered very slowly over 18–24 hours.
Gastric or gastrostomy (G) tube	G-tubes are used most commonly and are placed through the abdominal wall directly into the stomach. Often referred to as a *PEG tube* or *skin-level button device*. Used long term (i.e., more than 3 months).
Gastrojejunal (GJ) or transjejunal tube	GJ-tubes are similar to G-tubes because they enter the stomach directly through the abdominal wall. There are two feeding ports; one into the stomach and the other into the small intestine for children who cannot tolerate feeds into the stomach. Feedings must be given slowly over 18–24 hours. Typically used long term.
Jejunal tube	J-tubes are not very common in children and are placed directly into the small intestine. Feedings must be given slowly over 18–24 hours. Typically used long term.

Note. Adapted from Feeding Tube Awareness Foundation (n.d.).

impulsivity, communication delays, or medical problems that affect the ability to fall and stay asleep (Durand, 2014). CSHCN may also experience nighttime tooth grinding, which may result in jaw pain, headaches, or other dental conditions (Durand, 2014). More serious sleep problems such as narcolepsy or cataplexy may also be present (Durand, 2014). Safe and comfortable positioning for a CSHCN can also be a challenge for caregivers, resulting in loss of sleep for the caregivers. Some CSHCN may need assistance from an occupational therapy practitioner regarding daily sleep habits and routines and positioning; the practitioner can also suggest environmental modifications such as room temperature, bedding choices, and use of technology around bedtime (AOTA, 2017b).

Medical Equipment Needs

Children with neuromotor, orthopedic, or musculoskeletal problems often require specific positioning and support systems (Bobzien et al., 2015) to engage in meaningful activities. Some children may need specialized seating systems during feeding to offer postural support for safe feeding experiences (Korth & Rendell, 2015). Along with specialized seating for feeding, adaptive bathing systems are often necessary because standard bathtubs and showers do not provide an environment that is conducive to the child and caregiver.

Safe sleeping practices are also important when working with this population. Depending on the complexity of the child's health condition, a physician may prescribe a hospital-style bassinet or crib (U.S. Food and Drug Administration, 2017). Some CSHCN require specialized seating systems in both the family's automobile and school bus for safe transportation. Like other specialized seating systems, car seats require consideration of the child's overall medical diagnoses, muscle tone, development, and cognitive skills (Complex Child, 2011). Specialized seating for safe transportation may include medical car seats, adaptive boosters with reclining options, harness-style vests, or car beds (Indiana University School of Medicine, n.d.).

The need for specialized seating systems creates opportunities for occupational therapy practitioners to train caregivers and other team members on how to safely use these systems to support the child's occupational engagement. However, when recommending specialized seating systems, practitioners must consider the family's space within the home for positioning equipment as well as their perceptions of the equipment (Korth & Rendell, 2015).

In addition to specialized seating systems, many CSHCN have lifelong medical needs resulting in the need for home medical devices (Elias et al., 2012). Some children who were born prematurely have chronic conditions such as bronchopulmonary dysplasia and require supplemental oxygen (National Organization of Rare Diseases, 2018). Supplemental oxygen can be delivered via a nasal cannula or a face mask (Bobzien et al., 2015). However, a child with severe respiratory problems may also have apnea and require the use of a continuous positive airway pressure (CPAP) machine that provides oxygen and air through a face mask under continuous pressure (Bobzien et al., 2015).

Some children with more critical and complex needs may need a ventilator for respiratory support or home dialysis (Lowry & Shaw, 2013). Respiratory disorders can result in life-threatening consequences; thus, CSHCN often have monitors that provide alerts to potential problems (Bobzien et al., 2015). An apnea monitor is one example of a device that has an alarm that sounds when the heart rate or breathing slows or stops (U.S. National Library of Medicine, 2017). Pulse oximeters are also commonly used with CSHCN to monitor the amount of oxygen that the red blood cells carry (Johns Hopkins Medicine, n.d.). Like an apnea monitor, a pulse oximeter will sound an alarm to alert caregivers when there is not enough oxygen in the blood (Johns Hopkins Medicine, n.d.).

BEST PRACTICES

To best meet the needs of CSHCN, family-centered practices should be used to promote the organization and delivery of a variety services to address the child and family's strengths and their priorities to meet the child's social, emotional, and developmental needs (DHHS, 2013). Occupational therapy practitioners would do well to demonstrate a basic understanding of the family's day-to-day life; doing so allows the practitioner to address the family's needs in a sensitive, respectful, and purposeful way (Eddy, 2013). Positive outcomes have been reported with family-centered services when interventions are individualized and designed to best meet the needs of the child and family (Kingsley & Mailloux, 2013).

Initiate the Evaluation Process

The evaluation process should be comprehensive and include gathering essential information from all professionals involved with the child (Bobzien et al., 2015). The evaluation process begins with the occupational profile, which provides the occupational therapist with data through interview and record review to fully understand the child's skills within the context of the child's environment (Frolek Clark & Kingsley, 2013). Every child with complex needs has unique developmental differences (Bobzien et al., 2015), and depending on the child's needs, selecting appropriate evaluation methods is critical to a well-rounded view of the child. Exhibit 37.1 reviews some considerations for the occupational therapist when planning the evaluation.

Many CSHCN have acute or chronic pain that should be assessed and reassessed throughout the occupational therapy process. Being adept at reading a child's pain cues is important. Children with pain may demonstrate a wide variety of behaviors such as generalized irritability, restlessness, lethargy, anorexia, and sleep disturbances (Eddy, 2013). They may also demonstrate facial changes such as grimacing or biting as well as postural changes such as drawing up their knees (Eddy, 2013).

In addition to interviews, observation of the child throughout the evaluation process will help the occupational therapy practitioner learn how the child conveys their needs (Bobzien et al., 2015). For a list of assessment tools that are frequently used to evaluate child development

and participation, see Appendix F, "Examples of Assessments for Early Childhood (Birth–5 Years)."

Provide Evidence-Based Interventions

Ongoing knowledge about the effectiveness of interventions is critical. For example, when addressing feeding interventions, occupational therapy practitioners need to consider the different evidence-based approaches to feeding and select the best intervention to target the child's specific feeding needs (Howe & Wang, 2013). A systematic review by Novak and Honan (2019) found that interventions that focused on a partnership between the practitioner and parent to build capacity provided strong evidence of effectiveness. Parents value training that builds capacity to improve their child's skills (Kingsley & Mailloux, 2013). Communication with families is a critical component to family-centered services and when determining the effectiveness of interventions.

Use of assistive technology

Many CSHCN may benefit from the use of assistive technology (AT) to meet a variety of needs. *AT* can be defined as any item, device, or piece of equipment; durable medical equipment; system such as communication aids; or mobility aid that enhances an individual's functional mobility (Assistive Technology Act of 2004, P.L. 108-364). AT can be used in the home or school environment and may be as simple as modified eating utensils or more complicated such as eye-gaze technologies. When considering the use of AT, implementing a collaborative approach across all disciplines involved with the child should be considered (AOTA, 2016a). AT for infants and toddlers is often underutilized and not included in their individualized family service plan (IFSP). Best practices for early intervention providers state, "AT should be available for children of all ages and abilities, be considered during the development of every child's IFSP, and be available for daily use" (Long, 2015, p. 183).

Transition to Preschool

CSHCN are at a higher risk of poor educational outcomes as they transition to the school environment because of lack of academic readiness skills (O'Connor et al., 2014). Additionally, CSHCN experience more limitations regarding

---

EXHIBIT 37.1.   Evaluation Considerations

- **Prepare ahead of time:** Review the assessment tool using the manual for guidance on how to adapt the assessment, score, and interpret findings. Be aware that not all assessments allow adaptations for CSHCN.
- **Coordinate time and day:** Communicate with the child's parents to determine when the child is at their best in terms of sleep, comfort, endurance level, and medication schedule.
- **Consider positioning:** Ensure the child is positioned in a comfortable and safe position during assessment. This will support the child's ability to attend to tasks and demonstrate skills related to attention, concentration, and gross and fine motor skills.
- **Be aware of the child's activity tolerance:** CSHCN can easily become overstimulated and unable to participate at their full capacity. It is important to pace the flow of the assessment depending on the child's tolerance.
- **Interpret your assessment:** Be considerate of parents when reporting the results of the assessment. CSHCN may score significantly lower than their same-age peers; thus, focusing on the child's functional abilities and needs rather than the age level of the child's skill level can help with parent perspective.

Note. CSHCN = children with special health care needs.
Source. Adapted from Bobzien et al. (2015).

school attendance than their same-age peers (Houtrow et al., 2012). Some CSHCN live below the poverty line and lack participation in key developmental activities, which places them at an increased risk for negative outcomes later in life (Houtrow et al., 2012).

Occupational therapy practitioners are key team members throughout the transition process. Practitioners working in preschools can help "adjust the school demands to match the student's strengths and abilities, including participating in classroom activities, socializing with peers, and engaging in pre-academic tasks" (AOTA, 2018, para. 6). To avoid a disconnect between early intervention teams and preschool teams, good collaboration among all team members, including parents, teachers, therapists, and health care providers is essential (DHHS, 2013; Orentlicher et al., 2014). During the transition process, practitioners must maintain family-centered practice and acknowledge that this may be a stressful time for families. Parents are often fearful of the transition process and even more so when they have a CSHCN. Listening to the family's concerns and helping them work through barriers during the transition process can help achieve satisfactory outcomes (Orentlicher et al., 2014). There may be cultural and language barriers to overcome to alleviate parent stress, build trust, and to fully address the CSHCN.

Practitioners play an important role in preparing the educational environment to meet the child's needs. Teachers and administrators may express uncertainty regarding having the CSHCN in their classroom. During the transition, the child's educational team may need increased communication and additional classroom supports to provide education, listen to concerns, and provide additional direct services to meet the child's needs (Orentlicher et al., 2017).

School Health Plans

Health support services in the preschool environment are a significant need for CSHCN (O'Connor et al., 2014). *School nurses* play an essential role and are considered health care experts within the educational environment (AAP Council on School Health, 2016). The school nurse assists in coordinating the child's health needs between home and school and is responsible for the individualized health plans for children who have health care needs that may affect their ability to participate in a healthy and safe academic setting (National Association of School Nurses, 2016).

The individualized education program (IEP) may include an *individualized health plan* (IHP) that includes the child's health-related barriers to learning, recommended accommodations, personnel training needs, and the outcomes or goals of the plan to promote the child's health and enhance the child's academic achievement (DHHS, 2013; National Association of School Nurses, 2018). This is especially true for CSHCN because their school day may be affected because of their health care needs. Adequate health care support and training of staff are essential, and this can be done through good communication and by building strong partnerships with families (AAP Council on School Health, 2016; DHHS, 2013). School nurses are part of the child's team, and occupational therapy practitioners should collaborate regarding how to best optimize the educational environment and daily routines to support participation.

Ongoing Data Collection

Providing evidence to support the efficacy of occupational therapy when working with special populations is critical. Finding ways to accurately measure outcomes should be part of everyday practice (Schaaf, 2015). Occupational therapy practitioners should acknowledge that CSHCN may demonstrate slower than average progress toward occupational therapy goals and shared outcomes compared to other children because of their extensive medical needs. In the home environment, documentation of progress can be challenging when joint outcomes are addressed by multiple team members (Stoffel, n.d.). SOAP (*s*ubjective, *o*bjective, *a*ssessment, *p*lan) note documentation allows the practitioner to gather data related to parent involvement as subjective data and data related to the child's progress reported by the occupational therapist as objective data (Stoffel, n.d.). In the preschool environment, thorough documentation is needed to support the child's occupational engagement.

Data-driven decision making (DDDM) "provides a framework for reasoning through the occupational therapy process with a focus on utilization of data to guide and measure outcomes" (Schaaf, 2015, p. 2). Additionally, DDDM can help build capacity in families and empower other team members to address the child's ability to engage in occupation and participate across settings such as the home, community, and school (Henry & Lindsay, 2016). Another form of data collection in the school environment is known as *participation-focused, authentic, collaborative, and explicit* (PACE). PACE provides the occupational therapy practitioner with a vehicle to adhere to the Individuals With Disabilities Education Improvement Act of 2004 (IDEA; P. L. 108-446), supports meaningful participation identified by team members, including the child and parent, and allows the child to functionally participate within the school context and environment (Laverdure, 2018). Additionally, supports and barriers are addressed along with prioritization of the child's skills related to participation (Laverdure, 2018). For more information, see Chapter 6, "Best Practices in Data-Based Decision Making."

SUMMARY

CSHCN have many needs that affect occupational engagement. Meeting the needs of both the child and family embodies family-centered practice. Occupational therapy practitioners can best support CSHCN and their families by educating themselves on the strengths, priorities, and barriers the child and family experience daily. Communicating and collaborating with all team members is an essential component when working with this population.

REFERENCES

AAP Council on School Health. (2016). Role of the school nurse in providing school health services. *American Academy of Pediatrics, 137*(6). https://pediatrics.aappublications.org/content/pediatrics/137/6/e20160852.full.pdf

American Occupational Therapy Association. (2015). *Occupational therapy's role with children and youth* [Fact sheet]. https://www.aota.org/~/media/Corporate/Files/AboutOT/Professionals/WhatIsOT/CY/Fact-Sheets/Children%20and%20Youth%20fact%20sheet.pdf

American Occupational Therapy Association. (2016a). Assistive technology and occupational performance. *American Journal of Occupational Therapy, 70,* 7012410030. https://doi.org/10.5014/ajot.2016.706S02

American Occupational Therapy Association. (2016b). *Occupational therapy's distinct value: Mental health promotion, prevention, and intervention across the lifespan.* https://www.aota.org/~/media/Corporate/Files/Practice/MentalHealth/Distinct-Value-Mental-Health.pdf

American Occupational Therapy Association. (2017a). AOTA's societal statement on health literacy. *American Journal of Occupational Therapy, 71*(Suppl. 2), 7112410065. https://doi.org/10.5014/ajot.2017.716S14

American Occupational Therapy Association. (2017b). *Occupational therapy's role with sleep* [Fact sheet]. https://www.aota.org/~/media/Corporate/Files/AboutOT/Professionals/WhatIsOT/HW/Facts/Sleep-fact-sheet.pdf

American Occupational Therapy Association. (2018). *Transitions for children and youth: How occupational therapy can help.* https://www.aota.org/~/media/Corporate/Files/AboutOT/Professionals/WhatIsOT/CY/Fact-Sheets/Transitions.pdf

The Arc. (n.d.). *Home page.* https://thearc.org/

Assistive Technology Act of 2004. (2004). Pub. L. 108-364. 3.

Bobzien, J. L., Childress, D. C., & Raver, S. A. (2015). Infants and toddlers with cognitive and/or motor disabilities. In R. A. Raver & D. C. Childress (Eds). *Family-centered early intervention: Supporting infants and toddlers in natural environments* (pp. 255–283). Brookes.

Brehaut, J. C., Kohen, D. E., Garner, R. E., Miller, A. R., Lach, L. M., Klassen, A. F., & Rosenbaum, P. L. (2009). Health among caregivers of children with health problems: Findings from a Canadian population-based study. *American Journal of Public Health, 99,* 1254–1262. https://doi.org/10.2105/AJPH.2007.129817

Centers for Disease Control and Prevention. (2018a). *Data and statistics for cerebral palsy.* https://www.cdc.gov/ncbddd/cp/data.html

Centers for Disease Control and Prevention. (2018b). *Data and statistics on congenital heart defects.* https://www.cdc.gov/ncbddd/heartdefects/data.html

Centers for Disease Control and Prevention. (2018c). *Facts about Down syndrome.* https://www.cdc.gov/ncbddd/birthdefects/downsyndrome.html

Centers for Disease Control and Prevention. (2019). *Data and statistics on autism spectrum disorder.* https://www.cdc.gov/ncbddd/autism/data.html

Child Care Aware. (n.d.). *State by state resources.* https://www.childcareaware.org/resources/map/

Complex Child. (n.d.). *History and mission.* https://complexchild.org/about/history-and-mission/

Complex Child. (2011). *Car seats for children with special needs.* https://complexchild.org/articles/2011-articles/october/carseats/

Durand, V. M. (2014). *Sleep better: A guide to improving sleep for children with special needs.* Brookes.

Eddy, L. L. (2013). Enhancing quality of life for children with special healthcare needs. In L. L. Eddy (Ed.), *Caring for children with special healthcare needs and their families: A handbook for healthcare professionals* (pp. 149–159). Wiley-Blackwell. https://doi.org/10.1002/9781118783290.ch9

Elias, E. R., Murphy, N. A., & the Council on Children with Disabilities. (2012). Home care of children and youth with complex healthcare needs and technology dependencies. *Pediatrics, 129*(5), 996–1005. https://doi.org/10.1542/peds.2012-0606

Estrem, H. H., Pados, B. F., Park, J., Knafl, K. A., & Thoyre, S. M. (2017). Feeding problems in infancy and early childhood: Evolutionary concept analysis. *Journal of Advanced Nursing 73*(1), 56–70. https://doi.org/10.1111/jan.13140

Fabrizi, S. E., Ito, M. A., & Winston, K. (2016). Effect of occupational therapy–led playgroups in early intervention on child playfulness and caregiver responsiveness: A repeated-measures design. *American Journal of Occupational Therapy, 70*(2), 700220020p1. https://doi.org/10.5014/ajot.2016.017012

Feeding Tube Awareness Foundation. (n.d.). *Tube types.* https://www.feedingtubeawareness.org/tube-feeding-basics/tubetypes/

Fraker, C., & Walbert, L. (2003). *From NICU to childhood: Evaluation and treatment of pediatric feeding disorders.* Pro-Ed.

Frolek Clark, G., & Kingsley, K. (2013). *Occupational therapy practice guidelines for early childhood: Birth through 5 years.* AOTA Press.

Health Resources and Services Administration. (2019). *Children with special health care needs.* https://mchb.hrsa.gov/maternal-child-health-topics/children-and-youth-special-health-needs

Henry, D. A., & Lindsay, G. (2016). Empowering stakeholders through data-driven decision making. *SIS Quarterly Practice Connections, 1*(4), 6–8.

Houtrow, A., Jones, J., Ghandour, R., Strickland, B., & Newacheck, P. (2012). Participation of children with special health care needs in school and the community. *Academic Pediatrics, 12*(4), 326–334. https://doi.org/10.1016/j.acap.2012.03.004

Howe, T. H., & Wang, T. N. (2013). Systematic review of interventions used in or relevant to occupational therapy for children with feeding difficulties ages birth–5 years. *American Journal of Occupational Therapy, 67,* 405–412. https://doi.org/10.5014/ajot.2013.004564

Howe, T.-H., Hinojosa, J., & Sheu, C.-F. (2019). Latino-American mothers' perspectives on feeding their young children: A qualitative study. *American Journal of Occupational Therapy, 73,* 7303205110. https://doi.org/10.5014/ajot.2019.031336

Indiana University School of Medicine. (n.d.). *Special needs transportation: Child safety seats for children with special needs.* https://preventinjury.pediatrics.iu.edu/special-needs/child-restraint-options/

Individuals With Disabilities Education Improvement Act of 2004, Pub. L. 108-446, 20 U.S.C. §§ 1400–1482.

Johns Hopkins Medicine. (n.d.). *Pulse oximetry.* https://www.hopkinsmedicine.org/health/treatment-tests-and-therapies/pulse-oximetry

Kingsley, K., & Mailloux, Z. (2013). Evidence for the effectiveness of different service delivery models in early intervention services. *American Journal of Occupational Therapy, 67,* 431–436. https://doi.org/10.5014/ajot.2013.006171

Korth, K., & Rendell, L. (2015). Feeding intervention. In J. Case-Smith & J. C. O'Brien (Eds.), *Occupational therapy for children and adolescents* (7th ed., pp. 389–415). Elsevier/Mosby.

Kramer, J. M., Hwang, I. T., Levin, M., Acevedo-Garcia, G. D., & Rosenfeld, L. (2018). Identifying environmental barriers to participation: Usability of a health-literacy informed problem-identification approach for parents of young children with developmental disabilities. *Child: Care, Health & Development, 44*(2), 249–259. https://doi.org/10.1111/cch.12542

Kuo, D. Z., Cohen, E., Agrawal, R., Berry, J. G., & Casey, P. H. (2011). A national profile of caregiver challenges among more medically complex children with special health care needs. *Archives of Pediatric & Adolescent Medicine, 165,* 1020–1026. https://doi.org/10.1001/archpediatrics.2011.172

Laverdure, P. (2018). Collecting participation-focused evaluation data across the school environment. *SIS Quarterly Practice Connections, 3*(2), 5–7.

Leinwand, R., Cosbey, J., & Sanders, H. (2018). Better together: Team collaboration in early intervention. *SIS Quarterly Practice Connections, 3*(1), 7–9.

Lollar, D. J., Hartzell, M. S., & Evans, M. A. (2012). Functional difficulties and health conditions among children with special health needs. *Pediatrics, 129,* 714–722. https://doi.org/10.1542/peds.2011-0780

Long, T. M. (2015). Using appropriate behaviors to meet needs. In R. A. Raver & D. C. Childress (Eds.), *Family-centered early intervention: Supporting infants and toddlers in natural environments* (pp. 167–187). Brookes Publishing.

Lowry, N., & Shaw, P. (2013). Assessment and development of an interprofessional plan of care. In L. L. Eddy (Ed.), *Caring for children with special healthcare needs and their families: A handbook for healthcare professionals* (pp. 221–244). John Wiley & Sons.

March of Dimes. (2013). *Congenital heart defects and critical CHDs.* https://www.marchofdimes.org/complications/congenital-heart-defects.aspx

March of Dimes. (2016). *Fetal alcohol spectrum disorders.* https://www.marchofdimes.org/complications/fetal-alcohol-spectrum-disorders.aspx

March of Dimes. (2017). *Cleft lip and cleft palate.* https://www.marchofdimes.org/complications/cleft-lip-and-cleft-palate.aspx

Mayo Clinic. (2018). *Autism spectrum disorder.* https://www.mayoclinic.org/diseases-conditions/autism-spectrum-disorder/symptoms-causes/syc-20352928

McBean, A. L., & Schlosnagle, L. (2015). Sleep, health and memory: Comparing parents of typically developing children and parents of children with special health-care needs. *Journal of Sleep Research, 25*(1), 78–87. https://doi.org/10.1111/jsr.12329

McPherson, M., Arango, P., Fox, H., Lauver, C., McManus, M., Newacheck, P. W., . . . Strickland, B. (1998). A new definition of children with special health care needs. *Pediatrics, 102*(1), 137–139. https://doi.org/10.1542/peds.102.1.137

National Organization of Rare Diseases. (2018). *Bronchopulmonary Dysplasia.* https://rarediseases.org/rare-diseases/bronchopulmonary-dysplasia-bpd/

National Association of School Nurses. (2016). *The role of the 21st century school nurse* [Position Statement]. Author.

National Association of School Nurses. (2018). *IDEIA and section 504 teams: The school nurse as an essential team member* [Position Statement]. Author.

National Network of Libraries of Medicine. (n.d.). *Health literacy.* https://nnlm.gov/initiatives/topics/health-literacy

Novak, I., & Honan, I. (2019). Effectiveness of paediatric occupational therapy for children with disabilities: A systematic review. *Australian Occupational Therapy Journal, 66*(3), 258–273. https://doi.org/10.1111/1440-1630.12573

O'Connor, M., Howell-Meurs, S., Kvalsvig, A., & Goldfeld, S. (2014). Understanding the impact of special health care needs on early school functioning: A conceptual model. *Child: Care, Health and Development, 41*(1), 15–22. https://doi.org/10.1111/cch.12164

Orentlicher, M. L., Handley-More, D., Ehrenberg, R., Frenkel, M., & Markowitz, L. (2014). Interprofessional collaboration in schools: A review of current evidence. *Early Intervention & School Special Interest Section Quarterly, 21*(2), 1–3.

Orentlicher, M. L., Case, D., Podvey, M. C., Myers, C. T., Rudd, L. Q., & Schoonover, J. (2017). *What is occupational therapy's role in transition services and planning?* https://www.aota.org/~/media/Corporate/Files/Secure/Practice/Children/FAQ-What-is-OTs-Role-in-Transition-Services-and-Planning-20170530.pdf

PACER Center. (n.d.). *About PACER Center.* https://www.pacer.org/about/

Parent to Parent USA. (n.d.). *What is parent to parent?* https://www.p2pusa.org/parents

Park, J., Pados, B. F., & Thoyre, S. M. (2018). Systematic review: What is the evidence for side-lying position for feeding preterm infants? *Advances in Neonatal Care, 18*(4), 285–294. https://doi.org/10.1097/ANC.0000000000000529

Parker, S. E., Mai, C. T., Canfield, M. A., Rickard, R., Wang, Y., Meyer, R. E., . . . Correa, A. (2010). Updated national birth prevalence estimates for selected birth defects in the United States, 2004–2006. *Birth Defects Research. Part A, Clinical and Molecular Teratology, 88*(12), 1008–1016. https://doi.org/10.1002/bdra.20735

Pizur-Barnekow, K., Darragh, A., & Johnston, M. (2011). "I cried because I didn't know if I could take care of him": Toward a taxonomy of interactive and critical health literacy as portrayed by caregivers of children with special health care needs. *Journal of Health Communication, 16*(Suppl. 3), 205–221. https://doi.org/10.1080/10810730.2011.604386

Schaaf, R. C. (2015). Creating evidence for practice using data-driven decision making. *American Journal of Occupational Therapy, 69,* 6902360010. https://doi.org/10.5014/ajot.2015.010561

Stoffel, A. (n.d.). *Writing pediatric goals: How to document family involvement & developmental progress.* https://www.aota.org/Practice/Manage/Reimb/writing-pediatric-goals-family-involvment-developmental.aspx

Understood. (n.d.). *About us.* https://www.understood.org/about

U.S. Department of Health and Human Services, Health Resources and Services Administration, Maternal and Child Health Bureau. (2013). *National Survey of Children with Special Health Care Needs Chartbook 2009–2010.* https://mchb.hrsa.gov/cshcn0910/more/introduction.html

U.S. Food and Drug Administration. (2017). *Help keep sick child safe: Learn how to use a hospital crib.* https://www.fda.gov/consumers/consumer-updates/help-keep-sick-child-safe-learn-how-use-hospital-crib

U.S. National Library of Medicine. (2017). *MedlinePlus: Home apnea monitor use – infants.* https://medlineplus.gov/ency/patientinstructions/000755.htm

Zack, M. M., & Kobau, R. (2017). National and state estimates of the numbers of adults and children with active epilepsy – United States, 2015. *Morbidity and Mortality Weekly Report, 66*(31), 821.825. https://www.cdc.gov/mmwr/volumes/66/wr/mm6631a1.htm

Best Practices in Supporting Children With Autism Spectrum Disorder and Attention Deficit Hyperactivity Disorder

Lesly Wilson James, PhD, MPA, OTR/L, FAOTA; Ashley Stoffel, OTD, OTR/L, FAOTA; and Kris Pizur-Barnekow, PhD, OTR/L, IMH-E®

38

KEY TERMS AND CONCEPTS

- Advocacy
- Attention deficit hyperactivity disorder
- Autism spectrum disorder
- Autism spectrum disorder–specific screening
- Cognitive–Functional (Cog-Fun) intervention
- Cognitive Orientation to daily Occupational Performance Approach®
- Developmental monitoring
- Family-centered approach
- Learn the Signs. Act Early. program
- Metacognitive training
- Physical exercise
- Picture Exchange Communication System
- Universal screening

OVERVIEW

Autism spectrum disorder (ASD) and attention deficit hyperactivity disorder (ADHD) are among the most prevalent neurodevelopmental disorders (Ramtekkar, 2017). Teams of practitioners (i.e., developmental pediatricians, neurologists, psychologists, speech–language pathologists, occupational therapists) have diagnosed and provided recommendations for children with ASD and ADHD by gathering and reviewing information, interviewing the family, and observing the young child's behavior and development. (Note that there is a new saliva test that may be used in diagnosing ASD.) The *International Classification of Diseases* (10th rev., clinical modification; Centers for Medicare & Medicaid Services and National Center for Health Statistics, 2015), which is used for medical diagnosis and health care billing, assigned autism Code F84.0 and ADHD Code F90.9. The American Psychiatric Association's (APA; 2013) *Diagnostic and Statistical Manual of Mental Disorders* (5th ed.; *DSM–5*) provides definitions and expanded details about both diagnoses.

As early as age 2 years, a diagnosis of autism can be considered reliable, valid, and stable. (Centers for Disease Control and Prevention [CDC], 2020a). About 1 in 59 children has been identified with ASD, with boys four times more likely to be affected than girls, according to estimates from the CDC's Autism and Developmental Disabilities Monitoring (ADDM) Network. The ADDM Network has consistently noted over time that more non-Hispanic White children are being identified with ASD than non-Hispanic Black or Hispanic children, indicating that some children with ASD may not be receiving the services they need to reach their full potential (CDC, 2020a).

Research has identified increased estimated prevalence of ADHD among children and adolescents, from 6.1% to 10.2% between 1997 and 2016; boys are twice as likely to be diagnosed with ADHD (Guifeng et al., 2018). In 2016, 6.1 million children ages 2–17 years living in the United States were diagnosed with ADHD (CDC, 2019a). Out of 6 million children ages 2–5 years, 2 million were diagnosed with ADHD, with 388,000 children receiving treatement for it (CDC, 2019a). The APA (2013) stated in the *DSM–5* that 5% of children have ADHD (Guifeng et al., 2018). Occupational therapy practitioners are often an integral part of the early intervention (EI), preschool, community, and health care teams that provide services to young children with ASD and ADHD. (*Note. Occupational therapy practitioner* refers to both occupational therapists and occupational therapy assistants.)

Autism Spectrum Disorder

ASD is a developmental disability that can cause significant social, communication, and behavioral challenges (CDC, 2020b). The *DSM–5* presents two categories of symptoms: persistent deficits in social communication or interaction, and restricted, repetitive patterns of behavior. The earlier signs of ASD can be detected, the earlier the child can be evaluated by a medical specialist to determine a medical diagnosis (James et al., 2014). Surveillance and screening are two methods used to identify earlier potential risk for ASD among young children.

An educational diagnosis for ASD is best made through multidisciplinary team evaluation, and occupational therapists are typically asked to contribute to the diagnostic evaluation (Tomchek & Koenig, 2016). Early identification combined with intense and specific intervention leads to improved language skill development (Virués-Ortega, 2010), intelligence, and adaptive behavior (Dawson et al., 2010).

Children with ASD have multiple strengths and challenges that affect their occupational performance and limit participation. Cognitive (e.g., executive functioning), motor (e.g., balance, fine motor dexterity), social (e.g., interactions, social communication), and sensory (e.g., hyper- or hyporeactivity to sensations) difficulties may challenge occupations of play, rest and sleep, learning, and self-care. Functional performance of ADLs, including self-care activities such as eating, self-feeding, bathing, dressing, and toileting, are often a primary concern for parents of young children with ASD (Weaver, 2015).

Attention Deficit Hyperactivity Disorder

ADHD is characterized by deficits in attention, organization, activity levels, and impulse control and is classified into three subtypes: (1) inattentive presentation, (2) hyperactive–impulsive presentation, and (3) combined presentation (CDC, 2020c). (See Exhibit 38.1 for complete definitions). The *DSM–5* indicates that before a diagnosis there should be observation and a record of several inattentive or hyperactive–impulsive symptoms; several symptoms present in two or more settings (e.g., home, school, or work; with friends or relatives; in other activities); clear evidence that the symptoms interfere with or reduce the quality of social, school, or work functioning; and confirmation that the symptoms are not better explained by another mental disorder (e.g., a mood disorder, anxiety disorder, dissociative disorder, or personality disorder).

ADHD and the associated executive functioning deficits have the potential to affect all areas of occupation for a young child. ADHD can affect preschool performance, ADL participation, leisure and play, and peer and family social relationships (Cermak, 2018). Examples of responses of a young child with ADHD include disassociation between knowing what to do and doing it, decreased self-regulation, difficulty in unstructured or new situations, failure to continue or persist, decreased flexibility, failure to pay close attention to details, difficulty organizing tasks and activities, and excessive talking or fidgeting.

Distinct Value of Occupational Therapy

Occupational therapy practitioners are highly qualified, licensed professionals who have the training and expertise to support participation and engagement of young children and their families by addressing occupations such as ADLs, IADLs, rest and sleep, play, education, and social participation (AOTA, 2019). Practitioners are uniquely skilled to address participation challenges of children with ASD and ADHD in early childhood while also considering the lifelong effects that many of these children and families experience.

Occupational therapy practitioners can and should identify and share their distinct value when working with children with ASD and ADHD and their families. This might mean sharing information about occupational therapy education and professional development to show value on the interprofessional team. The education of occupational therapy practitioners includes key areas of influence for working with children with ASD and ADHD, including knowledge

---

EXHIBIT 38.1.   Types of ADHD Based on Symptoms

Inattention Presentation: Six or more symptoms of inattention for children up to age 16 years, or five or more for adolescents ages 17 years or older and adults; symptoms of inattention have been present for at least 6 months, and they are inappropriate for developmental level.

- Often fails to give close attention to details or makes careless mistakes in schoolwork, at work, or with other activities.
- Often has trouble holding attention on tasks or play activities.
- Often does not seem to listen when spoken to directly.
- Often does not follow through on instructions and fails to finish schoolwork, chores, or duties in the workplace (e.g., loses focus, side-tracked).
- Often has trouble organizing tasks and activities.
- Often avoids, dislikes, or is reluctant to do tasks that require mental effort over a long period of time (such as schoolwork or homework).
- Often loses things necessary for tasks and activities (e.g., school materials, pencils, books, tools, wallets, keys, paperwork, eyeglasses, mobile telephones).
- Is often easily distracted.
- Is often forgetful in daily activities.

Hyperactivity and Impulsivity Presentation: Six or more symptoms of hyperactivity-impulsivity for children up to ages 16 years, or five or more for adolescents ages 17 years or older and adults; symptoms of hyperactivity–impulsivity have been present for at least 6 months to an extent that is disruptive and inappropriate for the person's developmental level.

- Often fidgets with or taps hands or feet, or squirms in seat.
- Often leaves seat in situations when remaining seated is expected.
- Often runs about or climbs in situations where it is not appropriate (adolescents or adults may be limited to feeling restless).
- Often unable to play or take part in leisure activities quietly.
- Is often "on the go" acting as if "driven by a motor."
- Often talks excessively.
- Often blurts out an answer before a question has been completed.
- Often has trouble waiting their turn.
- Often interrupts or intrudes on others (e.g., butts into conversations or games).

Combined Presentation: When enough symptoms of both criteria inattention and hyperactivity-impulsivity have been present for the past 6 months.

Source. Reprinted from *Symptoms and Diagnosis of ADHD* by the Centers for Disease Control and Prevention, 2020c. https://www.cdc.gov/ncbddd/adhd/diagnosis.html

and training on child development, mental health, social and emotional learning, sensory integration and processing, and anatomy and neurology as well as activity, behavioral, and environmental analysis (AOTA, 2019).

ESSENTIAL CONSIDERATIONS

Occupational therapy practitioners provide individualized services to children and their families to support their health, well-being, and participation in life. The following section discusses family cultural diversity, disparity, and funding implications.

Disparities and Cultural Considerations

Existing literature highlights disparities in diagnosis and treatment for children with ASD and ADHD among variables such as racial and ethnic groups, geographic regions, and socioeconomic status. Most recent data from the Autism and Developmental Disabilities Monitoring Network continue to show disparities in ASD diagnosis, although disparities were smaller when compared with estimates from previous years, possibly because of more effective outreach to minority communities (Baio et al., 2018). Black and Hispanic children continue to be identified with ASD at a lower rate than White children (Baio et al., 2018). Even after diagnosis, Hispanic children are less likely to receive evidence-based interventions and specialty ASD treatments (Broder-Fingert et al., 2013; Magaña et al., 2013), and they experience disparities in access to services, such as receiving smaller doses of speech and occupational therapy than non-Hispanic White children (Angell et al., 2018; Irvin et al., 2012). Unmet therapy needs are especially high among Hispanic children with ASD in families with limited English proficiency (Zuckerman et al., 2017).

The most recent data on ADHD diagnosis reveal that the proportion of Black children who received an ADHD diagnosis was higher than for White children (Danielson et al., 2018). Other demographic factors in ADHD diagnosis were similar to previous estimates in that boys; non-Hispanic children; and children living in households with English as the primary language, in low-income households, with public insurance, or in the Midwest or South were more likely to have been diagnosed with ADHD than their counterparts (Danielson et al., 2018).

The existing literature and data on ASD and ADHD diagnosis and treatment reveal an important opportunity for occupational therapy to advocate for access to high-quality and evidence-based services for young children with ASD and ADHD across a variety of demographic factors. Screening, diagnosis, and intervention should consider these disparities and cultural impacts. Occupational therapy practitioners are key stakeholders in this process because they consider the participation and occupational performance of the child and family across contexts and environments.

Federal and State Policies and Funding Sources That Support ASD and ADHD Services

The Individuals With Disabilities Education Improvement Act of 2004 (IDEA; P. L. 108-446) is the federal legislation that provides EI (Part C) and preschool and school services for children needing special education and related services to benefit from their educational program. Each state has established an eligibility process to identify children with disabilities and provide access to services. Eligibility under IDEA Part C may have specific requirements (see Chapter 14, "Understanding Part C: Early Intervention Law and the Individualized Family Service Plan [IFSP] Process"), whereas eligibility under Part B is conducted through a multidisciplinary evaluation to identify educational disabilities and educational needs, resulting in an individualized education program (IEP) if eligible (see Chapter 18, "Understanding Preschool Laws and the Individualized Education Program Process"). A medical disability or condition does not always result in the need for special education services. Section 504 of the Rehabilitation Act of 1973 (P. L. 93-112) was designed to ensure that programs receiving federal funding, such as state EI systems and school districts, do not discriminate on the basis of disability in any program or activity. Children who need modifications or accommodations but not specialized instruction may be eligible for Section 504.

State insurance mandates for ASD are state laws that have been adopted by some states to require certain insurers to provide health care coverage for ASD. However, certain insurance plans may be exempted from the mandate. Some insurance plans do not cover habilitative services (e.g., teaching skills that a child has not developed) but focus only on rehabilitation (e.g., restoring skills after an injury or illness). Occupational therapy practitioners should be aware of these federal and state regulations and their impact on reimbursement for ASD and ADHD diagnostic and intervention services.

BEST PRACTICES

When occupational therapy practitioners use the *Occupational Therapy Practice Framework: Domain and Process* (4th ed.; *OTPF*; AOTA, 2020b) to guide the professional reasoning process as they serve young children diagnosed with ASD or ADHD and their families, they are engaging in best practice. The *OTPF* (AOTA, 2020b) describes occupational therapy's distinct value in developmental monitoring and identifying a need for developmental screening, evaluation, and intervention processes.

Monitor and Screen Children for ASD and ADHD

Developmental monitoring is an ongoing process of observing child development and checking for the presence of developmental milestones (CDC, 2019b). The CDC's (2019b) *Learn the Signs. Act Early.* (LTSAE) campaign promotes developmental monitoring for children ages 2 months–5 years (CDC, 2019b). This campaign assists parents with celebrating developmental milestones and identifying developmental concerns. If a parent has a concern, the LTSAE materials include resources that foster conversations with their child's physician about developmental and ASD-specific screening. *ASD-specific screening* involves use of a standardized screening instrument to identify red flags and refer for an ASD evaluation. Table 38.1 illustrates a sample of the therapeutic process in EI and early childhood settings

TABLE 38.1.   Therapeutic Process for Children With ASD and ADHD

PROCESS	EXAMPLES OF SCREENING AND ASSESSMENT TOOLS
Observation, monitoring, and surveillance	▪ Learn the Signs. Act Early. campaign (CDC, 2019b)
Screening	**General** ▪ Ages and Stages Questionnaire (3rd ed.; Squires, Bricker, & Potter, 2009) ▪ Ages and Stages Questionnaire—Social–Emotional (2nd ed.; Squires, Bricker, Twombly, & Potter, 2009) **ASD-specific** ▪ Modified Checklist for Autism in Toddlers—Revised (Robins et al., 2009) ▪ Screening Tool for Autism in Toddlers and Young Children (Stone & Ousley, 2008)
Occupational therapy and interprofessional assessments	**General** ▪ Canadian Occupational Performance Measure (Law et al., 2019) ▪ Pediatric Evaluation of Disability Inventory—Computer-Adaptive Test (2nd ed.; Haley et al., 2012) ▪ Miller Function and Participation Scales (Miller, 2006) ▪ Test of Playfulness (Okimoto et al., 2000) ▪ Bruininks–Oseretsky Test of Motor Proficiency (2nd ed.; Bruininks & Bruininks, 2005) **ASD-specific** ▪ Autism Diagnostic Observation Schedule (2nd ed.; Lord et al., 2012) **ADHD-specific** ▪ Behavior Rating Inventory of Executive Functioning (2nd ed.; Gioia et al., 2015)

Source. Adapted from Tomchek & Koenig (2016).

for a child diagnosed with ASD and ADHD. For an in-depth review of the level of evidence for types of evaluation instruments and interventions, refer to the *Occupational Therapy Practice Guidelines for Individuals With Autism Spectrum Disorder* (Tomchek & Koenig, 2016). Appendix F, "Examples of Assessments for Early Childhood (Birth–5 Years)," also provides a listing of various assessment tools commonly used by occupational therapists.

Part C: Early intervention

In EI settings, if the state allows screening, the child may be screened and monitored by the occupational therapist and other members of the EI team. They may use the CDC's (2019b) "Learn the Signs. Act Early." campaign materials to monitor development and identify concerns. If the occupational therapist hypothesizes that a child is at risk for ASD or ADHD, they should discuss this with the EI team (which includes the parents) and can administer screening instruments that would help identify red flags for these conditions.

Barger and colleagues (2018) recommended that early identification of developmental delays is optimized when developmental monitoring and screening are used in tandem. When a child demonstrates red flags after both processes, the child should be formally evaluated by the EI multidisciplinary team (e.g., adaptive, cognitive and learning, communication, physical, and social–emotional) to determine eligibility for EI services. Practitioners should then follow state procedures for referral to a developmental assessment clinic where targeted evaluation instruments for ASD are administered and recommendations about specific intervention processes are provided.

Community and early childhood preschools

In preschool settings, occupational therapy practitioners may implement multitiered support service processes.

First, they may assist the district or the teacher in **universal screening,** a process that identifies which students may be at risk for learning challenges. This is particularly important for children at risk for ASD and ADHD, because many children are not diagnosed until early childhood (Shaw et al., 2020). If a child is suspected of having an educational disability, their parents, the educational agency, or another state agency may request a full and individual initial evaluation to determine eligibility for special education. As a member of the educational team, the occupational therapist may conduct an occupational therapy evaluation to gather information used in the determination of eligibility for special education and related services.

Health care

Occupational therapists who work in hospitals and clinics are involved with children at risk for ASD and ADHD by serving on interprofessional diagnostic and intervention teams. In these practice settings, practitioners focus on understanding barriers to occupational performance secondary to ASD and ADHD (AOTA, 2020b) and designing evidence-based intervention plans. Common intervention approaches addressed in this chapter may also be used in hospital and clinic settings. Practitioners in health care in schools should strive to enhance communication between their agencies and the family to create a comfortable environment that facilitates the child's ability to meet outcomes.

Evaluate to Determine Strengths and Needs

Services provided to young children with ASD should follow the occupational therapy process, which includes evaluation, intervention, and targeting of outcomes (AOTA, 2020b). Evaluation should consist of a comprehensive occupational profile and analysis of the child's occupational performance. Review may include education records, medical records, parent interviews, teacher interviews, and observations. Intervention should include planning, which includes the development of an intervention plan or plan of care; implementation; and a review of the intervention, including reevaluating the plan and determining the need for continuing or discontinuing occupational therapy services. An analysis of the child's occupational performance, based on all of the data gathered, determines need for services and should occur before intervention is initiated.

Under IDEA, the decision for occupational therapy services is made by the individualized family service plan or IEP team, on the basis of the child's eligibility for EI or special education services and need for occupational therapy. EI should occur in the child's natural environment, including other siblings, caregivers, and parents for collaboration, coaching, or consultation on occupation-based interventions. Part B intervention should occur in the least restrictive environment, within the natural routines of the day. Health care services may occur in the hospital, clinic, or community, dependent on the payer source and child and family needs. Targeting of outcomes should consist of a review of the determinants of success for reaching established goals, a review to guide future actions with the child, and a program evaluation.

Intervene With Children Identified With ASD

The *Occupational Therapy Practice Guidelines for Individuals With Autism Spectrum Disorder* (Tomchek & Koenig, 2016), developed from systematic reviews of the literature, identified four main areas of occupational therapy intervention for persons with ASD: (1) social interaction, restricted and repetitive behaviors, play performance, and leisure participation; (2) sensory integration and sensory-based interventions for children from daily life activities and occupations; (3) occupational performance in daily routines; and (4) parent self-efficacy, family coping and resiliency (including spouse and children), and family participation in daily life routines.

Social interaction, restricted and repetitive behaviors, play performance, and leisure participation

Evidence strongly supports using group formats to deliver social skills training to improve social communication for individuals with ASD (Tomchek & Koenig, 2016). Improvement has been shown with "social competency, increasing self-esteem, social participation and increased frequency of social outings" (Tomchek & Koenig, 2016, p. 46). The use of the *Picture Exchange Communication System* (PECS; Flippin et al., 2010; Ganz et al., 2012), an augmentative and alternative communication device that promotes communication through the use of pictures, and joint attention training (e.g., Joint Attention, Symbolic Play, and Emotional Regulation; Kaale et al., 2012) to facilitate social communication skills has strong evidence support (Tomchek & Koenig, 2016).

For restricted and repetitive behaviors, there is moderate evidence supporting behavioral strategies that identify and manipulate antecedents that may cause the behavior and address ways to self-manage behaviors and the use of physical activity (Tomchek & Koenig, 2016). There is moderate evidence supporting Social Stories™ and recess interventions for improving recreational activities and engagement in leisure (Tomchek & Koenig, 2016). Additional Level I research on the interventions to support social interaction, restrictive and repetitive behaviors, play, performance, and leisure is needed, because these foundational skills affect performance and participation in various daily life activities.

Sensory integration and sensory-based interventions for children from daily life activities and occupations

There is mixed evidence to support sensory-based interventions, such as Snoezelen multisensory centers, sound therapies, dynamic seating, weighted vests, participation in linear movement, and the use of brushing, to support the occupational performance of ADLs and IADLs (Tomchek & Koenig, 2016). However, there is moderate evidence that supports the use of occupational therapy sensory integration using Goal Attainment Scaling to address individualized goal areas (Tomchek & Koenig, 2016). There is tremendous opportunity for Level I research and practice initiatives in these areas to support sensory-based interventions that affect ADLs and IADLs for young children with ASD.

Occupational performance in daily routines

Evidence to support improvement in play performance for children with ASD is limited (Tomchek & Koenig, 2016). Researchers have suggested that occupational therapy practitioners "cautiously implement play performance interventions" (e.g., adult modeling and prompting, social–pragmatic skills, DIR-Floortime®, water exercise swimming programs, child-led play-based interventions; Tomchek & Koenig, 2016, p. 52). Intervention approaches such as PECS and *Cognitive Orientation to daily Occupational Performance Approach*® (CO–OP Approach™; Dawson et al., 2017; Rodger, 2017), an intervention approach that incorporates the child in active goal setting and problem solving, offer evidence to support positive effects on daily routines of young children with ASD.

Parent self-efficacy, family coping and resiliency, and family participation in daily life routines

Moderate to strong evidence supports interventions to improve parental self-efficacy, confidence, and competence that affect daily routines of young children with ASD (Tomchek & Koenig, 2016). Coaching and cognitive problem solving approaches in a contextual intervention have been shown to be effective in "achieving parent-identified goals, increasing parenting competency, reducing parent stress, and increasing a child's participation in everyday activities" (Tomchek & Koenig, 2016, p. 59). Evidence provides moderate support of the CO–OP Approach to improve IADLs, with positive outcomes in skill development for such areas as "improving morning routines and utensil use" (Tomchek & Koenig, 2016, p. 59).

Wong and Kwan's (2010) Level I research suggests that early parent training and education may reduce parental stress; however, overall there is immense room for more evidence that supports the use of parent education, training, and coaching to reduce parental stress. Moderate evidence does support the use of parent education, training, and coaching to increase parental skill and knowledge, family coping and resilience, and quality of life (Tomchek & Koenig, 2016), which, in turn, affect the participation and performance of young children with ASD in ADLs and IADLs.

Interventions for Children Identified With ADHD

Occupational therapy practitioners can be instrumental in helping young children with ADHD and their families improve occupational performance of typical occupations, such as playing, learning, resting and sleeping, communicating with friends and family, and performing daily tasks such as brushing teeth and getting dressed.

Interventions targeting behavior

Behavioral and medication intervention or management and parent and family education and training are common practices for young children diagnosed with ADHD (CDC, 2019c). Intervention should consider both symptoms and skill as related to ADL participation of children diagnosed with ADHD (Cermak, 2018). The American Academy of Pediatrics recommends that ADHD intervention for preschool-age children include evidence-based behavioral therapy and maybe medication (CDC, 2019c). Occupational therapy practitioners work with families to provide education and training to enhance the child's compliance, coping skills, and so forth.

Cognitive-based interventions

The **Cognitive–Functional (Cog-Fun) intervention** is designed to address the functional implications of ADHD (Maeir et al., 2018). Cog-Fun promotes acquisition of executive strategies and self-efficacy in occupational performance through promoting executive strategy acquisition, enabling a therapeutic setting, and using environmental supports and procedural learning (Maeir et al., 2018). Cog-Fun has been effective with 5–7-year-olds with ADHD in improving occupational performance and executive functions (Maeir et al., 2014). Community-based Cog-Fun group intervention for preschoolers with ADHD implemented by occupational therapists significantly increased executive functioning as well as improvement on the Canadian Occupational Performance Measure (Law et al., 2019) and Goal Attainment Scaling (Rosenberg et al., 2015).

Metacognitive training can be incorporated into occupational therapy intervention to promote awareness and self-monitoring skills. Strategies might include those for planning; organizing time, materials, and ideas; prioritizing; shifting; practicing flexibility; and checking. Preschoolers and school-age children (ages 3–7 years) with ADHD who participated in a group metacognitive intervention to improve attention, self-regulation, and positive interactions demonstrated statistically significantly improved executive functions and parent ratings of executive functions (Tamm & Nakonezny, 2015; Tamm et al., 2012). Halperin and colleagues (2013) used a play-based cognitive enhancement intervention (i.e., group-based cognitive games and parent strategy training) with 4–5-year-old children and found significant improvement in ADHD severity (as rated by the ADHD Rating Scale–IV from pre- to posttreatment and 3 months later).

Family-centered approach and education

A model of practice for children with ADHD using a *family-centered approach* (a way of working with families that includes the family's priorities and recognizes that the family is the expert regarding their child) with emphasis on the child, task, and environment found statistically significant changes in scores on at least one subscale, and more than 50% of the children had statistically significant changes in scores on at least one ADHD rating scale (Chu & Reynolds, 2007). Although the study focused on older children (ages 5–10 years), the intervention included education of the parents and teachers about ADHD, sensory modulation techniques, adaptations of home and classroom environments and routines, integrated academic and behavior management strategies to promote engagement, and remediation of challenges to the child's daily living skills (e.g., self-care, handwriting).

Physical activities

A systematic review by Grassmann and colleagues (2017) found that 30 minutes of *physical exercise* reportedly improved the executive functions of children with ADHD. The authors suggested further studies to confirm these findings. Aerobic exercise was found to have a moderate to large effect on the symptoms of ADHD (e.g., attention, impulsivity, executive functions) and social anxiety (Archer & Kostrzewa, 2012). Self-regulation and coping skills are often addressed through programs such as the Alert Program (Williams & Shellenberger, 1996) and Zones of Regulation (Kuypers, 2011). These programs use visual images as well as cognitive and sensory strategies to enhance participation in natural routines. Evidence for stability balls and weighted vests is insufficient, with a lack of studies in natural settings.

Advocate for Occupational Therapy on Interprofessional Teams

Advocacy as an intervention approach when working with children and families is part of the occupational therapy process (evaluation, intervention, and outcome measurement) as described in the *OTPF* (AOTA, 2020b). Occupational therapy practitioners can and should advocate for consumer access to appropriate occupational therapy services that support families with children diagnosed with ASD and ADHD. The *OTPF* (AOTA, 2020b) and the *2020 Occupational Therapy Code of Ethics* (AOTA, 2020a) both support advocacy by the practitioner. Advocacy is critical for practitioners serving children at risk for or diagnosed with ASD or ADHD, because disparities in access to high-quality and evidence-based services exist.

When working on interprofessional teams, occupational therapy practitioners can advocate for children, families, and the profession by explaining that collaboration on a complementary team promotes the best outcomes for young children with diagnoses such as ASD and ADHD. As Muhlenhaupt and colleagues (2015) noted, "Best practices in early childhood teaming require a clear understanding of both core values and shared competencies of all team members in addition to a solid foundation of discipline-specific knowledge and skills" (p. 126). For example, literature outside of the profession specifies that occupational therapy is "indispensable" during interprofessional EI collaboration for enabling communication for children with ASD and their families (Hébert et al., 2014, p. 594).

SUMMARY

Information and resources related to ASD and ADHD continue to evolve. Even though these conditions are both highly prevalent neurodevelopmental disorders, early identification of these disorders is lacking, and disparities in diagnosis and access to quality occupational therapy services exist. Occupational therapy practitioners play a key role in developmental monitoring, screening, evaluation, and intervention for both disorders. Practitioners should advocate for access to high-quality and evidence-based services for young children with ASD and ADHD as well as service and funding updates.

RESOURCES

ASD

- **AOTA:** https://www.aota.org/Practice/Children-Youth/Autism.aspx
  Information to support practice, policy and advocacy, networking, and continuing education
  https://myaota.aota.org/shop_aota/product/900489U
  Autism Across the Lifespan: A Comprehensive Occupational Therapy Approach (4th ed.), edited by R. Watling & S. Spitzer, 2018, AOTA Press.
- **CDC:** https://www.cdc.gov/ncbddd/autism/index.html
  Information about ASD, screening, diagnostics, treatment, data and statistics, and current research
- **Early Childhood Technical Assistance Center:** https://ectacenter.org/topics/autism/autism.asp
  Information about early identification of ASD, evidence-based interventions, professional development, and more

ADHD

- **AOTA:** https://www.aota.org/Practice/Children-Youth/Evidence-based/EBP-SPSI.aspx
  Information about sensory processing and sensory integration to support ADHD intervention
- **CDC:** https://www.cdc.gov/ncbddd/adhd/index.html
  Information about ADHD, symptoms, diagnosis, treatment, data and statistics, and current research

REFERENCES

American Occupational Therapy Association. (2019). *AOTA practice advisory: Occupational therapy practitioners in early intervention.* https://www.aota.org/~/media/Corporate/Files/Practice/Children/Practice-Advisory-Early-Intervention.pdf

American Occupational Therapy Association. (2020a). 2020 occupational therapy code of ethics. *American Journal of Occupational Therapy, 74*(Suppl. 3), 7413410005. https://doi.org/10.5014/ajot.2020.74S3006

American Occupational Therapy Association. (2020b). Occupational therapy practice framework: Domain and process (4th ed.). *American Journal of Occupational Therapy, 74*(Suppl. 2), 7412410010. https://doi.org/10.5014/ajot.2020.74S2001

American Psychiatric Association. (2013). *Diagnostic and statistical manual of mental disorders* (5th ed.). American Psychiatric Publishing.

Angell, A., Empey, A., & Zuckerman, K. E. (2018). A review of diagnosis and service disparities among children with autism from racial and ethnic minority groups in the United States. In R. M. Hodapp & D. J. Fidler (Eds.), *International review of research in developmental disabilities* (Vol. 55, pp. 145–180). Elsevier.

Archer, T., & Kostrzewa, R. M. (2012). Physical exercise alleviates ADHD symptoms: Regional deficits and developmental trajectory. *Neurotoxicity Research, 21,* 195–209. https://doi.org/10.1007/s12640-011-9260-0

Baio, J., Wiggins, L., Christensen, D. L., Maenner, M. J., Daniels, J., Warren, Z., . . . Dowling, N. F. (2018). Prevalence of autism spectrum disorder among children aged 8 years—Autism and Developmental Disabilities Monitoring Network, 11 Sites, United States, 2014. *Morbidity and Mortality Weekly Report, 67*(6), 1–23. https://doi.org/10.15585/mmwr.ss6706a1

Barger, B., Rice, C., & Roach, A. (2018). Socioemotional developmental surveillance in young children: Monitoring and screening best identify young children that require mental health treatment. *Child and Adolescent Mental Health, 23,* 206–213. https://doi.org/10.1111/camh.12240

Broder-Fingert, S., Shui, A., Pulcini, C. D., Kurowski, D., & Perrin, J. M. (2013). Racial and ethnic differences in subspecialty service use by children with autism. *Pediatrics, 132,* 94–100. https://doi.org/10.1542/peds.2012-3886

Bruininks, R. H., & Bruininks, B. D. (2005). *Bruininks–Oseretsky Test of Motor Proficiency* (2nd ed.). Pearson.

Centers for Disease Control and Prevention. (2019a). *Data and statistics about ADHD.* https://www.cdc.gov/ncbddd/adhd/data.html

Centers for Disease Control and Prevention. (2019b). *Learn the Signs. Act Early. program.* https://www.cdc.gov/ncbddd/actearly/freematerials.html

Centers for Disease Control and Prevention. (2019c). *Treatment of ADHD.* https://www.cdc.gov/ncbddd/adhd/treatment.html

Centers for Disease Control and Prevention. (2020a). *Autism data visualization tool.* https://www.cdc.gov/ncbddd/autism/data/index.html

Centers for Disease Control and Prevention. (2020b). *What is autism spectrum disorder?* https://www.cdc.gov/ncbddd/autism/facts.html

Centers for Disease Control and Prevention. (2020c). *Symptoms and diagnosis of ADHD.* https://www.cdc.gov/ncbddd/adhd/diagnosis.html

Centers for Medicare and Medicaid Services & National Center for Health Statistics. (2015). *International classification of diseases* (10th rev., clinical modification). Author.

Cermak, S. A. (2018). Cognitive rehabilitation of children and adults with attention deficit hyperactivity disorder. In N. Katz &

J. Toglia (Eds.), *Cognition, occupation, and participation across the life span: Neuroscience, neurorehabilitation, and models of intervention in occupational therapy* (4th ed., pp. 189–217). AOTA Press.

Chu, S., & Reynolds, F. (2007). Occupational therapy for children with attention deficit hyperactivity disorder (ADHD), Part 1: A delineation model of practice. *British Journal of Occupational Therapy, 70,* 372–383. https://doi.org/10.1177/030802260707000902

Danielson, M. L., Bitsko, R. H., Ghandour, R. M., Holbrook, J. R., Kogan, M. D., & Blumberg, S. J. (2018). Prevalence of parent-reported ADHD diagnosis and associated treatment among U.S. children and adolescents, 2016. *Journal of Clinical Child & Adolescent Psychology, 47,* 199–212. https://doi.org/10.1080/15374416.2017.1417860

Dawson, D. R., McEwen, S. E., & Polatajko, H. J. (Eds.). (2017). *Cognitive Orientation to daily Occupation: Using the CO-OP Approach™ to enable participation across the lifespan.* AOTA Press.

Dawson, G., Roger, S., Munson, J., Smith, M., Winter, J., Greenson, J., . . . Varley, J. (2010). Randomized, controlled trial of an intervention for toddlers with autism: The Early Start Denver Model. *Pediatrics, 125,* e17–e23. https://doi.org/10.1542/peds.2009-0958

Flippin, M., Reszka, S., & Watson, L. R. (2010). Effectiveness of the Picture Exchange Communication System (PECS) on communication and speech for children with autism spectrum disorders: A meta-analysis. *American Journal of Speech-Language Pathology, 19,* 178–195. https://doi.org/10.1044/1058-0360(2010/09-0022)

Ganz, J. B., Davis, J. L., Lundy, E. M., Goodwyn, F. D., & Simpson, R. L. (2012). Meta-analysis of PECS with individuals with ASD: Investigation of targeted versus non-targeted outcomes, participant characteristics, and implementation phase. *Research in Developmental Disabilities, 33,* 406–418. https://doi.org/10.1016/j.ridd.2011.09.023

Gioia, G. A., Inquish, P. K., Guy, S. C., & Kenworthy, L. (2015). *Behavior Rating Inventory of Executive Function* (2nd ed.). PAR.

Grassmann, V., Alves, M. V., Santos-Galduroz, R. F., & Galduroz, J. C. (2017). Possible cognitive benefits of acute physical exercise in children with ADHD: A systematic review. *Journal of Attention Disorders, 21,* 367–371. https://doi.org/10.1177/1087054714526041

Guifeng, X., Lane, S., Buyun, L., Binrang, Y., & Wei, B. (2018). Twenty-year trends in diagnosed attention-deficit/hyperactivity disorder among US children and adolescents, 1997–2016. *JAMA Network Open, 1,* e181471. https://doi.org/10.1001/jamanetworkopen.2018.1471

Haley, S., Coster, W., Dumas, H. M., Fragala-Pinkham, M. A., & Moed, R. (2012). *Pediatric Evaluation of Disability Inventory—Computer Adaptive Test (PEDI-CAT)* (2nd ed.). Pearson.

Halperin, J. M., Marks, D. J., Bedard, A. C. V., Chacko, A., Curchack, J. T., Yoon, C. A., & Healey, D. M. (2013). Training executive, attention, and motor skills: A proof-of-concept study in preschool children with ADHD. *Journal of Attention Disorders, 17,* 711–721. https://doi.org/10.1177/1087054711435681

Hébert, M. L. J., Kehayia, E., Prelock, P., Wood-Dauphinee, S., & Snider, L. (2014). Does occupational therapy play a role for communication in children with autism spectrum disorders? *International Journal of Speech-Language Pathology, 16,* 594–602. https://doi.org/10.3109/17549507.2013.876665

Individuals With Disabilities Education Improvement Act of 2004, Pub. L. 108-446, 20 U.S.C. §§ 1400–1482.

Irvin, D. W., McBee, M., Boyd, B. A., Hume K., & Odom S. L. (2012). Child and family factors associated with the use of services for preschoolers with autism spectrum disorder. *Research in Autism Spectrum Disorder, 6,* 565–572. https://doi.org/10.1016/j.rasd.2011.07.018

James, L. W., Pizur-Barnekow, K. A., & Schefkind, S. (2014). Online survey examining practitioners' perceived preparedness in the early identification of autism. *American Journal of Occupational Therapy, 68,* e13–e20. https://doi.org/10.5014/ajot.2014.009027

Kaale, A., Smith, L., & Sponheim, E. (2012). A randomized controlled trial of preschool-based joint attention intervention for children with autism. *Journal of Child Psychology and Psychiatry, 53,* 97–105. https://doi.org/10.1111/j.1469-7610.2011.02450.x

Kuypers, L. (2011). *The zones of regulation.* Think Social.

Law, M., Baptiste, S., Carswell, A., McColl, M., Polatajko, H., & Pollock, N. (2019). *Canadian Occupational Performance Measure* (5th ed., rev.) COPM, Inc.

Lord, C., Rutter, M., DiLavore, P. C., Risi, S., Gotham, K., & Bishop, S. (2012). *Autism Diagnostic Observation Schedule* (2nd ed.). Western Psychological Services.

Maeir, A., Bar-Ilan, R. T., Kastner, L., Fisher, O., Levanon-Erez, N., & Hahn-Markowitz, J. (2018). An integrative Cognitive–Function (Cog-Fun) intervention model for children, adolescents, and adults with ADHD. In N. Katz & J. Toglia (Eds.), *Cognition, occupation, and participation across the lifespan* (4th ed., pp. 335–351). AOTA Press.

Maeir, A., Fisher, O., Bar-Ilan, R. T., Boas, N., Berger, I., & Landau, Y. E. (2014). Effectiveness of Cognitive–Functional (Cog-Fun) occupational therapy intervention for young children with attention deficit hyperactivity disorder: A controlled study. *American Journal of Occupational Therapy, 68,* 268–276. https://doi.org/10.5014/ajot.2014.011700

Magaña, S., Lopez, K., Aguinaga, A., & Morton, H. (2013). Access to diagnosis and treatment services among Latino children with autism spectrum disorders. *Intellectual and Developmental Disabilities, 51,* 141–153. https://doi.org/10.1352/1934-9556-51.3.141

Miller, L. J. (2006). *Miller Function and Participation Scales.* Pearson.

Muhlenhaupt, M., Pizur-Barnekow, K., Schefkind, S., Chandler, B., & Harvison, N. (2015). Occupational therapy contributions in early intervention: Implications for personnel preparation and interprofessional practice. *Infants & Young Children, 28*(2), 123–132. https://doi.org/10.1097/IYC.0000000000000031

Okimoto, A. M., Bundy, A., & Hanzlik, J. (2000). Playfulness in children with and without disability: Measurement and intervention. *American Journal of Occupational Therapy, 54,* 73–82. https://doi.org/10.5014/ajot.54.1.73

Ramtekkar, U. P. (2017). *DSM–5* changes in attention deficit hyperactivity disorder and autism spectrum disorder: Implications for comorbid sleep issues. *Children, 4*(8), 62. https://doi.org/10.3390/children4080062

Rehabilitation Act of 1973, Pub. L. 93-112, 29 U.S.C. §§ 701–796l.

Robins, D., Fein, D., & Barton, M. (2009). *Modified Checklist for Autism in Toddlers—Revised.* https://www.m-chat.org/reference/mchatDOTorg.pdf

Rodger, S. A. (2017). Using the CO–OP Approach™: Autism spectrum disorder. In D. R. Dawson, S. E. McEwen, & H. J. Polatajko (Eds.), *Cognitive Orientation to Daily Occupation: Using the CO–OP Approach to enable participation across the lifespan* (pp. 61–74). AOTA Press.

Rosenberg, L., Maeir, A., Tochman, A., Dahan, I., & Hirsch, I. (2015). Effectiveness of a cognitive–functional group intervention among preschoolers with attention deficit hyperactivity disorder: A pilot study. *American Journal of Occupational Therapy, 69,* 6903220040. https://doi.org/10.5014/ajot.2015.014795

Squires, J., Bricker, D., & Potter, L. (2009). *Ages & Stages Questionnaires, Third Edition (ASQ-3) user's guide.* Brookes.

Squires, J., Bricker, D., Twombly, E., & Potter, L. (2009). *ASQ technical report.* https://agesandstages.com/products-pricing/asqse-2/

Stone, W. L., & Ousley, O. Y. (2008). *Screening Tool for Autism in Toddlers and Young Children (STAT): User's manual.* Vanderbilt University.

Tamm, L., & Nakonezny, P. A. (2015). Metacognitive executive function training for young children with ADHD: A proof-of-concept study. *Attention Deficit and Hyperactivity Disorders, 7,* 183–190. https://doi.org/10.1007/s12402-014-0162-x

Tamm, L., Nakonezny, P. A., & Hughes, C. W. (2012). An open trial of a metacognitive executive function training for young children with ADHD. *Journal of Attention Disorders, 18,* 551–559. https://doi.org/10.1177/1087054712445782

Tomchek, S., & Koenig, K. (2016). *Occupational therapy practice guidelines for individuals with autism spectrum disorder.* AOTA Press.

Virués-Ortega, J. (2010). Applied behavior analytic intervention for autism in early childhood: Meta-analysis, meta-regression and dose–response meta-analysis of multiple outcomes. *Clinical Psychology Review, 30,* 387–399. https://doi.org/10.1016/j.cpr.2010.01.008

Weaver, L. L. (2015). Effectiveness of work, activities of daily living, education, and sleep interventions for people with autism spectrum disorder: A systematic review. *American Journal of Occupational Therapy, 69,* 6905180020. https://doi.org/10.5014/ajot.2015.017962

Williams, M. S., & Shellenberger, S. (1996). *"How does your engine run?" A leader's guide to the Alert Program for self-regulation.* Therapy Works.

Wong, V. C. N., & Kwan, Q. K. (2010). Randomized controlled trial for early intervention for autism: A pilot study of the Autism 1-2-3 Project. *Journal of Autism and Developmental Disorders, 40,* 677–688. https://doi.org/10.1007/s10803-009-0916-z

Zuckerman, K. E., Lindly, O. J., Reyes, N. M., Chavez, A. E., Macias, K., Smith, K. N., & Reynolds, A. (2017). Disparities in diagnosis and treatment of autism in Latino and non-Latino White families. *Pediatrics, 139,* e20163010. https://doi.org/10.1542/peds.2016-3010

Best Practices Supporting Families of Children With Prenatal Substance Exposure and Postnatal Trauma

39

Yvonne Swinth, PhD, OTR/L, FAOTA, and Jennifer S. Pitonyak, PhD, OTR/L, SCFES

KEY TERMS AND CONCEPTS

- Abandonment
- Abuse
- Adverse childhood experiences
- Adverse Childhood Experiences Study
- Alcohol-related birth defect
- Alcohol-related neurodevelopmental disorder
- Attachment
- Co-regulation
- Developmental trauma
- Epigenetics
- Family coaching
- Fetal alcohol spectrum disorders
- Fetal alcohol syndrome
- Healthy attachment
- Infant massage
- Life course health development
- Man-made traumas
- Multitiered systems of support
- Natural traumas
- Neglect
- Neonatal abstinence syndrome
- Neurobehavioral disorder associated with prenatal alcohol exposure
- Opioid use disorder
- Perinatal risks
- Prenatal cannabis exposure
- Prenatal risks
- Prenatal substance exposure
- Prenatal tobacco exposure
- Promoting First Relationships
- Routine-based interventions
- School Mental Health Toolkit
- Systems effects
- Trauma
- Trauma-informed care

OVERVIEW

For years, occupational therapy practitioners have addressed the needs of infants and children with prenatal substance exposure and postnatal trauma and their families. (*Note. Occupational therapy practitioner* refers to both occupational therapists and occupational therapy assistants.) With the emerging and increased understanding of the effects of prenatal substance exposure and postnatal trauma on developing infants and children, such as the impact on brain development, regulation, physical development, and psychosocial needs, as well as the effect on family interactions, practitioners can more thoroughly assess the needs of this population and provide interventions that better support development, occupational engagement, and the establishment of healthy roles, habits, and routines of children and their families.

Prenatal Substance Exposure

Prenatal substance exposure is the exposure of the fetus to opioids, alcohol, nicotine, or other toxic or illicit substances in utero because of maternal use. The use of substances such as opioids and alcohol during pregnancy is a significant public health problem in the United States. The Centers for Disease Control and Prevention (CDC; n.d.-d) reported that opioid use disorder among pregnant women more than quadrupled in the period from 1999 to 2014. Abuse of opioids is a growing crisis for health care, social services, education, and other systems. Infants, children, and youths with a history of perinatal exposure to opioids, alcohol, and other substances are at risk for a number of problems, including neurodevelopmental disorders, postnatal trauma, and struggling family systems.

Prenatal opioid exposure

Opioid use disorder is defined in the *Diagnostic and Statistical Manual of Mental Disorders* (5th ed.; *DSM–5;* American Psychiatric Association [APA], 2013) as a chronic, problematic pattern of opioid use that results in clinically significant impairment, including reducing or giving up other occupational activities because of opioid use (CDC, n.d.-c). When infants are exposed in utero to opioids and other drugs, they may experience withdrawal during the neonatal period. These signs and symptoms of withdrawal in a neonate, which are attributed to prenatal exposure because of maternal substance abuse during pregnancy, are described as *neonatal abstinence syndrome* (NAS; ICD-10Data.com, 2018).

Substance withdrawal among neonates was first documented in the 1870s in case reports of morphine-exposed infants and had a high mortality rate until the mid-20th century (Grossman & Berkwitt, 2019). Opioid exposure other than morphine was not prominent until the 1950s, when heroin and prenatal methadone exposure were first documented among infants. Prenatal opioid exposure has continued to evolve, with infants experiencing withdrawal from a variety of prescription and nonprescription opioids (Grossman & Berkwitt, 2019). Both the increased treatment of women during pregnancy for substance use disorders and the hospitalization of infants experiencing substance withdrawal in the neonatal intensive care unit (NICU) have helped lessen infant mortality related to neonatal substance exposure and withdrawal (Grossman & Berkwitt, 2019).

The clinical manifestation of NAS generally appears within 36 hours of birth and may vary on the basis of the substance of exposure, dose, and polysubstance use (Grossman & Berkwitt, 2019; Kaltenbach & Jones, 2016); however, common signs of withdrawal include irritability, tremors, hypertonicity, poor feeding, disturbed sleep, and loose stools (Edwards & Brown, 2016; Grossman & Berkwitt, 2019). The Finnegan Neonatal Abstinence Scoring System (FNASS) categorizes signs and symptoms of withdrawal into three types of disturbances: (1) central nervous system; (2) metabolic, vasomotor, and respiratory; and (3) gastrointestinal (Finnegan et al., 1975). Autonomic dysregulation may present as sweating, respiratory distress, yawning, and sneezing (Grim et al., 2013; Grossman & Berkwitt, 2019; Jensen, 2014). Infants with NAS often experience neonatal morbidities consistent with prematurity and low birthweight, such as difficulties feeding and overresponsiveness to both external and internal stimuli (Grim et al., 2013; Grossman & Berkwitt, 2019; Jensen, 2014). Therefore, infants with NAS are at increased risk of experiencing problems with ***attachment*** (e.g., enduring emotional bond connecting one person to another that may not be reciprocal) and subsequent challenges with emotional and behavioral regulation (Maguire, 2014).

Prenatal alcohol exposure

Fetal alcohol spectrum disorders (FASDs) are a group of conditions that describe the growth and other neurodevelopmental problems that may occur with prenatal exposure to alcohol, such as abnormal facial features, small head size, atypical growth, attention and other behavior challenges, and a range of other related intellectual, developmental, and medical problems (CDC, n.d.-b). ***Fetal alcohol syndrome*** (FAS) describes the most involved of the FASDs. Persons with FAS may have abnormal facial features, atypical growth, and central nervous system problems that contribute to significant problems with learning and social relationships.

Fetal alcohol effects was the term previously used to describe a person with less-widespread effects of prenatal alcohol exposure; however, in 1996, the Institute of Medicine (IOM) replaced this term with two new conditions: (1) alcohol-related neurodevelopmental disorder (ARND), and (2) alcohol-related birth defects (ARBDs; CDC, n.d.-b). ***ARND*** describes individuals who experience intellectual and developmental problems, particularly with learning, as a result of prenatal alcohol exposure. In contrast, ***ARBD*** is the term used to describe individuals with impairments of body structures and functions, often the heart, kidneys, or bones, as a result of prenatal alcohol exposure.

Another FASD condition was introduced in 2013 in the *DSM–5*: ***neurobehavioral disorder associated with prenatal alcohol exposure*** (ND–PAE). Individuals with ND–PAE display problems in three areas: (1) thinking and memory, (2) behavior, and (3) ADLs (APA, 2013). To be diagnosed

with ND–PAE, the individual must have been exposed prenatally to greater than the minimal levels of alcohol—currently 13 drinks by the mother in any 30-day period (CDC, n.d.-b). According to the CDC (n.d.-b), the exact prevalence of FASDs is unknown. CDC studies have found a range from 0.2 to 1.5 infants with FAS for every 1,000 live births in some regions of the United States; however, some researchers estimate that the prevalence of FASDs in the United States may be as high as 1–5 per 100 school children (May et al., 2014, 2018).

FASDs are lifelong developmental conditions; however, research has shown that early intervention treatment services may improve outcomes, including these protective factors:

- Diagnosis before age 6 years,
- Stable home environment as a school-age child,
- Violence-free home environment, and
- Special education and social services support (Streissguth et al., 2004).

Prenatal exposure to other substances

Prenatal exposure to cannabis, tobacco, and other drugs are also linked with infant and childhood morbidity. Although more research is needed to understand the health and developmental effects of prenatal exposure to cannabis, the National Academies of Sciences, Engineering, and Medicine (NASEM; 2017) summarized current evidence indicating that ***prenatal cannabis exposure*** is linked to lower birthweight and cited one study that found a relationship between prenatal cannabis exposure and risk of preterm birth (Gunn et al., 2016). It is of note that the NASEM committee did not identify any fair- to good-quality systematic review studies assessing the potential association between prenatal cannabis exposure and other intellectual, developmental, or health outcomes into childhood (NASEM, 2017).

In comparison with cannabis, there is significant evidence documenting the health and developmental effects of perinatal tobacco exposure on children. ***Prenatal tobacco exposure*** is associated with preterm birth, low birth weight, and birth defects of the mouth and lip (CDC, n.d.-d). Studies also describe the increased risk of sudden infant death syndrome with both prenatal and postnatal tobacco exposure (CDC, n.d.-e; National Cancer Institute, 2019).

Postnatal Trauma

Trauma is defined as a psychological, emotional, neurological, or physical response to a deeply distressing or disturbing experience (Center for Treatment of Anxiety and Mood Disorders, n.d.). In adults, trauma is often talked about in terms of posttraumatic stress disorder (PTSD). However, the sequelia of PTSD does not consistently "fit" the experiences of individuals who experienced an early childhood trauma. From 1995 to 1997, a study was conducted at Kaiser Permanente involving more than 17,000 health maintenance organization members from southern California. Participants receiving physical exams completed confidential surveys regarding their childhood experiences and current health status and behaviors. This study became known as the ***Adverse Childhood Experiences (ACE) Study*** (CDC, n.d.-f). **ACEs** are traumatic events occurring during childhood and linked to health problems, mental illness, education problems, and difficulty with future jobs. This study found a correlation between ACEs and risk factors for disease and poorer later-life health and well-being (CDC, n.d.-f). Figure 39.1, the ACE Pyramid, represents the conceptual framework for the ACE Study.

As a result of the ACE Study, there has been an increased understanding of and discussion about **developmental trauma,** which may also be referred to as *chronic interpersonal trauma* or *complex trauma.* Developmental trauma is the result of abandonment, abuse, and neglect during the first 3 years of a child's life that disrupts cognitive, neurological, and psychological development and attachment to adult caregivers (IOM & National Research Council, 2014). It is often inflicted on infants and children unconsciously and most often without malicious intent by adult caregivers who are unaware of children's social and emotional needs (Weinhold & Weinhold, 2013).

In addition to **abandonment, abuse,** and **neglect,** defined as "the failure of a parent or other person with responsibility for the child to provide needed food, clothing, shelter, medical care, or supervision to the degree that the child's health, safety, and well-being are threatened with harm" [Child Welfare Information Gateway, 2019, p. 2]), other risk factors may include **prenatal risks,** such as exposure to drugs or alcohol or a stressful pregnancy; **perinatal risks,** such as a difficult or complicated birth or early or extended hospitalization; **systems effects,** such as homelessness, poverty, or multiple foster placements (the "Social Conditions/Local Context" tier in Figure 39.1); and **natural** or **man-made traumas,** such as war, car accidents, or floods. These traumas occur whenever both internal and external resources are inadequate to cope with an external threat (van der Kolk & Ducey, 1989). For additional information on ACEs and postnatal trauma, see Chapter 12, "Early Childhood Mental Health."

The ACE Pyramid (Figure 39.1) recognizes the impact generational embodiment and historical trauma may have on early development. This emerging area of research is also referred to as **epigenetics** and is gaining increased attention in the field of child development. Through the study of epigenetics, there is increasing evidence that environmental influences and children's experiences affect the expression of their genes. Researchers believe that the DNA that makes up humans' genes accumulates chemical marks that determine how the gene influences one's behavior and responses. Additionally, researchers believe that epigenetics may be intergenerational (Murgatroyd & Spengler, 2011; Yehuda & Lehrner, 2018). Awareness of this area of research can help occupational therapy practitioners understand the interplay between nature and nurture during infant and child development. This may result in better occupational profiles, which, in turn, may result in evaluations, intervention plans, and intervention implementation that best meet the needs of the child and family.

Impact on Brain Development and Developmental Milestones

Research and literature addressing infants and children who have had adverse experiences speaks to a significant impact on brain development, which, in turn, affects developmental milestones, attachment, regulation, learning, and more (Fraser et al., 2019; Purvis et al., 2013; Ryan et al., 2017). See Chapter 11, "Brain Development in the Early Years," for more information on brain development in early childhood.

Infants and children who have not experienced developmental trauma experience safe, predictable, loving interactions with caregivers, which support their brain development. Children with traumatic experiences have changes in brain structures, neurochemistry, and genetic expression (Purvis et al., 2013). The trauma affects three main areas of the brain: (1) brain stem, (2) amygdala, and (3) prefrontal lobe. At a young age, children with adverse experiences have an overdeveloped lower brain (i.e., brain stem), and they learn that the world is unpredictable. As a result, these children often live in a state of hyperarousal and high alert, with high amounts of cortisol in their system and poor insulin receptors. They may not feel safe, even in safe environments, relying on fight, flight, or freeze responses to manage their environment. As the brain continues to develop, they may not develop important neural pathways (Purvis et al., 2013).

Trauma experiences also affect the development of the amygdala, further increasing the state of hyperarousal. The amygdala is sensitive to any threat, and over time a fear response is triggered with less and less stress, resulting in fight, flight, or freeze tactics and the continued overdevelopment of the brain stem. Important development of neural pathways to the prefrontal cortex is interrupted, causing the child to lose control of their emotions (Siegel & Bryson, 2012). Children who have experienced trauma may not develop executive functions and problem-solving skills and may have poor emotional regulation.

FIGURE 39.1. ACE pyramid.

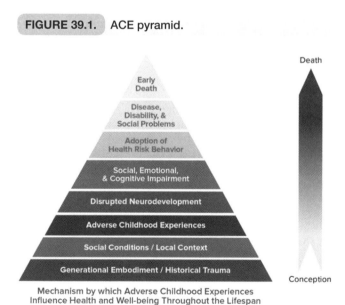

Mechanism by which Adverse Childhood Experiences Influence Health and Well-being Throughout the Lifespan

Source. Reprinted from *About the CDC-Kaiser ACE Study,* by the Centers for Disease Control and Prevention, n.d.-a https://www.cdc.gov/violenceprevention/childabuseandneglect/acestudy/about.html.

In addition, developmental trauma results in a stronger left hemisphere, which supports logical, literal, linear, and linguistic processing. The right hemisphere, which is connected to emotions, sensations, and the "big picture," is weakened, so children may struggle with emotions, sensations, and social situations. Thus, although a neurotypical infant or child moves from a neurological emphasis on survival to increasing emphasis on social–emotional and cognitive development, a child who has developmental trauma continues to focus on survival and, as a result, may have fewer neural pathways established to support social–emotional and cognitive development, which could affect occupational performance at home, in the community, and at school (Fraser et al., 2019).

ESSENTIAL CONSIDERATIONS

Occupational therapy practitioners working with these populations often move from becoming *trauma aware* to *trauma sensitive* to *trauma responsive* and finally *trauma informed* (Trauma Informed Oregon, 2018). This section is designed to help practitioners increase awareness and sensitivity to infants and children with developmental trauma and their families. It is beyond the scope of this chapter to fully prepare practitioners for trauma-informed care (TIC). However, we anticipate that as practitioners apply the principles discussed, they will begin their journey from being trauma responsive to becoming more trauma informed.

Many professionals working with these children and families lack awareness of the impact of developmental trauma on development, attachment, behavior, and state regulation (Fraser et al., 2019). Awareness involves understanding and discussing issues of TIC. Becoming trauma sensitive means developing a foundational knowledge of TIC as well as developing an infrastructure and process within the practice setting to meet the needs of this population. At this point, the practice setting and occupational therapy practitioners can become trauma responsive by gathering information about policies and trauma-informed practices and creating a plan for implementing TIC. Finally, practitioners become trauma informed through advanced training, implementation of principles, and ongoing data collection regarding services. As part of this process, differential diagnosis from other developmental conditions is important so that the approach to assessment and intervention considers the unique factors of TIC.

Trauma-Informed Care

The CDC, along with the Substance Abuse and Mental Health Services Administration, has defined six *TIC* principles: (1) safety, (2) trustworthiness, (3) peer support, (4) collaboration, (5) empowerment, and (6) cultural competence (CDC, 2018). It is important when working with infants and young children to understand the impact of trauma on the nervous system (Sanders & Hall, 2018). Occupational therapy practitioners should shift the emphasis of their assessment and intervention from "What is wrong?" to "What has happened?" Challenging behaviors should be seen as the result of poor self-regulation and an overdeveloped brain stem. Additionally, the occupational therapy assessment and intervention plan should address the needs of family and caregivers. This should include evaluating the awareness of principles of TIC, attachment, training that may be needed, and accommodations or adaptions needed to support the infant or child.

Cook et al. (2005) described seven domains of impairment among children exposed to developmental trauma: (1) attachment, (2) biology, (3) affect regulation, (4) dissociation, (5) behavioral control, (6) cognition, and (7) self-concept. Occupational therapy scope of practice includes many of these domains, and it is within the domain of occupational therapy for practitioners to provide developmental, preventive, and health promotion services to infants and children who have experienced developmental trauma and their families. When services are provided to this population in early years, there is increased likelihood that some of the adverse impacts of the developmental trauma can be overcome. Additionally, strategies can be learned and implemented that prevent further trauma, promote healthy development, and are consistent with infant mental health initiatives.

Theoretical Framework for Evaluation and Intervention: Life Course Approach

Substantial evidence links early life experiences with chronic health conditions across the life course, and contemporary models of health seek to explain the complex, biopsychosocial influences of factors such as trauma and adversity on health and development (Bronfenbrenner, 2005; Halfon & Forrest, 2018; Halfon et al., 2014). One such framework, *life course health development* (LCHD), examines the transactions among the developmental origins of health, biological and behavioral adaptation, and contextual influences to explain how health develops and why disparities in health exist (Halfon & Forrest, 2018; Halfon & Hochstein, 2002; Halfon et al., 2014). The LCHD framework has emerged from a set of theories, conceptual models, and empirical evidence informing this complex, relational, dynamic framework of health development and is grounded in epigenetics, neurodevelopment, and life course epidemiology (Halfon & Forrest, 2018).

LCHD is a useful framework for understanding the lifelong implications of prenatal substance exposure and postnatal trauma. Principles of the LCHD framework include concepts of unfolding, complexity, timing, and plasticity. *Unfolding* posits that health development continuously evolves over the life course, shaped by prior experiences and contextual influences (Halfon & Forrest, 2018). Children and youths with prenatal substance exposure and postnatal trauma often demonstrate varied and unexpected behavioral responses with stressful contextual influences or new life stages.

The principle of complexity acknowledges the multidimensional etiology of developmental trauma, in that influences such as prenatal substance exposure are usually coupled with other adversity, such as abuse and neglect, repeated separations from parents and caregivers, and poverty—among many other factors. Timing is another principle of LCHD, acknowledging that there are sensitive or critical periods of development that, if disrupted, may lead to poorer health outcomes. This principle of LCHD is reflected in the health outcomes of children and youths with prenatal substance exposure and postnatal trauma, given that evidence indicates that exposure to childhood adversity is associated with outcomes such as delays in cognitive development, chronic conditions such as asthma, differences in cortisol levels, and other somatic complaints (Oh et al., 2018). Similarly, children with a history of NAS are more likely to be evaluated for developmental delay, meet criteria for a disability, and qualify for special education and therapy services (Fill et al., 2018).

Finally, given growing understanding of the neurobiological implications of trauma and adversity, the LCHD principle of plasticity is particularly relevant for children and youths with prenatal substance exposure and postnatal trauma. Although trauma and adversity affect brain structure and function, neurobiological adaptability is possible and allows behavior and health development changes across the life course that support improved health and occupational outcomes (Gupta et al., in press; Halfon & Forrest, 2018).

BEST PRACTICES

This section is organized into two themes: (1) evaluation and intervention for management of NAS, and (2) evaluation and intervention to address developmental trauma. Best practices in interventions for children with prenatal substance exposure and related developmental trauma vary by age; developmental considerations; the environment in which intervention is provided; and other factors, such as the type of adversity experienced. For both infants and children, an ecological approach should be used whenever possible. This requires the occupational therapy practitioner to consider not only direct intervention with the child and family but also services on behalf of the child, such as advocacy and education, as well as other approaches at a systems level, such as those that support promotion and prevention. The *Occupational Therapy Practice Framework: Domain and Process* (4th ed.; *OTPF;* American Occupational Therapy Association [AOTA], 2020) should guide the scope of services as well as the occupational therapy process when practitioners are working with each child and family.

Evaluate the Infant With Neonatal Abstinence Syndrome and Family

The evaluation process for an infant with NAS may vary across practice settings, with the age of the child, and according to their developmental and occupational needs. Although the occupational therapy evaluation centers around developing an occupational profile of the infant and their caregivers and analyzing occupational performance (AOTA, 2014), regardless of practice setting, therapists need to be knowledgeable about screening tools and assessments used by other medical team members to document withdrawal. For example, the previously mentioned FNASS has been considered the gold standard for assessing opioid-exposed infants since the 1970s and measures 21 different signs of withdrawal (Finnegan et al., 1975). However, neonatal nurseries have recently adopted the eat, sleep, console approach, which assesses the infant's functioning in the context of withdrawal (Grossman et al., 2017). Additionally, NICU teams use a number of neonatal assessment

instruments to assess and describe infant behavior, such as the Assessment of Preterm Infant Behavior (APIB; Als et al., 1982). The APIB and similar instruments require training and certification to administer, which reflects the importance of continued professional development for occupational therapists working with infants with NAS and other preterm high-risk needs.

In general, the occupational therapy evaluation of an infant with NAS includes assessment of the following areas: medical considerations, physiological stability, neurobehavioral organization, reflexes, motor organization and posture, engagement with people and the environment, parents' and caregivers' routines, and their knowledge and skills for child rearing (Grossman & Berkwitt, 2019; Oostlander et al., 2019; Vergara & Bigsby, 2004). Occupational therapists may use a variety of assessment methods to gather data, such as medical record review and consultation with the primary nurse, standardized assessments, observation, and caregiver and family interviews. It is particularly important for therapists to expand their evaluation approach to include the family and information about any responsibilities and routines that the birth mother or other caregivers might have related to their own recovery process, work, or other essential occupations. Therapists working with infants with NAS and other preterm high-risk needs should also be aware of the impact of postpartum anxiety and mood disorders on parent and caregiver behavior and occupational performance, take these needs into consideration during evaluation of the infant and family, and make appropriate referrals to services and resources.

Provide Effective Interventions for Neonatal Abstinence Syndrome

Although pharmacological treatment is used in as many as 91% of cases of NAS (Grossman & Berkwitt, 2019) to achieve short-term improvement in withdrawal signs, it may prolong withdrawal, and its long-term impact on growth and development is unknown. Nonpharmacological treatment is therefore the desired approach for managing withdrawal signs, supporting caregiver–infant bonding, and providing overall developmental care (Grossman & Berkwitt, 2019; Oostlander et al., 2019). As such, a recent scoping review (Oostlander et al., 2019) described occupational therapy management strategies for infants with NAS, considering interventions directed at person-related and environmental factors that promote regulation as well as those interventions that foster infant mental health through support of the caregiver–infant dyad relationship.

Promoting regulation

Approaches for promoting autonomic stability and regulation include positioning, swaddling, handling, strategies for temperature stability, and use of other sensory input (Oostlander et al., 2019; Vergara & Bigsby, 2004). Occupational therapists can evaluate infant responses to prone, supine, and side-lying positions and create a positioning plan in the NICU and at home. Swaddling may also be used as a strategy to facilitate regulation and promote longer periods of sleep, and occupational therapy practitioners can instruct caregivers and other team members in use of slow, gentle handling to help avoid overstimulation (Jensen, 2014; Oostlander et al., 2019).

Although nursing may provide strategies for temperature stability in the NICU, occupational therapy practitioners can also support caregivers in the use of strategies such as kangaroo care, a method of newborn care where infants are held chest-to-chest and skin-to-skin with a caregiver (Maguire, 2014; Neu & Robinson, 2010; World Health Organization [WHO], 2014), for temperature stability and regulation. Furthermore, the infant's response to oral, vestibular, and tactile input should also be assessed at rest and during feeding, diapering, bathing, and other occupational activities.

Before touching or moving an infant with NAS in the NICU, it is best practice to assess vital signs and then monitor the infant for changes in vital signs with touch, movement, or other sensory input. The occupational therapy practitioner can use the intervention strategy of containment by first gently placing a hand on the infant's stomach, head, or bottom to slowly introduce tactile input before a movement transition (Neu & Robinson, 2010). If the infant is not overstimulated by movement, then slow, gentle rocking in a linear plane may also support regulation. Furthermore, facilitating oral stimulation with a pacifier or encouraging the infant to mouth their hands is another sensory strategy that may support regulation and subsequent participation in bonding and other early infant occupations, such as diapering and bathing.

Best practices for supporting infants with NAS also include implementation of environmental modifications to decrease overstimulation and support regulation. Occupational therapy practitioners can consult with the medical team in the NICU and with caregivers at home about adjusting lighting and sound in the immediate environment. In addition to decreasing noise, practitioners can evaluate how the use of music or sounds with a consistent rhythm and tempo may help facilitate regulation. Infants with NAS, similar to those with prematurity who have had long stays in the NICU, may have difficulty establishing day–night sleep patterns and can benefit from environmental modifications such as room-darkening shades during naps and nighttime sleep.

Fostering relational attachment

Beyond interventions focused on decreasing overstimulation in the environment and supporting infant regulation, best practices include approaches that support caregiver–infant dyad relationships. When a parent or other infant caregiver is present, it is best practice to enable that person to engage in bonding and providing care activities such as feeding, diapering, and bathing. The occupational therapy practitioner should attempt to schedule therapy sessions during times when the infant is awake and participating in early occupational routines, to instruct caregivers in strategies for infant regulation and environmental modifications.

Difficulty with feeding is a common problem of infants experiencing withdrawal. Although the occupational therapy process with infants and young children with feeding difficulties is beyond the scope of this chapter, there are several specific considerations for best practice with infants with NAS. Evidence indicates that infants with NAS may

have decreased symptoms of withdrawal when given small, frequent, high-calorie feedings (Grim et al., 2013; Oostlander et al., 2019). Occupational therapy practitioners with expertise in infant feeding can assist parents and caregivers in establishing a feeding routine that acknowledges the infant's feeding cues and is responsive to any signs of distress with feeding.

Furthermore, given the demonstrated health benefits of and opportunity for enhanced maternal–infant attachment through breastfeeding given the situation of maternal substance abuse and NAS, WHO (2014, p. 15) recommends that "mothers with substance use disorders should be encouraged to breastfeed unless the risks clearly outweigh the benefits" and offers guidance on risk assessment and strategies for reducing exposure to substances through breastfeeding. If breastfeeding is desired by the mother but determined to be risky because of the mother's level of use of substances or other factors, the occupational therapy practitioner can support a routine for pumping breastmilk (Pitonyak, 2014) so that the milk supply is established; if and when breastfeeding is indicated, the infant can be fed at the breast or fed expressed breastmilk by bottle. In general, practitioners can support early feeding by implementing previously discussed strategies to decrease overstimulation and promote regulation during the feeding routine.

Relationship-based programs

Beyond routine-based interventions for feeding, sleeping, diapering, bathing, and other early occupations, several established relationship-based programs exist for supporting infant mental health. One such program is ***Promoting First Relationships*** (PFR), a curriculum that promotes children's social–emotional development through relational responsiveness and nurturing (Kelly et al., 2008). PFR uses a video feedback approach in which the practitioner provides intervention grounded in attachment theory and principles of reflective practice (Kelly et al., 2008).

Several randomized controlled trials have been conducted studying the effectiveness of PFR with families of young children who have experienced adversity such as abuse, neglect, and impermanency in early relationships (Hash et al., 2019; Oxford et al., 2016; Pasalich et al., 2016; Spieker et al., 2014, 2018). These studies found that PRF was associated with improved parental sensitivity, changed parental knowledge of the child's socioemotional needs, improved child behavior, and a reduction in foster care placement (Hash et al., 2019; Oxford et al., 2016; Pasalich et al., 2016; Spieker et al., 2014, 2018). Occupational therapy practitioners working with young children with a history of prenatal substance exposure can receive training in PFR and implement this curriculum with parents and caregivers who need support for and education about establishing strong relationships with young children.

Finally, ***infant massage*** is an intervention that supports infant regulation as well as the caregiver–infant relationship. Evidence supports a relationship between infant massage, when used for attachment and positive infant–caregiver interactions, and a variety of health and developmental outcomes (Field, 2014). Occupational therapy practitioners who are interested should pursue training to become certified infant massage instructors.

Evaluate the Child for Developmental Trauma

The evaluation process when occupational therapists work with a child with developmental trauma and the family should start with an occupational profile. In some settings this may include screening for ACEs. On the basis of the information gathered, the therapist should select methods and measures to best analyze occupational performance, including underlying client factors. Often, for this population, methods and measures address fine and gross motor skills, sensory processing and self-regulation, behavior, executive functioning, participation in home activities appropriate for the child's developmental age, and environmental factors such as family and caregiver support and knowledge about developmental trauma. Cognitive function in areas such as attention and transitioning between activities also should be addressed (Fraser et al., 2019).

Provide Effective Interventions for Developmental Trauma

TIC interventions for children who have experienced developmental trauma are similar to approaches with infants with NAS. Promoting regulation; fostering attachment; and addressing routine-based interventions that support occupational performance in the home, the community, and early intervention settings is the focus of occupational therapy practitioners working with this population. Practitioners should also be prepared to work with the family to support the application of strategies in the home as well as to ensure the family understands the unique needs of this population through education and coaching strategies. These interventions are grounded in infant mental health, which is defined as the social and emotional well-being that occurs within supportive and nurturing relationships and includes emotional regulation as well as close and secure attachment.

Emotional regulation

When children are exposed to trauma, they may have an overdeveloped brain stem and have a difficult time with emotional regulation. They may be difficult to console, have difficulty with self-soothing, have poor arousal, and be easily emotionally triggered. Co-regulation and accommodations and adaptations to support regulation should be used during therapy as well as taught to caregivers. *Co-regulation* is warm, responsive interactions that provide support for children to modulate their feelings and behaviors (Gillespie, 2015). For infants, as discussed earlier, this may include swaddling and "wearing" the child when in the community rather than placing the child in a stroller. Implementing other sensory strategies, such as playing soothing music, using firm touch, and limiting busy visual stimuli, may also help with regulation. Attention should be given to helping the infant learn that they have a caregiver who is loving, predictable, and safe. Practices such as a set feeding schedule or letting the baby "cry it out" are not beneficial for children with developmental trauma. Instead, feeding on demand and responding when the infant cries helps build connection, which, in turn, prevents the overdevelopment of the brain stem.

As the infant develops, the occupational therapy practitioner and caregiver continue to provide co-regulation but also work to help the child begin to develop emotional regulation. This may include providing a consistent and structured environment. Because children who have experienced trauma are often fear driven, developing trust-driven practices such as predictability in responses helps them "feel that their environment and relationships are safe and predictable" and in turn "learn to trust others and develop healthy emotions and behaviors" (Purvis et al., 2013, p. 363).

Supporting sensory needs also helps with the development of self-regulation. Several researchers have documented the need to address self-regulation and sensory processing with this population (Fraser et al., 2019; Purvis et al., 2013). Opportunities to promote participation in sensory-rich environments to support play and participation should be sought. Although research is limited regarding the outcomes of specific approaches, occupational therapy practitioners may consider using specific therapeutic interventions, such as Ayres Sensory Integration® (Smith Roley et al., 2007) or a sensory processing approach, during therapy sessions. Emphasis should be on helping with ongoing brain development, including opportunities for developing and strengthening healthy neural pathways from the brain stem, up through the amygdala, and to the prefrontal cortex. Data should be collected to ensure the strategies used result in the intended outcomes. See Chapter 33, "Best Practices in Supporting Social, Emotional, and Self-Regulation Skills (Social–Emotional Skills)" for more information on self-regulation.

Cognitive approaches

Many children who have experienced trauma have difficulties with cognitive function in areas such as attention, organization, planning, and transitioning between activities (Fraser et al., 2019). Early intervention that takes these needs into consideration may decrease some of these challenges. Some children with ACEs can have a fixed mindset, resulting in negative self-talk and difficulty trying new tasks. Using tools such as those from the Big Life Journal (https://biglifejournal.com/) can help these children develop a growth mindset during early years and into adolescence.

Foster attachment

Fostering healthy attachment supports the healing of this population. *Healthy attachment* enables both the child and the caregiver to experience personal and interpersonal behaviors that build trust. The brain develops in the context of relationships, so services that help caregivers read and respond to the child's cues, that encourage interactions, and that support healthy relationships will help build attachment. These services may include engaging in play activities such as imitation, encouraging exploration, and encouraging the child to try new things. Many of the approaches to support attachment described earlier work with this population as well.

When working with children with ACEs and their families, occupational therapy practitioners should seek opportunities to model, support, and teach healthy attachment strategies. Using a framework such as the Circle of Security (https://www.circleofsecurityinternational.com/), which helps caregivers understand a child's emotional needs, supports the child in handling emotions and enhances the development of self-esteem. Other programs, such as the Halo Project (www.haloprojectokc.org), have specific interventions to support the development of attachment.

Routine-based interventions

Routine-based interventions are opportunities for the child to learn through repeated interactions with the environment distributed over time. Using routine-based interventions can help the occupational therapy practitioner embed developmental interventions into daily routines and scaffold the skill as needed. This can support ongoing, healthy brain development, enable family coping, and prevent the ongoing impact of the developmental trauma on engagement in skills and activities. Routine-based interventions also are more functional and meaningful for the child and caregivers. They also can help caregivers with behaviors at home. Often there is a higher rate of mastery and self-confidence when routine-based interventions are used.

Family coaching

Although direct services with the infant or child are important and a critical part of occupational therapy services with this population, *family coaching* should also be considered as part of the occupational therapy intervention plan. Coaching is built on the belief that participants have the answers to the challenges they are facing. It allows the family and occupational therapy practitioner to build on family strengths, collaboratively learn and implement new skills, and overcome challenges. This approach is gaining increased attention in "supporting caregiver–therapist collaboration in planning and evaluating intervention addressing occupational performance deficits" (Kraversky, 2019, p. CE-1).

Occupational therapy practitioners may use intervention approaches such as DIRFloortime® (Greenspan & Wieder, 2006) or Trust-Based Relational Intervention (Purvis et al., 2013) to support these families. Emphasis should be on reframing behavior, connecting, supporting self-regulation, using routine-based approaches, and supporting family interactions. Educating family members about developmental trauma to increase awareness and understanding may also be part of the coaching process. Practitioners may also work with caregivers and others to advocate the child's needs outside of the home.

Communicate with professionals

Many infants and children with prenatal substance exposure and postnatal trauma and their families receive services from more than one professional. They may be seeing physicians, counselors, nutritionists, speech therapists, and other medical professionals. They may be involved in the foster care system or in community services. Occupational therapy practitioners need to determine what other professionals are part of the child's intervention team and seek opportunities to communicate and collaborate across professions. It is important to prioritize consistency in services, what is communicated to caregivers, and intervention approaches with this population.

Advocate for the Prevention of ACEs and Childhood Trauma

Parallel to the growing practice of screening for ACEs to better identify and treat those with trauma is the need to prevent ACEs and the resulting, complex impact on health and well-being. The CDC (n.d.-f) identified a number of focuses for health promotion and prevention that align with the scope of occupational therapy, such as providing access to quality care and education in early childhood and enhancing parenting skills to promote healthy child development. Promotion and prevention priorities such as these seek to break the cycle of adversity and trauma and attempt to mediate upstream exposure to social determinants such as poverty and level of education.

Therefore, in addition to direct intervention approaches using remediation or adaptation to enable occupational performance of clients with developmental trauma, occupational therapy practitioners can provide services focused on promotion of health and wellness and prevention of ACEs and subsequent development trauma, consistent with the variety of approaches to intervention identified in the *OTPF* (AOTA, 2020). Several of the intervention programs shared in this chapter align with health promotion and prevention approaches, such as infant massage and PFR (Kelly et al., 2008). Additional examples of occupational therapy–developed promotion and prevention approaches include Every Moment Counts (https://everymomentcounts.org/), a mental health promotion initiative consisting of model programs and toolkits supporting youth participation at school, at home, and in the community. Additionally, training for caregivers, provided either face to face or web based, has been shown to decrease children's behavioral problems and trauma symptoms (Razuri et al., 2017). Occupational therapy practitioners have much to offer such programs.

Finally, AOTA's (n.d.) *School Mental Health Toolkit* is a resource designed to guide service provision for mental health promotion, prevention, and intervention for children and youths in school and community settings. Resources and services are aligned with the public health approach to mental health, which emphasizes mental health promotion for all children and youths, regardless of whether they are identified as having a disability. The public health model of occupational therapy services to promote mental health among children and youths consists of *multitiered systems of support* (Bazyk, 2011, 2019). *Tier 1* includes universal services promoting mental health for whole populations. *Tier 2* consists of targeted prevention and early intervention for children and youths at risk of mental health conditions. *Tier 3* services are intensive individualized interventions for children and youths with existing mental health conditions.

SUMMARY

It is clear that occupational therapy practitioners are critical members of the team addressing the needs of infants and children with prenatal substance exposure and postnatal trauma and their families. Intervening early for this population not only supports the development of the child but also may prevent further trauma and promotes occupational engagement in the home, community, school, and, eventually, work environments. It may be necessary to seek advanced training and connect with other professionals serving this population if the occupational therapy practitioner desires to implement TIC (Fraser et al., 2019).

RESOURCES

- **AOTA School Mental Health Toolkit:** https://bit.ly/2S16C2t
  Includes a variety of resources for occupational therapy practitioners to use when addressing the mental health of school-aged children.
- **Big Life Journal:** https://biglifejournal.com/
  Has a variety of resources that help children ages 4–15+ years and their families develop a growth and resilient mindset so they can face life's challenges with confidence.
- **National Child Traumatic Stress Network's Child Trauma Toolkit for Educators:** https://bit.ly/334HC0S
  Provides resources and information for educators to best address the needs of children who have experienced trauma so they can participate in school.
- **Community Resilience Initiative:** https://criresilient.org/
  Includes opportunities for training to address trauma and resilience; provides additional resources for intervention and a framework for building a community response to address the needs of this population.
- **Every Moment Counts:** https://everymomentcounts.org/
  Focuses on reframing mental health as a positive state of functioning; resources include programs, tip sheets, and videos.
- **Massachusetts Advocates for Children's Helping Traumatized Children Learn:** https://bit.ly/307AQW9
  Helps educators and administrators develop school initiatives to support the academic performance of children traumatized by family violence so that they can succeed in school
- **Preventing Adverse Childhood Experiences (ACEs): Leveraging the Best Available Evidence:** https://bit.ly/3i51LYE
  Offers guidance for professionals on the best available evidence for preventing ACEs and helping families create and sustain safe, stable, and nurturing relationships.
- **Promoting First Relationships:** https://pfrprogram.org
  Promotes children's social–emotional development through responsive, nurturing caregiver–child relationships.
- *The Heart of Learning: Compassion, Resiliency, and Academic Success* (Wolpow et al., 2009)
  Provides information on how to work with and support the learning of children who have been adversely affected by trauma.

REFERENCES

Als, H., Lester, B. M., Tronickm, E. Z., & Brazelton, T. B. (1982). Manual for the Assessment of Preterm Infants' Behavior (APIB). In H. E. Fitzgerald, B. M. Lester, & M. W. Yogman (Eds.), *Theory and research in behavioral pediatrics* (pp. 36–63). Kluwer Academic/Plenum.

American Occupational Therapy Association. (n.d.). *School mental health toolkit.* https://www.aota.org/Practice/Children-Youth/Mental%20Health/School-Mental-Health.aspx

American Occupational Therapy Association. (2020). Occupational therapy practice framework: Domain and process (4th ed.). *American Journal of Occupational Therapy, 74*(Suppl. 2), 7412410010. https://doi.org/10.5014/ajot.2020.74S2001

American Psychiatric Association. (2013). *Diagnostic and statistical manual of mental disorders* (5th ed.). American Psychiatric Publishing.

Bazyk, S. (Ed.). (2011). *Mental health promotion, prevention, and intervention with children and youth: A guiding framework for occupational therapy.* AOTA Press.

Bazyk, S. (2019). Best practices in school mental health. In G. Frolek Clark, J. Rioux, & B. Chandler (Eds.), *Best practice in school occupational therapy* (2nd ed., pp. 153–160). AOTA Press.

Bronfenbrenner, U. (2005). *Making human beings human: Bioecological perspectives on human development.* Sage.

Center for Treatment of Anxiety and Mood Disorders. (n.d.). *What is trauma?* https://centerforanxietydisorders.com/what-is-trauma/

Centers for Disease Control and Prevention. (n.d.-a). *About the CDC–Kaiser ACE Study.* https://www.cdc.gov/violenceprevention/childabuseandneglect/acestudy/about.html

Centers for Disease Control and Prevention. (n.d.-b). *Fetal alcohol spectrum disorders (FASDs): Basics about FASDs.* https://www.cdc.gov/ncbddd/fasd/facts.html

Centers for Disease Control and Prevention. (n.d.-c). *Module 5: Assessing and addressing opioid use disorder (OUD).* https://www.cdc.gov/drugoverdose/training/oud/accessible/index.html

Centers for Disease Control and Prevention. (n.d.-d). *Reproductive health: Substance use during pregnancy.* https://www.cdc.gov/reproductivehealth/maternalinfanthealth/substance-abuse/substance-abuse-during-pregnancy.htm

Centers for Disease Control and Prevention. (n.d.-e). *Smoking during pregnancy.* https://www.cdc.gov/tobacco/basic_information/health_effects/pregnancy/index.htm

Centers for Disease Control and Prevention. (n.d.-f). *Violence prevention: Prevention strategies.* https://www.cdc.gov/violenceprevention/childabuseandneglect/prevention.html

Centers for Disease Control and Prevention (2018). *Preventing adverse childhood experiences.* https://www.cdc.gov/violenceprevention/childabuseandneglect/aces/fastfact.html

Child Welfare Information Gateway. (2019). *Definitions of child abuse and neglect.* U.S. Department of Health and Human Services, Children's Bureau. https://www.childwelfare.gov/topics/systemwide/laws-policies/statutes/define/

Cook, A., Spinazzola, J., Ford, J., Lanktree, C., Blaustein, M., Cloitre, M., . . . van der Kolk, B. (2005). Complex trauma in children and adolescents. *Psychiatric Annals, 35,* 390–398. https://doi.org/10.3928/00485713-20050501-05

Edwards, L., & Brown, L. F. (2016). Nonpharmacologic management of neonatal abstinencesyndrome: An integrative review. *Neonatal Network, 35,* 305–313. https://doi.org/10.1891/0730-0832.35.5.305

Field, T. (2014). *Touch* (2nd ed.). MIT Press.

Fill, M.-M. A., Miller, A. M., Wilkinson, R. H., Warren, M. D., Dunn, J. R., Schaffner, W., & Jones, T. F. (2018). Educational disabilities among children born with neonatal abstinence syndrome. *Pediatrics, 142,* e20180562. https://doi.org/10.1542/peds.2018-0562

Finnegan, L. P., Connaughton, J. F., Kron, R. E., & Emich, J. P. (1975). Neonatal abstinence syndrome: Assessment and management. *Addictive Diseases, 2*(1–2), 141–158.

Fraser, K., MacKenzie, D., & Versnel, J. (2019). What is the current state of occupational therapy practice with children and adolescents with complex trauma? *Occupational Therapy in Mental Health, 35,* 317–338. https://doi.org/10.1080/0164212X.2019.1652132

Gillespie, L. (2015). The role of co-regulation in building self-regulation skills. *Young Children, 70*(3), 94–96.

Greenspan, S., & Wieder, S. (2006). *Engaging autism: Using the Floortime approach to help children relate, communicate, and think.* Da Capo Press.

Grim, K., Harrison, T. E., & Wilder, R. T. (2013). Management of neonatal abstinence syndrome from opioids. *Clinics in Perinatology, 40,* 509–524. https://doi.org/10.1016/j.clp.2013.05.004

Grossman, M., & Berkwitt, A. (2019). Neonatal abstinence syndrome. *Seminars in Perinatology, 43,* 173–186. https://doi.org/10.1053/j.semperi.2019.01.007

Grossman, M. R., Berkwitt, A. K., Osborn, R. R., Xu, Y., Esserman, D. A., Shapiro, E. D., & Bizzarro, M. J. (2017). An initiative to improve the quality of care of infants with neonatal abstinence syndrome. *Pediatrics, 139,* e20163360. https://doi.org/10.1542/peds.2016-3360

Gunn, J. K. L., Rosales, C. B., Center, K. E., Nunez, A., Gibson, S. J., Christ, C., & Ehiri, J. E. (2016). Prenatal exposure to cannabis and maternal and child health outcomes: A systematic review and meta-analysis. *BMJ Open, 6,* e009986. https://doi.org/10.1136/bmjopen-2015-009986

Gupta, J., Lynch, A., Pitonyak, J., Rybski, D., & Taff, S. (in press). Enhancing occupational potential and health: Addressing early adversity and social exclusion using a life course health development approach. In N. Pollard, S. Kantartzis, & H. Van Bruggen (Eds.), *Manifesto for occupational therapy: Occupation-based social inclusion.* Whiting & Birch.

Halfon, N., & Forrest, C. B. (2018). The emerging theoretical framework of life course health development. In N. Halfon, C. B. Forrest, R. M. Lerner, & E. Faustman (Eds.), *The handbook of life course health development* (pp. 19–43). Springer.

Halfon, N., & Hochstein, M. (2002). Life course health development: An integrated framework for developing health, policy, and research. *Milbank Quarterly, 80,* 433–479. https://doi.org/10.1111/1468-0009.00019

Halfon, N., Larson, K., Lu, M., Tullis, E., & Russ, S. (2014). Life-course health development: Past, present and future. *Maternal and Child Health, 18,* 344–365. https://doi.org/10.1007/s10995-013-1346-2

Hash, J. B., Oxford, M. L., Fleming, C. B., Ward, T. M., Spieker, S. J., & Lohr, M. J. (2019). Impact of a home visiting program on sleep problems among young children experiencing adversity. *Child Abuse & Neglect, 89,* 143–154. https://doi.org/10.1016/j.chiabu.2018.12.016

ICD10Data.com. (2018). *Neonatal withdrawal symptoms from maternal use of drugs of addiction.* https://www.icd10data.com/ICD10CM/Codes/P00-P96/P90-P96/P96-/P96.1

Institute of Medicine & National Research Council. (2014). *New directions in child abuse and neglect research.* National Academies Press.

Jensen, C. L. (2014). Improving outcomes for infants with NAS. *Clinical Advisor, 17*(6), 85–92.

Kaltenbach, K., & Jones, H. E. (2016). Neonatal abstinence syndrome: Presentation and treatment considerations. *Journal of Addiction Medicine, 10,* 217–223. https://doi.org/10.1097/ADM.0000000000000207

Kelly, J. F., Zuckerman, T., Sandoval, D., & Buehlman, K. (2008). *Promoting first relationships* (2nd ed.). NCAST-AVENUW Publications.

Kraversky, D. G. (2019) Occcupational performance coaching as an ultimate facilitator. *OT Practice, 24*(11), CE-1–CE-8.

Maguire, D. (2014). Care of the infant with neonatal abstinence syndrome: Strength of the evidence. *Journal of Perinatal & Neonatal Nursing, 28,* 204–211. https://doi.org/10.1097/JPN.0000000000000042

May, P. A., Baete, A., Russo, J., Elliott, A. J., Blankenship, J., Kalberg, W. O., . . . Hoyme, H. E. (2014). Prevalence and characteristics of fetal alcohol spectrum disorders. *Pediatrics, 134,* 855–866. https://doi.org/10.1542/peds.2013-3319

May, P. A., Chambers, C. D., Kalberg, W. O., Zellner, J., Feldman, H., Buckley, D., . . . Hoyme, H. E. (2018). Prevalence of fetal alcohol spectrum disorders in 4 US communities. *JAMA, 319,* 474–482. https://doi.org/10.1001/jama.2017.21896

Murgatroyd, C., & Spengler, D. (2011). Epigenetics of early child development. *Frontiers in Psychiatry, 2,* 16. https://doi.org/10.3389/fpsyt.2011.00016

National Academies of Sciences, Engineering, and Medicine. (2017). *The health effects of cannabis and cannabinoids: The current state of evidence and recommendations for research.* National Academies Press.

National Cancer Institute. (2019). *Smoking & your baby.* https://women.smokefree.gov/pregnancy-motherhood/quitting-while-pregnant/smoking-your-baby

Neu, M., & Robinson, J. (2010). Maternal holding of preterm infants during the early weeks after birth and dyad interaction at six months. *Journal of Obstetric, Gynecologic & Neonatal Nursing, 39,* 401–414. https://doi.org/10.1111/j.1552-6909.2010.01152.x

Oh, D. L., Jerman, P., Marques, S. S., Koita, K., Boparai, S. K. P., Harris, N. B., & Bucci, M. (2018). Systematic review of pediatric health outcomes associated with childhood adversity. *BMC Pediatrics, 18,* 83. https://doi.org/10.1186/s12887-018-1037-7

Oostlander, S. A., Falla, J. A., Dow, K., & Fucile, S. (2019). Occupational therapy management strategies for infants with neonatal abstinence syndrome: Scoping review. *Occupational Therapy in Health Care, 33*(2), 197–226. https://doi.org/10.1080/07380577.2019.1594485

Oxford, M. L., Spieker, S. J., Lohr, M. J., & Fleming, C. B. (2016). Promoting First Relationships®: Randomized trial of a 10-week home visiting program with families referred to child protective services. *Child Maltreatment, 21,* 267–277. https://doi.org/10.1177/1077559516668274

Pasalich, D. S., Fleming, C. B., Oxford, M. L., Zheng, Y., & Spieker, S. J. (2016). Can parenting intervention prevent cascading effects from placement instability to insecure attachment to externalizing problems in maltreated toddlers? *Child Maltreatment, 21,* 175–185. https://doi.org/10.1177/1077559516656398

Pitonyak, J. S. (2014). Occupational therapy and breastfeeding promotion: Our role in societal health. *American Journal of Occupational Therapy, 68,* e90–e96. https://doi.org/10.5014/ajot.2014.009746

Purvis, K. B., Cross, D. R., Dansereau, D. F., & Parris, S. R. (2013). Trust-Based Relational Intervention (TBRI): A systemic approach to complex developmental trauma. *Child & Youth Services, 34,* 360–386. https://doi.org/10.1080/0145935X.2013.859906

Razuri, E. B., Howard, A. R. H., Purvis, K. B., & Cross, D. R. (2017). Mental state language development: The longitudinal roles of attachment and maternal language. *Infant Mental Health Journal, 38*(3), 329–342. https://doi.org/10.1002/imhj.21638

Ryan, K., Lane, S. J., & Powers, D. (2017). A multidisciplinary model for treating complex trauma in early childhood. *International Journal of Play Therapy, 26*(2), 111–123. https://doi.org/10.1037/pla0000044

Sanders, M. R., & Hall, S. L. (2018). Trauma-informed care in the newborn intensive care unit: promoting safety, security and connectedness. *Journal of Perinatology, 38*(1), 3–10. https://doi.org/10.1038/jp.2017.124

Siegel, D. J., & Bryson, T. P. (2012). *The whole-brain child: 12 revolutionary strategies to nurture your child's developing mind.* Scribe.

Smith Roley, S., Mailloux, Z., Miller-Kuhaneck, H., & Glenn, T. (2007). Understanding Ayres Sensory Integration®. *OT Practice, 12*(7), CE1–CE8.

Spieker, S. J., Oxford, M. L., & Fleming, C. B. (2014). Permanency outcomes for toddlers in child welfare two years after a randomized trial of a parenting intervention. *Children and Youth Services Review, 44,* 201–206. https://doi.org/10.1016/j.childyouth.2014.06.017

Spieker, S. J., Oxford, M. L., Fleming, C. B., & Lohr, M. J. (2018). Parental childhood adversity, depressive symptoms, and parenting quality: Effects on toddler self-regulation in child welfare services involved families. *Infant Mental Health Journal, 39,* 5–16. https://doi.org/10.1002/imhj.21685

Streissguth, A. P., Bookstein, F. L., Barr, H. M., Sampson, P. D., O'Malley, K., & Young, J. K. (2004). Risk factors for adverse life outcomes in fetal alcohol syndrome and fetal alcohol effects. *Developmental and Behavioral Pediatrics, 5,* 228–238. https://doi.org/10.1097/00004703-200408000-00002

Trauma Informed Oregon. (2018). *Trauma Informed Care Screening Tool.* https://traumainformedoregon.org/roadmap-trauma-informed-care/screening-tool/

van der Kolk, B. A., & Ducey, C. P. (1989). The psychological processing of traumatic experience: Rorschach patterns in PTSD. *Journal of Traumatic Stress, 2,* 259–274. https://doi.org/10.1002/jts.2490020303

Vergara, E. R., & Bigsby, R. (2004). *Developmental & therapeutic interventions in the NICU.* Brookes.

Weinhold, B., & Weinhold, J. (2013). *What is developmental trauma?* https://weinholds.org/what-is-developmental-trauma-2/

Wolpow, R., Johnson, M. M., Hertel, R., & Kincaid, S. O. (2009). *The heart of learning: Compassion, resiliency, and academic success.* http://www.k12.wa.us/CompassionateSchools/HeartofLearning.aspx

World Health Organization. (2014). *Guidelines for the identification and management of substance use and substance use disorders in pregnancy.* Author.

Yehuda, R., & Lehrner, A. (2018). Intergenerational transmission of trauma effects: Putative role of epigenetic mechanisms. *World Psychiatry, 17,* 243–257. https://doi.org/10.1002/wps.20568

Appendixes

Appendix A. Guidelines for Occupational Therapy Services in Early Intervention and Schools

The primary purpose of this document is to provide guidelines for the provision of occupational therapy services in early intervention (EI) and school settings. This document is intended for an internal audience (e.g., occupational therapists, occupational therapy assistants, students in occupational therapy programs) as well as external audiences (e.g., school staff and administrators, regulatory and policymaking bodies, accreditation agencies) who seek clarification of occupational therapy's role related to these settings. Occupational therapy practitioners[1] often are supervised by people unfamiliar with occupational therapy practices; the principles (e.g., level of expected performance) included in these guidelines and other American Occupational Therapy Association (AOTA) documents can be used to enhance their knowledge about the profession.

Approximately 25% of occupational therapists and 18% of occupational therapy assistants work in EI and school settings (AOTA, 2015a). Occupational therapy practitioners work with children and youth, parents, caregivers, educators, team members, and district and agency staff to facilitate children's and youth's ability to participate in their *occupations,* which are daily life activities that are purposeful and meaningful to the person (AOTA, 2014b). Occupations are based on meaningful social or cultural expectations or peer performance. Examples include social interactions with peers on the playground, literacy activities (e.g., writing, reading, communicating, listening), eating school lunch, opening locker combination to access books and coat, ability to drive car to school. Occupational therapy practitioners apply their knowledge of biological, physical, social, and behavioral sciences to evaluate and intervene with people across the life span when physical, adaptive, cognitive, behavioral, social, and mental health concerns compromise occupational engagement.

Occupational therapy practitioners provide services to young children and families in EI and to students, families, and educational staff in preschool and school settings to support engagement and participation in daily living activities (e.g., activities of daily living, instrumental activities of daily living, education, work, play, leisure, rest and sleep, and social participation; AOTA, 2014b). These guidelines provide information about occupational therapy practice in schools, including the influences (e.g., legislative, professional, environmental, contextual) and roles that occupational therapy practitioners may assume. Each section outlines guidelines related to these factors for occupational therapy practitioners. The variability in policy and practices across states and school districts results indifferences in how occupational therapy service delivery is implemented in each state.

Influences on Early Intervention and School Practice

Legislation and Regulatory Influences

Occupational therapy practitioners working in EI and schools must adhere to federal, state, and local education policies unless they conflict with occupational therapy state regulations (e.g., licensure). If inconsistencies occur, practitioners must work with employment agencies or district administrators to align policies to eliminate conflict. To ensure adherence to legislation and regulatory requirements in providing occupational therapy services, practitioners in EI and schools have a responsibility to

- Make recommendations for services in accordance with federal, state, and local policies and procedures related to EI and school practice, in both general and special education (see Table A.1 for examples of relevant legislation);
- Apply information from state occupational therapy practice acts and rules (licensure) to service delivery in EI and schools; and
- Understand state regulations for Medicaid cost recovery and other payment sources and adhere to professional codes of ethics and billing requirements.

Navigating the nuances of the vast regulatory landscape and keeping up with changes to each law can be a daunting challenge, especially for practitioners new to EI or school practice settings. Practitioners must make educating themselves and keeping up with regulatory changes a priority. AOTA provides leadership and resources that can assist practitioners with staying current on legislation that affects practice.

---

[1]*Occupational therapy practitioners* refers to both occupational therapists and occupational therapy assistants. The *occupational therapist* is responsible for all aspects of occupational therapy service delivery and is accountable for the safety and effectiveness of the occupational therapy service delivery process. *Occupational therapy assistants* deliver occupational therapy services under the supervision of and in partnership with an occupational therapist (AOTA, 2014a).

Table A.1.   Legislative Influences on Occupational Therapy Practice in EI and Schools

LAW	INFLUENCE ON OCCUPATIONAL THERAPY SERVICES
Individuals With Disabilities Education Improvement Act of 2004 (IDEA), Parts B and C	Part B mandates access to occupational therapy as a related service for eligible students with disabilities ages 3–21 years if services are needed for a student to benefit from special education. Part B is administered through state education agencies. Part C is voluntary at the state level and lists occupational therapy as a primary service for infants and toddlers ages 0–3 years who are experiencing developmental delays or have identified disabilities. Part C services may be administered through state education agencies, state health and human services agencies, or a combination.
Every Student Succeeds Act of 2015 (ESSA), a reauthorization of the Elementary and Secondary Education Act of 1965	ESSA ensures equal opportunity for all students in Grades K–12 and builds on previous legislation focusing on educational achievement. Bill includes occupational therapy as "specialized instructional support personnel" (SISP). SISPs should be included in state, local, and schoolwide planning activities as well as certain school-wide interventions and supports. ESSA is administered through state and local education agencies.
Section 504 of the Rehabilitation Act Amendments of 2004; Americans With Disabilities Act Amendments Act of 2008 (ADAA)	These civil rights statutes prohibit discrimination on the basis of disability for places that are open to the general public (ADAA) or programs receiving federal funds (504). Disability is defined more broadly than in IDEA. Children who are not eligible for special instruction under IDEA may be eligible under Section 504 or the ADAA for services including environmental adaptations and other reasonable accommodations.
Medicaid (Title XIX of the Social Security Act of 1965)	Medicaid is a federal–state matching program that provides medical and health services for low-income children and adults. Occupational therapy is an optional service under state Medicaid plans but is mandatory for children and youth under the federal Early Periodic Screening, Diagnosis, and Treatment (EPSDT) program. Although state Medicaid programs do not cover the costs of providing all services under IDEA in schools (e.g., services on behalf of the child), costs associated with providing medically necessary occupational therapy services provided directly to the child in EI and school settings can be reimbursed by Medicaid for students who are enrolled in the Medicaid program.
Family Educational Rights and Privacy Act of 1974 (FERPA) and Health Insurance Portability and Accountability Act of 1996 (HIPAA)	FERPA is a federal law that protects the privacy of education records, including health records, for children with disabilities in programs under IDEA Parts B and C. The law applies to all EI programs and schools that receive funds under an applicable program of the U.S. Department of Education. Service providers, school districts, and educational agencies billing Medicaid are also subject to HIPAA rules under protected health information provisions.
Improving Head Start for School Readiness Act of 2009	Head Start and Early Head Start are federal programs that provide comprehensive child development services to economically disadvantaged children ages 0–5 years, including children with disabilities, and their families. Early Head Start serves children up to age 3; Head Start serves children ages 3 and 4. Occupational therapy may be provided in these settings under the Head Start requirements or under IDEA.
Assistive Technology Act of 2004 (Tech Act)	The Tech Act promotes access to assistive technology to enable people with disabilities to more fully participate in education, employment, and daily activities.
Healthy, Hunger-Free Kids Act of 2010	The National School Breakfast and Lunch Programs are required to provide food substitutions and modifications of school meals for students whose disabilities restrict their diets, as determined by their health care provider.
State education codes and rules	In compliance with IDEA Part B, state education codes and rules must include policies and procedures for administration of instruction and for special education. Local education agencies further define these policies for their specific school communities.

(Continued)

Table A.1. Legislative Influences on Occupational Therapy Practice in EI and Schools *(Cont.)*

LAW	INFLUENCE ON OCCUPATIONAL THERAPY SERVICES
State Part C EI	If state chooses to use federal funds for EI services (Part C), it must provide statewide, comprehensive, coordinated, multidisciplinary, interagency EI systems with a designated lead agency. The lead agency determines policies and procedures for implementation and monitoring within the state.
State practice acts and rules (licensure)	Practice acts and rules provide stipulations for occupational therapy service delivery, including evaluation, intervention, documentation, and supervision of occupational therapy assistants. Ethical and behavioral expectations for professional conduct are often included.

Note. EI = early intervention.

Individuals With Disabilities Education Improvement Act (IDEA; Pub. L. 108–446) Part C programs, which serve infants and toddlers and their families, may seek reimbursement for occupational therapy services from Medicaid or Medicaid managed care programs available in their state and from the family's private insurance. States vary in their agreements with third-party payers for reimbursement of EI services. Some states require the family to pay a portion of the cost of Part C services, typically determined according to a sliding scale based on family income, whereas others (known as "birth mandate states") cover all costs except those that can be billed to Medicaid. In all cases, compliance with documentation requirements is critical for facilitating optimum reimbursement for Part C programs.

States provide public schools the opportunity to receive Medicaid reimbursement for the costs of providing occupational therapy services to eligible school-age children under Part B of IDEA. Reimbursable services typically include occupational therapy evaluations and services provided directly to the child. As in IDEA Part C programs, documenting services so that Medicaid requirements are met is essential to ensure that public schools realize available Medicaid revenue under state laws.

Professional Influences

In addition to adhering to state regulatory requirements (licensure), occupational therapy practitioners are guided by several professional documents (e.g., AOTA, 2013, 2014a, 2014b, 2015b, 2015c). The *Occupational Therapy Practice Framework: Domain and Process* (3rd ed.; AOTA, 2014b) articulates occupational therapy's distinct role and contributions to participation through engagement in occupation. Occupational therapy practitioners use the *Framework* to guide them in their practice, including service delivery (e.g., approaches to intervention may include creating skills, restoring movement, maintaining safe access, modification of the environment, prevention of back injury through backpack awareness). Providing client-centered delivery of services using evidence-based practices (EBP) is inherent to occupational therapy practice. In addition to providing individual services to the child or youth, the occupational therapy practitioner may focus on family structure and resources; specific groups or populations (e.g., co-teaching in general education classroom), the school system or district (e.g., serving on curriculum or playground committees), and the community (e.g., school health and wellness initiatives). Early intervention programs through Part B of the IDEA and the school programs through Part C of the IDEA provide a structure to these effective practice guidelines.

Guidelines for ensuring consistency with professional practice are as follows:

- The occupational therapist and occupational therapy assistant must demonstrate professional role performance and conduct aligned with AOTA official documents, state occupational therapy regulations, and best available evidence.
- The occupational therapist conducts evaluations aligned with current evidence and best practices across the home, preschool, school, and community environments (e.g., evaluate child in natural environment using observation and input from parents and others; identify priorities, concerns, and resources from the family [Part C] or from the day care, education, or transition team [Part B].
- During the evaluation, the occupational therapist must identify the child's performance in his or her occupations, the affordances and barriers to successful engagement, and expectations for the child's development and participation and synthesize information to develop a working hypothesis.
- In collaboration with the team, the occupational therapist identifies the young child's current performance and identifies priorities and concerns of the parent or caregiver to develop family or child outcomes (Part C) or identify the priorities and concerns of parents and school staff to develop goals for the school-age child (Part B).
- The occupational therapist must determine service recommendations on the basis of individual need, as indicated by the occupational therapy evaluation and data shared during the team process.
- The occupational therapist, with input from the occupational therapy assistant, develops an occupational therapy intervention plan (e.g., occupation-based goals, intervention approach, methods of service delivery) that provides a framework for the implementation of the individualized education program (IEP) and individualized family service plan (IFSP).

- The occupational therapist and occupational therapy assistant demonstrate service delivery aligned with current evidence and best practices across the home, preschool, school, and community environments (e.g., provide intervention in the natural environment to facilitate child development and skill building [Part C] and in the least restrictive environment (LRE) to enhance the child's benefit from education [Part B]; provide assistance to teachers to enhance the participation of children in school activities and routines, including provision of strategies for improving performance in these activities; use assistive technologies (AT), universal design for learning (UDL) principles, and environmental modifications).
- The occupational therapist and occupational therapy assistant apply knowledge of risk factors affecting growth, development, learning, and engagement in meaningful occupations during interventions to support health and participation.
- The occupational therapist and occupational therapy assistant monitor and document progress toward annual goals in accordance with organizational and professional (e.g., state licensure regulations, AOTA) requirements and measure outcomes.
- The occupational therapist determines the need for ongoing or discontinuation of services or for referral to other professional.

Environmental and Contextual Influences

Services under the Every Student Succeeds Act of 2015 (ESSA; Pub. L. 114–195) are provided to educational staff and children in general education, whereas IDEA requires services to be provided in the natural environment for infants and toddlers (Part C) or in the LRE for children and youth (Part B). When providing services, occupational therapy practitioners must understand the climate, culture, beliefs, and values of the family or school (Frolek Clark, 2013). Occupational therapy service delivery is influenced by the environment (e.g., social and physical) and context (e.g., cultural, personal, temporal, virtual), including where children and youth live (e.g., homes), learn (e.g., community, day care, classroom, music room), play (e.g., playgrounds, gymnasium), socialize (e.g., hallways, cafeteria), take care of needs (e.g., bathroom), and work (e.g., locations in the community). Exploring the dynamic connections among the student, occupations or activities, and the environment are critical during service delivery. Guidelines for addressing environment and context include the following elements:

- The occupational therapy practitioner must be knowledgeable about the systems that influence practice (e.g., state lead agency, education agencies, community organizations, medical providers) and establish access to community resources.
- The occupational therapy practitioner must understand the procedures and practices of the EI system, including those of the lead agency; the model of service delivery in the home; the definition of developmental delay; and the source of reimbursement (e.g., birth mandate state, third-party payer, payer of last resort; Part C).
- The occupational therapy practitioner must understand and apply principles of family-centered practice (e.g., empowering parents; building relationships; encouraging involvement in decision making; building on informal community support systems; being respectful of the family's culture, beliefs, and attitudes; Part C).
- The occupational therapy practitioner must understand the procedures and practices of the local education agency (e.g., multitier systems of support, UDL, bullying prevention), curriculum standards (e.g., developmental sequences, program of studies, standards of learning, adapted curricula, and high-stakes testing), and special education process (Part B).
- The occupational therapy practitioner must form effective partnerships with team members (e.g., parents, teachers) and the medical community to effectively identify children who may be at risk for a substantial developmental delay (Part C) or a child with a disability (Part B).
- The occupational therapy practitioner must provide interventions based on EBP for early intervention, school, and community settings (e.g., coaching families, social emotional development, safe transportation, driving).
- The occupational therapy practitioner must understand expectations at the district, classroom, and agency level (e.g., classroom routines, curriculum, literacy practices, AT, building rules; Part B).
- The occupational therapy practitioner must understand opportunities for students' postsecondary transition goals of function in education and employment, independent living, and social inclusion in communities.

Roles of Occupational Therapy Practitioners

Occupational therapy practitioners assume many roles during service delivery in EI and school settings. As described in the Professional Influence section, occupational therapy practitioners provide services to groups (e.g., students at risk for academic or behavior problems) and populations (e.g., general education classes in school; school district staff) as well as individuals.

With the passage of the ESSA, the role of specialized instructional support personnel (SISP), including occupational therapy practitioners, includes schoolwide interventions and supports. Additionally, IDEA's inclusion of early intervening services (EIS) allows SISPs to support general education children (kindergarten through grade 12) who are at risk in academic and behavioral areas and offer professional development and training to teaching staff. Contributions by occupational therapy practitioners to response to intervention (RTI) frameworks and multitiered systems of support (MTSS) demonstrate occupational therapy practitioners' role in working at the system level (e.g., school district, building, classroom levels). Table A.2 provides examples of the roles for occupational therapy practitioners.

As service providers in EI and school settings under IDEA, occupational therapy practitioners fulfill role responsibilities including service provision to children and youth, families, teams, organizations, and communities. Table A.3 lists the core

Table A.2.   Examples of Occupational Therapy Practitioner Roles Under ESSA (General Education)

ROLE AND DESCRIPTION	GENERAL
Consultation	▪ Stakeholders to be consulted regarding the development of State Accountability Plans, which are replacing the annual yearly progress (AYP). ▪ Assist with information about assessment of schools and development of alternative academic achievement standards for students with the most severe cognitive disabilities.
Schoolwide systems of support	▪ Provide services to support at-risk students. ▪ Improve student performance through schoolwide programs (e.g., positive behavioral interventions and supports, RTI, MTSS, antibullying strategies). ▪ Implement schoolwide positive behavioral interventions and supports, including coordination with similar activities carried out under IDEA, in order to improve academic outcomes and school conditions for student learning.
Professional development and training	▪ Provide professional development, preparation, and training programs with teachers and other staff.

Note. ESSA = Every Student Succeeds Act of 2015; IDEA = Individuals With Disabilities Education Improvement Act; MTSS = multi-tiered systems of support; RTI = response to intervention.

Table A.3.   Examples of Occupational Therapy Practitioner Roles in Part C and Part B of IDEA

ROLE AND DESCRIPTION	FOR BOTH PART C AND PART B UNLESS SPECIFIED
Evaluator (primarily the occupational therapist role; under the supervision of the occupational therapist, an occupational therapy assistant may assist in data collection).	▪ Under IDEA Child Find, identify children who are suspected of having a disability. ▪ Serve as an evaluator for the team to determine each child's eligibility under IDEA Part C or Part B (special education). ▪ Serve as an evaluator under IDEA to determine each child's strengths and needs, including need for occupational therapy (Part C, as an EI service; Part B, as a related service). ▪ Document referral source, reason for services, dates of services for data gathering and planning, and results of evaluation (report). ▪ Serve as an evaluator for children's assistive technology needs ▪ Conduct reevaluations to determine child's strengths and ongoing needs. **Part C: Early Intervention** ▪ Identify the family's concerns, priorities, and resources during the evaluation of the child. ▪ Gather relevant data to address the functional needs of the child related to adaptive development, adaptive behavior, and play and sensory, motor, and postural development. ▪ Synthesize information and collaborate with family to identify possible outcomes and need for services. **Part B: Preschool and School** ▪ Provide educational and behavioral evaluations, services, and supports to enhance general education instruction for students at risk (K–12). ▪ Solicit input from child, family, school personnel, and others. ▪ Gather relevant functional, developmental, and academic information (e.g., conduct interviews, review existing evaluation information; use assessment tools and strategies; observe child across relevant contexts) to obtain reliable information about what the child knows and can perform academically, developmentally, and functionally. ▪ Synthesize information and collaborate with family and educational staff to identify goals and need for services.

(Continued)

Table A.3. Examples of Occupational Therapy Practitioner Roles in Part C and Part B of IDEA *(Cont.)*

ROLE AND DESCRIPTION	FOR BOTH PART C AND PART B UNLESS SPECIFIED
Service coordinator for children and family (Part C) (only occupational therapist role)	▪ Demonstrate leadership by serving as service coordinator. ▪ Collaborate with families to enable them to receive the services and rights under Part C. ▪ Accurately interpret and communicate evaluation findings collaboratively with family members. ▪ Coordinate all evaluations, the development and review of the IFSP, all services on the IFSP, any funding sources, and development of a transition plan within the established timelines and procedures. ▪ Engage in collaborative decision making and problem solving with IFSP team.
Case manager for students (Part B) (only occupational therapist role)	▪ Demonstrate leadership by serving as case manager. ▪ Synthesize evaluation findings and, in collaboration with the IEP team, identify and prioritize meaningful educational goals. ▪ Engage in collaborative decision making and problem solving with IEP team. ▪ Collaborate to develop and implement comprehensive transition plans.
Service provider	▪ Design and implement interventions that are congruent with expectations in the setting and culture. ▪ Embed therapy interventions into the context of child's environments and routines. ▪ Gather data to determine the effectiveness of the intervention and guide changes to the intervention. ▪ Document performance changes and service provision (e.g., daily logs, progress notes, intervention plans, reports) in commonly understood and meaningful terms. ▪ Use modifications, adaptations, and assistive technology, as needed, to enhance developmental, functional, or academic skills. ▪ Document services ethically and accurately for third-party payers. ▪ Provide mental health promotion, prevention, and intervention services to children and youth. ▪ Demonstrate knowledge of evidence-based research in this area. ▪ Use knowledge of current research when planning intervention approaches and strategies. **Part C: Early Intervention** ▪ Actively participate with the team in the development of the IFSP in accordance with the priorities and preferences of the family and child (the occupational therapy assistant provides input under the supervision of the occupational therapist). ▪ Occupational therapist designs the intervention to meet the stated IFSP outcomes; the occupational therapist or the occupational therapy assistant implements intervention and strategies. ▪ Assist in the transition of child to community or Part B programs. **Part B: Preschool and School** ▪ Actively participate with the team in the development of the IEP to document the child's strengths and needs, prioritize goals, and determine services (occupational therapy assistant provides input under the supervision of the occupational therapist). ▪ Occupational therapist designs the intervention to meet the child's IEP goals; the occupational therapist or the occupational therapy assistant implements intervention and strategies. ▪ Support student's achievement of postsecondary transition goals of function, education and employment, independent living, and social inclusion in communities.
Collaborative team member	▪ Form partnerships and work collaboratively with others to contribute to the understanding of the nature and extent of the child's strengths and needs. ▪ Demonstrate effective communication and interpersonal skills (e.g., active listening, collaboration, coaching). ▪ Actively participate in team decisions (e.g., eligibility, transition, behavior needs) using clinical reasoning (the occupational therapy assistant provides input under the supervision of the occupational therapist). ▪ Promote inclusion of the child within the home, school and community settings.

(Continued)

Table A.3. Examples of Occupational Therapy Practitioner Roles in Part C and Part B of IDEA *(Cont.)*

ROLE AND DESCRIPTION	FOR BOTH PART C AND PART B UNLESS SPECIFIED
Educator and trainer	▪ Build the capacity of relevant stakeholders and teams through instruction, technical assistance, and training. ▪ Educate family, children, school staff, and administration (e.g., resources, inservice, presentations, serving on committee). ▪ Conduct trainings addressing strategies to best support children in natural environments and to empower families. ▪ Educate EI teams on family-centered principles that empower families and respect families' culture, beliefs, and attitudes. ▪ Educate school personnel on schoolwide programs (e.g., UDL, mental health, self-regulation).
Resource (Consultant)	▪ Provide technical assistance to teams, family, and community as necessary. ▪ Assist the EI team in identifying resources for families (e.g., transportation options, child development). ▪ Promote the child's access to school environments, instruction, and social communities. ▪ Promote national, state, and local priorities for the participation and education of all children and school improvement. ▪ Serve on committees and teams to address school and community challenges (e.g., evidence-based curriculum, accessible community participation, social community engagement, mental health and fitness). ▪ Assist administrators and policy makers with the development of systemwide educational supports and programs.
Advocate	▪ Advocate for schoolwide initiatives that promote learning, health, wellness, and engagement (e.g., multitiered systems of support, also known as RTI; playground safety; mental health; ergonomics; fitness). ▪ Promote understanding of diversity. ▪ Advocate for access to occupational therapy services, when appropriate, for children and families in EI; teachers and children in general education; and children in special education programs and educational staff. ▪ Provide guidance on the developments in educational, social, and health care policy and research that affect EI and school therapy services.
Leader	▪ Supervise occupational therapy assistants (only an occupational therapist role). ▪ Supervise professional students and school personnel who implement occupational therapy recommendations. ▪ Participate in the mentorship process to build knowledge and skills in the practice area. ▪ Address trends in occupational therapy service provision by gathering, synthesizing, and evaluating data (only an occupational therapist role). ▪ Educate others on the role of occupational therapy in this setting. ▪ Assume personal responsibility for professional development. ▪ Promote development of job descriptions, recruitment, orientation, and professional development for occupational therapy practitioners. ▪ Manage workload and needs related to the job description.
Researcher	▪ Conduct program evaluation to determine effectiveness. ▪ Design or assist in research studies in this setting.

Note. EI = early intervention; IEP = individualized education program; IFSP = individualized family service plan; RTI = response to intervention; UDL = universal design for learning.

responsibilities of all practitioners working in these practice settings; however, because of the difference in procedures and practices, the roles and responsibilities vary by state and school district. Because of the level of analysis and decision making required, only an occupational therapist may fill the evaluator, service coordinator, and case coordinator roles. Although agencies may create service coordinator or case coordinator positions and hire occupational therapy assistants in those capacities, such employees are not typically working as occupational therapy practitioners. The other roles may be filled by an occupational therapist or occupational therapy assistant in accordance with agency and state policy.

Summary

In EI and school settings, occupational therapy practitioners use their expertise to enhance participation in activities and occupations for children and youth. Occupational therapy practitioners also provide resources for and build the capacity of families, caregivers, and education staff. The guidelines presented in this document serve to empower occupational therapy practitioners working in EI and school settings with the resources to achieve positive outcomes and demonstrate the distinct value of their practice in these settings.

References

American Occupational Therapy Association. (2013). Guidelines for documentation of occupational therapy. *American Journal of Occupational Therapy, 67*(Suppl.), S32–S38. https://doi.org/10.5014/ajot.2013.67S32

American Occupational Therapy Association. (2014a). Guidelines for supervision, roles, and responsibilities during the delivery of occupational therapy services. *American Journal of Occupational Therapy, 68*(Suppl. 3), S16–S22. PubMed https://doi.org/10.5014/ajot.2014.686S03

American Occupational Therapy Association. (2014b). Occupational therapy practice framework: Domain and process (3rd ed.). *American Journal of Occupational Therapy, 68*(Suppl. 1), S1–S48. https://doi.org/10.5014/ajot.2014.682006

American Occupational Therapy Association. (2015a). *2015 salary and workforce survey: Executive summary.* Retrieved from http://www.aota.org/Education-Careers/Advance-Career/Salary-Workforce-Survey.aspx

American Occupational Therapy Association. (2015b). Occupational therapy code of ethics (2015). *American Journal of Occupational Therapy, 69*(Suppl. 3), 6913410030. https://doi.org/10.5014/ajot.2015.696S03

American Occupational Therapy Association. (2015c). Standards of practice for occupational therapy. *American Journal of Occupational Therapy, 69*(Suppl. 3), 6913410057. https://doi.org/10.5014/ajot.2015.696S06

Americans With Disabilities Act Amendments Act of 2008, Pub. L. 110–325, 122 Stat. 3553.

Assistive Technology Act of 2004, Pub. L. 108–364, 118 Stat. 1707.

Elementary and Secondary Education Act of 1965, Pub. L. 89–10, 20 U.S.C. § 6301 et seq.

Every Student Succeeds Act of 2015, Pub. L. 114–195, 114 Stat. 1177.

Family Educational Rights and Privacy Act of 1974, 20 U.S.C. § 1232g, 34 CFR Part 99.

Frolek Clark, G. (2013). Best practices in school occupational therapy interventions to support participation. In G. Frolek Clark & B. E. Chandler (Eds.), *Best practices for occupational therapists in schools* (pp. 95–106). Bethesda, MD: AOTA Press.

Health Insurance Portability and Accountability Act of 1996, Pub. L. 104–191, 110 Stat. 1936.

Healthy, Hunger-Free Kids Act of 2010, Pub. L. 111–296, 124 Stat. 3183.

Improving Head Start for School Readiness Act of 2007, Pub. L. 110–134, 121 Stat. 1363, 42 USC 9801 et seq.

Individuals With Disabilities Education Improvement Act of 2004, Pub. L. 108–446, 20 U.S.C. § 1400 et seq.

Rehabilitation Act Amendments of 2004, 29 U.S.C. §794.

Social Security Act of 1965, Pub. L. 89–97, 79 Stat. 286, Title XIX.

Resources

For information on rights and privacy rules related to IDEA, refer to the following sites:
- DaSy Center. http://dasycenter.org/category/privacyguidance/
- United States Department of Education. http://www2.ed.gov/policy/gen/guid/fpco/ferpa/index.html
- United States Department of Health and Human Services. http://www.hhs.gov/hipaa/for-professionals/faq/513/does-hipaa-apply-to-an-elementary-school/index.html

For EBP, refer to the following documents, which were designed to share current research:
- Bazyk, S. (2013). *Mental health promotion, prevention, and intervention with children and youth.* Bethesda, MD: AOTA Press.
- Bazyk, S., & Arbesman, M. (2013). *Occupational therapy practice guidelines for mental health promotion, prevention, and intervention for children and youth.* Bethesda, MD: AOTA Press.
- Chandler, B. (2010). *Early childhood: Occupational therapy services for children birth to three.* Bethesda, MD: AOTA Press.
- Frolek Clark, G., & Chandler, B. (2013). *Best practices for occupational therapy services in schools.* Bethesda, MD: AOTA Press.
- Frolek Clark, G., & Kingsley, K. (2013). *Occupational therapy practice guidelines for early childhood: Birth through 5 years.* Bethesda, MD: AOTA Press.
- Frolek Clark, G., & Handley-More, D. (2017). *Best practices for documenting occupational therapy services in schools.* Bethesda, MD: AOTA Press.
- Jackson, L. (2007). *Occupational therapy services for children and youth under IDEA.* Bethesda, MD: AOTA Press.
- Hanft, B., & Shepherd, J. (2016). *Collaborating for student success.* Bethesda, MD: AOTA Press.
- Tomchek, S., & Koenig, K. P. (2016). *Occupational therapy practice guidelines for individuals with autism spectrum disorder.* Bethesda, MD: AOTA Press.

Authors

Gloria Frolek Clark, PhD, OTR/L, BCP, SCSS, FAOTA
Patricia Laverdure, OTD, OTR/L, BCP
Jean Polichino, OTR, MS, FAOTA

for

The Commission on Practice
Kathleen Kannenberg, MA, OTR/L, CCM, *Chairperson*

Adopted by the Representative Assembly Coordinating Council (RACC) for the Representative Assembly, 2017

Revised by the Commission on Practice 2017

Note. This revision replaces the 2011 document *Occupational Therapy Services in Early Childhood and School-Based Settings,* previously published and copyrighted in 2011 by the American Occupational Therapy Association in the *American Journal of Occupational Therapy, 65,* S46–S54. https://doi.org/10.5014/ajot.2011.65S46

Citation. American Occupational Therapy Association. (in press). Guidelines for occupational therapy services in early intervention and schools. *American Journal of Occupational Therapy, 71*(Suppl. 2), 7112410010. https://doi.org/10.5014/ajot.2017.716S01

Appendix B. Evidence-Based Practice and Occupational Therapy

Elizabeth G. Hunter, PhD, OTR/L, and Deborah Lieberman, MHSA, OTR/L, FAOTA

Evidence-based practice (EBP) is an important component of occupational therapy practice. It is crucial for occupational therapy practitioners[1] to stay current on research in the field, particularly in their practice area. EBP is tripartite in that it relies on (1) research evidence, (2) practitioner expertise, and (3) client needs and preferences (see Figure B.1). All 3 components need to be included to provide best practice with a goal of efficiency and effectiveness. In schools, instruction is individualized and changes regularly; therefore, a strong foundation in which interventions are effective and supported by research is critical.

TYPES OF EVIDENCE

The best research evidence is usually found in peer-reviewed published research studies that have been conducted using sound methodology (Sackett et al., 2000). To provide EBP, practitioners need to recognize different types of evidence and understand that they provide stronger or weaker evidence. A magazine article (e.g., *OT Practice, SIS Quarterly Practice Connections*) reporting on a certain intervention may not be the strongest evidence if it is based solely on opinion. Findings from a group or program trying to sell a product may not be unbiased because they may really be marketing a product rather than conducting rigorous research. Findings from research funded by a group that will benefit from the outcomes may not be considered strong evidence and may have a high risk of bias.

The goal is to find unbiased, well-designed, well-conducted research that is published in a peer-reviewed journal. Peer-reviewed journals, such as the *American Journal of Occupational Therapy (AJOT)*, rely on outside, unbiased peer reviewers who do not stand to benefit from the findings of the research. This is the gold standard in

research in terms of reporting research findings. Only studies that pass peer review will be published in a peer-reviewed journal. These are the data needed when conducting EBP.

There are many types and methods of research. All well-designed, peer-reviewed research publications are useful and informative for one reason or another. For decision making, it is important to feel certain that the study's outcomes are the result of the intervention being tested. The gold standard in assessing an intervention's efficacy is the randomized controlled trial (RCT), a study design in which participants are randomized into 2 or more groups. The groups receive different interventions, often standard of care (e.g., methods accepted by qualified practitioners) in 1 group and the intervention being tested in the other.

When the study has the appropriate number of participants, randomizing minimizes the risk of selection bias. In a perfect world, the participants and the people doing the assessments would not know which participants were in which group (double-blind study). Such a study is not always feasible in all settings or with all interventions; regardless, the RCT is considered the highest level of scientific evidence. Having said that, practitioners should not be hesitant to consider lower level evidence to answer their specific focus questions, recognizing that lower level evidence is at risk for various biases and limitations, including the research design, and the findings need to be looked at with that in mind.

Qualitative research is often not included in analyses of scientific evidence and systematic reviews of interventions, but the findings from qualitative studies can provide important foundational understanding of factors such as client experiences and understanding events, among other issues. This knowledge can improve how a practitioner provides services and care. When looking for evidence to support an intervention, however, the experimental design is the first line of information.

ANALYZING EVIDENCE

Once a practitioner locates evidence, they have some work to do in terms of analyzing, appraising, and understanding the findings of a study. Three major factors—level of evidence, risk of bias, findings and outcomes—need to be assessed and are described next.

---

[1]*Occupational therapy practitioner* refers to both the occupational therapist and the occupational therapy assistant. The American Occupational Therapy Association (AOTA; 2014a, p. S18) states, "The occupational therapist is responsible for all aspects of occupational therapy service delivery and is accountable for the safety and effectiveness of the occupational therapy service delivery process" and "must be directly involved in the delivery of services during the initial evaluation and regularly throughout the course of intervention. . . . The occupational therapy assistant delivers safe and effective occupational therapy services under the supervision of and in partnership with the occupational therapist."

FIGURE B.1. *Evidence-based practice* is the use of the best available research evidence combined with the practitioner's expertise and the client's needs and preferences.

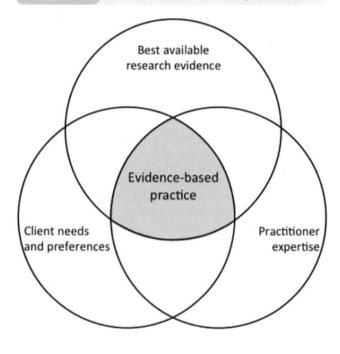

Level of Evidence

As we have discussed, different research designs have different levels of evidence. Level I studies, such as RCTs, are the gold standard. As one considers the lower levels of evidence in the hierarchy, the innate risk of bias increases. Therefore, identifying the study design is the first step in analyzing the evidence and beginning the process of assessing the trustworthiness of the findings and the application to practice. The levels of evidence are as follows:

- **Level 1A:** Systematic review of homogeneous RCTs (similar population, intervention, etc.), with or without meta-analysis
- **Level 1B:** Well-designed individual RCT (not a pilot or feasibility study with a small sample size)
- **Level 2A:** Systematic review of cohort studies
- **Level 2B:** Individual prospective cohort study, low-quality RCT (e.g., less than 80% follow-up or low number of participants, pilot and feasibility studies), ecological studies, and two-group nonrandomized studies
- **Level 3A:** Systematic review of case-control studies
- **Level 3B:** Individual retrospective case-control study, one-group nonrandomized pretest–posttest study, cohort studies
- **Level 4:** Case series (and low-quality cohort and case-control study)
- **Level 5:** Expert opinion without explicit critical appraisal (Howick et al., 2016).

Risk of Bias

Bias in research is a systematic error or deviation from true results, often resulting from limitations in study methods and procedures. Bias can cause something to be overestimated or underestimated. Either way, bias makes it very hard to trust research results. Better designed and conducted studies are more likely to end up with results that are unlikely to be false or misleading.

Bias can come from selection (characteristics of the participant group), performance (whether study participants and personnel know who is receiving which intervention), and detection (whether the assessor knows which participant is assigned to which group), as well as from how results are reported, whether all participants remained in the study from beginning to end, and others. It is important for practitioners to read research articles critically, assess the study design, and look for a very detailed description of the study procedures and outcomes.

Findings and Outcomes

The final step in evaluating the evidence is to assess the study for the significance of the findings. It is necessary to understand whether the findings were in fact statistically significant (e.g., were the outcomes significantly different between groups?). If the findings were not significantly different, occupational therapy practitioners should question implementing the intervention. Descriptions such as "the intervention resulted in a small improvement" and other vague statements such as "the intervention improved" are not very useful in evaluating the difference between the efficacy of interventions and determining whether to use the intervention in practice.

SYNTHESIZING EVIDENCE

The final step for a practitioner in terms of deciding which research to incorporate into practice is synthesizing all of the evidence. *Synthesizing the evidence* means looking at the level of evidence (study design), the risk of bias (study limitations), and the study results and merging the information. A practitioner may review 1 study or, even better, more than 1 study testing the intervention of interest. For example, 2 or more RCTs increases the strength and level of certainty of a given intervention. Having multiple studies to evaluate assists the occupational therapy practitioner in deciding whether the level of evidence is strong enough to implement the intervention in practice. Table B.1 provides information to evaluate the strength of the evidence for the intervention being reviewed.

Thankfully, practitioners can consider numerous systematic reviews related to different interventions, practice conditions, or populations. The benefit of finding a good-quality systematic review is that the authors have already reviewed, appraised, and synthesized specific studies and provided guidance on critical practice questions. Practitioners can evaluate single studies or multiple studies, or they can use existing systematic reviews to evaluate to what degree they can trust the findings and how sure they are that an intervention has the best available evidence to incorporate it into school practice.

TABLE B.1.   Strength of Evidence (Level of Certainty)

STRENGTH OF EVIDENCE	DESCRIPTION
Strong	▪ Two or more Level I studies ▪ The available evidence usually includes consistent results from well-designed, well-conducted studies. The findings are strong, and they are unlikely to be called into question by the results of future studies. ▪ All studies have moderate to low risk of bias.
Moderate	▪ At least 1 Level I high-quality study or multiple moderate-quality studies (Level II, Level III, etc.) ▪ The available evidence is sufficient to determine the effects on health outcomes, but confidence in the estimate is constrained by such factors as • The number, size, or quality of individual studies. • Inconsistency of findings across individual studies. As more information (other research findings) becomes available, the magnitude or direction of the observed effect could change, and this change may be large enough to alter the conclusion related to the usefulness of the intervention. ▪ The studies have moderate to low risk of bias.
Low	▪ Small number of low-level studies, flaws in the studies, etc. ▪ The available evidence is insufficient to assess effects on health and other outcomes of relevance to occupational therapy. Evidence is insufficient because of • The limited number or size of studies • Important flaws in study design or methods • Inconsistency of findings across individual studies • Lack of information on important health outcomes. Many of these studies will have high risk of bias. More information may allow estimation of effects on health and other outcomes of relevance to occupational therapy.

Source: U.S. Preventive Services Task Force (2016).

EDUCATION PRACTICE: EVIDENCE-BASED INTERVENTIONS

Occupational therapy practitioners working in schools must also be knowledgeable about how *evidence-based interventions* are defined in education law. The Every Student Succeeds Act (2015–2016; Pub. L. 114–95) defines the term *evidence based,* when used with respect to a state, local educational agency, or school activity, as an activity, strategy, or intervention that

(i) demonstrates a statistically significant effect on improving student outcomes or other relevant outcomes based on—
  (I) strong evidence from at least 1 well-designed and well-implemented experimental study;
  (II) moderate evidence from at least 1 well-designed and well-implemented quasi-experimental study; or
  (III) promising evidence from at least 1 well-designed and well-implemented correlational study with statistical controls for selection bias; or
(ii) (I) demonstrates a rationale based on high quality research findings or positive evaluation that such activity, strategy, or intervention is likely to improve student outcomes or other relevant outcomes; and
  (II) includes ongoing efforts to examine the effects of such activity, strategy, or intervention. (§ 8101[21])

Table B.2 outlines the U.S. Department of Education's (2016) recommendations for identifying evidence across 4 different levels.

The Individuals With Disabilities Education Improvement Act of 2004 (Pub. L. 108–446) uses the term *scientifically based research* but does not define it. According to the No Child Left Behind Act of 2001 (Pub. L. 107–110), which was later replaced by ESSA, *scientifically based research*

(A) Means research that involves the application of rigorous, systematic, and objective procedures to obtain reliable and valid knowledge relevant to education activities and programs; and
(B) (i) Employs systematic, empirical methods that draw on observation or experiment;
  (ii) Involves rigorous data analyses that are adequate to test the stated hypotheses and justify the general conclusions drawn;
  (iii) Relies on measurements or observational methods that provide reliable and valid data across evaluators and observers, across multiple measurements and observations, and across studies by the same or different investigators;
  (iv) Is evaluated using experimental or quasi-experimental designs in which individuals, entities, programs, or activities are assigned to different conditions and with appropriate controls to evaluate the effects of the condition of interest, with a preference for random-assignment

TABLE B.2.   U.S. Department of Education (2016) Criteria Recommended in ESSA for the Identification of Evidence

LEVEL	DESCRIPTION
Strong	• One well-designed and well-implemented experimental study (e.g., RCT) • Statistically significant and positive effect of the intervention on student outcome or other relevant outcome • Not overridden by statistically significant and negative evidence for the same intervention in other studies • Has a large, multisite sample • Has a sample that overlaps with the populations (i.e., the types of students served) and settings (e.g., rural, urban) proposed to receive the intervention
Moderate	• Must have at least 1 well-designed and well-implemented quasi-experimental study of the intervention • Shows a statistically significant and positive effect of the intervention on student outcome or other relevant outcome • Not overridden by statistically significant and negative evidence for the same intervention in other studies • Has a large, multisite sample • Has a sample that overlaps with the populations (i.e., the types of students served) and settings (e.g., rural, urban) proposed to receive the intervention
Promising evidence	• At least 1 well-designed and well-implemented correlational study with statistical controls for selection bias on the intervention • Shows a statistically significant and positive (i.e., favorable) effect of the intervention on student outcome or other relevant outcome • Not overridden by statistically significant and negative (i.e., unfavorable) evidence for that intervention from findings
Demonstrates a rationale	• Includes a well-specified logic model that is informed by research or an evaluation that suggests how the intervention is likely to improve relevant outcomes • An effort to study the effects of the intervention, ideally producing promising evidence or higher, that will happen as part of the intervention or is underway elsewhere (e.g., another state education agency, local education agency, or research organization) to inform stakeholders about the success of that intervention

Note. ESSA = Every Student Succeeds Act (2015–2016); RCT = randomized controlled trial.

experiments, or other designs to the extent that those designs contain within-condition or across-condition controls;

(v) Ensures that experimental studies are presented in sufficient detail and clarity to allow for replication or, at a minimum, offer the opportunity to build systematically on their findings; and

(vi) Has been accepted by a peer-reviewed journal or approved by a panel of independent experts through a comparably rigorous, objective, and scientific review. (No Child Left Behind Act of 2001, 20 U.S.C. § 1411[e][2][C][xi])

Taking this a step further, the Council for Exceptional Children (CEC; 2014) has developed explicit standards for categorizing the evidence base of practices in special education. These indicators and criteria apply to studies that examine practice or programs on student outcomes. Eight quality indicators are used to assess the evidence for various intervention and program practices:

1. **Context and setting**. The study provides sufficient information regarding the critical features of the context or setting.
2. **Participants**. The study provides sufficient information to identify the population of participants to which results may be generalized and to determine or confirm whether the participants demonstrated the disability or difficulty of focus.
3. **Intervention agent**. The study provides sufficient information regarding the critical features of the intervention agent.
4. **Description of practice**. The study provides sufficient information regarding the critical features of the practice (intervention), such that the practice is clearly understood and can be reasonably replicated.
5. **Implementation fidelity**. The practice is implemented with fidelity.
6. **Internal validity.** The independent variable is under the control of experimenter. The study describes the services provided in control and comparison conditions and phases. The research design provides sufficient evidence that the independent variable causes change in the dependent variable or variables. Participants stayed with the study, so attrition is not a significant threat to internal validity.
7. **Outcome measures/dependent variables**. Outcome measures are applied appropriately to gauge the effect of the practice on study outcomes. Outcome measures demonstrate adequate psychometrics.
8. **Data analysis**. Data analysis is conducted appropriately. The study reports information on effect size. (CEC, 2014, pp. 3–6)

Several research groups have published EBP documents that identify specific practices that have met the evidence threshold (e.g., National Professional Development Center on Autism Spectrum Disorder, What Works

Clearinghouse). Many of the models place stronger emphasis on research that has replicated studies of manualized or operationalized interventions (Cook & Cothren Cook, 2011). Occupational therapy practitioners working in schools must be familiar with evidence within the occupational therapy profession and the education–special education profession.

USE IN PRACTICE

Differences in the interpretation of EBP among occupational therapy practitioners and other members of the service delivery team may cause misunderstandings, because each team member is expected to adhere to the EBP standards set forth by their practice setting (Scheibel & Watling, 2016). Occupational therapy practitioners cannot continue to use interventions that they learned 15 years ago or that were presented at a conference but have no evidence base. They must implement current EBP into their daily practice, gather data, and use the data to make decisions about the effectiveness of the decisions (AOTA, 2017; Hanft & Shephard, 2016). Some practitioners are unsure how to incorporate research into their practice. Torres et al. (2012) authored a guide for special educators on implementing EBP. Torres et al. authored a guide for special educators on implementing EBP. Their step-by-step process is as follows:

1. Determine the student's, environment's, and instructor's characteristics
2. Search sources of EBPs
3. Select applicable EBP
4. Identify essential components of the EBP
5. Implement the EBP in the cycle of effective instruction
6. Monitor implementation fidelity
7. Progress monitor student outcomes
8. Adapt the EBP if necessary
9. Make data-driven decisions and return to previous steps as needed.

OCCUPATIONAL THERAPY RESOURCES

The American Occupational Therapy Association (AOTA) has developed a repository of EBP resources for practitioners, educators, researchers, and students. AOTA collaborates with teams of researchers to conduct systematic reviews and develop Practice Guidelines. The systematic reviews are published in *AJOT* and as Practice Guidelines. Also, critically appraised summaries are published on AOTA's website. The Evidence-Based Practice section of AOTA's website (https://bit.ly/2AQcbbQ) provides many different resources and tools to remain current and provide services that are informed and guided by evidence.

A journal club may be an efficient and effective way for a group of occupational therapy practitioners to explore and evaluate evidence. The Journal Club Tool Kit provides step-by-step instructions and templates that can help practitioners set up and run different types of journal clubs. For additional sources for EBP, see Table 41.3 in Chapter 41, "Best Practices in School Occupational Therapy Interventions to Support Participation."

SUMMARY

All occupational therapy practitioners have a professional responsibility to use evidence-based interventions. Gaining experience in EBP is a process and skill that is developed with time, perseverance, and experience. Many resources are available that can enhance practitioners' familiarity and experience with accessing and evaluating research to support the provision of EBP in the school setting.

REFERENCES

American Occupational Therapy Association. (2017). Guidelines for occupational therapy services in early childhood and schools. *American Journal of Occupational Therapy, 71*(Suppl. 2), 7112410010. https://doi.org/10.5014/ajot.2017.716S01

Cook, B., & Cothren Cook, S. (2011). Unraveling evidence-based practices in special education. *Journal of Special Education, 47,* 71–82. https://doi.org/10.1177/002246691142087.

Council for Exceptional Children. (2014). *Standards for evidence-based practice in special education.* Retrieved from https://www.cec.sped.org/~/media/Files/Standards/Evidence%20based%20Practices%20and%20Practice/EBP%20FINAL.pdf

Every Student Succeeds Act, Pub. L. No. 114–95, 129 Stat. 1802 (2015–2016).

Hanft, B., & Shepherd, J. (2016). *Collaborating for student success* (2nd ed.). Bethesda, MD: AOTA Press.

Howick, J., Chalmers, I., Glasziou, P., Greenhalgh, T., Heneghan, C., Liberati, A., . . . Hodgkinson, M.; OCEBM Levels of Evidence Working Group. (2016). *The Oxford levels of evidence 2.* Oxford, England: Oxford Centre for Evidence-Based Medicine. Retrieved from https://www.cebm.net/index.aspx?o=5653

Individuals With Disabilities Education Improvement Act of 2004, Pub. L. 108–446, 20 U.S.C. §§ 1400–1482.

No Child Left Behind Act of 2001, Pub. L. 107–110, 20 U.S.C. §§ 6301–8962. (2002)

Sackett, D. L., Straus, S. E., Richardson, W. S., Rosenberg, W., & Haynes, R. B. (2000). *Evidence-based medicine: How to practice and teach EBM* (2nd ed.). New York: Churchill Livingstone.

Scheibel, G., & Watling, R. (2016). Collaborating with behavior analysts on the autism service delivery team. *OT Practice, 21*(7), 15–19.

Torres, C., Farley, C. A., & Cook, B. G. (2012). A special educator's guide to successfully implementing evidence-based practices. *TEACHING Exceptional Children, 47,* 85–93. https://doi.org/10.1177/0040059914553209

U.S. Department of Education. (2016). *Non-regulatory guidance: Using evidence to strengthen education investments.* Retrieved from https://ed.gov/policy/elsec/leg/essa/guidanceuseseinvestment.pdf

U.S. Preventive Services Task Force. (2016). *Grade definitions.* Retrieved from https://www.uspreventiveservicestaskforce.org/Page/Name/grade-definitions

Appendix C. AOTA Occupational Profile Template

APPENDIX C. AOTA OCCUPATIONAL PROFILE TEMPLATE

"The occupational profile is a summary of a client's occupational history and experiences, patterns of daily living, interests, values, and needs" (AOTA, 2014, p. S13). The information is obtained from the client's perspective through both formal interview techniques and casual conversation and leads to an individualized, client-centered approach to intervention.

Each item below should be addressed to complete the occupational profile. Page numbers are provided to reference a description in the *Occupational Therapy Practice Framework: Domain and Process, 3rd Edition* (AOTA, 2014).

Client Report	**Reason the client is seeking service and concerns related to engagement in occupations**	Why is the client seeking service, and what are the client's current concerns relative to engaging in occupations and in daily life activities? (This may include the client's general health status.)
	Occupations in which the client is successful (p. S5)	In what occupations does the client feel successful, and what barriers are affecting his or her success?
	Personal interests and values (p. S7)	What are the client's values and interests?
	Occupational history (i.e., life experiences)	What is the client's occupational history (i.e., life experiences)?
	Performance patterns (routines, roles, habits, & rituals) (p. S8)	What are the client's patterns of engagement in occupations, and how have they changed over time? What are the client's daily life roles? (Patterns can support or hinder occupational performance.)

What aspects of the client's environments or contexts does he or she see as:

		Supports to Occupational Engagement	Barriers to Occupational Engagement
Environment	**Physical (p. S28) (e.g., buildings, furniture, pets)**		
	Social (p. S28) (e.g., spouse, friends, caregivers)		
Context	**Cultural (p. S28) (e.g., customs, beliefs)**		
	Personal (p. S28) (e.g., age, gender, SES, education)		
	Temporal (p. S28) (e.g., stage of life, time, year)		
	Virtual (p. S28) (e.g., chat, email, remote monitoring)		
Client Goals	**Client's priorities and desired targeted outcomes: (p. S34)**	Consider: occupational performance—improvement and enhancement, prevention, participation, role competence, health and wellness, quality of life, well-being, and/or occupational justice.	

ADDITIONAL RESOURCES

For a complete description of each component and examples of each, refer to the *Occupational Therapy Practice Framework: Domain and Process, 3rd Edition*.

American Occupational Therapy Association. (2014). Occupational therapy practice framework: Domain and process (3rd ed.). *American Journal of Occupational Therapy, 68*, S1–S48. https://doi.org/10.5014/ajot.2014.682006

The occupational profile is a requirement of the *CPT®* occupational therapy evaluation codes as of January 1, 2017. For more information visit www.aota.org/coding.

Appendix D. Occupational Therapy Intervention Plan

Client Information

Name:	DOB:	School/Grade:
Parents:	Phone:	
Diagnosis or Conditions:		
Precautions:		

Intervention Goals: *Areas of Occupations to be Addressed:*

☐ ADLs ☐ IADLs ☐ Education ☐ Leisure ☐ Play ☐ Rest/Sleep ☐ Social Participation ☐ Work

Intervention Approaches: Check/Describe

☐ Create/promote ☐ Establish/Restore ☐ Maintain ☐ Modify ☐ Prevent

Types of Interventions: Check/Describe

☐ Occupations & Activities ☐ Preparatory Methods & Tasks ☐ Education & Training ☐ Advocacy ☐ Group

Service Delivery Mechanisms

Frequency:	Duration:
Location of services:	Provider(s):

Discharge Plan (criteria for discharge)

Outcome Measures (check)

☐ Occupational Performance ☐ Prevention ☐ Health & Wellness ☐ Quality of life
☐ Participation ☐ Role Competence ☐ Well-Being ☐ Occupational Justice

Developed by:

Date Developed: **Date Revised:**

Source. From *Best Practices for Documenting Occupational Therapy Services in Schools* by G. Frolek Clark & D. Handley-More, p. 76. Bethesda, MD: AOTA Press. Copyright © 2017 by the American Occupational Therapy Association. Reprinted with permission.

Appendix E. AOTA Resources for Practitioners and Families

AOTA RESOURCE	AOTA WEBSITE LINK	PURPOSE
Building Play Skills for Healthy Children & Families	https://bit.ly/37vuvpV	Provides tips for families to promote play skills
Childhood Occupations Toolkit	https://bit.ly/2zoTOlG	Provides tips for families on everyday routines and illustrates occupational therapy's role to professional partners
Enjoying Halloween With Sensory Challenges (also available in Spanish)	https://bit.ly/3fmoU8f	Provides tips for families on enjoying Halloween for children with sensory challenges
Establishing Bath Time Routines for Children (also available in Spanish)	https://bit.ly/2XTBANV	Provides tips for families on bath time routines
Establishing Bedtime Routines for Children (also available in Spanish)	https://bit.ly/37r1Imc	Provides tips for families on bedtime routines
Establishing Mealtime Routines for Children	https://bit.ly/30zKPEz	Provides tips for families on mealtime routines
Establishing Morning Routines for Children	https://bit.ly/2BTrR1o	Provides tips for families on morning routines
Establishing Toileting Routines for Children (also available in Spanish)	https://bit.ly/3dUGhwA	Provides tips for families on toileting routines
Establishing Tummy Time Routines to Enhance Your Baby's Development	https://bit.ly/2AnjBXk	Provides tips for families on promoting tummy time
Evidence-Based Practice & Research	https://bit.ly/3fvGpnO	Provides literature and other resources for occupational therapy practitioners to incorporate evidence-based practices
How to Pick a Toy: Checklist for Toy Shopping	https://bit.ly/2UH24QO	Provides tips for families on selecting toys (includes a checklist)
Living With an Autism Spectrum Disorder (ASD): The Preschool Child	https://bit.ly/2MY4zcV	Provides tips for supporting preschool-age children with ASD
Living With an Autism Spectrum Disorder (ASD): Supporting a Smooth Transition to Preschool	https://bit.ly/2MQb01F	Provides tips for supporting a smooth transition to preschool for children with ASD
Video: *Make Play an Important Part of Your Family's Day*	https://bit.ly/30wxME2	Video for parents on the importance of play

Note. Practitioners who are members of AOTA may access the above resources and many more at https://www.aota.org/Practice/Children-Youth.aspx. Evidence-based resources are available to members at https://www.aota.org/Practice/Children-Youth/Evidence-based.aspx

Appendix F. Examples of Assessments for Early Childhood (Birth–5 Years)

DOMAIN OF OCCUPATIONAL THERAPY	ASSESSMENT TOOLS AND AUTHOR
Occupations ▪ ADLs ▪ IADLs ▪ Health management ▪ Rest and sleep ▪ Education ▪ Work ▪ Play ▪ Leisure ▪ Social participation	*Everyday activities* ▪ Adaptive Behavior Assessment System (3rd ed.; Harrison & Oakland, 2015) ▪ Asset-Based Context Matrix (Wilson & Mott, 2006) ▪ Canadian Occupational Performance Measure (Law et al., 2019) ▪ Miller Function and Participation Scales (Miller, 2006) ▪ Pediatric Evaluation of Disability Inventory Computer Adaptive Test (Haley et al., 2012) ▪ Preschool Activity Card Sort (Berg & LaVesser, 2006) ▪ Routines-Based Interview (McWilliam, 2009) ▪ Scales of Independent Behavior—Revised (Bruininks et al., 1996) ▪ Short Child Occupational Profile (Bowyer et al., 2008) ▪ Vineland Adaptive Behavior Scales (Sparrow et al., 2005) ▪ WeeFIM II (Uniform Data System for Medical Rehabilitation, 2003) *ADLs and IADLs* ▪ Brief Assessment of Mealtime Behavior in Children (Hendy et al., 2013) ▪ Brief Autism Mealtime Behavior Inventory (Lukens & Linscheid, 2008) ▪ Eating Profile (Nadon et al., 2011) ▪ PEACH screening tool for early intervention (Campbell & Kelsey, 1994) ▪ Pre-Feeding Skills (Morris & Klein, 2000) ▪ Roll Evaluation of Activities of Life (Roll & Roll, 2013) ▪ Screening Tool of Feeding Problems for children (Seiverling et al., 2011) *Play and leisure* ▪ Revised Knox Preschool Play Scale (Knox, 2008) ▪ Test of Playfulness (Skard & Bundy, 2008) ▪ Transdisciplinary Play-Based Assessment (2nd ed.; Linder, 2008) *Social participation (also social–emotional for performance skills)* ▪ Evaluation of Social Interaction (Fisher & Griswold, 2010) ▪ Miller Function and Participation Scales (Miller, 2006) *Sleep and rest* ▪ Bedtime Routines Questionnaire (Henderson & Jordan, 2010) ▪ Behavioral Evaluation of Disorders of Sleep Scale (Schrek et al., 2003) ▪ Parental Interactive Bedtime Behaviour Scale (Morrell & Cortina-Borja, 2002) ▪ Pediatric Sleep Questionnaire Sleep-Related Breathing Disorder Scale (Chervin et al., 2000) ▪ Sleep and Settle Questionnaire (Matthey, 2001) ▪ Tayside Children's Sleep Questionnaire (McGreavey et al., 2005)
Client factors ▪ Body functions ▪ Body structures ▪ Values, beliefs, and spirituality	▪ Assisting Hand Assessment (Krumlinde-Sundholm et al., 2007) ▪ Behavior Rating Inventory of Executive Function (Gioia et al., 2015) ▪ Quality of Upper Extremity Skills Test (cerebral palsy and traumatic brain injury specific; DeMatteo et al., 1992)

(Continued)

Performance skills
- Motor skills
- Process skills
- Social interaction skills

Screening
- Ages & Stages Questionnaires (3rd ed.; Squires & Bricker, 2009)
- Ages & Stages Questionnaires: Social Emotional (2nd ed.; Squires et al., 2015)
- Developmental Indicators for the Assessment of Learning (Mardell & Goldenberg, 2019)

Screening and evaluation: Specific diagnoses
- Autism Diagnostic Observation Schedule (2nd ed.; Lord et al., 2012)
- Callier–Azusa Scale (for children with deaf-blindness; Callier Center for Communication Disorders, 1978)
- Developmental Assessment for Individuals With Severe Disabilities (Dykes & Murzek, 2018)
- Every Move Counts (Korsten et al., 1993)
- Functional Vision and Learning Media Assessment Kit (American Printing House for the Blind, 2003)
- Gross Motor Function Classification System (for children with cerebral palsy; Palisano et al., 2007)
- Gross Motor Function Measure (for children with cerebral palsy; Hanna et al., 2008)
- Manual Ability Classification System (cerebral palsy–specific; Eliasson et al., 2006)
- Modified Checklist for Autism in Toddlers—Revised (Robins et al., 2009)
- Oregon Project for Preschoolers With Visual Impairment Skills Inventory (Southern Oregon Education Service District, 2019)
- Screening Tool for Autism in Toddlers and Young Children (Stone & Ousley, 2008)

Evaluation: Multiple developmental domains
- Assessment, Evaluation and Programming System for Infants and Children (2nd ed.; Bricker, 2002)
- Battelle Developmental Inventory—3 (Newborg, 2020)
- Bayley Scales of Infant and Toddler Development (4th ed.; Bayley & Aylward, 2019)
- Brigance Inventory of Early Development—III (Brigance & French, 2013)
- Carolina Curriculum for Infants and Toddlers With Special Needs (3rd ed.; Johnson-Martin, Attermeier, & Hacker, 2004)
- Carolina Curriculum for Preschoolers With Special Needs (Johnson-Martin, Hacker, & Attermeier, 2004)
- Creative Curriculum® for Infants and Twos (Dodge et al., 2015)
- Creative Curriculum® for Preschool (Dodge et al., 2010)
- Developmental Assessment of Young Children (Voress & Maddox, 2013)
- Early Learning Accomplishment Profile (Glover et al., 2002)
- Griffith Mental Development Scales (Green et al., 2015)
- Hawaii Early Learning Profile (Vort Corporation, 2019)
- HighScope Infant–Toddler Curriculum (HighScope, 2002)
- HighScope Preschool Curriculum (Epstein & Hohmann, 2012)
- Miller Function and Participation Scales (Miller, 2006)
- Pediatric Evaluation of Disability Inventory Computer Adaptive Test (Haley et al., 2012)
- Transdisciplinary Play-Based Assessment (2nd ed.; Linder, 2008)

Evaluation: Motor
- Alberta Infant Motor Scales (Piper & Darrah, 1994)
- Beery–Buktenica Developmental Test of Visual–Motor Integration (Beery et al., 2010)
- Bruininks–Oseretsky Test of Motor Proficiency (Bruininks, 2005)
- Movement Assessment Battery for Children (Henderson et al., 2007)
- Oral Motor Assessment Scale (Ortega et al., 2009)
- Peabody Development Motor Scales (Folio & Fewell, 2000)
- Test of Gross Motor Development (3rd ed.; Ulrich, 2019)
- Test of Infant Motor Performance (Campbell et al., 2002)
- Test of Visual–Motor Skills (Martin, 2010)

(Continued)

Evaluation: Process
- Developmental Test of Visual Perception (Hammill et al., 2013)
- Motor-Free Visual Perception Test (Colarusso & Hammill, 2015)
- Sensory Processing Measure—Preschool Home Form (Ecker et al., 2010)
- Sensory Profile 2 (Dunn, 2014)
- Test of Visual Perceptual Skills (Martin, 2017)

Evaluation: Social interaction skills
- Child Behavioral Checklist Preschool (Achenbach & Rescoria, 2000)
- Preschool and Kindergarten Behavior Scales (2nd ed.; Merrell, 2003)
- Social–Emotional Assessment/Evaluation Measure (Squires et al., 2014)
- Social Responsiveness Scale (Constantino & Gruber, 2012)
- Social Skills Improvement System: Rating Scales (Gresham & Elliott, 2008)

Performance patterns
- Habits
- Rituals
- Roles
- Routines

- Asset-Based Context Matrix (Wilson & Mott, 2006)
- Canadian Occupational Performance Measure (Law et al., 2019)
- Routines-Based Interview (McWilliam, 2009)
- Short Child Occupational Profile (Bowyer et al., 2008)

Context
- Cultural
- Personal
- Physical
- Social
- Temporal
- Virtual

- Asset-Based Context Matrix (Wilson et al., 2006)
- Canadian Occupational Performance Measure (Law et al., 2019)
- Children's Assessment of Participation and Enjoyment (King et al., 2004)
- Early Childhood Environmental Rating Scale—Revised (Harms et al., 2015)
- Home Observation for Measurement of the Environment (Caldwell & Bradley, 2016)
- Short Child Occupational Profile (Bowyer et al., 2008)
- Test of Environmental Supportiveness (Bundy, 1999)

Note. ADLs = activities of daily living; IADLs = instrumental activitie of daily living.

RESOURCES

Berry, D., Bridges, L., & Zaslow, M. (2004). *Early Childhood Measure Profiles.* https://www.childtrends.org/wp-content/uploads/2013/09/2004-32EarlyChildhoodMeasuresProfiles1.pdf

Ringwalt, S. (2008). *Developmental screening and assessment instruments with emphasis on social and emotional development for young children ages birth through five.* https://ectacenter.org/~pdfs/pubs/screening.pdf

REFERENCES

Achenbach, T., & Rescoria, L. (2000). *Child Behavioral Checklist Preschool (Preschool CBLC).* ASEBA.

American Printing House for the Blind. (2003). *Functional Vision and Learning Media Assessment Kit.* Author.

Bayley, N., & Aylward, G. (2019). *Bayley Scales of Infant and Toddler Development* (4th ed.). NCS Pearson.

Beery, K. E., Buktenica, N. A., & Beery, N. A. (2010). *Beery–Buktenica Developmental Test of Visual–Motor Integration: Administration, scoring, and teaching manual.* (6th ed.). Pearson.

Berg, C., & LaVesser, P. (2006). Preschool Activity Card Sort. *OTJR: Occupational, Participation, and Health, 26,* 143–151. https://doi.org/10.1177/153944920602600404

Bowyer, P. L., Kramer, J., Ploszaj, A., Ross, M., Schwartz, O., Kielhofner, G., & Kramer, K. (2008). *The Short Child Occupational Profile (SCOPE), Version 2.2.* University of Illinois at Chicago.

Bricker, D. (2002). *Assessment, Evaluation and Programming System for Infants and Children: Birth to Three Years and Three to Six Years* (2nd ed.). Brookes.

Brigance, A., & French, B. (2013). *Brigance Inventory of Early Development.* Curriculum Associates.

Bruininks, R. H. (2005). *Bruininks–Oseretsky Test of Motor Proficiency.* AGS.

Bruininks, R. H., Woodcock, R. W., Weatherman, R. F., & Hill, B. K. (1996). *SIB–R: Scales of Independent Behavior—Revised.* Riverside.

Bundy, A. C. (1999). *Test of Environmental Supportiveness (TOES).* Colorado State University.

Caldwell, B. M., & Bradley, R. H. (2016). *Home Observation for Measurement of the Environment: Administration manual.* Family & Human Dynamics Research Institute, Arizona State University.

Callier Center for Communication Disorders. (1978). *Callier–Azusa Scale.* https://calliercenter.utdallas.edu/evaluation-treatment/callier-azusa-scale/

Campbell, M. K., & Kelsey, K. S. (1994). The PEACH Survey: A nutrition screening tool for use in early intervention programs. *Journal of the American Dietetic Association, 94,* 1156–1158. https://doi.org/10.1016/0002-8223(94)91139-8

Campbell, S. K., Wright, B. D., & Linacre, J. M. (2002). Development of a functional movement scale for infants. *Journal of Applied Measurement, 3,* 190–204.

Chervin, R., Hedger, K., Dillon, J. E., & Pituch, K. J. (2000). *Pediatric Sleep Questionnaire (PSQ): Validity and reliability of scales for sleep-disordered breathing, snoring, sleepiness, and behavioral problems.* Sleep Medicine, 1, 21–32.

Colarusso, R., & Hammill, D. D. (2015). *MVPT-4: Motor-Free Visual Perception Test.* Academic Therapy Publications.

Constantino, J. N., & Gruber, C. P. (2012). *Social Responsiveness Scale (SRS).* Western Psychological Services.

DeMatteo, C., Law, M., Russell, D., Pollock, N., Rosenbaum, P., & Walter, S. (1992). *QUEST: Quality of Upper Extremity Skills Test.* McMaster University, Neurodevelopmental Clinical Research Unit.

Dodge, D. T., Berke, K., Rudick, S., Baker, H., Colker, L. J., Dombro, A. L., . . . Sanders, S. (2015). *The Creative Curriculum® for Infants, Toddlers & Twos* (3rd ed.). Teaching Strategies.

Dodge, D., Colker, L., & Heoman, C. (2010). *The Creative Curriculum* for Preschool* (6th ed.). Teaching Strategies.

Dunn, W. (2014). *Sensory Profile 2.* San Antonio: Pearson.

Dykes, M. K., & Murzek, D. W. (2018). *Developmental Assessment for Individuals With Severe Disabilities (DASH 3).* Western Psychological Services.

Ecker, C., Parham, L., Kuhaneck, H., Henry, D., & Glennon, T. (2010). *Sensory Processing Measure—Preschool Home Form.* Western Psychological Services.

Eliasson, A. C., Krumlinde-Sundholm, L., Rosblad, B., Beckung, E., Arner, M., Ohrvall, A. M., & Rosenbaum, P. (2006). The Manual Ability Classification System (MACS) for children with cerebral palsy: Scale development and evidence of validity and reliability. *Developmental Medicine and Child Neurology, 46,* 549–554. https://doi.org/10.1017/S0012162206001162

Epstein, A., & Hohmann, M. (2012). *High Scope Preschool Curriculum.* High Scope Press.

Fisher, A. G., & Griswold, L. A. (2010). *Evaluation of Social Interaction.* Three Star Press.

Folio, M. R., & Fewell, R. R. (2000). *Peabody Developmental Motor Scales: Examiner's manual.* Pro-Ed.

Gioia, G. A., Esquith, P. K., Guy, S. C., & Kenworthy, L. (2015). *Behavior Rating Inventory of Executive Functioning* (2nd ed.). Psychological Assessment Resources.

Glover, M. E., Preminger, J. L., & Sanford, A. R. (2002). *Early Learning Accomplishment Profile (E-LAP).* Kaplan Early Learning Center, Chapel Hill Training Outreach Project.

Green, E., Stroud, L., Bloomfield, S., Cronje, J., Foxcroft, C., Hurter, K., . . . Venter, D. (2015). *Griffith Mental Developmental Scales* (3rd ed.). Hogrefe.

Gresham, F. M., & Elliott, S. N. (2008). *Social Skills Improvement System: Rating scales manual.* NCS Pearson.

Haley, S. M., Coster, W. J., Dumas, H. M., Fragala-Pinkam, M. A., & Moed, R. (2012). *Pediatric Evaluation of Disability Inventory Computer Adaptive Test.* http://www.pedicat.com

Hammill, D., Pearson, N., & Voress, J. (2013). *Developmental Test of Visual Perception* (3rd ed.). Pro-Ed.

Hanna, S. E., Bartlett, D. J., Rivard, L. M., & Russell, D. J. (2008). Reference curves for the Gross Motor Function Measure: Percentiles for clinical description and tracking over time among children with cerebral palsy. *Physical Therapy, 88,* 596–607. https://doi.org/10.2522/ptj.20070314

Harms, T., Clifford, R., & Cryer, D. (2015). *Early Childhood Environmental Rating Scale—Revised* (3rd ed.). Teachers College, Columbia University.

Harrison, P., & Oakland, T. (2015). *Adaptive Behavior Assessment System* (3rd ed.). Psychological Corporation.

Henderson, J. A., & Jordan, S. S. (2010). Development and preliminary evaluation of the Bedtime Routines Questionnaire. *Journal of Psychopathology and Behavioral Assessment, 32,* 271–280. https://doi.org/10.1007/s10862-009-9143-3

Henderson, S. E., Sugden, D. A., & Barnett, A. L. (2007). *Movement Assessment Battery for Children—2.* Harcourt Assessment.

Hendy, H. M., Seiverling, L., Lukens, C. T., & Williams, K. E. (2013). Brief Assessment of Mealtime Behavior in Children: Psychometrics and association with child characteristics and parent responses. *Children's Health Care, 42,* 1–14. https://doi.org/10.1080/02739615.2013.753799

High Scope. (2002). *High Scope Infant–Toddler Curriculum.* High Scope Press.

Johnson-Martin, N., Attermeier, S., & Hacker, B. (2004). *Carolina Curriculum for Infants and Toddlers With Special Needs.* Brookes.

Johnson-Martin, N., Hacker, B., & Attermeier, S. (2004). *Carolina Curriculum for Preschoolers With Special Needs.* Brookes.

King, G., Law, M., King, S., Hurley, P., Hanna, S., Kertoy, M., . . . Young, N. (2004). *Children's Assessment of Participation and Enjoyment and Preferences for Activities of Children.* Harcourt Assessment.

Knox, S. (2008). Development and current use of the Revised Knox Preschool Play Scale. In L. Parham & L. Fazio (Eds.), *Play in occupational therapy for children* (2nd ed., pp. 55–70). Elsevier.

Korsten, J. E., Dunn, D. K., Foss, T. V., & Francke, M. K. (1993). *Every Move Counts: Sensory-based communication techniques.* Pro-Ed.

Krumlinde-Sundholm, L., Holmefur, M., Kottorp, A., & Eliasson, A.C. (2007). The Assisting Hand Assessment: Current evidence of validity, reliability, and responsiveness to change. *Developmental Medicine and Child Neurology, 49,* 259–264. https://doi.org/10.1111/j.1469-8749.2007.00259.x

Law, M., Baptiste, S., Carswell, A., McColl, M., Polatajko, H., & Pollock, N. (2019). *Canadian Occupational Performance Measure.* CAOT Publications.

Linder, T. (2008). *Transdisciplinary Play-Based Assessment* (2nd ed.). Brookes.

Lord, C., Rutter, M., DiLavore, P. C., Risi, S., Gotham, K., & Bishop, S. (2012). *Autism Diagnostic Observation Schedule* (2nd ed.). Western Psychological Services.

Lukens, C. T., & Linscheid, T. R. (2008). Development and validation of an inventory to assess mealtime behavior in children with autism. *Journal of Autism and Developmental Disorders, 38,* 342–352. https://doi.org/10.1007/s10803-007-0401-5

Mardell, C., & Goldenberg, D. S. (2019). *Developmental Indicators for the Assessment of Learning* (4th ed.). Pearson.

Martin, N. A. (2010). *Test of Visual–Motor Skills* (3rd ed.). Academic Therapy Publications.

Martin, N. A. (2017). *Test of Visual–Perceptual Skills* (4th ed.). Western Psychological Services.

Matthey, S. (2001). Sleep and Settle Questionnaire for parents of infants: Psychometric properties. *Journal of Paediatrics and Child Health, 37,* 470–475. https://doi.org/10.1046/j.1440-1754.2001.00703.x

McGreavey, J. A., Donnan, P. T., Pagliari, H. C., & Sullivan, F. M. (2005). The Tayside Children's Sleep Questionnaire: A simple tool to evaluate sleep problems in young children. *Child: Care, Health and Development, 31,* 539–544. https://doi.org/10.1111/j.1365-2214.2005.00548.x.

McWilliam, R. (2009). *Routines-Based Interview and observations.* Siskin Children's Institute.

Merrell, K. W. (2003). *Preschool and Kindergarten Behavior Scales* (2nd ed.). Pro-Ed.

Miller, L. J. (2006). *Miller Function and Participation Scales manual.* Harcourt Assessment.

Morrell, J., & Cortina-Borja, M. (2002). The developmental changes in strategies parents employ to settle young children to sleep, and their relationship to infant sleeping problems, as assessed by a new questionnaire: The Parental Interactive Bedtime Behaviour Scale. *Journal of Analytical Psychology, 11,* 17–41. https://doi.org/10.1002/icd.251

Morris, S. E., & Klein, M. D. (2000). *Pre-feeding skills: A comprehensive resource for mealtime development* (2nd ed.). Academic Press.

Nadon, G., Feldman, D. E., Dunn, W., & Gisel, E. (2011). Association of sensory processing and eating problems in children with autism spectrum disorders. *Autism Research and Treatment, 2011,* 541926. https://doi.org/10.1155/2011/541926

Newborg, J. (2020). *Battelle Developmental Inventory—3.* Riverside Assessments.

Ortega, A., Ciamponi, A., Mendes, F., & Santos, M. (2009). Assessment scale of the oral motor performance of children and adolescents with neurological damages. *Journal of Oral Rehabilitation, 36,* 653–659. https://doi.org/10.1111/j.1365-2842.2009.01979.x

Palisano, R., Rosenbaum, P., Bartlett, D., & Livingston, M. (2007). *Gross Motor Function Classification System: Expanded and revised.* McMaster University.

Piper, M. C., & Darrah, J. (1994). *Motor assessment of the developing infant.* Saunders.

Robins, D. L., Fein, D., & Barton, M. (2009). *Modified Checklist for Autism in Toddlers—Revised.* https://www.m-chat.org/reference/mchatDOTorg.pdf

Roll, K., & Roll, W. (2013). *The REAL: The Roll Evaluation of Activities of Life.* Pearson.

Schrek, K., Mulick, J., & Rojahn, J. (2003). Development of the Behavioral Evaluation of Disorders of Sleep Scale. *Journal of Children and Family Studies, 12,* 349–359. https://doi.org/10.1023/A:1023995912428

Seiverling, L., Hendy, H. M., & Williams, K. (2011). The Screening Tool of Feeding Problems applied to children (STEP–CHILD): Psychometric characteristics and associations with child and parent variables. *Research in Developmental Disabilities, 32,* 1122–1129. https://doi.org/10.1016/j.ridd.2011.01.012

Skard, G., & Bundy, A. C. (2008). Test of Playfulness. In L. D. Parham & L. S. Fazio (Eds.), *Play in occupational therapy for children* (2nd ed., pp. 71–93). Mosby.

Southern Oregon Education Service District. (2019). *Oregon Project for Preschoolers With Visual Impairment Skills Inventory.* Author.

Sparrow, S., Cicchetti, D., & Balla, D. (2005). *Vineland Adaptive Behavior Scales* (2nd ed.). AGS.

Squires, J., & Bricker, D. (2009). *Ages & Stages Questionnaires®* (3rd ed). Brookes.

Squires, J., Bricker, D., & Twombly, E. (2015). *Ages & Stages Questionnaires®: Social Emotional* (2nd ed.). Brookes.

Squires, J., Bricker, D., Waddell, M., Funk, K., Clifford, J., & Hoselton, R. (2014). *Social–Emotional Assessment/Evaluation Measure (SEAM) Research Edition.* Baltimore: Brookes.

Stone, W. L., & Ousley, O. Y. (2008). *Screening Tool for Autism in Toddlers and Young Children (STAT): User's manual.* Vanderbilt University.

Ulrich, D. (2019). *Test of Gross Motor Development* (3rd ed). Pro-Ed.

Uniform Data System for Medical Rehabilitation. (2006). *The WeeFIM II™ System clinical guide: Version 6.0.* UDS-MR.

Voress, J., & Maddox, T. (2013). *Developmental Assessment of Young Children (DAYC-2).* Western Psychological Services.

Vort Corporation. (2019). *Hawaii Early Learning Profile (HELP).* Author.

Wilson, L., & Mott, D. (2006). Asset-Based Context Matrix: An assessment tool for developing contextually-based child outcomes. *CASEtools, 4*(6), 1–12.

Appendix G. Sample Early Intervention Team Report

Early Intervention Team Evaluation Report
Date of Report: December 18, 2019

Child's Name: Dani Perez   **Date of Birth:** April 15, 2017   **Age:** 20 months
Parents/Caregivers: Jose and Ariana Perez   **Address:** 23345 Woodpine St., Dadel, KS

A. REFERRAL AND BACKGROUND INFORMATION
The following information was obtained through parent interview and review of medical records.

Referral: Dr. Jon Williams, MD, referred Dani to early intervention on November 15, 2019, for services because of encephalitis, spasticity, and seizures.

Health: Dani is followed annually by Dr. Powers, a neurologist. She passed her newborn hearing screen, and Dr. Williams checks her vision at well-baby checks. Ariana states Dani was hospitalized with encephalitis when she was 15 months old. She has been hospitalized several times over the past 4 months (once for 6 days) because of viral respiratory infections and poor weight gain. A nasogastric (NG) tube was placed when Dani was hospitalized and was unable to eat. Dani is currently tube fed twice daily—at noon and during the night. When contacted, Dr. Williams states his goal is to remove Dani's NG tube in the next 4 months if she continues to gain weight. She is being weaned off her seizure medication because she has had no seizure activity for 6 months. Her electroencephalograph (EEG) did not show additional seizures, so medications are being decreased. When she was hospitalized in October, an occupational therapist provided the parents with developmental information and home exercises. Dani did not seem well enough for direct intervention at that time.

Other: The family lives an hour from the hospital, so Dani's hospitalizations have been stressful for them. Support from friends and family has allowed Ariana to be at the hospital, but she hates to be away from her son, 6-month-old Carlo, and her husband. The family speaks English to their children but Spanish with friends and family.

B. FAMILY ROUTINES, INTERESTS, CONCERNS, AND PRIORITIES
Routines and Activities:
- Dani lives at home with her parents, brother, and paternal grandmother (Rosa). She sleeps in a crib in a room she shares with her brother, Carlo.
- In the mornings, Ariana feeds Carlo and Dani, then leaves for work.
- During the week, when the parents are working, Rosa is home with Dani and Carlo.
- Dani is tube fed twice a day, at 10 a.m. and 10 p.m. The family prepares soft foods for Dani, and they are trying to get her to eat different textures.
- Rosa reads to the children while they lie on the floor or sit in small, supportive chairs.
- Rosa puts them down for naps around 2:00 p.m., and they both sleep until 4 p.m., when they are fed a small snack.
- The parents arrive home at 5:30 p.m., and Ariana helps Rosa make supper while Jose plays with the children.
- Ariana puts Carlo to bed at 7:30 p.m., and Dani goes to bed at 8 p.m. Either parent gives Dani her 10 p.m. feeding, then they go to bed around 10:30 p.m.

Interests and Preferences:
- Dani likes riding in the car, looking at books, playing games such as peekaboo, playing with toys that make sounds and light up, and being with her family.

Dani's Developmental Growth Across Domains

DOMAIN	DEVELOPMENTAL AGE	PERFORMANCE
Adaptive	6–9 months	Dani is unable to assist in dressing, bathing, or eating because of her physical challenges. Dani eats primarily pureed foods but will eat some mashed table foods (bananas, beans). She does not finger feed herself. Using a small cup, she can drink 1 ounce of PediaSure.
Cognitive (learning)	9 months	Dani likes to look at pictures in books and to bang and shake toys (after they are placed in her hand). She will turn to her name and smile.
Communication	5–6 months	Dani smiles, laughs, and squeals. Her parents feel she is trying to talk and heard *ma-ma* once before her last hospitalization. Dani uses wide arm gestures to communicate with her family.
Physical: fine motor	4 months	Dani likes to bat hanging toys, look at books, and bang toys, especially those that light up or make sounds. If objects are placed in her hand, she will shake them but must be closely monitored for eye safety. Her limited movements significantly impede participation in all daily life skills.
Large motor	7 months	Dani is able to roll across the room to access toys. When placed in a supported chair, she can maintain head control but maintains propped sitting for 3 minutes. Tightness in her arms prevents her from maintaining a hands and knees position or belly crawling. She loves when adults hold her in standing position.
Social–emotional	7 months	Dani enjoys playing with her family but is wary of strangers. She is not around other children much because of her health. Being around Carlos puts a smile on her face.

Family Concerns:
- Ariana's greatest concern for Dani is her health and eating. She wants Dani to gain weight and eat more types of foods.
- Mealtimes are challenging because Dani refuses food; changing her clothing or moving her is difficult because she is so "stiff."
- Ariana does not sleep well because she is afraid Dani will become ill again and have to go back to the hospital.

Family Priorities:
Dani's mom has prioritized the following concerns to be addressed immediately by the team:
- Would like Dani to eat more food so she gains weight and can stop the night feeding
- Would like Dani to be able to eat more table foods with rest of the family at mealtimes
- Would like Dani to be able to let people know what she wants
- Would like Dani to be able to play with other children when she is healthier.

C. CHILD'S STRENGTHS AND CHALLENGES (DEVELOPMENT INFORMATION)
Dani's health, hearing, and vision are being monitored by her pediatrician. Developmental assessment included observations, interview with Dani's mother, and use of the Early Learning Accomplishment Profile (Glover et al., 2002) as the primary source for estimated developmental age in months. Dani's physical and communication challenges affect her performance across all domains. Dani's performance is shown in the table above.

D. ANALYSIS AND SUMMARY
Dani is a sweet and determined young girl with a strong and involved family. Her health is being monitored by her pediatrician. The family's priorities include the areas of eating, communication, and playing with toys.

Analysis:
- Dani's strengths include social interactions with her family, and she enjoys looking at books.
- Her challenges include eating foods and motor and communication skills because of spasticity.

Summary of Needs:
Dani would benefit from early intervention, including skilled occupational therapy services to address feeding and motor concerns. The occupational therapist found muscle tightness; poor feeding; and difficulties with fine motor, large motor, and social interaction skills. Support from the speech therapist is also recommended to enhance communication, both receptive (understanding) and expressive (vocalizations). Specialized instruction and family services coordination from the early childhood teacher are needed to monitor overall development and provide the parents with education and coaching to support Dani's development at home.

Signature of Evaluators:
Mickey Jones, MEd, FSC/Special Instruction Provider
Rachi Powers, MS, OT/R
Thomas Sanchez, CCC-SLP

Appendix H. Sample Initial Preschool Team Evaluation Report

Preschool Evaluation Team Report

Child Name: Bobby Doe **Date of Birth:** March 24, 2016 **Date of Report:** March 10, 2020
Parents: John and Jane Doe **Child's Age:** 3.11 months **Preschool:** Apple Valley Head Start Early Childhood Center

Evaluators: Jani Theronz (teacher), Alex King (occupational therapist), Jacki French (speech therapist), Maggie Booton (school psychologist)

Purpose of Evaluation: Bobby was referred by his parent and teacher for an evaluation to determine his eligibility for special education and related services.

Record Review: Bobby lives at home with his parents and older sibling. On the school district's child questionnaire, Bobby's mother indicated Bobby was born full term at 40 weeks gestation and weighed 8 pounds, 8 ounces. He has attended preschool 4 mornings per week since this fall.

Interview: His parents indicated Bobby loves to be around people. He cares about others and wants people to be happy. Their main concern is with Bobby's overall development. They want him to be on track in all areas and will do whatever Bobby needs to ensure that is the case. In addition, Bobby's behavior (aggressiveness, impulsivity, noncompliance) and communication (speaking, listening, answering questions) are the main challenges to being able to successfully manage Bobby both at home and preschool. He lives at home with his parents and older sibling. Bobby's parents are hopeful he will be able to continue to attend preschool and receive support services if he is eligible.

Observation of Academic and Functional Performance: The Team Assessment of Preschoolers in Routines (TAPIS; Parks, 2012) was used as an observation tool during Bobby's preschool classroom observation over a period of 2 weeks (February

ROUTINE	LEVEL OF PARTICIPATION	STRENGTHS AND INTERESTS	ADAPTATIONS NEEDED	INTERVENTION TARGETS
Arrival and Dismissal	③2 1	Negotiates curbs or steps	Hand held to increase safety	Increase ability to remain with group for personal safety
Bathroom	3②1	Manipulates most clothing on his own	Close adult proximity and supervision	Increase ability to remain in own space and follow adults' directions for safety
Circle	3②1	Enjoys music and movement activities	"Cube" chair close to teacher, positive behavioral support system	▪ Attend to group directions ▪ Take turns
Small group	3②1		Seated near teacher with additional space from nearby peers	Increase conventional knowledge (e.g., colors, rote and 1:1 counting, sorting, patterning, opposites)

(Continued)

ROUTINE	LEVEL OF PARTICIPATION	STRENGTHS AND INTERESTS	ADAPTATIONS NEEDED	INTERVENTION TARGETS
Play	3②1		▪ Close proximity of adults ▪ Problem solving visuals and facilitation ▪ Priming for desired interactions	▪ Initiate, maintain, and complete interactive play with peers ▪ Increase ability to identify and solve problems in play with others
Outside	3②1	Independently accesses a variety of equipment to climb, slide, and jump	Close proximity to adult	Increase ability to follow rules and expectations for safety
Snack	3②1		▪ Cues to clear mouth ▪ Cues to take a turn, leave some for others	▪ Chew and clear mouth before taking in more food ▪ Pass and exchange items with peers
Transitions	3②1		▪ Prewarning for transition ▪ Use of visuals ▪ Close proximity of an adult	Increase ability to follow rules and expectations for safety

Note. Level of participation: 3 = independent or full participation; 2 = support needed; 1 = constant or intensive support needed. Value in bold is the score Bobby was given.

20–March 5, 2020). The tool looks at functional participation, strengths, adaptations, and potential intervention targets to increase participation.

The following observations are organized by Bobby's routines. Examples of peer performance are in *italics*.

Arrival and Dismissal: Bobby arrives at school on the bus. Although he is able to independently ambulate to and from the classroom, he requires adult close proximity and his hand held by another student to stay with the group. When he brings his belongings, he is typically able to manage them by placing them on his coat hook, and he can access his folder and place it in the appropriate spot. He is observed to zip a threaded zipper, take off his coat, and unfasten most fasteners. When greeted by a familiar adult, Bobby typically responds to the greeting by looking at the person, smiling, and saying, "Hi." *Peers generally establish eye contact to gain joint attention with others, initiate and respond to greeting and departure phrases, and ambulate independently between environments with close supervision or hand holding.*

Bathroom: Given verbal cues from an adult to address related behavioral concerns, Bobby is able to follow the basic toileting and handwashing routines. On occasion, he needs to change clothes after using the toilet. Usually, these accidents occur when he does not get his pants down far enough before using the toilet. During these clothing changes, Bobby is noted to independently take off long pants or elastic-waisted jeans and shoes, then put on clean clothes and shoes. Throughout the school day, Bobby indicates when he needs to go the bathroom and is typically able to take care of these routines *at the same rate as his peers.*

Circle Time (Whole-Group Instruction): Bobby sits in a cube chair near the teacher during large-group (circle time) activities. He benefits from visuals depicting expected actions, such as *sit, stand up,* and *give,* and an individualized positive reinforcement system to increase his on-task behavior and safe choices while in close proximity to his peers. Bobby seems to prefer music and movement activities at this routine time. He participates in choral responses to songs and familiar stories. When in the role of the "helper of the day," Bobby seems to enjoy making choices for the group, such as the order of the songs, how the class will move to transition, and so forth. He is noted to seem proud when he is "caught" sitting in his space and demonstrating the ability to be ready for group routines. *Peers are able to sit independently for 10–15 minutes while participating in the group.*

Small Group: During cutting activities, Bobby places school scissors (self-opening) in his right hand with his thumb down. He requires multiple adult cues (e.g., modeling, verbal, physical hand placement, hand over hand) to snip paper. He has not independently placed scissors correctly in his hand or cut in a forward motion to cut paper in half. During drawing activities, Bobby uses a right-handed functional grasp (tripod or four-finger) to imitate horizontal and vertical lines, and he copies drawing a face. However, Bobby often refuses to participate in drawing and cutting activities (e.g., says, "No!" and turns away, tries to leave the area). During class, Bobby does not draw shapes such as circles, crosses, or squares consistently, and he does not yet copy any letters of his name. During structured small-group games, Bobby requires cues to remain with the group and to take a turn or exchange materials with peers. He can match 8 of 14 colors when presented with one color at a time and is able to match 9 of 12 common pictures of animals and objects to play a bingo game. He correctly labels the colors *blue* and *black* and uses number words when asked to count; however, he is not yet able to count items meaningfully or count by rote in sequence. *His peers can independently position scissors correctly on their hand and cut on a thick line, copy a cross, copy their name, label most common animals and objects and 10 colors, and count 10 objects in a row.*

Play and Centers: Bobby seems to prefer active, self-directed play at preschool. He uses strong imaginary play skills to interact with others on his preferred topics. He likes to pretend to be the driver of the truck on the playground and "buckles" each of the truck passengers in their seat before turning the key and "driving." When playing with the doll-house and figures, he is noted to imitate activities (e.g., using the figures to cook) and gives directions when in the role of the father. Bobby prefers to explore building, blocks, and dramatic play instead of art or games during the center-time routine. Across all activities, Bobby often experiences difficulties taking turns, solving simple problems, and following adult directions for safety. This limits his ability to access learning activities with his same-age peers. During the evaluation, he was noted to hit, kick, slap, bite, throw objects, spit, and run away while in the school environment and to need assistance solving a problem within classroom and school expectations for safety. He has also been observed to hoard toys even if a peer requests one of the toys. For example, Bobby took all of the toy cars and put them under an object. When a peer asked him for a car, he said, "No!" and would not share one of the cars. Additionally, Bobby was not observed to follow one- or two-step directions from an adult to ensure his safety or the safety of others within his environment. Bobby requires a structured, positive behavioral support system to increase his successful participation and access learning. *Peers generally understand the rules, express anger with words, share toys, and take turns.*

Snack: Bobby readily accesses a variety of containers and packages to serve himself snack at school. He often has second and third helpings of food and seems to like a variety of foods and textures. He is able to pour water from a child-sized pitcher and on most days drinks more than one cup of water. He has been observed to prefer having the snack basket and water pitcher closest to him at the table and to need encouragement to share them with others at the table. He seems to like helping during this routine by passing out items to others. He often overstuffs his mouth, taking in additional food before swallowing and clearing his mouth first. He benefits from cues to slow down and reassurance he can have more if he is hungry and if others take a second serving, too. *Peers independently eat their food and may need reminders not to overstuff their mouth.*

Outside Play: Bobby is able to jump in a forward motion, run while avoiding obstacles in his environment, and climb playground equipment independently. He is able to kick and throw a ball at a target and is beginning to catch and bounce a large playground ball. Bobby has been observed to initiate interactions with peers in the classroom; however, the majority of his attempts are directives rather than requests. For example, when he wanted a peer to ride in the play car with him on the playground, he said, "Get in my car right now!" in a harsh tone instead of asking the peer whether they wanted to ride in the car. Socially, he has difficulty if a peer does not respond the way he wants them to respond. For example, when Bobby wanted a peer to get in the back of the play car on the playground and they did not want to go in the back, he raised his voice at the peer, saying "No, boy!" and pulled him to the back of the car. *Peers are able to jump, gallop, climb, run around objects in the environment, and hop on one foot and then the other; socially, they take turns, cooperate with peers for imaginative play, do not require constant adult supervision, and negotiate conflicts.*

Transitions: During transitions and across the school day, Bobby benefits from close adult proximity and clear expectations. When presented with frequent, positive feedback (visuals, verbal feedback, a highly motivating item) to remain with the group and in his own space, Bobby is more likely to be successful. Wait time during transitions is another challenging time for Bobby. He benefits from opportunities to help by carrying and holding materials or performing a "special job" as well as from strategic placement in the line (at the beginning or end) with his hand held by an adult or trained peer model. *Peers generally manage transitions with minimal adult supervision by waiting their turn and moving to the appropriate areas when directed by the adult.*

FORMAL AND INFORMAL MEASURES

Vision: Bobby's vision was screened by his pediatrician and passed. No concerns.
Hearing: Bobby passed his screening by a district audiologist. No concerns.
Health: The school nurse met with Bobby's parents. He has seasonal allergies. No health concerns.
Programming Needs: The Assessment, Evaluation, and Programming System for Infants and Children (AEPS®; Bricker, 2002) is a criterion-referenced, curriculum-based assessment for young children from birth to age 6 years. Bobby's performance across six developmental areas was assessed on March 2, 2020, while he played and engaged in typical, age-appropriate activities. His parents reported on his performance at home. Area goal scores reflect Bobby's performance based on the observations and parent report. The cutoff score represents the predicted score of peers in each domain. Numbers in bold indicate scores at or below the cutoff for his age (i.e., below average).

AEPS LEVEL 2 (37–60 MONTHS)

DOMAIN	AREA GOAL SCORE	CUTOFF SCORE
Fine motor (emergent writing, bilateral coordination)	**3**	3
Gross motor (balance and mobility, ball skills)	6	5.5
Adaptive (mealtime, dressing skills, personal hygiene)	**8**	8
Cognitive (includes play, problem solving, recalling events, concepts, categorizing, premath and phonological awareness)	**3**	14
Social–communication (production of words, phrases, and sentences; social–communicative interactions, including asking and answering questions)	8	9
Social (interaction with others, interaction with the environment, participation)	**10**	13.5

ANALYSIS OF PERFORMANCE

Bobby has many positive skills as well as areas that are challenging. According to the speech–language pathologist, his ability to answer *wh* questions (e.g., *why, what, where*) is interfering with his performance. During everyday routines, he primarily used gestures or answered questions with the same phrase. He uses directives rather than requests, which interferes with social communications. According to the occupational therapist, Bobby's difficulty with manipulating small objects and tools (e.g., scissors, pencil, crayon) and with visual–motor skills (e.g., drawing, staying on the line) interferes with his task completion in the classroom. Skills such as attending to the task, turn taking, and problem solving are challenging to Bobby.

SUMMARY

A summary of the team evaluation is included in the matrix below. Skilled occupational therapy and speech therapy to enhance Bobby's performance at preschool will be discussed at his upcoming individualized education program meeting.

Strengths
Playground skills
Recognizes his accomplishments
Curious
Imaginative play ideas
Is curious

Interests
Music and movement activities
Cars
Building
Dramatic play
Likes structure

Concerns
Following directions for safety
Social–interactive play skills
Social problem-solving skills
Conventional knowledge
Aggression

Potential Intervention Targets
Problem solving
Conversational skills
Use hands to manipulate objects
    and tools
Increase conventional knowledge

Appendix I. Sample Occupational Therapy Evaluation in Health Care

Stephanie L. de Sam Lazaro, OTD, OTR/L

Occupational Therapy Evaluation Report

Client Name: Aron Jones **Client Date of Birth:** 6/18/2018 **Date of Referral:** 5/25/2019
Date of Report: 6/3/2019 **Setting:** Outpatient clinic
Diagnosis: Developmental delay **Precautions/Medical History:** Born full term, no complications

Reason for Referral to Occupational Therapy: Concerns about motor skills, particularly fine motor skills, and their impact on play and child's ability to sit for extended periods of time.

Therapist: Tiffany Williams, OTR/L

Occupational Profile: Aron is 11 months and 15 days old. He was born full term with no significant medical history or complications. He lives at home with his parents and two older siblings (ages 6 and 4 years). He is happy, loves to explore, and is described as a "daddy's boy." He spends daytime hours at a home day care that his 4-year-old sister attends in the afternoons and his 6-year-old sister attends after school. His parents describe him as active and say that he crawled before he could sit independently. He pulls to stand, cruises along furniture, and pushes chairs and stools around. He also walks with one-handed help from an adult. Aron sits to play for very short periods (less than 2 minutes) but is more interested in moving around his environment and being near the older children at day care and his siblings at home. His parents brought their concerns about his fine motor development (e.g., does not finger feed or manipulate toys in play because his fingers are fisted) to their pediatrician at his 6-month well-child visit, and he was referred for an evaluation to occupational therapy.

Assessments Performed: The Peabody Developmental Motor Scales (2nd ed.; PDMS-2; Folio & Fewell, 2000) was used to assess Aron's fine and large motor skills at the outpatient clinic with his father present. The majority of children assessed with this tool receive a score between 85 and 115. The average score for children on this test is 100. Aron's father was interviewed during the evaluation, and informal observation of Aron's play and exploration skills in the clinic session were conducted.

Analysis of Occupational Performance: Aron willingly participated in activities presented by the therapist but needed redirection to play with toys (e.g., by other children present in the gym). His father reported this was typical and that Aron is interested in other children. Aron's father reported they have several gates all over their home to keep Aron away from his siblings' small toys. Aron pulls items into his palm or fist rather than using any isolated finger movements (e.g., uses whole hand to grasp toy rings, blocks, and cereal pieces). He is not yet using his thumb and finger pads to grasp items, and did not pick up the cup by the handle with one hand but did pick up the cup with two hands. He rolls over in both directions, moves in and out of sitting and standing with support, and gets down from standing in a controlled manner. He cruises along surfaces with one-handed support and was observed to push a toy cart with toys 10 feet. His large motor quotient score was 95, and his fine motor quotient score was 80.

Evaluation Summary and Analysis: The results of the PDMS-2 and caregiver report are consistent with each other. Aron scores in the average range for large motor skills and in the low average–below average range for fine motor skills. A discrepancy between large and fine motor skills was noted. Performance deficits were identified in the area of play. Low clinical decision making was required for this evaluation. Recommend outpatient occupational therapy once per week for 3 months to address fine motor skills to support play, ADL development (e.g., eating), and skill acquisition. Risks and benefits of services were shared with caregivers. Because of Aron's active nature, without intervention, there is risk that he may fall further behind in play and ADL participation because of his limited participation in fine motor play at this time.

Skilled Occupational Therapy Statement: Aron would benefit from skilled occupational therapy services to increase attention, fine motor grasp and manipulation, and interactive play skills to support participation and engagement in play and self-feeding. Occupational therapy services are also needed to provide education to caregivers to support Aron in home and community settings and connect caregivers with any external resources.

Signature/Date: Tiffany Williams, OTR/L 6/3/19

Appendix J. Occupational Therapy Telehealth Practices in Early Childhood

Stephanie Parks, PhD, OT/L, and Gloria Frolek Clark, PhD, OTR/L, BCP, FAOTA

The American Occupational Therapy Association (AOTA) supports the use of synchronous and asynchronous information and communication technology for occupational therapy evaluation, consultation, prevention and therapeutic services to clients (AOTA, 2018). Often this practice method is referred to as *telehealth,* but similar terms such as *tele-intervention, tele-therapy,* or *tele-practice* are also used. In education systems including early childhood special education services, terms such as *distance learning, e-learning,* and *remote instruction* may be used to describe the use of various technologies to facilitate practitioner–student and student–student communication and learning (e.g., non-traditional classroom environments). Regardless of the terminologies, when using video conferencing to provide services to young children and families, occupational therapy practitioners are required to follow professional standards of practice, including the *2020 Occupational Therapy Code of Ethics* (AOTA, 2020a) and *Standards of Practice for Occupational Therapy* (AOTA, 2015).

STATE AND PAYOR REQUIREMENT FOR TELEHEALTH

Occupational therapy practitioners are required to follow the regulations regarding this area of practice. Guidance is provided by AOTA (2018) and other documents.

- *State requirements.* Some state occupational therapy practice acts limit or do not allow telehealth. Most states require that the occupational therapy practitioner who delivers telehealth be licensed in their home state and the state in which the client resides. (Updates regarding changes in coverage of services and requirements due to the COVID-19 pandemic can be found on AOTA's website at https://bit.ly/2Jbpuuw.)
- *Payors.* Occupational therapy practitioners are required to understand reimbursement of telehealth services. There are limitations by specific payors (which may be waived in a time of crisis, such as a pandemic). For example, during the COVID-19 pandemic, legal requirements were waived to remove barriers to care.
- *Services.* When providing services under the Individuals with Disabilities Education Improvement Act (IDEA; 2004), occupational therapy practitioners must understand the rules of the Family Education Rights and Privacy Act (FERPA; 1974) and the Health Insurance Portability and Accountability Act (HIPAA; 1996) if billing to Medicaid or insurance is occurring. For example, FERPA covers recorded video (and photos) that are part of the child's record, but it does not address live recorded video. Recording and maintaining sessions would be considered part of the child's educational record and must be handled as such. (See FERPA's FAQs at https://bit.ly/3e65xkn and https://bit.ly/3jJASdz for more information on photos and videos).
- *Consent to treat.* Clients should be informed about the risks, benefits, and their rights (especially if any of the session is recorded). Risks may include potential loss of client privacy or confidentiality, possible malfunction of the equipment, modifications in assessment administration and scoring, or the occupational therapy practitioner's lack of knowledge and skills in equipment use (AOTA, 2018).
- *Privacy and confidentiality.* Occupational therapy practitioners should have clear policies about confidentiality of all communications, transmissions, storage of recordings, and disposal of recordings that comply with HIPAA.
- *Provider competence.* Occupational therapy practitioners must be competent and the equipment should be of sufficient quality (AOTA, 2018). A plan of action should be in place in case the equipment malfunctions or services are disrupted.

BENEFITS AND LIMITATIONS OF TELEHEALTH

Telehealth allows occupational therapy practitioners to build on family strengths and resources while working with the child in a natural environment and routine. Rather than using "therapy equipment," practitioners should embrace the naturally occurring materials and activities (e.g., eating, dressing, play, chores) within the home.

Benefits and Limitations for Families

Although most of the research appears to be in lower levels of research design (e.g., Levels III, IV, or V of evidence) parents appear to be highly satisfied with telehealth as a service model (Zylstra, 2013). A recent study by Wallisch and colleagues (2019) surveyed parents of children with autism spectrum disorder who were under 7 years of age and who received occupational therapy via a 12-week, telehealth-delivered service model. Three major themes emerged in parents' perceptions:

1. The model fit within family's daily life and helped meet the family's needs.
2. A feeling of partnership and collaborative relationship was strong as the parents and occupational therapy practitioners worked together.
3. Learning new strategies and problem-solving situations increased the parent's confidence and empowerment.

The overall comfort and competence of the family must be considered in telehealth. Occupational therapy practitioners must consider whether the family is competent with technology and electronic communication or has any sensory loss that would interfere with their ability to use telehealth (e.g., hearing, cognition, motor, vocal). Sometimes e-helpers (i.e., in-person support staff, also called *extenders*) is needed. The family may not be comfortable discussing concerns with the e-helper present, so other options may be necessary.

Overall, there is no large, Level III or higher, randomized, multi-site study that demonstrates the effectiveness of telehealth. The satisfaction surveys vary in how the questions were asked, leaving some concern about their reliability (Zylstra, 2013).

Benefits for Agencies and Practitioners

Benefits of telehealth include
- Assisting with provider shortages, especially in rural areas;
- Helping with transportation challenges (e.g., time distance, and cost of travel);
- Decreasing costs;
- Improving access to specific providers and specialists;
- Preventing delays in services; and
- Sharing expertise among practitioners (Carson, 2012a, 2012b).

Telehealth allows occupational therapy practitioners to view the environment to discuss safety and modifications with the family. They can observe the child during the actual routine (e.g., eating lunch while in the family's high chair).

Despite its benefits, caution must be used with telehealth so that this is not "pushed" out without proper training and adherence to state and federal laws. Confidentiality policies must be in place. Practitioners must be properly licensed and trained in service delivery using telehealth.

CONSIDERATIONS FOR OCCUPATIONAL THERAPY EVALUATION

The purpose of the evaluation process is to determine what the family and child wants and needs to do; what the family and child can do; identifying family concerns, resources, and priorities; identifying supports and barriers to the child's health, well-being, and participation (AOTA, 2020b). The occupational therapist begins the evaluation process by gathering the occupational profile and then collecting, interpreting, and analyzing data to identify strengths and specific needs and barriers.

The reliability and validity of specific assessment tools must be considered when using telehealth services (Royeen et al., 2020). E-helpers may assist with the administration of the assessment tools by following the therapist's directions. Sending assessment materials prior to the evaluation is recommended, depending upon the tool used.

CONSIDERATIONS FOR OCCUPATIONAL THERAPY INTERVENTION

Occupational therapy interventions should be carefully planned considering the effectiveness, safety, family and child outcomes, technology available, compliance with laws and regulations, and practitioner's knowledge and skills. Intervention may be directly with the child and family present; consultation with a remote provider, child, and family; indirect with the provider and the family (child not present); and many other scenarios. Not all will be reimbursed by payer sources.

During any service delivery, documentation and data collection must be performed. The family should be given choices of ways to contribute to the data collection process (e.g., individualized data sheet taped to the refrigerator, videotape, photos), as they will be participating in the routine activity targeted for intervention and reporting on its effectiveness. For example, families can videotape the routine or activity to share during the telehealth session. By reviewing the video together, practitioners can offer timely feedback. If possible, use other family members as "videographers" to observe and document progress.

TELEHEALTH RESOURCES FOR EARLY CHILDHOOD

In addition to AOTA documents, early childhood technical centers have provided various resources. These include resources developed for the COVID-19 pandemic, but they have very practical information for telehealth in general:

- *Planning for the use of video conferencing during the COVID-19 pandemic:* Early intervention home visits (https://bit.ly/2ENx1O3) and preschool special education and early care and education (https://bit.ly/39QjrVs) documents include key questions for reimbursement; resources for equipment, software, licensing, and bandwidth services; practitioner and coach skill sets; video-conferencing applications; and relevant resources.
- *Early Childhood Technical Assistance Center.* Their document, *Use of Tele-intervention in Early Intervention (IDEA Part C): Strategies for Providing Services Under the COVID-19 Public Health Emergency* (https://bit.ly/2X-oEdXw) provides resources for consideration during the pandemic including practice and effectiveness of telehealth, specific telehealth resources addressing Early Intervention, Medicaid, insurance, and HIPAA policy information.

REFERENCES

American Occupational Therapy Association. (2015). Standards of practice for occupational therapy. *American Journal of*

Occupational Therapy, 69(Suppl. 3), 6913410057. https://doi.org/10.5014/ajot.2015.696S06

American Occupational Therapy Association. (2018). Telehealth in occupational therapy. *American Journal of Occupational Therapy, 72*(Suppl. 2), 1–18.

American Occupational Therapy Association. (2020a). 2020 occupational therapy code of ethics. *American Journal of Occupational Therapy, 74*(Suppl. 3), 7413410005. https://doi.org/10.5014/ajot.2020.74S3006

American Occupational Therapy Association. (2020b). Occupational therapy practice framework: Domain and process (4th ed.). *American Journal of Occupational Therapy, 74*(Suppl. 2), 7412410010. https://doi.org/10.5014/ajot.2020.74S2001

Cason, J. (2012a). An introduction to telehealth as a service delivery model within occupational therapy. *OT Practice, 17*, CE1–CE8.

Cason, J. (2012b). Telehealth opportunities in occupational therapy through the Affordable Care Act. *American Journal of Occupational Therapy, 66*, 131–136. https://doi.org/10.5014/ajot.2012.662001

Family Education Rights and Privacy Act of 1974, 20 U.S.C. §1232g.

Health Insurance Portability and Accountability Act of 1996, Pub. L. 104-191, 110 Stat. 1938.

Individuals with Disabilities Education Act of 2004, 20 U.S.C. 1412.

Royeen, L., Little, L., Olson, L., & Kramer, P. (2020). Evaluation in emerging practice settings: Primary care, telehealth, and group- and population-based evaluation. In P. Kramer & N. Grampurohit (Eds.), *Hinojosa and Kramer's evaluation in occupational therapy: Obtaining and interpreting data* (5th ed., pp. 1671–86). North Bethesda, MD: AOTA Press.

Wallish, A., Little, L., Pope, E., & Dunn, W. (2019). Parent perspectives of an occupational therapy telehealth intervention. *International Journal of Telerehabilitation, 11*(1), 15–22. https://doi.org/10.5195/ijt.2019.6274

Zylstra, S. E. (2013). Evidence for the use of telehealth in pediatric occupational therapy. *Journal of Occupational Therapy, Schools, & Early Intervention, 6*, 326–355.

Index

Note: Page numbers in *italics* indicate figures, tables, and exhibits.

A

abandonment, 349
Able Play, 61
abuse, 349
academic performance, observation of, 393–395
academic preparation, for early childhood practice, 24–26, *25, 26*
accessibility, 74
accountability, 7, 47
  expectation about, 47–48
Accreditation Council for Occupational Therapy Education (ACOTE), 24, *25,* 31
ACE(s). *See* adverse childhood experiences (ACEs)
Acquaviva, Jane, 6
acquired brain injuries (ABIs), 215–216
acquired conditions, 215–223
  acute phase of, 221–222
  age-specific considerations with, 219
  best practices for, 220–223
  brain injuries as, 215–217
  burns as, 217
  cancer as, 217–218
  chronic phase of, 222–223
  compensatory training for, 222
  defined, 199, 215
  evaluation in health care settings of, 199–200
  family adjustment and setting expectations for, 219–220
  habilitation *vs.* rehabilitation for, 219
  health care interventions for, 215–223
  interprofessional coordination of care for, 219
  medical complications and precautions with, 220–221
  mental health conditions as, 218
  and neuroplasticity, 219
  payment sources for, 220
  physical trauma injuries as, 218
  restoring function with, 222
  spinal cord injuries as, 217

acquired diagnoses. *See* acquired conditions
acquired hearing loss, 309
activities
  in early childhood team report, 391
  evaluation in health care setting of, 202
  in preschool, 176
activities of daily living (ADLs), 235–240
  assessment tools for, 237, *237,* 385
  defined, 235
  dressing and undressing as, 236, 239–240
  evaluation of, *237,* 237–238
  family partnerships for, 238
  grooming and hygiene as, 236, 239–240
  in health care setting, *210*
  in natural context, 238
  overview of, 235
  sleep and rest as, 236–237, *237,* 240
  toileting as, 235–236, 238–239
activity analysis, for early intervention, *139,* 141
adaptations
  for literacy development, 112–113
  for visual impairments, 323
adaptive equipment, for feeding, 251
adaptive leadership, 42–43
ADOS–2 (Autism Diagnostic Observation Schedule–2), 28
Advancing Equity in Early Childhood Education (NAEYC), 18
adverse childhood experiences (ACEs)
  defined, 40, *101,* 349
  prevalence of, *101*
  prevention of, 40, 354
  resources on, 355
  risks related to, 40, 100, *101*
Adverse Childhood Experiences (ACE) Pyramid, 349, *349*
Adverse Childhood Experiences (ACE) Study, 348–349
advocacy
  for autism spectrum disorder and ADHD, 342–343

collaboration and, *72,* 75
history of, 4
for inclusion and natural environments, 18
by occupational therapy assistants, 35–36
in preschool, 176
for prevention of adverse childhood experiences and childhood trauma, 354
role of occupational therapy practitioners in, 27, *368*
for social participation, 286
Aetna, *194*
Affordable Care Act (ACA, 2010), 193
aftercare services, 4
Ages and Stages Questionnaire, *294*
age-specific considerations, with acquired conditions, 219
Ages & Stages Questionnaires, *134*
Alberta Infant Motor Scales, *134, 276*
albinism, *322*
alcohol, prenatal exposure to, 91, 348
alcohol-related birth defects (ARBDs), 348
alcohol-related neurodevelopmental disorder (ARND), 348
Alert Program, 296
Allen, Edgar, 4
alphabet knowledge, *111*
amblyopia, 320, *322*
American Montessori International (AMI), *15*
American Montessori Society (AMS), *15*
American Occupational Therapy Association (AOTA), *15*
  accountability expectations of, 47
  early childhood resources of, 43, *44*
  resources for practitioners and families of, 383
American Physical Therapy Association (APTA), *15*
American Sign Language (ASL), *313*
American Speech-Language-Hearing Association (ASHA), *15*

Americans with Disabilities Act Amendments Act (ADAA, 2008), *362*

amygdala, impact of postnatal trauma on, 349

analysis, in early childhood team report, 392

analysis of performance, in team evaluation report, 396

annual performance report (APR), 157

annual performance report (APR) indicators, *80*

annual progress report, 186–187

antiepileptic drugs (AEDs), nutrition with, 246

apnea monitor, 332

applied behavioral analysis provider, *208*

The Arc, 4, *330*

arrival, in team evaluation report, 393, 394

ask questions, in PAUSE method, 102, 103

assessment
authentic, 131–132, *139,* 139–140, 168, 284
of communication, 284
criterion-referenced, 133
defined, 47, 129, 130
documentation of, 149
for early intervention, 121–123, *122,* 124–125, 129–135, *134*
functional, 131–132
functional behavioral, 293
in initial evaluation, 397
norm-referenced, 133
ongoing, 170
of social participation, 284, 385

Assessment, Evaluation, and Programming System for Infants and Children (AEPS), *134,* 395–396

Assessment of Preterm Infant Behavior (APIB), 351

assessment tools, 385–387
for activities of daily living, 237, *237,* 385
for cognitive development, 259, *259*
for eating and feeding skills, 250
for fine motor coordination, 267, *267*
in health care setting, *203,* 204
for large motor coordination, 275, *276*
for play, 303–304, *304,* 385
for preschool, 168, *169*
for visual impairment, 321–323, *323*
for visual-motor coordination, 267, *267*

Asset-Based Context Matrix, *134*

Assisting Hand Assessment, *267*

assistive technology (AT), 55–61
adaptation for child's use of, 59
for children with special health care needs, 333
collaborative decision-making tools for, 57–58
for communication needs, 59–60
defined, 55
determining need for, 57–58
and early intervention and preschool, 56
federal laws supporting, 55–56
funding sources for, 60
interdisciplinary approach to, 57
for literacy development, 112–113
myths regarding, 55, *56*
ongoing research needs for, 60
for play, 58
power mobility needs for, 58–59
in professional guidelines, 364
resources on, 61
for self-care routines, 58
switches in, 59, 60
underuse of, 55
and universal design, 57
uses of, 56
for visual impairments, 323

Assistive Technology Act (Tech Act, 2004), 55–56, *363*

associational systems, 90

Association for Childhood Education International (ACEI, CEI, CE International), *15*

Association for Children with Learning Disabilities, 4

Association of State and Tribal Home Visiting Initiatives (ASTHVI), *15*

Association of University Centers on Disabilities (AUCD), 5

Associations of Service Providers Implementing IDEA Reforms in Education (ASPIRE), 7

associative play, *303*

AT Consideration Flowchart, 58

attachment
for developmental trauma, 353–354
with neonatal abstinence syndrome, 348, 352

attention, 258
selective, 93

attention deficit hyperactivity disorder (ADHD), 337–343
advocacy for, 342–343
cognitive and literacy skills with, 260
defined, 338
and delays in development of social skills, 292
diagnosis of, 338, *338*
disparities and cultural considerations with, 339

early intervention for, 340
epidemiology of, 337
evaluation of, 340–341
family-centered approach and education for, 342
family coping and resiliency with, 341–342
family participation in daily life routines with, 341–342
federal and state policies and funding sources for, 339
health care for, 340
interventions for, 342
leisure participation with, 341
monitoring and screening for, 339–340, *340*
occupational performance in daily routines with, 341
parent self-efficacy with, 341–342
physical activities for, 342
play performance with, 341
preschool for, 340
resources on, 343
restricted and repetitive behaviors with, 341
sensory integration and sensory-based interventions for, 341
social interaction with, 341
subtypes of, 338, *338*
types of, 338, *338*
value of occupational therapy for, 338–339

audiogram, 310, *311*

auditory receptors, 92

auditory system, development of, 92

Auditory Verbal (AV) therapy, *313*

augmentative and alternative communication (AAC), 59–60, 281, 286–287

authentic approach, to data gathering, 53

authentic assessment
for early intervention, 131–132, *139,* 139–140
for preschool, 168
for social participation, 284

Autism and Developmental Disabilities Monitoring (ADDM) Network, 337

Autism Collaboration, Accountability, Research, Education and Support (Autism CARES) Act (2019), 29

Autism Diagnostic Observation Schedule-2 (ADOS-2), 28

Autism Society of America, 4

autism spectrum disorder (ASD), 337–343
advocacy for, 342–343
cognitive development with, 260

defined, 337
and delays in development of social skills, 292, 293
diagnosis of, 337
disparities and cultural considerations with, 339
early intervention for, 340
evaluation of, 340–341
family-centered approach and education for, 342
family coping and resiliency with, 341–342
family participation in daily life routines with, 341–342
federal and state policies and funding sources for, 339
health care considerations and impact on participation of, *331*
health care for, 340
interventions for, 341–342
leisure participation with, 341
monitoring and screening for, 339–340, *340*
nutrition with, 244–245
occupational performance in daily routines with, 341
parent self-efficacy with, 341–342
physical activities for, 342
play performance with, 341
preschool for, 340
resources on, 343
restricted and repetitive behaviors with, 341
sensory integration and sensory-based interventions for, 341
social interaction with, 341
value of occupational therapy for, 338–339
autism spectrum disorder (ASD)-specific screening, 339–340, *340*
autonomic dysreflexia (AD), 220
autonomic nervous system (ANS), development of, 91
autonomy, *33*
avoidant/restrictive food intake disorder (ARFID), 245
Ayres Sensory Integration, for developmental trauma, 353

B
background information, in early childhood team report, 391
backward chaining, for dressing, grooming, and hygiene, 239
bacterial meningitis, 217
balance, *278*
baseline data, 48
bathing, 236, 239–240
in health care setting, *210*
bathroom, in team evaluation report, 393, 394

Battellle Developmental Inventory, *134, 323*
Bayley Scales of Infant and Toddler Development
in early intervention, *134*
to evaluate cognitive development, *259*
to evaluate fine and visual-motor skills, *267*
to evaluate large motor skills, *276*
to evaluation social-emotional skills, *294*
in health care setting, *203*
Beery-Buktenica Developmental Test of Visual Motor Integration, *267*
behavioral difficulties, literacy and, 109
behavioral interventions, for ADHD, 342
behavioral modification, for toilet training, 238–239
behavioral regulation, 291
behavior approach, *19*
Behavior Rating Inventory of Executive Function, *259*
beliefs, assessment tools for, 385
beneficence, *33*
bias, risk of, 372
Big Life Journal, 355
bilateral coordination, *269*
billing for services, 182, 194–196, *195*, 226
bimanual intensive therapy (BIT), 268, 277
Binet, Alfred, 3
biomechanical theory, in health care setting, *211*
birth defects, alcohol-related, 348
birth mandate, 121, 363
birthweight, and delays in development of social skills, 292
BIT (bimanual intensive therapy), 268, 277
Blindness. *See also* visual impairments
legal, 319
ocular, *324*
blood pressure, with acquired conditions, 220
BlueCross BlueShield, *194*
body functions, assessment tools for, 385
body structures, assessment tools for, 385
bone-anchored hearing aid, 311–312
bone density decrease, with acquired conditions, 221
brain development, 89–95
of autonomic nervous system, 91
and cognitive development, 94
collaboration across systems to support, 94

core concepts of, 90–91
cutting-edge science to enhance, 94–95
defined, 89
of emotions, 93–94
identify needs and make referrals related to, 94
impact of maternal nutrition and extreme stress on, 90
impact of postnatal trauma on, 349–350
in utero, 90–91
and motor development, 93
prenatal exposure to toxicants and, 91
resources on, 95
of selective attention, 93
of sensory systems and sensory processing, 91–93
brain injuries, 215–217
acquired, 215–216
classification of, 216
due to pediatric stroke, 216
due to tumors and infections, 216–217
nontraumatic, 216
traumatic, 216
brain tumors, 216
breastfeeding, for neonatal abstinence syndrome, 352
Brigance Early Childhood Screens III, *294*
Brigance Inventory of Early Development-III, *134*
Brown v. Board of Education of Topeka (1954), 5
Bruininks-Oseretsky Test of Motor Proficiency, *169, 276*
Buddhism, dietary practices and restrictions in, *248*
Bureau of Education for the Handicapped, 5
burns, 217
businesses, collaboration with, 74

C
Caldwell, Bettye, 3
Callier-Azusa Scale, *323*
Canadian Occupational Performance Measure (COPM), 51–52, *203, 267, 275*
cancer, 217–218
cannabis, prenatal exposure to, 348
capacity building, 66–67
in early intervention, 138
for transitions, 83
caregiver education and coaching
for sleep, 240
for toileting, 238
caregiver report, on eating and feeding skills, 250

CareToy, 268, 276

Carolina Curriculum, *259*

car seats, for children with special health care needs, 332

casein-free diet, for autism spectrum disorder, 245

case manager
  on interprofessional team, *208*
  role of occupational therapy practitioner as, *367*

categorization, 320

CEI (Association for Childhood Education International), *15*

CE International (Association for Childhood Education International), *15*

Center for Applied Special Technology, 57, 61

Center for IDEA Early Childhood Data Systems, *16*

Center for Parent Information and Resource, 61

Center for Technology and Disability, 61

Centers for Medicare & Medicaid Services, *194*

central nervous system (CNS), 90

cerebral palsy
  fine and visual-motor coordination with, 268
  health care considerations and impact on participation of, *331*
  large motor coordination with, 277, *277*
  nutrition with, 246–247

cerebral visual impairment (CVI), 319–320, *322, 324*

certainty, level of, 372, *373*

certified diabetes educator (CDE), 246

chaining strategies, for dressing, grooming, and hygiene, 239

Chandler, Barbara, 7

checklists, 50–51, *51, 52*

chemical burns, 217

Child Behavioral Checklist–Preschool, *294*

Child Care Aware of America, *15, 330*

Child Care Services Association (CCSA), *15*

Child-Centered AT Plan, 58

child-centered evaluation, for preschool, 167

child education, on acquired conditions, 222, 223

child-family relationships, in early intervention, 142

Child Find system, 121, 132, 159, 166, 183

child-focused care, 7

child outcome(s)
  documentation of, *148,* 148–149
  measurement for early intervention of, 123, 125

Child Outcomes Summary (COS)
  for early intervention, 123, 125, 135, *148,* 149
  for preschool, 169–170

Child Outcomes Summary Form (COSF), for early intervention, 135

Childhood Daily Occupations Toolkit, 141

childhood stroke, 216

Children and Youth SIS, 7

children at risk, programs for, 14

The Children's Bureau, 3, 4

children's medical services (CMS), partnering with, *26*

children with disabilities
  cognitive development of, 260
  early perspectives on, 3
  in special education process, 159

children with special health care needs (CSHCN), 329–334
  assistive technology for, 333
  coordinating with health care providers for, 330
  data collection on, 334
  defined, 329
  evaluation of, 333, *333*
  evidence-based interventions for, 333
  home nursing care for, 329
  impact on daily occupations for, 330–332, *331*
  medical equipment needs of, 332
  nutrition for, 244–247, 331, *332*
  play and leisure for, 331
  school health plans for, 334
  sleep and rest for, 331–332
  social participation by, 331
  support for family of, 329–330, *330*
  transition to preschool by, 333–334

child saving movement, 4

Child Trauma Toolkit for Educators, 355

choice boards, 286

choice making, 285

Choose My Plate Program, 243, *244*

chronic interpersonal trauma. *See* developmental trauma

Church of Latter Day Saints, dietary practices and restrictions in, *249*

Cigna Health, *194*

Circle of Security, 354

circle time, in team evaluation report, 393, 394

cleft lip and palate, health care considerations and impact on participation of, *331*

client-centered care, 64

client-centered goals, in health care setting, 204

client factors
  assessment tools for, 385
  in health care setting, 202–203

close supervision, 32

coaching
  caregiver, 238
  in early intervention, *139,* 140
  family, 354
  in home setting, 73
  occupational performance, 238
  parent, 7, 211, 240, 268
  in preschool, 177–178, *178*
  for transitions, 82, *82*

COAST format, 229

cochlear implant (CI), 311, *312*

Code of Ethics, 33, *33,* 56, 225

coding, 194–196, *195*

cognition
  defined, 94
  with hearing loss, 315

cognitive approaches, for developmental trauma, 353

cognitive-based interventions, for ADHD, 342

cognitive development, 257–261
  attention and, 258
  of children with disabilities, 260
  collaboration with preschool team on, 261
  evaluation for, 259, *259*
  foundations of, 94
  imitation and, 258
  interventions to facilitate, 260–261
  literacy and, 258–259
  memory and, 258
  parent education on, 260–261
  perceptual functions and, 258
  of premature infants, 260
  problem solving and, 258
  temperament and, 257–258

Cognitive–Functional (Cog–Fun) intervention, 342

Cognitive Orientation to daily Occupational Performance (CO–OP) approach, 27, 211, 341

cognitive process theories, in health care setting, 211

cognitive skills, defined, 257

collaboration, 71–77
  advantages of, 71
  and advocacy, 75
  communication and, 76, *76*
  communication logs for, 74
  at community level, *72,* 74, *74*
  conceptual framework for, 71, *72*
  conflict resolution in, 76, *76*
  data to guide decision-making and evaluate effectives in, 75
  defined, 71

in early intervention, 138–139
for evaluation in health care
    settings, 200–201
factors that influence, 71
with family, *72*
in health care interventions for
    developmental conditions, 209
in health care setting, *73*
in home setting, 72–73, *73*
in inpatient health care, 71–72
interprofessional, 7, *28*, 74–75, *75*,
    139
intraprofessional, *73*, 73–74
between occupational therapy
    practitioners in different practice
    settings, *73*, 73–74
at organizational level, *72*
in outpatient health care, 72
overview of, 71
at policy level, *72*, 75
in preschool setting, 72, *73*, 174, 176
priorities of care and, 75
relationships and partnerships in, 75
self-examination in, 76
within settings, 71–73
Situation-Background-Assessment-
    Recommendation strategy for,
    74, *74*
for social participation, 286–287
at systems level, *72*
technology to promote, 76
Tuckman's Model for, 75
collaborative approach, 71
collaborative decision-making tools,
    for assistive technology, 57–58
collaborative interventions, on
    cognitive development, 261
collaborative partnerships, with
    educational staff, 167
collaborative team member, role of
    occupational therapy practitioner
    as, *367*
collaborative team model
    for nutrition, 253
    for visual impairment, 321
colors, rapid naming of, *111*
communication, 281–287
    assessment of, 284
    assistive technology for, 59–60
    augmentative and alternative,
        59–60, 281, 286–287
    choice making for, 285
    and collaboration, 76, *76*
    development of, 281–283, *282*
    early indicators of delays in or
        disorders of, 283
    early literacy development and, 287
    essential considerations for,
        281–283
    functional communication training
        for, 285

with hearing loss, 312, *313*
inclusive services for, 286
interprofessional, 26
interventions for, *284*, 284–287
occupation-centered practice and,
    283
overview of, 281
peer-mediated social strategies for,
    286
resources on, 287
responding, modeling, and
    scaffolding for, 285
routines for, 284–285
and social-emotional reciprocity,
    282–283
and social participation, 281
visual supports in, 285–286
communication logs, 74
communication strategies, for
    evaluation in health care settings,
    200–201
communities of practice (CoPs), 43
community
    defined, 141
    transition from home to, 84
    transition from hospital to, 83
    transition to IDEA Part B from, 80,
        80
community health care teams,
    communication with, 201
community integration, of early
    intervention, *139*, 141
Community Mental Health Act
    (1963), 5
community partnering, *72*, 74, *74*
Community Resilience Initiative, 355
community safety and participation,
    in health care setting, *210*
community settings
    collaboration in, *72*, 74, *74*
    occupational therapy assistants in,
        34
compensatory education, 14
compensatory training, for acquired
    conditions, 222
complementary feeding, 250–251
Complex Child, *330*
complexity, in life course health
    development framework, 350
complex trauma. *See* developmental
    trauma
comprehensive commercially
    available curricula, *19*
comprehensive system of personnel
    development, for early
    intervention, 120–121
concepts of print, *111*
concerns, in team evaluation report,
    396
confidentiality
    in health care settings, 226

of records, 181–182
with telehealth, 399
conflict resolution, 76, *76*
congenital hearing loss, 309
congenital heart defects, health care
    considerations and impact on
    participation of, *331*
consent to treat, and telehealth, 399
constipation, 238
constraint-induced movement
    therapy (CIMT), 268, 277
constructive play, 303
consultation
    in preschool, 177–178, *178*
    roles of occupational therapy
        practitioners in, *366*, *368*
contact note, 35, *146*
contact reports, 185, *186*
    in health care settings, *228, 230, 231*
context
    assessment tools for, 387
    in family partnerships, 64
    of play, 304–305
    in preschool, 174
contextual influences
    on occupational therapy services in
        early intervention and schools,
        364–365
    on play, 302
continuous positive airway pressure
    (CPAP) machine, 332
contracts, for early intervention, 120
co-occupation(s)
    play as, 301
    for preschool, 178
co-occupational engagement, 99
cooperative play, *303*
coordination, *28*, 278
Coping with and Caring for Infants
    with Special Needs Program, 277
core competencies, from professional
    early childhood organizations,
    26–27, *27*
co-regulation
    defined, 291–292
    for developmental trauma, 353
core life skills, 95
cortical visual impairment (CVI),
    319–320, *322, 324*
Cortical Visual Impairment Range,
    323
Council for Exceptional Children
    (CEC), 14, *15*, 23, 374
counselor, *208*
Coventry, *194*
CPT codes. *See* Current Procedural
    Terminology (CPT) codes
create, in preschool intervention, 175
credentialing, 193–194
crippled children, 4
crippled children's centers, 5

criterion-reference assessments, for early intervention, 133
critical periods, in life course health development framework, 350–351
Crohn's disease, nutrition with, 246
cross-disciplinary competencies, 17
Cued Speech (CS), *313*
cultural competency, in family partnerships, 66
cultural considerations
  with autism spectrum disorder and ADHD, 339
  with hearing loss, 312
cultural context, assessment tools for, 387
cultural reciprocity, in family partnerships, 66
cultural responsivity, in early intervention, 138
culturally appropriate evaluation practice, for Part C services, 131
culturally competent practice, leadership in, 41
Current Procedural Terminology (CPT) codes
  in billing for services, 182
  in documentation, 226, *227*
  in evaluation, *195,* 195–196
  in treatment, 196, *196*
Cuyahoga County Council for the Retarded Child, 4
CVI (cortical/cerebral visual impairment), 319–320, *322, 324*

D
daily notes, *146*
dairy, *244*
data analysis, for early intervention, 142
data-based decision making, 47–54
  and accountability expectations, 47–48
  and collaboration, 75
  data collection methods for, 48–52, *48–52*
  defined, 47
  determination of fidelity of implementation in, 53–54.*54*
  documentation in, 47
  gathering data during evaluation for, 52–53, *53*
  gathering data during evidence-based interventions for, 53
  overview of, 47
data collection, 48–53
  best practices for, 52–54
  Canadian Occupational Performance Measure for, 51–52
  checklists or rubrics with standards in, 50–51, *51, 52*

for children with special health care needs, 334
  to determine fidelity of implementation, 53–54, *54*
  on early intervention, 142
  during evaluation, 52–53, *53*
  during evidence-based interventions, 53
  goal attainment scaling in, 50, *50*
  for hearing loss, 315
  mastery monitoring in, *49,* 49–50
  performance-based measurement in, *48,* 48–49
  on play, 306
  for preschool, 178
data-driven decision making (DDDM), for children with special health care needs, 334
data teams, 42
deaf and hard of hearing (d/HH) individuals. *See* hearing loss
deaf-blindness, 324–325, *325*
Deaf culture, 312
deafness. *See* hearing loss
decision making, data-based, 47–54
delayed toileting skills, 235–236
delivery of services, 6–7
demographic information, in health care settings, 228
De Morsier's syndrome, *322*
denial of service, 197–198
developmental, individual-difference, relationship based (DIR)/Floortime™, *211,* 295, 354
Developmental Assessment for Individuals with Severe Disabilities, *323*
Developmental Assessment of Young Children, *134, 259, 294*
developmental conditions
  defined, 207
  health care interventions for, 207–212
developmental considerations, with transitions, 81–82
developmental disabilities and delays, 121, 130, 159
  cognitive development with, 260
  defined, 199
  evaluation in health care settings of, 199–200
  literacy with, 109
developmental growth, in early childhood team report, 392, *392*
Developmental Indicators for the Assessment of Learning, *169*
developmental information, in early childhood team report, 392, *392*
developmental milestones, impact of postnatal trauma on, 349–350
developmental monitoring, 339

developmental pediatrician, *208*
developmental perspective, 283
developmental progress, documentation of, 147
developmental trauma
  ACE Pyramid for, 349, *349*
  Adverse Childhood Experiences (ACE) Study of, 348–349
  advocacy for prevention of, 354
  defined, 349
  evaluation of, 353
  impact on brain development and developmental milestones of, 349–350
  interventions for, 353–354
  life course approach to, 350–351
  resources on, 355
  risk factors for, 349
  trauma-informed care for, 350
developmentally appropriate occupations, and occupational therapy assistants, 35
developmentally appropriate practice (DAP), 13, 17, *17*
Developmentally Appropriate Practice Position Statement (NAEYC), 13
dexterity, *269*
d/HH (deaf and hard of hearing) individuals. *See* hearing loss
diabetes, nutrition with, 246
dialysis, 332
dietary customs and practices, 247, *248–249*
Dietary Reference Intakes (DRIs), 243
diffuse axonal injury (DAI), 216
digestive diseases and conditions, nutrition with, 246
digestive enzyme supplements (Peptizyde, Neo-Digestin), for autism spectrum disorder, 245
digits, rapid naming of, *111*
DIR (developmental, individual-difference, relationship based)/Floortime™, *211,* 295, 354
discharge from services
  for developmental conditions in health care setting, 212
  documentation of, 188
discharge planning
  for acquired conditions, 223
  in health care setting, 204
  for preschool, 176, 185
discharge report, *146*
  in health care settings, *228,* 230
discontinuation, of early intervention, 142
discontinuation report, in health care settings, 230
dismissal, in team evaluation report, 393, 394

disparities, with autism spectrum disorder and ADHD, 339
displaced families, early intervention with, 138
distal relationships, 100–101
distance learning, 399
diversity, 18
Division for Early Childhood (DEC)
    on best practices, 14
    on core competencies, *27*
    description of, *15*
    on recommended practices, 17, 23
    on role of occupational therapy practitioners, 27
documentation
    of child outcomes, *148,* 148–149
    in data-based decision making, 47
    defined, 145
    of developmental progress, 147
    of early intervention, 145–152, *146*
    education-based, 183
    electronic, 182
    of evaluation, assessment, and reevaluation, *146,* 149
    of family engagement, *147,* 147–148
    fundamentals of, 181, *182*
    of health care intervention for acquired condition, 223
    of health care services and outcomes, 197, 225–232
    health literacy in, 226
    in home care, 227, *228, 230*
    of implementation, 150
    in inpatient hospital settings, 226–227, *228, 230*
    of intervention, 150–152
    in NICUs, 226, *228, 230*
    of occupational therapy outcomes, 152
    in outpatient settings, 227, *228, 230*
    and payment, 197
    point-of-service, 148
    for preschool, 181–189, *182*
    of progress toward outcomes, 150–151, *152*
    of services by occupational therapy assistants, 35
    of skilled occupational therapy, *146,* 146–147
    of supervision, 32
    tips for, *146*
double-blind study, 371
Down syndrome
    health care considerations and impact on participation of, *331*
    nutrition with, 246–247
    dressing, 236, 239–240
    in health care setting, *210*
dual language learners (DLLs), 111
duration, 48
duration chart, 51, *52*

dysautonomia, 220
dysphagia
    due to cerebral palsy, 247
    swallow study for, 253
Dysphagia Disorder Survey, 250

E
Early Child Outcomes (ECOs), 188
early childhood education (ECE), 4–5, 13
early childhood inclusion, 18
early childhood outcomes, for preschool, 161
Early Childhood Personnel Center (ECPC), *16,* 17, 27, *27,* 43
early childhood practice
    educational preparation for, 24–26, *25, 26*
    value and role of occupational therapy practitioners in, 27
early childhood practitioners, resources for, *8*
early childhood programs and services
    history of, 3–7
    preparing for future of, 8–9
early childhood special education (ECSE), 13–14
early childhood team report, 391–392
Early Childhood Technical Assistance (ECTA) Center, *16,* 119
Early Head Start, 14
early intervention (EI), 13–14
    activity analysis and environmental modifications for, *139,* 141
    assistive technology in, 56
    for autism spectrum disorder and ADHD, 339, 340
    child and family outcome measurement for, 123, 125, 135
    coaching in, *139,* 140
    collaboration in, 138–139
    community integration of, *139,* 141
    contracts and interagency agreements for, 120
    cultural responsivity in, 138
    data collection and analysis on, 142
    definition of developmental delay for, 121
    discontinuation of, 142
    with displaced families, 138
    documentation of, 145–152, *146*
    eligibility criteria for, 130, 132
    environmental and contextual influences on, 364–365
    family partnerships in, 68, 69
    family service coordinator for, 121, 124, 130
    financial requirements for, 120
    flexibility to serve children beyond age 3 years and birth mandate in, 121

guidelines for occupational therapy services in, 361–369
history of, 119
IFSP development, review, and evaluation in, 123, 125
integration of everyday items and activities in, *139,* 140
interventions in, 137–142, *139*
laws and process of, 119–126, *122*
lead agency designation in, 120, 145
legislation and regulatory influences on, 361–363, *362–363*
natural environments for, 124, 137, 138, *139,* 139–140
occupational performance analysis for, 133, *134*
occupational profile for, 132–133
occupational therapy role in, 130
occupations in, 361
overview of, 119
payment sources for, 139
Person-Environment-Occupation-Performance model for, 138
personnel standards and personnel development system for, 120–121
procedural safeguards for, 123
professional influences on, 363–364
providing service in context of team in, 125–126
providing service in natural environments in, 124
public awareness and Child Find for, 121, 132
reevaluation of, 135, 149
referral for, 132
relationship-based practices in, *139,* 141–142
roles of occupational therapy practitioners in, 365–368, *366–368*
routines-based approach to, *139,* 140–141
screening, evaluation, and assessment in, 121–125, *122,* 129–135, *134*
self-efficacy in, 138
service coordination for, 121
service delivery for, 123
strengths-based approach to, 137
supervision and monitoring of, 120
transition to preschool from, 84, 124, 126
Early Intervention and Schools SIS, 7
Early Learning Accomplishment Profile, *134, 259*
early learning and development standards, 17
early learning guidelines (ELGs), 17
early literacy development, 110
early literacy learning, 110
Early Screening Inventory, *169*

Eastern Orthodox Christianity, dietary practices and restrictions in, *248*
Easterseals, 4, 5
eating. *See also* nutrition
  for children with special health care needs, 244–247, 331, *332*
  defined, 243
  interventions to support healthy, 250–253
eating skills, evaluation of, 250
ecological systems theory, 64
Ecology of Human Performance (EHP), 64, *65*
Edinburgh Postnatal Depression Scale, *134*
education
  on acquired conditions, 222, 223
  compensatory, 14
  early childhood, 4–5, 13
  free appropriate public, 6
  interprofessional, 23
  leadership in, 41
  in preschool, 176
  special (*See* special education (SPED))
education-based documentation, state practice act *vs.*, 183
education evaluation, 167
Education for All Handicapped Children Act (1975), 6, 7
Education of the Handicapped Act (1970), 5–6
education requirements, for occupational therapy assistants, 31
education settings, occupational therapy assistants in, 34
educational preparation, for early childhood practice, 24–26, *25, 26*
educator, role of occupational therapy practitioner as, *368*
effective, collaborative partnerships, with educational staff, 167
e-learning, 399
electrical burns, 217
electronic documentation platforms, 182
electronic health care records (EHR), 226
Elementary and Secondary Education Act (ESEA, 1965), 5, *5, 6, 362, 366*
eligibility criteria
  for Part C services, 130, 132
  for special education, 159
embedded approach, to data gathering, 53
embedded learning opportunities (ELOs), *19*
  in preschool, 176–177, *177*
emergent literacy development, 110, 283

emotion(s), development of, 93–94
emotional regulation, 291
  for developmental trauma, 353
emotional skills, 291–297
  best practices for, 293–296, *294, 296*
  defined, 291
  delays in development of, 292–293
  essential considerations for, 292–293
  evaluation of, 293–294, *294*
  evidence-based interventions for, 294–296, *296*
  outcome and goal language for, 296, *296*
  overview of, 291–292
encephalitis, 217
entry-level requirements, in educational preparation, 24, *25*
enuresis, nocturnal, 239
environmental factors, in preschool, 174
environmental influences, on occupational therapy services in early intervention and schools, 364–365
environmental modifications
  for early intervention, 141
  for neonatal abstinence syndrome, 352
  in professional guidelines, 364
  for visual impairments, 323
epigenetics, 349, *349*
epilepsy
  health care considerations and impact on participation of, *331*
  nutrition with, 246
equality, 18
establish, in preschool intervention, 175, *175*
ethical practice, 197
ethics, 26
  Code of, 33, *33*, 56, 225
evaluate, in PAUSE method, 102, 104
evaluation codes, *195*, 195–196
evaluation report, 184
  in health care settings, 229
evaluation(s)
  for autism spectrum disorder and ADHD, 340–341
  child-centered, 167
  of children with special health care needs, 333, *333*
  culturally and linguistically appropriate, 131
  defined, 47, 129, 130, 195
  for developmental trauma, 353
  documentation of, *146,* 149
  for early intervention, 121–123, *122,* 124–125, 129–135, *134*
  education, 167
  family-centered, 131, *131*

in health care settings, 199–204
  of hearing loss, 312–314
  of large motor coordination, 275, *276*
  for neonatal abstinence syndrome, 351
  occupational therapy assistant assisting with, 35
  of play, 302–304, *303, 304*
  for preschool, 165–170
  role of occupational therapy practitioner in, *366*
  of social skills, 293–294, *294*
  for special education, 159
  telehealth for, 400
  of visual impairments, 321–323, *323*
Every Moment Counts, 163, 354, 355
Every Student Succeeds Act (ESSA, 2015)
  accountability expectations in, 47
  on criteria for identification of evidence, 373, *374*
  on guidelines for occupational therapy services in early intervention and schools, *362,* 364, 365
  history of, 9
  multitiered systems of support in, 162
everyday items and activities
  assessment tools for, 385
  in early intervention, *139,* 140
everyday leadership, 43
evidence
  analysis of, 371–372
  findings and outcomes based on, 372
  guidelines for identification of, 373–374, *374*
  levels of, 372
  risk of bias in, 372
  strength of, 372, *373*
  synthesis of, 372, *373*
  types of, 371
evidence-based interventions, 373–375, *374*
  data gathering during, 53
  defined, 373
  by occupational therapy assistants, 35
evidence-based practice (EBP), 371–375
  analyzing evidence in, 371–372
  course objectives for, *28*
  defined, 371, *372*
  in education law, 373–375, *374*
  in professional guidelines, 363
  resources on, 375
  synthesizing evidence in, 372, *373*
  types of evidence in, 371
  use in practice of, 375
executive functioning skills, 110
  with hearing loss, 315

Expanded Child-Centered AT Plan, 58
exploratory play, 303
expressive language, 281
extended school year (ESY), 161
extreme stress, maternal, 90

F
familiar sounds audiogram, 310, *311*
family(ies)
   adjustment to acquired conditions
      by, 219–220
   with autism spectrum disorder,
      341–342
   checking in with, 105
   of children with special health care
      needs, 329–330, *330*
   collaboration with, *72*
   displaced, 138
   diversity of, 147–148
   transition supports for, 79
family capacity building, 66–67
   in early intervention, 138
   for transitions, 83
family-centered approach
   for ADHD, 342
   to transitions, *82*, 82–83
family-centered care, 7, 63
Family-Centered Care Project, 6
family-centered goals, 67
family-centered practice, 23, *28*
   for early intervention, 131
   implementation of, 64–66
family-centered services, for
   transitions, 81–83, *82*
family coaching, for developmental
   trauma, 354
family concerns, in early childhood
   team report, 391–392
family-directed assessment, for Part
   C services, 130–131
family education
   on acquired conditions, 222, 223
   for ADHD, 342
Family Educational Rights and
   Privacy Act (FERPA, 1974), 73–74,
   145, 181–182, *362*, 399
family engagement
   documentation of, *147*, 147–148
   leadership in, 41
family outcome measurement, for
   early intervention, 123, 125
family partnerships, 63–69
   for activities of daily living, 238
   cultural competence and reciprocity
      in, 66
   defined, 63
   in early intervention, 68, 69
   embedding interventions in family
      routines in, 65–66
   family capacity building in, 66–67
   family-centered goals in, 67

family resources and supports in, 67
   how practice models changed over
      time to address, 63–64
   implementation of, 64–66
   listening to parent concerns in, 66
   in outpatient clinic, 68
   overview of, 63
   participatory practice in, 63
   positive, 63
   for preschool, 68, 166–167, 178
   relational practice in, 63
   with siblings, 65
   strength-based approach in, 66–67, *67*
   in telehealth, 69
   theoretical perspectives that inform,
      64, *65*
family-practitioner relationships, in
   early intervention, 142
family priorities, in early childhood
   team report, 392
family resources, 67
family routines
   in early childhood team report, 391
   embedding interventions in, 65–66
family service coordinator, for early
   intervention, 121, 124, 130
family supports, 4, 67
fear circuitry, 95
fecal incontinence, 238
federal laws, 26, 33–34
   supporting assistive technology,
      55–56
federal policies
   on autism spectrum disorder and
      ADHD, 339
   and occupational therapy services
      in early intervention and schools,
      361–362, *362–363*
feedback, for cerebral palsy, *277*
feeding. *See also* nutrition
   for children with special health care
      needs, 244–247, 331, *332*
   complementary, 250–251
   defined, 243
   social implications during, 252
feeding difficulties, due to neonatal
   abstinence syndrome, 352
feeding on demand, and cognitive
   development, 260
feeding skills, evaluation of, 250
feeding tubes, 252, 331, *332*
fetal alcohol effects, 348
fetal alcohol spectrum disorder (FASD)
   defined, 348
   and delays in development of social
      skills, 292
   diagnostic criteria for, 348
   effects of, 348
   evaluation for, 351
   health care considerations and
      impact on participation of, *331*

impact on brain development and
   developmental milestones of, 91,
   348
interventions for, 351–352
life course approach to, 350–351
protective factors for, 348
resources on, 355
fidelity, *33*
   of implementation, 53–54, *54*
fieldwork, in educational preparation,
   24–25
fieldwork educators, 24
financial requirements, for early
   intervention, 120
findings, evidence-based, 372
fine motor activities, 269, 269–270
fine motor coordination, 265–270
   additional interventions to enhance,
      269, 269–270
   assessment tools for, 267, *267*
   with cerebral palsy, 268
   defined, 265
   development of, 265, *266*
   evidence-based interventions for,
      267–268
   occupational profile for, 266–267,
      267
   overview of, 265
fine motor delay, 265
Finnegan Neonatal Abstinence
   Scoring System (FNASS), 348, 351
First Chance projects, 5
first-degree burns, 217
First Step Screening Test for
   Evaluating Preschoolers, *169*
food allergies, 247
food groups, 243, *244*
food modifications, 251–252
forced choice, of foods, 252
formal measures, in team evaluation
   report, 394
forward chaining, for dressing,
   grooming, and hygiene, 239
free appropriate public education
   (FAPE), 6, 158
frequency, 48
frequency chart, 51, *51*
Froebel, Friedrich, 13
function object use, 320
Function Scheme: Functional Skills
   Assessment, *323*
fruits, *244*
function object use, 320
Function Scheme: Functional Skills
   Assessment, *323*
functional assessment, for early
   intervention, 131–132
functional behavioral assessment
   (FBA), 293
functional communication training
   (FCT), 285

Functional Evaluation for Early Technology form, 58

Functional Feeding Assessment–Modified, 250

functional IFSP outcomes, 149–150, *150*

Functional Independence Measure for Children (Wee-FIM), *203, 237, 267, 275, 276*

functional mobility, in health care setting, *210*

functional performance, observation of, 393–395

functional play, 303

Functional Vision and Learning Media Assessment Kit, *323*

funding sources

for assistive technology, 60

for autism spectrum disorder and ADHD, 339

fussy eating, 243, 253

G

G (gastric/gastrostomy) tube, *332*

Galloway, Cole, 58

gastric (G) tube, *332*

gastroesophageal reflux disease (GERD), nutrition with, 246

gastrojejunal (GJ) tube, *332*

gastrostomy (G) tube, *332*

general supervision, 32

gestures, 283

Get Ready intervention, 112, 261

Glasgow Coma Scale (GCS), 216

gluten-free/casein-free (GFCF) diet, for autism spectrum disorder, 245

Goal Attainment Scaling (GAS), 50, *50, 75, 267, 275, 276*

goal line, *48*, 48–49

goal(s), 48

family-centered, 67

in health care settings, 229, *230*

Goals-Activity-Motor Enrichment program, 277

Go Baby Go, 58–59

grains, *244*

grasp pattern development, 265, *266*

Griffiths Mental Development Scales, *259*

grooming, 236, 239–240

in health care setting, *210*

Gross Motor Function Classification System, 275, *276*

Gross Motor Function Measure, 275, *276*

group interventions, in preschool, 176

Guidelines for Documentation of Occupational Therapy (AOTA), 225

Guidelines for Occupational Therapy in Early Intervention and Schools (AOTA), 27

Guidelines for Occupational Therapy Services in School Systems (AOTA), 6

gustatory receptors, 92

gustatory system, development of, 92

H

habilitation, 193, 219

habit(s)

assessment tools for, 387

defined, 203

to support mealtime, 252

hair care, 236, 239–240

halal foods, *248*

Halo Project, 354

Handicapped Children's Early Education Assistance Act (1968), 5

handwriting intervention, in Head Start, 268

handwriting tasks, 110

Handwriting Without Tears–Get Set for School program, 112

Hanft, Barbara, 6

haram foods, *248*

hard of hearing. *See* hearing loss

Hawaii Early Learning Inventory for Preschoolers, *169*

Hawaii Early Learning Profile, *134, 323*

Head Start program

handwriting intervention In, 268

history of, 5, 6

literacy learning support from, 112

multicultural principles for, 18, *18*

purpose of, 14, *16*

transition to kindergarten from, 81

Head Start Research-Based Developmentally Informed intervention, 261

health care

accountability expectations for, 48

for autism spectrum disorder and ADHD, 340

defined, 207

health care delivery, key concepts in, 208, *208*

health care interventions

for acquired conditions, 215–223

for developmental conditions, 207–212

health care needs. *See* children with special health care needs (CSHCN)

health care providers, coordination with, 330

health care services

coding and billing for, 194–196, *195*

commitment to ethical practice for, 197

communication with medical home provider on, 197

credentialing for, 193–194

denials of payment for, 197–198

documentation of, 197, 225–232

goals of, 197

in managed care organizations, 194, *194*

medical necessity of, 193

payer requirements for, 194, 197

health care settings

collaboration in, *73*

defined, 225

evaluation in, 199–204

evaluation of social skills in, 293–294

occupational therapy assistants in, 34

occupational therapy role in, *208,* 208–209

referral for, 225–226

Health Insurance Portability and Accountability Act (HIPAA, 1996)

on documentation of early intervention services and outcomes, 145

on documentation of health care services and outcomes, 225, 226

influence on occupational therapy practice of, *362*

on interprofessional collaboration, 73–74

on protected health information, 193

and telehealth, 399

health literacy, 147, *147*, 226

with children with special health care needs, 330

health needs. *See* children with special health care needs (CSHCN)

Health Net Federal Services, *194*

health promotion, in preschool intervention, 175

health screening, in team evaluation report, 395

Healthy, Hunger-Free Kids Act (2010), *363*

healthy working alliance, 101

hearing aids, 310–312, *312*

hearing loss, 309–316

acquired, 309

cognitive and executive functioning with, 315

communication approaches for, 312, *313*

conductive, *310*

congenital, 309

cultural considerations for, 312

data collection for, 315

diagnosis of, 310, *311*

disabilities and delays with, 309

evaluation of, 312–314

fluctuating *vs.* stable, *310*
hearing devices and technology for, 310–312, *312*
interventions for, 314–315, *315,* 316
mild, *310*
mixed, *310*
moderate, *310*
overview of, 309
postlingual, 309–310
prelingual, 309
profound, *310*
screening for, 309, 395
sensorineural, *310*
severe, *310*
social and play skills for, 314
sudden *vs.* progressive, *310*
symmetrical *vs.* asymmetrical, *310*
types and causes of, 309–310, *310*
unilateral *vs.* bilateral, *310*
vestibular dysfunction and sensory processing with, 314–315, 316
with visual impairment, 324–325, *325*
hearing test, 310, *311*
hemianopsia, 320
hemorrhagic stroke, 216
HighScope curriculum, *19*
HighScope Educational Research Foundation, 14, *15*
HIPAA. *See* Health Insurance Portability and Accountability Act (HIPAA, 1996)
hippotherapy, 277
history of early childhood programs and services, 3–7
  in 1950s: forget and hide, 5
  in 1960s: screen and segregate, 5, *5*
  in 1970s: identify and help, 5–6
  in 1980s: train and deliver, 6–7
  in 1990s: collaboration and accountability, 7
  in 2000–2010: family-centered, child-focused collaborative partnerships, 7
  in 2010–present: participation, parent coaching, interprofessional collaboration, 7, *8*
home
  transition from hospital to, 83
  transitions to IDEA Part B from, 80, *80*
home-based parent coaching, for fine and visual-motor development, 268
home care, documentation in, 227, *228, 230*
home environment, and literacy, 110–111
home health care teams, communication with, 201

home health services, 209
home medical devices, for children with special health care needs, 332
home nursing, for children with special health care needs, 329
home settings
  collaboration in, 72–73, *73*
  health care interventions for developmental conditions in, 209
  occupational therapy assistants in, 34
hospital, transition to home and community from, 83
hospital teams, communication with, 200
Humana Group, *194*
hygiene, 236, 239–240
  in health care setting, *210*
hypotension, orthostatic, 220
hypothesis(es)
  formulation and testing of, 167
  in health care settings, 201
  working, 52–53

I

imitation, 258
implementation
  documentation of, 150
  fidelity of, 53–54, *54*
implementation review, 151–152
implicit learning, for cerebral palsy, *277*
Improving Head Start for School Readiness Act (2009), *362*
inclusion, early childhood, 18
inclusive practices, in preschool, 162
inclusive services, for social participation, 286
individualized education program (IEP)
  and accountability expectations, 48
  assistive technology in, 56
  for children with special health care needs, 334
  collaboratively developed, 184–185, *185*
  components of, 160
  development of, 159–160
  evaluation of social skills in, 293
  goals of, 169, 184, *185*
  implementation of, 175
  and occupational therapy assistants, 33–34
  progress report to family on, 185–186, *187*
  in transitions, *80,* 81
individualized education program (IEP) progress note, 185–186, *187*
individualized family service plan (IFSP)
  and accountability expectations, 48

assistive technology in, 56
defined, 133–135, 137
development, review, and evaluation of, *122,* 123, 125, 133–135
documentation of, 145, 147, *147*
evaluation of social skills in, 293
and occupational therapy assistants, 33–34
individualized family service plan (IFSP) outcomes, 149–151, *150–152*
individualized family service plan (IFSP) review, 149
individualized health plan (IHP), for children with special health care needs, 334
Individuals with Disabilities Education Act (IDEA, 1986)
  and accountability expectations, 48
  on assistive technology, 56
  history of, 6, 7, 9
  and leadership, 39
  and occupational therapy assistants, 33
  on scientifically based research, 373
  and special education, 13
  transitions under, 79–81, *80*
Individuals with Disabilities Education Act (IDEA, 1986) Part B
  on annual progress report, 186–187
  for autism spectrum disorder and ADHD, 339
  on billing for services, 182
  on coaching and consultation, 177, *178*
  on collaboration, 174, 176
  on confidentiality of records, 181–182
  on developing partnership with parents, 178
  on discharge planning, 176, 188
  on documentation, 181–189, *182*
  on early childhood outcomes, 161, 188
  on embedded learning opportunities, 176–177, *177*
  on environmental factors, 174
  evaluation and eligibility for, 159
  evaluation of social skills under, 293
  extended school year under, 161
  and free appropriate public education, 158
  on inclusive practices, 162
  individualized education program under, 159–160, 175, 184–186, *185, 187*
  influences on occupational therapy practice of, *362*
  on initiating services, 182–183

on interventions, 173–179
laws and IEP process under,
    157–163
least restrictive environment under,
    160–161, 176
and local education agency,
    158–159
on multitiered systems of support,
    162–163, 165, 166, 173–174
on occupational therapy
    intervention plan, 175, 185, *185*
on occupational therapy outcomes,
    188
on occupational therapy practice
    framework, *175*, 175–176
on ongoing data collection, 178
overview of, 157–158, *158*
performance indicators under, 158,
    158
procedural safeguards under, 161
on reevaluation report, 187–188
reimbursement for, 363
related services under, 160
resources on, 178–179
roles of occupational therapy
    practitioners in, *366–368*
on screening and evaluation,
    165–170, 183–184
on service delivery in natural
    context and routines, 176–177
and special education process,
    159–161
on state practice act, 183
transition planning under, 161–162,
    188
transitions from home or
    community to, 80, *80*
transitions from Part C to, 79–80,
    80
on universal design for learning,
    174, *174*
Individuals with Disabilities
    Education Act (IDEA, 1986)
    Part C
    for autism spectrum disorder and
        ADHD, 339
    on child and family outcome
        measurement, 123, 125
    on contracts and interagency
        agreements, 120
    on definition of developmental
        delay, 121
    documentation under, 145–152, *146*
    early intervention law and process
        of, 119–126
    evaluation of social skills under, 293
    on family service coordination, 124
    on financial requirements, 120
    on flexibility to serve children
        beyond age 3 years and birth
        mandate, 121

history of, 119
on IFSP development, review, and
    evaluation, 123, 125
influences on occupational therapy
    practice of, *362*
interventions under, 137–142, *139*
on lead agency designation, 120, 145
overview of, 119
to Part B from, 79–80, *80*
on personnel standards and
    personnel development system,
    120–121
on procedural safeguards, 123
on providing service in context of
    team, 125–126
on providing service in natural
    environments, 124
on public awareness and Child
    Find, 121
reimbursement for, 363
roles of occupational therapy
    practitioners in, *366–368*
on screening, evaluation, and
    assessment, 121–123, *122*,
    124–125, 129–135, *134*
on service coordination, 121
on service delivery, 123
state eligibility criteria for, 130–131
on supervision and monitoring, 120
on transition, 124, 126
transitions from hospital to, 79
infant massage, for neonatal
    abstinence syndrome, 352
infant mental health (IMH), and
    transitions, 81–82
infectious diseases, acquired brain
    injury due to, 216–217
inflammatory bowel disease (IBD),
    nutrition with, 246
informal measures, in team
    evaluation report, 394
informed clinical opinion, 130
initial evaluation
    in health care example, 397–398
    in health care settings, *228*, 228–229
initial team evaluation report,
    sample, 393–396
initiation of services, documentation
    requirements for, 182–183
inpatient health care, collaboration
    in, 71–72
inpatient hospital settings
    documentation in, 226–227, *228*,
        230
    health care interventions for
        developmental conditions in,
        208–209
instrumental activities of daily living
    (IADLs), assessment tools for, 385
Intellectual and Developmental
    Disabilities Research Centers, 5

Intentional Relationship Model
    (IRM), 104–105
interagency agreements, for early
    intervention, 120
interdisciplinary approach, to
    assistive technology, 57
interdisciplinary standardized care
    plans, 72
interdisciplinary team, for evaluation
    in health care settings, 200–201
interdisciplinary therapeutic feeding
    teams, 244
interests
    in early childhood team report, 391
    in team evaluation report, 396
internal validity, 374
International Classification of
    Diseases (ICD) codes, 182,
    194–195
interoception
    development of, 93
    and toileting skills, 236
interprofessional collaboration,
    74–75
    with acquired conditions, 219
    communication strategies for, 74, *74*
    at community level, 74, *74*
    course objectives for, *28*
    for developmental conditions in
        health care setting, 207, *208*
    in early intervention, 139
    history of, 7
    with occupational therapy
        assistants, 34
    at policy level, 75
interprofessional collaborative
    practice (IPCP), 26, 27, *27*, 39
interprofessional communication, 26
interprofessional concepts, with
    course objectives, 27, *28*
interprofessional education (IPE), 23,
    25–26, *26*
interprofessional practice, 25–26, *26*
intervention goals, 185
intervention plan
    in early intervention, *146*, 150
    in health care settings, *228*, 229, *230*
    in preschool, 175
    template for, *381*
intervention targets, in team
    evaluation report, 396
intervention(s)
    approaches to, 185
    for autism spectrum disorder and
        ADHD, 341–342
    for children with special health care
        needs, 333
    for cognitive development, 260–261
    for communication, *284*, 284–287
    for developmental trauma, 353–354
    documentation of, 150–152

early (*see* early intervention (EI))
embedded in family routines, 65–66
to facilitate literacy, 260–261
for fine and visual-motor coordination, 267–268
group, 176
handwriting, 268
health care, 207–212, 215–223
for healthy eating, 250–253
for hearing loss, 314–315, *315,* 316
for large motor coordination, 275–277
oral-motor, 251
peer-mediated, 286
for postnatal trauma, 353–354
for prenatal substance exposure, 351–352
in preschool, 173–179
sensory-based, 296, 341
for social skills, 294–296, *296*
to support occupations in preschool, 176
telehealth, 399, 400
types of, 185
for visual impairments, 323–324, *324*
for visual–motor coordination, 267–270, *269*
interview
routines-based, 133, *134*
in team evaluation report, 393
intraprofessional collaboration, *73,* 73–74
irritable bowel syndrome (IBS), nutrition with, 246
ischemic stroke, 216
Islam, dietary practices and restrictions in, *248*

J
Jainism, dietary practices and restrictions in, *248*
jejunal tube, *332*
joint attention, 258
joint preservation, with acquired conditions, 221
Judaism, dietary practices and restrictions in, *249*
justice, *33*

K
Kaiser Permanente, *194*
kangaroo care
and cognitive development, 261
for neonatal abstinence syndrome, 352
for sleep and rest, 240
to support caregiver-infant attachment, 294
Kids in Transition to School (KITS), 112, 261

Kielhofner's Model of Human Occupation, 27, 28
kindergarten
transition from Head Start to, 81
transition from preschool to, 81, 84–85
Knox Preschool Play Scale, revised, *134*
kosher foods, *249*

L
language
defined, 281
expressive, 281
pragmatic, 281
receptive, 281
language decoding, 258
large motor coordination, 273–278
additional interventions for, 277, *278*
with cerebral palsy, 277, *277*
defined, 273
development of, 273–274, *274*
evaluation of, 275, *276*
evidence-based interventions for, 275–277
overview of, 273
large motor delay, 273
late referral, 80–81
lead agency, for early intervention, 120, 145
leadership, 39–44
adaptive (social), 42–43
best practices for, 41–43
in cultural competency, 41
defined, 39
and demographics of workforce, 39–40
in education, 41
essential considerations for, 40–41
everyday, 43
in family engagement, 41
and interprofessional collaborative practice, 29
in mental health, 40
by occupational therapy assistants, 35–36, *36*
overview of, 39–40
in physical health, 40
in poverty, 40–41
relevant background for, 40
resources on, 43, *44*
role of occupational therapy practitioners in, *368*
technical, 41–42
Leadership Education in Neurodevelopmental and Related Disabilities (LEND) programs, 5, 27–29
Learn the Signs. Act Early. (LTSAE) campaign, 100, 339
learning
promotion of, 111–113

with visual impairment, 320
learning activities
additional opportunities for, 27–29
in educational preparation, 24, *25*
learning difficulties, literacy with, 112
Learning Disabilities Association of America (LDAA), 4
Learning Media Assessment, for visual impairments, 322–323
least restrictive environment (LRE), 160–161, 176, 364
Leber's congenital amaurosis, *322*
legal blindness, 319
legislative influences, on occupational therapy services in early intervention and schools, 361–362, *362–363*
leisure activities. *See* play
Let's Participate! Project, 57, 61
letters, rapid naming of, *111*
level of certainty, 372, *373*
licensure, influences on occupational therapy practice of, *363*
life course health development (LCHD), 350–351
lifelong learning, by occupational therapy assistants, 36
life skills, core, 95
lighting, for visual impairments, 323
linguistically appropriate evaluation practice, for Part C services, 131
Listening and Spoken Language (LSL) therapy, *313*
literacy, 109–113
adaptations and assistive technology for, 112–113
and behavioral difficulties, 109
defined, 258
with developmental disabilities and delays, 109
development of, 110, 258–259
in dual language learners, 111
emergent, 283
evidence-based interventions to facilitate, 260–261
formal opportunities for, 112
and handwriting concerns, 110
health, 147, *147,* 226
influence of home environment on, 110–111
informal opportunities for, 112
occupational therapy role in, 110
overview of, 109–110
predictors of achievement of, 110, *111*
in preschoolers at risk for learning difficulties, 112
in preschoolers with low socioeconomic status, 111, 112

in preschoolers with special needs, 112
promotion of, 111–113
and reading difficulties, 109
resources on, 113
and social participation, 287
stages of, 110
literacy development, 258–259
early, 110
emergent, 110
pre-, 110
literacy learning, early, 110
literacy-rich environments, 112
literacy skills, 109
local education agency (LEA), 157, 158–159
local policies, and occupational therapy services in early intervention and schools, 361–362, *362–363*
long-term memory, 258
low-FODMAP diet, 246
low vision. *See also* visual impairments
defined, 319
ocular, *324*

M
magnification, for visual impairments, 323
maintain, in preschool intervention, 175, *175*
Malaguzzi, Loris, 13
maltreatment, and delays in development of social skills, 292, 293
managed care, 194, *194*
managed care organizations (MCOs), 194, *194*
man-made trauma, 349
manual guidance, for cerebral palsy, *277*
Massachusetts Advocates for Children's Helping Traumatized Children, 355
massage
and cognitive development, 260–261
for neonatal abstinence syndrome, 352
and social skills, 295
mastery monitoring, *49,* 49–50
material modification, for dressing, grooming, and hygiene, 239–240
material(s), play, 305
Maternal, Infant, and Early Childhood Home Visiting (MIECHV), *15*
Maternal and Child Health Bureau, 3, 5
Maternal and Child Health Services programs, 4

Maternal–infant attachment, with neonatal abstinence syndrome, 352
maternal nutrition, and brain development, 90
maternal stress, and brain development, 90
meaningful activities, for cerebral palsy, *277*
meaningfulness, during play, 301
measurable IFSP outcomes, 149–150, *150*
Measurement of Engagement, Independence, and Social Relationships (MEISR), *134*
meats, *244*
mediated approach, to data gathering, 53
media use, and sleep, 240
Medicaid
billing for services with, 182
for early intervention, 120
influences on occupational therapy practice of, *362*
reimbursement from, 363
medical complications and precautions, with acquired conditions, 220–221
medical equipment, for children with special health care needs, 332
medical home provider, communication with, 197
medical necessity, 193
Medicare
National Correct Coding Initiative (NCCI) of, 196
reimbursement from, 182
Medicare Catastrophic Coverage Act (1988), 7
memory, 258
meningitis
bacterial, 217
viral, 216–217
mental health, 99–105
checking in with family for, 105
children at risk for concerns about, 99–100
co-occupational engagement in, 99
defined, 99
development of, 99
Intentional Relationship Model for, 104–105
leadership in, 40
overview of, 99–100
PAUSE method for, 102–104
play and, 302, 305
reflective supervision for, 104
relationships in, 100–102, *101*
resources and activities on, 105
role of occupational therapy in, 100
mental health conditions, 218

mental retardation, 5
mental status, changes in, 220–221
mentors, 24
metacognitive training, 342
methylphenidate (Ritalin), appetite loss due to, 245
microphthalmia, *322*
Military Child Education Coalition (MCEC), *15*
Miller Assessment for Preschoolers, *259*
Miller Function and Participation Scales, *134, 169, 294*
mindfulness, 295
minimum supervision, 32
Model of Co-Occupation, 27
Model of Human Occupation (MOHO), 27, 28
modeling
of play, 305
for social participation, 285
for transitions, 82, *82*
modifiers, 196
modify, in preschool intervention, 175
monitoring activities
for autism spectrum disorder and ADHD, 339–340, *340*
for early intervention, 120
Montessori, Maria, 13
Montessori approach, *19*
Mormonism, dietary practices and restrictions in, *249*
mother infant transaction program, 268
motor acquisition theories, in health care setting, 211, *211*
motor commands, 93
motor coordination
fine and visual–, 265–270
large, 273–278
motor development, 93, 273
motor planning, *278*
motor skills
assessment tools for, 386, 387
play and, 306
with visual impairment, 320
motor systems, 90
Movement Assessment Battery for Children, *169*
Multicultural Principles for Head Start Programs (Office of Head Start), 18, *18*
multidisciplinary evaluation and assessment, for early intervention, 129, 130
multisensory integration, development of, 92–93
multitiered systems of support (MTSS)
future of, 9

for preschool, 162–163, 165, 166, 173–174
for prevention of adverse childhood experiences and developmental trauma, 354
roles of occupational therapy practitioners in, 365
myelination, 90

N
name, writing of, *111*
nasal chemoreceptors, 92
nasoduodenal (ND) tube, *332*
nasogastric (NG) tube, *332*
nasojejunal (NJ) tube, *332*
National Association for Bilingual Education (NABE), *15*
National Association for Family, School, and Community Engagement (NAFSCE), *16*
National Association for Family Child Care (NAFCC), *16*
National Association for the Education of Young Children (NAEYC), 13, 14, *16*, 17, *17*, 18
National Association on Mental Illness (NAMI), *16*
National Black Child Development Institute (NBCDI), *16*
National Board Certification of Occupational Therapy (NBCOT), 31
National Center for Pyramid Model Innovations, *16*
National Child Traumatic Stress Network, 355
National Correct Coding Initiative (NCCI), 196
National Early Literacy Panel (NELP), 110
National Head Start Association (NHSA), *16*
National Provider Identifier (NPI), 193–194
National Society for Autistic Children, 4
National Society for Crippled Children, 4
national technical assistance centers, 14
natural context
activities of daily living in, 238
play in, 303
for preschool, 176
natural environments
advocacy for, 18
for early intervention, 124, 137, 138, *139*, 139–140
for transitions, 83
for visual impairment, 321
natural trauma, 349

naturalistic instruction, *19*
neglect, 349
Neo-Digestin (digestive enzyme supplement), for autism spectrum disorder, 245
neonatal abstinence syndrome (NAS)
advocacy for prevention of, 354
best practices for, 351–354
defined, 347–348
essential considerations with, 350–351
evaluation of, 351
interventions for, 351–352
life course approach to, 350–351
resources on, 355
neonatal intensive care unit (NICU)
documentation in, 226, *228*, *230*
health care interventions for developmental conditions in, 208
neonatal abstinence syndrome in, 351–352
transition to home from, 83
network building, 43
neural circuits, 90
neural development, 89
neurobehavioral disorder associated with prenatal alcohol exposure (ND-PAE), 348
neurodevelopment, 89–95
of autonomic nervous system, 91
and cognitive development, 94
collaboration across systems to support, 94
core concepts of, 90–91
cutting-edge science to enhance, 94–95
defined, 89
of emotions, 93–94
identify needs and make referrals related to, 94
impact of maternal nutrition and extreme stress on, 90
in utero, 90–91
and motor development, 93
overview of, 89
prenatal exposure to toxicants and, 91
resources on, 95
of selective attention, 93
of sensory systems and sensory processing, 91–93
neurodevelopmental disorder, alcohol-related, 348
neurodevelopmental perspective, 89
neurodevelopmental theories, in health care setting, 211
neurological disorders, nutrition with, 246–247
neuron(s), 90
neuroplasticity, 90, 217, 219

Newborn Individualized Developmental Care and Assessment Program (NIDCAP), 260
No Child Left Behind Act (2001), 373–374
nocturnal enuresis, 239
nonmaleficence, *33*
nontraumatic brain injuries, 216
norm-referenced assessments, for early intervention, 133
North American Reggio Emilia Alliance (NAREA), *16*
numbers, rapid naming of, *111*
nurse(s)
on interprofessional team, *208*
school, 334
nutrition, 243–253
adaptive equipment for, 251
with autism spectrum disorder, 244–245
with avoidant/restrictive food intake disorder, 245
for children with special health care needs, 244–247, 331, *332*
collaborative team model for, 253
complementary feeding for, 250–251
with diabetes, 246
dietary customs and practices for, 247, *248–249*
Dietary Reference Intakes for, 243
with digestive diseases, 246
with epilepsy, 246
evaluation of eating and feeding skills for, 250
feeding tubes for, 252
with food allergies, 247
food groups for, 243, *244*
food modifications for, 251–252
habits and routines to support, 252
interdisciplinary therapeutic feeding teams for, 244
interventions to support healthy eating for, 250–253
maternal, 90
with neurological disorders, 246–247
oral-motor interventions for, 251
overview of, 243
with phenylketonuria, 245–246
with pickiness, 243, 253
positioning for, 251
registered dietitian nutritionists for, 244, 253
resources on, 253
self-determination and force choice for, 252
with sensory issues, 247
social implications of, 252
swallow study for, 253
nystagmus, *322*

O

obesity, 40
object adaptations, for visual
    impairments, 323
object constancy, 320
object permanence, 320
object(s), rapid naming of, *111*
observation(s)
    of academic and functional
        performance, 393–395
    in child's environment and routines,
        168
    of eating and feeding skills, 250
    of play, 303, *303*
    for visual impairment, 321
occupation(s)
    assessment tools for, 385
    defined, 133
    in early intervention and school
        settings, 361
    in health care setting, 202, 210, *210*
    impact of special health care needs
        on, 330–332, *331, 332*
    interventions to support, 176
    play as, 304–306
    in preschool, 176
    and transitions, 83
occupational-centered practice, 283
occupational deprivation, 40
occupational performance analysis
    for early intervention, 133, *134*
    in health care setting, 201–204, *203,*
        229
    in initial evaluation, 397
    for preschool, 167–168, 184
occupational performance coaching,
    for activities of daily living, 238
occupational performance in daily
    routines, with autism spectrum
    disorder, 341
occupational profile
    for early intervention, 132–133
    for fine and visual–motor
        coordination, 266–267, *267*
    in health care setting, 201, *202,* 229
    in initial evaluation, 397
    for large motor coordination, 275
    for play, 302–303
    for preschool, 167, 184
    template for, 377–379, *378*
    for visual impairment, 321
occupational therapists (OTs),
    educational preparation for,
    23–29
occupational therapy assistants
    (OTAs)
    advocacy by, 35–36
    AOTA Code of Ethics for, 33, *33*
    assisting with screening and
        evaluations by, 35
    benefits of, 31–32

building strong relationships with,
    32–33
    in community settings, 34
    documentation by, 35
    educational preparation for, 23–29
    education requirements for, 31
    in education settings, 34
    evidence-based interventions by, 35
    in health care settings, 34
    in home settings, 34
    knowledge of federal, state, and
        local laws and policies by, 33–34
    leadership skills in, 35–36, *36*
    lifelong learning by, 36
    overview of, 31–32
    role of, 34, 35, *36*
    supervision of, 32–33
Occupational Therapy Code of Ethics
    (AOTA), 33, *33,* 56, 225
occupational therapy evaluation. *See
    also* evaluation(s)
    in health care setting, 199–204
    for preschool, 166, 184
occupational therapy intervention.
    See also intervention(s)
    documentation of, 185–187, *186,*
        187
    implementation of, 175
occupational therapy intervention
    plan, *146,* 185
    for developmental conditions in
        health care setting, 209–210, *210*
    in health care settings, *228,* 229, *230*
occupational therapy outcomes,
    documentation of, 152, 188
occupational therapy practice
    framework, for preschool, *175,*
    175–176
*Occupational Therapy Practice
    Framework: Domain and Process*
    (OTPF, AOTA), 7, 27, 201, 363
occupational therapy practitioners
    defined, 13
    on interprofessional team, *208*
    roles in early intervention and
        schools of, 365–368, *366–368*
occupation-based assessment
    practices, 284
occupation-based models, 27
ocular blindness, *324*
ocular low vision, *324*
ocular vision impairment, 319, *324*
Office of Economic Opportunity, 5
Office of Head Start, 18
Office of Special Education Programs
    (OSEP)
    history of, 5
    indicators and outcomes of, 81, 158,
        158
    and preschool laws, 157–158
olfactory system, development of, 92

ongoing assessment, for preschool,
    170
ongoing data collection, for
    preschool, 178
onlooker play, *303*
ophthalmologist, *208*
opioid exposure, prenatal, 347–348
opioid use disorder, 347
optic nerve atrophy, *322*
optic nerve hypoplasia, *322*
optometrist, *208*
oral hygiene, 236, 239–240
oral language, *111*
Oral Motor Assessment Scale, 250
Oral–motor interventions, 251
Oregon Project for Preschool
    Children Who Are Blind or
    Visually Impaired, *323*
Organisation Mondiale Pour
    L'Education Préscolaire (OMEP),
    16
organizational level, collaboration
    at, *72*
orientation, 320
orientation and mobility (O & M)
    instructor, 321
orthopedic precautions, with
    acquired conditions, 221
orthostatic hypotension, 220
orthotist, *208*
Oscar Health, *194*
outcomes
    based on evidence, 372
    child, 123, 125, 135, *148, 149,*
        169–170
    documentation of, 152, 188
    early child, 188
    for emotional skills, 296, *296*
    evidence-based, 372
    family, 123, 125
    functional IFSP, 149–150, *150*
    in occupational therapy
        intervention plan, 185
    of play, 304, *304*
    for preschool, 188
    for self-regulation skills, 296, *296*
    with special education, 161
    for transitions, 81
outpatient clinic
    collaboration in, 72
    communication with health care
        team in, 201
    documentation in, 227, *228, 230*
    family partnerships in, 68
    health care interventions for
        developmental conditions in, 209
outside play, in team evaluation
    report, 394, 395
overstimulation, in neonatal
    abstinence syndrome, 351–352
oxygen, supplemental, 332

P

PACER Center, 61, *330*
parallel play, *303*
parasympathetic responses, 91
parent coaching
  for developmental conditions, 211
  for fine and visual-motor
    development, 268
  history of, 7
  for sleep, 240
parent education, on cognitive
  development, 260–261
parent self-efficacy, with autism
  spectrum disorder, 341–342
parent storytelling, 67
Parent to Parent USA, *330*
parent–child interaction therapy
  (PCIT), 295
parent(s)
  on interprofessional team, *208*
  listening to concerns of, 66
parental consent, 225
Parents Interactions With Infants
  (PIWI), *26*
pareve foods, *249*
participation, 7
participation-based IFSP outcomes,
  149–150, *150*
participation-focused, authentic,
  collaborative, and explicit (PACE)
  data collection, 334
participatory practice, in family
  partnerships, 63
partnerships
  and collaboration, 75
  family, 63–69
Patient Protection and Affordable
  Care Act (ACA, 2010), 193
PAUSE method, 102–104
payer requirements, 194
payment, 193–198
  coding and billing for, 194–196,
    195, 196
  communication with medical home
    provider and, 197
  credentialing and, 193–194
  denials of, 197–198
  documentation and, 197
  for early intervention, 139
  ethical practice and, 197
  in managed care organizations, 194,
    194
  overview of, 193
  varying requirements for, 194, 197
payment sources
  for acquired conditions, 220
  for health care interventions for
    developmental conditions, 209
  in health care settings, 226
payor requirement, for telehealth,
  399

Peabody Developmental Motor
  Scales-2 (PDMS-2)
  in early intervention, *134*
  for fine and visual-motor skills, *267*
  in health care settings, *203*
  in initial evaluation, 397
  for large motor coordination, *276*
  in preschool evaluation, *169*
PEAT's (Physical Environment and
  Assistive Tools) Suite, 61
Pediatric Evaluation of
  Developmental Inventory (PEDI),
  134, 203, 237
Pediatric Evaluation of Disability
  Inventory, *169, 276, 294*
Pediatric Functional Independence
  Measure II (WeeFIM), *203, 237,
  267, 275, 276*
Pediatric Interest Profiles, *304*
pediatric stroke, 216
peer-mediated intervention, for
  social participation, 286
peer-mediated social strategies, 286
Peptizyde (digestive enzyme
  supplement), for autism spectrum
  disorder, 245
perceive, in PAUSE method, 102–103
perceptual functions, 258
performance analysis, in team
  evaluation report, 396
performance-based measurement,
  48, 48–49
performance patterns
  assessment tools for, 387
  evaluation in health care setting of,
    203–204
performance skills
  assessment tools for, 386–387
  evaluation in health care setting of,
    203
perinatal postpartum depression, *101*
perinatal risks, of postnatal trauma,
  349
perinatal stroke, 216
peripheral nervous system (PNS), 90
Perry Preschool Project, 14
personal care, 236, 239–240
personal context, assessment tools
  for, 387
personal device care, in health care
  setting, *210*
personal factors, in preschool, 174
personal frequency modulation
  system, 312
Person-Environment-Occupation
  (PEO) model, 277
Person-Environment-Occupation-
  Participation (PEOP) model, 27,
  210–211, 259
personnel development system, for
  early intervention, 120–121

personnel preparation, 23–29
  best practices for, 26–29
  essential considerations for, 24–26
  overview of, 23
personnel shortages, 40
personnel standards, for early
  intervention, 120–121
phenylalanine (Phe), in
  phenylketonuria, 245–246
phenylketonuria (PKU), nutrition
  with, 245–246
philanthropy, 4
phonological awareness, *111*
phonological memory, *111*
physical activities, for ADHD, 342
physical context, assessment tools
  for, 387
Physical Environment and Assistive
  Tools (PEAT's) Suite, 61
physical exercise, for ADHD, 342
physical health, leadership in, 40
physical skills. *See* fine motor
  coordination; large motor
  coordination
physical therapist, *208*
physical trauma injuries, 218
physician, on interprofessional team,
  208
Physicians Mutual, *194*
picky eating, 243, 253
Picture Exchange Communication
  System (PECS), 341
Pidgin Signed English (PSE), *313*
Plan-Do-Review format, 14
plan of care
  for developmental conditions in
    health care setting, 209–210, *210*
  in early intervention, *146*, 150
  in health care settings, *228, 229, 230*
plasticity, in life course health
  development framework, 351
play, 301–306
  adapting context of, 304–305
  adapting materials for, 305
  assessment tools for, 303–304, *304,
    385*
  assistive technology for, 58
  associative, *303*
  benefits of, 301–302
  during caregiving routines, 302
  for children with special health care
    needs, 331
  constructive, 303
  contextual influences on, 302
  as co-occupation, 301
  cooperative, *303*
  defined, 301
  desired outcomes of, 304, *304*
  enhancing self-care through, 306
  enhancing social interactions
    through, 305

exploratory, 303
functional, 303
in health care setting, *210*
impact of delays and disabilities on, 302
as learning opportunity, 301–302
meaningfulness during, 301
and mental health, 302, 305
modeling of, 305
in natural contexts and routines, 303
observation of, 303, *303*
as occupation, 304–306
occupational profile for, 302–303
onlooker, *303*
overview of, 301
parallel, *303*
pretend, 305
progress monitoring of, 306
promoting motor skills through, 306
prompting of, 305
social, 303, *303*
solitary, *303*
symbolic, 303, 305
in team evaluation report, 394, 395
with toys and objects, 303, *303*
Play Assessment Scale, *304*
play-based assessment, for early intervention, 131–132
play materials, 305
play outcomes, 304, *304*
play performance, with autism spectrum disorder, 341
play skills
with hearing loss, 314
with visual impairment, 320
point-of-service documentation, 148
policy level, collaboration at, *72,* 75
positioning
for feeding, 251
for neonatal abstinence syndrome, 351–352
positioning equipment, for feeding, 251
positioning systems, for children with special health care needs, 332
positive behavior interventions and supports (PBIS), 162, 293, 295
postlingual hearing loss, 309–310
postnatal trauma, 347–355
ACE Pyramid for, 349, *349*
ACE Study of, 348–349
advocacy for prevention of, 354
defined, 348
developmental, 349
evaluation of, 353
impact on brain development and developmental milestones of, 349–350
interventions for, 353–354

life course approach to, 350–351
overview of, 347
resources on, 355
risk factors for, 349
trauma-informed care for, 350
postpartum depression (PPD)
perinatal, *101*
and relationships, *101*
posttraumatic stress disorder (PTSD), 348
poverty, leadership in, 40–41
power mobility needs, for assistive technology, 58–59
practice frameworks, 27
pragmatic language, 281
praxis, *278*
preferences, in early childhood team report, 391
pre-kindergarten, universal, 14
prelingual hearing loss, 309
preliteracy development, 110
premature infants, cognitive development of, 260–261
prematurity, retinopathy of, *322*
prenatal alcohol exposure, 348
prenatal cannabis exposure, 348
prenatal risks, of postnatal trauma, 349
prenatal substance exposure, 347–355
to alcohol, 348
defined, 347
evaluation of, 351
interventions for, 351–352
life course approach to, 350–351
to opioids, 347–348
to other substances, 348
overview of, 347
resources on, 355
prenatal tobacco exposure, 348
prenatal toxicant exposure, 91
preschool
annual progress report for, 186–187
assistive technology in, 56
for autism spectrum disorder and ADHD, 339, 340
billing for services in, 182
Child Find system for, 159, 166, 183
for children with special health care needs, 333–334
coaching and consultation for, 177, *178*
collaboration for, 72, *73*, 174, 176
confidentiality of records for, 181–182
discharge planning for, 176, 188
documentation for, 181–189, *182*
early childhood outcomes in, 161, 188
embedded learning opportunities in, 176–177, *177*

environmental factors in, 174
evaluation and eligibility for, 159
extended school year for, 161
family partnerships for, 68, 166–167, 178
fine and visual-motor coordination in, 268
and free appropriate public education, 158
in health care setting, *210*
inclusive practices in, 162
individualized education program for, 159–160, 175, 184–186, *185, 187*
initiating services in, 182–183
intervention in, 173–179
large motor coordination in, 276–277
laws and IEP process for, 157–163
least restrictive environment for, 160–161, 176
and local education agency, 157, 158–159
multitiered systems of support for, 162–163, 165, 166, 173–174
occupational therapy intervention plan for, 175, 185, *186*
occupational therapy outcomes for, 188
occupational therapy practice framework for, *175,* 175–176
ongoing data collection for, 178
overview of, 157–158, *158*
performance indicators for, 158, *158*
procedural safeguards for, 161
reevaluation report for, 187–188
referral for special education evaluation for, 183–184
related services in, 160
resources on, 178–179
screening and evaluation for, 165–170, 183–184
service delivery in natural context and routines for, 176–177
social skills in, 295
and special education process, 159–161
and state practice act, 183
supports for, 166
transition from early intervention to, 84, 124, 126
transition planning from, 161–162, 188
transition to kindergarten from, 81, 84–85
universal, 14
universal design for learning in, 174, *174*
Preschool Activity Card Sort, *237*
Preschool and Kindergarten Behavior Scales, *294*

preschool grants program, 157
preschool performance indicators, 158, *158*
preschool programs, 173
preschool setting, collaboration in, 72, *73*
preschool teacher, on interprofessional team, *208*
President's Panel on Mental Retardation, 4
pretend play, 305
prevent, in preschool intervention, 175, *175*
primary memory, 258
primitive reflexive movements, 273
print knowledge, *111*
prior authorization, in health care settings, 227–228, *228*
prior written notice, 161
priorities, of care, 75
privacy, with telehealth, 399
Privacy Rule, 145, 193
problem solving, 258
procedural safeguards
    for early intervention, 123
    for preschool, 161
procedural visual supports, for social participation, 286
process skills, assessment tools for, 386, 387
professional influences, on occupational therapy services in early intervention and schools, 363–364
professional intervention plan, 150
professional organizations, 14, *15–16*
professionalism, *28*
    apply knowledge from, 26–27, *27*
programming needs, in team evaluation report, 395
progress monitoring, 48–50, *48–50*
    for developmental conditions in health care setting, 212
    of play, 306
progress report, *146*
    in health care settings, *228*, 230, *231*
progress toward outcomes, documentation of, 150–151
promote, in preschool intervention, 175
Promoting First Relationships (PFR), 352, 355
prompting, of play, 305
proprioceptive system, development of, 92
proprioceptors, 92
protected health information (PHI), 145, 193
proteins, *244*
Protestants, dietary practices and restrictions in, *249*

provider competence, with telehealth, 399
proximal development, zone of, 14
proximal relationships, 100–101
pruning, 90
public awareness, of early intervention, 121
public education, free appropriate, 6, 158
Public Protection of Maternity and Infancy Plan, 4
pulse oximeters, 332

Q
Qigong massage, 276
qualitative research, 371
Quality Indicators for Assistive Technology (QIAT), 60, 61
Quality of Upper Extremity Skills Test, *267*

R
radiation burns, 217
randomized controlled trial (RCT), 371
rapid naming of letters and digits, *111*
rapid naming of objects and colors, *111*
Rapid Toileting Training (RTT) method, 238
Read It Again prekindergarten (RIA-PreK) program, 112, 261
reading readiness, *111*
receptive language, 281
record review, in team evaluation report, 393
record(s), confidentiality of, 181–182
reduplicated and variegated babbling, 282
reevaluation
    documentation of, 149
    for early intervention, 135, 149
    in health care settings, *228*
    for preschool, 170
reevaluation report, 187–188
referral
    in early childhood team report, 391
    for health care settings, 225–226
    for preschool evaluation, 166
referral sources, for early intervention, 132
reflective practices, 99
reflective supervision, 104
reflexive movements, primitive, 273
Reggio Emilia approach, 13, *16, 19*
registered dietitian nutritionists (RDNs), 244, 253
regulation, for neonatal abstinence syndrome, 351–352

regulatory influences, on occupational therapy services in early intervention and schools, 361–362, *362–363*
rehabilitation, 219
Rehabilitation Act (1973), Section 504 of, 6, 159, *362*
reimbursement. *See* payment
related services, 160
relational attachment, for neonatal abstinence syndrome, 352
relational practice, in family partnerships, 63
relationship building, in context, 42–43
relationship theories, in health care setting, 211
relationship-based practices, in early intervention, *139*, 141–142
relationship-based programs, for neonatal abstinence syndrome, 352
relationship-centered practices, 99
relationship(s)
    and collaboration, 75
    defined, 100
    factors influencing, *101*, 101–102
    in mental health, 100–102, *101*
    proximal and distal, 100–101
religion-based dietary practices and restrictions, 247, *248–249*
religious activities, in health care setting, *210*
remediation, in preschool intervention, 175
remote instruction, 399
repetition, for cerebral palsy, *277*
repetitive behaviors, with autism spectrum disorder, 341
research
    on assistive technology, 60
    bias in, 372
    role of occupational therapy practitioners in, *368*
    scientifically based, 373–374
    types and methods of, 371
Research-Based Developmentally Informed program, 112
residential schools and institutions, 3
resilience, 95
resource(s)
    allocation of, 75
    of AOTA, 43, *44*, 383
    on assistive technology, 61
    on autism spectrum disorder and ADHD, 343
    on brain development, 95
    for early childhood practitioners, *8*
    early social, 4
    on evaluation in health care setting, 204

for evaluation in health care settings, 204
on evidence-based practice, 375
family, 67
on leadership, 43, *44*
on literacy, 113
on mental health, 105
on nutrition, 253
on occupational therapy services in early intervention and schools, 370
on preschool, 178–179
role of occupational therapy practitioner as, *368*
on social participation, 287
on telehealth, 400
resource-based interventions, in family partnerships, 67
response to intervention (RTI) framework, 365
responsibilities, 26
responsiveness, initiation of, 43
rest
  assessment tools for, 385
  best practices to support, 236–237, *237,* 240
  by children with special health care needs, 331–332
restore, in preschool intervention, 175
restoring function, with acquired conditions, 222–223
restricted and repetitive behaviors, with autism spectrum disorder, 341
retinitis pigmentosa, *322*
retinopathy of prematurity, *322*
Revised Knox Preschool Play Scale, *134, 304*
Ritalin (methylphenidate), appetite loss due to, 245
rituals, assessment tools for, 387
roles
  assessment tools for, 387
  in health care setting, 203
  in interprofessional practice, 26
  of occupational therapy practitioners, 365–368, *366–368*
Roll Evaluation of Activities of Life, *237*
Roman Catholicism, dietary practices and restrictions in, *249*
routine supervision, 32
routine(s)
  assessment tools for, 387
  in early childhood team report, 391
  in health care setting, 203
  social, 284–285
  to support mealtime, 252
  and transitions, 83
routines-based approach, to early intervention, *139,* 140–141

routines-based interventions, for developmental trauma, 354
routines-based interview, for early intervention, 133, *134*
rubrics, 50–51, *52*
RUMBA format, 229

S

safety, in health care setting, *210*
scaffolding, for social participation, 285
Scale for Assessment of Family Enjoyment Within Routines (SAFER), 140–141
Scales of Independent Behavior– Revised Personal Living subscale, *237*
Schedule for Oral Motor Assessment, 250
scheduling, of health care interventions for developmental conditions, 209
school health plans, for children with special health care needs, 334
School Mental Health Toolkit (AOTA), 40, 354, 355
school nurses, 334
school settings
  environmental and contextual influences on, 364–365
  guidelines for occupational therapy services in, 361–369
  legislation and regulatory influences on, 361–363, *362–363*
  occupations in, 361
  professional influences on, 363–364
schoolwide positive behavior support (SWPBS), 295
schoolwide systems of support, roles of occupational therapy practitioners in, *366*
school year, extended, 161
scientifically based research, 373–374
scoliosis, with acquired conditions, 221
screening
  for autism spectrum disorder and ADHD, 339–340, *340*
  defined, 129
  for early intervention, 121–123, *122,* 124–125, 129–135, *134*
  history of, 5
  occupational therapy assistant assisting with, 35
  for performance skills, 386
  for preschool, 165–170
screening report, 183
seating systems, for children with special health care needs, 332
secondary settings, health care interventions for developmental conditions in, 207

second-degree burns, 217
Section 504, of Rehabilitation Act (1973), 6, 159, *362*
segregation, 5
seizure disorders, health care considerations and impact on participation of, *331*
selective attention, development of, 93
self, therapeutic use of, 102
self-care routines, assistive technology for, 58
self-care skills, play and, 306
self-determination, of food choices, 252
self-efficacy, in early intervention, 138
self-evaluation, 76
self-feeding, in health care setting, *210*
self-regulation skills, 291–297
  defined, 292
  delays in development of, 292–293
  evaluation of, 293–294, *294*
  evidence-based interventions for, 294–296, *296*
  outcome and goal language for, 296, *296*
  overview of, 291–292
sensitive periods, in life course health development framework, 350–351
sensory-based interventions
  for autism spectrum disorder, 341
  for social, emotional, and self-regulation skills, 296
sensory-friendly events, 74
sensory integration
  for autism spectrum disorder, 341
  for developmental trauma, 353
  for social, emotional, and self-regulation skills, 296
sensory processing
  development of, 91–93
  with hearing loss, 314–315
sensory processing approach, for developmental trauma, 353
sensory processing disorder, nutrition with, 247
Sensory Processing Measure– Preschool, *294*
Sensory Profile 2, *134, 294*
sensory-rich environments, for developmental trauma, 353
Sensory Stories, 212
sensory strategies, 296
sensory systems
  defined, 90
  development of, 91–93
septo-optic dysplasia, *322*
service competency, 32

service coordinator
  for early intervention, 121, 124
  role of occupational therapy
    practitioner as, *367*
service delivery
  for early intervention, 123
  mechanisms for, 185
service provider, role of occupational
    therapy practitioner as, *367*
service(s), in telehealth, 399
Services for Crippled Children
    programs, 4
session treatment notes, in health
    care settings, 230, *231*
SETT (Student, Environments, Tasks,
    and Tools) framework, 58
Seventh-Day Adventists, dietary
    practices and restrictions in, *249*
Sheppard-Towner Maternity and
    Infancy Protection Act (1921), 4
short-term memory, 258
Shriver, Eunice Kennedy, 4
siblings, partnering with, 65
Signed Exact English (SEE), *313*
sign language, *313*
Sikhism, dietary practices and
    restrictions in, *249*
Simon Technology Center, 58, 61
Situation-Background-Assessment-
    Recommendation strategy, for
    collaboration, 74, *74*
skilled occupational therapy,
    documentation of, *146,* 146–147
skilled occupational therapy statement,
    in initial evaluation, 397–398
skin-to-skin contact, 294
sleep
  assessment tools for, 385
  best practices to support, 236–237,
    237, 240
  by children with special health care
    needs, 331–332
  in health care setting, *210*
sleep challenges, 236–237
small groups, in team evaluation
    report, 393, 394–395
snack time, in team evaluation
    report, 394, 395
SOAP ("subjective, objective,
    assessment, and plan") notes, 35,
    147, 230, *231*
social behaviors, 291
social cognition, 291
social competence, 291
social context
  assessment tools for, 387
  of play, 305
Social–Emotional Assessment
    Measure, *294*
Social–Emotional Learning theory, in
    health care setting, *211*

social–emotional performance skills,
    assessment tools for, 385
social–emotional reciprocity,
    282–283
social–emotional skills, 291–297
  defined, 291
  delays in development of, 292–293
  evaluation of, 293–294, *294*
  evidence-based interventions for,
    294–296, *296*
  outcome and goal language for, 296,
    296
  overview of, 291–292
social implications, during feeding,
    252
social interactions
  with autism spectrum disorder, 341
  and play, 305
social interaction skills, assessment
    tools for, 386, 387
social knowledge, 291
social leadership, 42–43
social occupations, in health care
    setting, *210*
social participation, 281–287
  assessment of, 284
  assessment tools for, 385
  augmentative and alternative
    interventions for, 286–287
  by children with special health care
    needs, 331
  choice making for, 285
  defined, 281
  development of, 281–283, *282*
  early indicators of delays in or
    disorders of, 283
  early literacy development and, 287
  essential considerations for,
    281–283
  functional communication training
    for, 285
  inclusive services for, 286
  interventions for, *284,* 284–287
  occupation-centered practice and,
    283
  overview of, 281
  peer-mediated social strategies for,
    286
  resources on, 287
  responding, modeling, and
    scaffolding for, 285
  routines for, 284–285
  and social-emotional reciprocity,
    282–283
  visual supports in, 285–286
social play, 303, *303*
social power, 42
social routines, 284–285
Social Security Act (1935), 4, *362*
social skills, 291–297
  defined, 291

delays in development of, 292–293
evaluation of, 293–294, *294*
evidence-based interventions for,
    294–296, *296*
with hearing loss, 314
outcome and goal language for, 296,
    296
overview of, 291–292
with visual impairment, 320
Social Skills Improvement System, *294*
social skills interventions, for play,
    305
Social Stories™, 212, 295–296
social worker, *208*
socialization, 42
socioeconomic status (SES), and
    literacy, 111, 112
solitary play, *303*
somatosensory system, 92
spatial relationships, 320
spatial visual supports, for social
    participation, 286
special care nurseries. *See* neonatal
    intensive care unit (NICU)
special education (SPED)
  comparison of approaches to, *19*
  determining eligibility and need for,
    168–169
  early childhood outcomes with, 161
  evaluation and eligibility for, 159
  extended school year for, 161
  history of, 13–14
  individualized education program
    for, 159–160
  least restrictive environment for,
    160–161
  procedural safeguards for, 161
  process of, 159–161
  referral for evaluation for, 183–184
  related services for, 160
special health care needs. *See*
    children with special health care
    needs (CSHCN)
special interest section (SIS), 7
special needs, literacy with, 112
specialized instructional support
    personnel (SISP), 365
speech production, 281
speech therapist, *208*
SPEEDI (Supporting Play,
    Exploration, and Early
    Development Intervention), 268
spinal cord injuries (SCIs), 217
spiritual activities, in health care
    setting, *210*
spirituality, assessment tools for, 385
splinter skills, 283
state data, for preschool, 178
state education codes and rules, *363*
state-identified measurable result
    (SIMR), 81

state insurance mandates, for autism spectrum disorder and ADHD, 339

state laws, 26, 33–34

state Part C early intervention, *363*

state performance plan (SPP), 157

state performance plan (SPP) indicators, *80*

state policies
  on autism spectrum disorder and ADHD, 339
  and occupational therapy services in early intervention and schools, 361–362, *362–363*

state practice acts
  vs. education-based documentation, 183
  influences on occupational therapy practice of, *363*

state requirement, for telehealth, 399

Stay 'n Play Parents Interactions With Infants (PIWI), *26*

stool toileting refusal, 238

strabismus, 320, *322*

strategize, in PAUSE method, 102, 104

strengths-based approach, to early intervention, 137

strengths-based practice, in family partnerships, 66–67, *67*

strength(s)
  in early childhood team report, 392, *392*
  in motor evaluation, *278*
  in team evaluation report, 396

stress
  maternal, 90
  and transitions, 82

stroke
  childhood, 216
  defined, 216
  hemorrhagic, 216
  ischemic, 216
  pediatric, 216
  perinatal, 216

Student, Environments, Tasks, and Tools (SETT) framework, 58

Sturge-Weber syndrome, *322*

substance exposure, prenatal. *See* prenatal substance exposure

substance use disorder (SUD), and relationships, *101*

summary of needs, in early childhood team report, 392

supervision
  close, 32
  defined, 32
  documentation of, 32
  of early intervention, 120
  general, 32
  and leadership, 42

methods of, 32
  minimum, 32
  of occupational therapy assistants, 32–33
  routine, 32

supervision log, 32

supplemental oxygen, 332

support systems, for children with special health care needs, 332

Supporting Play, Exploration, and Early Development Intervention (SPEEDI), 268

swaddling, for neonatal abstinence syndrome, 351

swallow study, 253

switch, for assistive technology, 59, 60

symbolic play, 303, 305

sympathetic nervous system responses, 91

Synactive Development Theory, 211

system of payment, for early intervention, 120

systems effects, on postnatal trauma, 349

systems level, collaboration at, *72*

T

tactile cues, 323

tactile receptors, 91–92

tactile system, development of, 91–92

task modification, for dressing, grooming, and hygiene, 239–240

taste receptors, 92

teacher of the visually impaired (TVI), 321

Team Assessment of Preschoolers in Routines (TAPIR), 393–395

team development, 42

team evaluation report, sample, 393–396

team report, sample early childhood, 391–392

team(s) and teamwork
  best practices for, 26
  for early intervention, 125–126

Tech Act (Technology Related Assistance for Individuals with Disabilities Act, 1988), 55–56, *363*

technical assistance centers, 14

technical leadership, 41–42

technology, to promote collaboration, 76

Technology Related Assistance for Individuals with Disabilities Act (Tech Act, 1988), 55–56, *363*

Technology to Improve Kids' Educational Success Project, 58, 61

telehealth, 399–400
  benefits and challenges of, 76, 399–400

defined, 76
  family partnerships in, 69
  for occupational therapy evaluation, 400
  for occupational therapy intervention, 400
  to promote collaboration, 76
  resources on, 400
  state and payor requirement for, 399

tele-intervention, 399

tele-practice, 399

tele-therapy, 399

temperament, 257–258

temperature stability, for neonatal abstinence syndrome, 352

temporal context, assessment tools for, 387

temporal visual supports, for social participation, 286

Test of Infant Motor Performance, *276*

Test of Playfulness, *304*

texture modifications, for feeding, 251–252

theoretical models, 27

therapeutic use of self, 102

therapy balls, 296

therapy clinic settings, health care interventions for developmental conditions in, 209

therapy log, 185

thermal burns, 217

third-degree burns, 217

30 Million Word Gap, 110–111

Tier I supports, 112

Tier II supports, 112

timing, in life course health development framework, 350–351

tobacco, prenatal exposure to, 348

toilet training, 235, 238–239

toileting, 235–236, 238–239
  in health care setting, *210*

toileting readiness skills, 235

toileting skills, delayed, 235–236

tool use, *269*

tooth brushing, 236, 239–240

Total Communication (TC), *313*

toxicants, prenatal exposure to, 91

toys
  adapting, 305
  observation of play with, 303, *303*

trainer, role of occupational therapy practitioner as, *368*

training
  history of, 6
  in preschool, 176

Training Occupational Therapists in Education Management Systems (TOTEMS), 6

transdisciplinary mode, 73

transfer of learning, for cerebral palsy, *277*

transition conference, *80*
transition notification, *80*
transition plan, 80, *80*
transition planning, to preschool, 161–162
transition report, *146*
transition supports, 79
transition(s), 79–85
　building capacity for, 83
　childhood occupations and routines in, 83
　defined, 79
　developmental considerations with, 81–82
　documentation of, 188
　from early intervention to preschool, 84, 124, 126
　effect of stress on, 82
　family-centered approach to, *82*, 82–83
　family-centered services for, 81–83, *82*
　from Head Start to kindergarten, 81
　from home or community to Part B, 80, *80*
　from home to community settings, 84
　from hospital to home and community, 83
　from hospital to Part C, 79
　under IDEA, 79–81, *80*
　natural environments in, 83
　near 3rd birthday, 80–81
　Office of Special Education Programs indicators and outcomes for, 81
　overview of, 79
　from Part C to Part B, 79–80
　preparing for future, 83
　from preschool, 81, 84–85, 170
　to preschool, 161–162
　across settings, 83–85
　in team evaluation report, 394, 395
transjejunal tube, *332*
trauma, 347–355
　ACE Pyramid for, 349, *349*
　Adverse Childhood Experiences (ACE) Study of, 348–349
　advocacy for prevention of, 354
　defined, 348
　developmental (chronic interpersonal, complex) (*See* developmental trauma)
　essential considerations with, 350–351
　evaluation of, 353
　impact on brain development and developmental milestones of, 349–350
　interventions for, 353–354
　life course approach to, 350–351

　overview of, 347
　physical, 218
　postnatal, 347–355
　resources on, 355
　risk factors for, 349
　trauma-informed care for, 350
trauma-informed care (TIC), 350, 353–354
traumatic brain injuries (TBIs), 216
treatment codes, 196, *196*
TriCare East, *194*
TriCare West, *194*
Trust-Based Relational Intervention, 354
Tuckman's Model, 75

U
ulcerative colitis, nutrition with, 246
understand, in PAUSE method, 102, 103–104
Understood, *330*
undressing, 236, 239–240
unfolding, in life course health development framework, 350
United Cerebral Palsy Association, 4
United Healthcare, *194*
United Nations Children's Fund (UNICEF), *16*
universal design, 57
Universal Design for Learning (UDL), 57, 174, *174*
universal pre-kindergarten, 14
universal preschool, 14
universal screening, for autism spectrum disorder and ADHD, 340
University Affiliated Facilities for the Mentally Retarded (UAF), 5
University Centers for Excellence in Developmental Disabilities (UCEDDs), 5
Usher syndrome, *322*

V
validity, internal, 374
values
　assessment tools for, 385
　in core competencies, 26
vegetables, *244*
ventilator, 332
veracity, *33*
verbal cues, 323
vestibular areflexia, 316
vestibular dysfunction, with hearing loss, 314–315, 316
vestibular receptors, 92
vestibular system, development of, 92
video modeling, for developmental conditions in health care setting, 211–212
Vineland Adaptive Behavior Scales, *169, 237*

viral meningitis, 216–217
virtual context, assessment tools for, 387
Vision 2025 (AOTA), 8, 18, 38
vision loss. *See* visual impairments
visual acuity, 265
visual impairments, 319–326
　assistive technology and adaptation of environment and objects for, 323
　collaborative teaming for, 321
　conditions and diagnoses of, 319–320, 321, *322*
　cortical or cerebral, 319–320, *322*
　with deafness, 324–325, *325*
　early signs of, 321, *322*
　epidemiology of, 319
　evaluation of, 321–323, *323*
　impact on participation and development of, 320
　interventions for, 323–324, *324*
　learning with, 320
　motor skills with, 320
　ocular, 319
　overview of, 319–320
　play skills with, 320
　resources on, 325–326
　social skills with, 320
visual–motor activities, *269*, 269–270
visual–motor coordination, 265–270
　additional interventions to enhance, *269*, 269–270
　assessment tools for, 267, *267*
　with cerebral palsy, 268
　defined, 265
　development of, 265–266, *266*
　evidence-based interventions for, 267–268
　occupational profile for, 266–267, *267*
　overview of, 265
visual–motor delay, 265
visual–motor integration, 265
visual perception, 265
visual processing, *111*, 265
visual receptors, 92
visual scanning, 323
visual schedule, for dressing, grooming, and hygiene, 239
visual stimulation, 323–324
visual supports, for social participation, 285–286
Visual Supports Checklist, 61
visual system, development of, 92
visual task schedules, for dressing, grooming, and hygiene, 239
vocalizations, development of early, 282–283
Vygotsky, Lev, 14

W
Wee-FIM (Functional Independence Measure for Children), *203, 237, 267,* 275, *276*
weight bearing, with acquired conditions, 221
weighted vests, 296
Weikart, David, 14

wetting alarms, 239
whole-group instruction, in team evaluation report, 393, 394
workforce, 39–40
working hypothesis, 52–53
working memory, 258
World Health Organization (WHO), *16*

World Organization for Early Childhood Education, *16*
writing name, *111*

Z
Zero to Three (ZTT), *16,* 105
zone of proximal development, 14